Chemoradiation in Cancer Therapy

Cancer Drug Discovery and Development

Beverly A. Teicher, Series Editor

Oncogene-Directed Therapies, edited by *Janusz Rak,* 2003
Cell Cycle Inhibitors in Cancer Therapy: *Current Strategies,* edited by *Antonio Giordano and Kenneth J. Soprano,* 2003
Chemoradiation in Cancer Therapy, edited by *Hak Choy,* 2003
Fluoropyrimidines in Cancer Therapy, edited by *Youcef M. Rustum,* 2003
Targets for Cancer Chemotherapy: ***Transcription Factors and Other Nuclear Proteins,*** edited by *Nicholas B. La Thangue and Lan R. Bandara,* 2002
Tumor Targeting in Cancer Therapy, edited by *Michel Pagé,* 2002
Hormone Therapy in Breast and Prostate Cancer, edited by *V. Craig Jordan and Barrington J. A. Furr,* 2002
Tumor Models in Cancer Research, edited by *Beverly A. Teicher,* 2002
Tumor Suppressor Genes in Human Cancer, edited by *David E. Fisher,* 2001
Matrix Metalloproteinase Inhibitors in Cancer Therapy, edited by *Neil J. Clendeninn and Krzysztof Appelt,* 2001
Farnesyltransferase Inhibitors in Cancer, edited by *Saïd M. Sebti and Andrew D. Hamilton,* 2001
Platinum-Based Drugs in Cancer Therapy, edited by *Lloyd R. Kelland and Nicholas P. Farrell,* 2000
Apoptosis and Cancer Chemotherapy, edited by *John A. Hickman and Caroline Dive,* 1999
Signaling Networks and Cell Cycle Control: ***The Molecular Basis of Cancer and Other Diseases,*** edited by *J. Silvio Gutkind,* 1999
Antifolate Drugs in Cancer Therapy, edited by *Ann L. Jackman,* 1999
Antiangiogenic Agents in Cancer Therapy, edited by *Beverly A. Teicher,* 1999
Anticancer Drug Development Guide: ***Preclinical Screening, Clinical Trials, and Approval,*** edited by *Beverly A. Teicher,* 1997
Cancer Therapeutics: ***Experimental and Clinical Agents,*** edited by *Beverly A. Teicher,* 1997

CHEMORADIATION IN CANCER THERAPY

Edited by

HAK CHOY, MD

Department of Radiation Oncology,
Vanderbilt University Medical Center,
Nashville, Tennessee

HUMANA PRESS
TOTOWA, NEW JERSEY

To my wife Sunny and my children Natalie, Alex, and Megan, whose love and support make my work possible.

999 Riverview Drive, Suite 208
Totowa, New Jersey 07512
www.humanapress.com

Production Editor: Adrienne Howell.

Cover illustration: Figure 4 from Chapter 12, "Combined Modality Therapy in Locally Advanced Breast Cancer," by Silvia C. Formenti and Matthew Volm.

Cover design by Patricia F. Cleary.

This publication is printed on acid-free paper. ∞
ANSI Z39.48-1984 (American National Standards Institute)
Permanence of Paper for Printed Library Materials

For additional copies, pricing for bulk purchases, and/or information about other Humana titles, contact Humana at the above address or at any of the following numbers: Tel.:973-256-1699; Fax: 973-256-8341; Email: humanapr.com; or visit our Website: http://humanapress.com

Printed in the United States of America. 10 9 8 7 6 5 4 3 2 1

Library of Congress Cataloging-in-Publication Data

Chemoradiation in cancer therapy/edited by Hak Choy.
p. ; cm. — (Cancer drug discovery and development)
ISBN 1-58829-028-X(alk. paper) 1-59259-325-9 (e-book)
1. Cancer—Adjuvant treatment. 2. Cancer—Chemotherapy. 3. Cancer—Radiotherapy. I. Choy, Hak. II. Series.
[DNLM: 1. Neoplasms—drug therapy. 2. Neoplasms--radiotherapy. 3. Combined Modality Therapy. QZ 266 C5174 2003]
RC271.A35 C445 2003
616.99'406--dc21

2002027347

Preface

As the treatment of cancer continues to evolve, clinicians are constantly seeking new and innovative strategies to expand the use of currently available treatment modalities. Among the different strategies to improve therapy, the combining of chemotherapeutic drugs with radiation has perhaps had the strongest impact on current solid tumor treatment practice. This combination has been in use for many decades, but now has become a common treatment option in many clinical settings. This is particularly true for concurrent chemoradiotherapy, which in many recent clinical trials has been shown to be superior to radiotherapy alone in controlling local–regional disease and in improving patient survival. Combining chemotherapeutic drugs with radiotherapy has a strong biologic rationale. Such agents reduce the number of cells in tumors undergoing radiotherapy by their independent cytotoxic action and by rendering tumor cells more susceptible to killing by ionizing radiation. An additional benefit of combined treatment is that chemotherapeutic drugs, by virtue of their systemic activity, may also act on metastatic disease. Most drugs have been chosen for combination with radiotherapy based on their known clinical activity in particular disease sites. Alternatively, agents that are effective in overcoming resistance mechanisms associated with radiotherapy could be chosen. There have been recent clinical successes of concurrent chemoradiotherapy using traditional drugs, such as cisplatin and 5-FU, but these studies have led to extensive research on exploring newer chemotherapeutic agents for their interactions with radiation. A number of new potent chemotherapeutic agents, including taxanes, nucleoside analogs, and topoisomerase inhibitors, have entered clinical trial or practice. Preclinical testing has shown that they are potent enhancers of radiation response and thus might further improve the therapeutic outcome of chemoradiotherapy. Also, there are rapidly emerging molecular targeting strategies aimed at improving the efficacy of chemoradiotherapy. All these important aspects of combined modality therapy in solid tumors are discussed in this book, particularly for tumors that historically have had a poor prognosis and few treatment options.

Curry and Curran review the literature on the combined modality treatment of patients with malignant glioma, focusing on the data from prospective randomized trials, and discuss future directions in research to improve outcome for patients affected by this disease. It is clear that any one systemic agent or multiagent regimen will not have substantial effects on altering the natural history of malignant glioma. A significant improvement in survival will be realized only when improvements in local–regional control are combined with progress in the systemic management of the disease. Specific opportunities to improve surgical and radiotherapy approaches to this disease need to be explored concurrently with development of novel agents targeted to modify the biologic response of these tumors to chemotherapy and radiation. However, novel approaches when combining standard cytotoxic chemotherapy agents with new cytotoxic and cytostatic agents and improved radiotherapy techniques are promising in promoting decreased radioresistance, toxicities, and possibly increased overall survival of head and neck cancer. Outside of an academic setting, cisplatin and 5-FU still remain the standard of treatment. Though more aggressive, as mentioned in Drs. Eng and Vokes' chapter, these drugs have overall demonstrated improved response rates in locally advanced and recurrent disease. Newer agents will continue to be discovered and provide a basis for further consideration in the treatment of head and neck cancer.

It is apparent that significant progress has been made in improving the outcome of treatment for stage III nonsmall-cell lung cancer, even though there is still a long way to go before victory can be declared. It is clear that radiation alone and surgery alone are inadequate for most stage III disease. Preoperative radiation therapy alone is of limited benefit. Postoperative radiation is controversial, but there may be a limited role in resected N2 patients. For selected stage III cases (N2), there may be a role for surgery after chemoradiation, but this conclusion awaits the outcome of a major phase III study. For inoperable stage III disease, combined modality now appears to be the new standard of care. Concurrent chemoradiation seems to be superior to sequential chemoradiation, but combined sequential followed by concurrent chemoradiation remains under investigation as does consolidative chemotherapy after concurrent chemoradiation. The best results combining chemotherapy with radiation therapy were also seen in limited-stage small-cell lung cancer. At this time, standard treatment for patients with limited-stage small-cell lung cancer is early concurrent twice-daily radiation therapy of 1.8 Gy fractions for a total dose of 45 Gy and platinum-based chemotherapy.

As discussed by Brahmer et al., newer chemotherapy regimens emerge for the treatment of small-cell lung cancer, and these regimens are currently undergoing evaluation for combining chemo- and radiation therapy. As far as esophageal cancer goes, results from surgery alone or primary chemoradiation are equivalent, and both can be offered as options for patients with locally advanced esophageal cancer. The optimal treatment may be based on individual patient selection criteria such as the ability to undergo major surgery, histology, and the location of the tumor. The fact that local recurrence is high despite primary chemoradiation, provides a rationale for tri-modality therapy that includes surgery following preoperative chemoradiation.

The major advance in the treatment of local–regional gastric carcinoma had been the new standard of adjuvant chemoradiotherapy following a curative resection. Laparoscopy is more or less established as a staging procedure prior to surgery. Staging with endoscopic ultrasonography has improved. New strategies will include the use of preoperative approaches and incorporation of new agents. Similar to the carcinoma of the esophagus, the use of molecular markers to predict response and survival is needed. Investigative efforts are underway to further improve the results of multimodality therapy of colorectal carcinoma. In addition to phase III trials discussed in Chapter 14, other studies are incorporating novel chemotherapeutic agents to improve systemic control and radiosensitization, to optimize physical delivery of radiation, and to perform risk stratification with current molecular and genetic techniques. Chronomodulation may have a role in combined modality therapy for colorectal cancer by affecting higher response rates and less stomatitis and neuropathy in metastatic colorectal carcinoma and may become a viable option for treatment of primary disease.

The inferior results with radiotherapy alone compared to cystectomy in patients with muscle-invasive disease have prompted a large number of trials adding systemic chemotherapy to radiotherapy in an attempt to increase local control and eliminate micrometastatic disease frequently present at the time of diagnosis of muscle-invasive disease.

As discussed by Dr. Roth, it is not easy to directly compare surgical series with trials of bladder-sparing approaches. A number of confounding factors can potentially complicate the interpretation of trials of chemoradiotherapy, including the effect of the TURBT on the natural history of this disease, the errors of clinical staging both before and after chemotherapy/radiotherapy, and the endpoints utilized to determine efficacy. Nonetheless, his approach can certainly be offered to patients who are not surgical candidates because of medical co-morbidities, or the occasional patient who refuses surgical intervention. Recent studies in a variety of gynecologic malignancies have convincingly demonstrated that concurrent chemotherapy can significantly improve the outcome of some patients who require radiation therapy for treatment of their disease. Despite the fact that controversies persist about the indications for chemoradiation and ideal drug regimens, the fundamental value in patients with loco–regionally advanced cervical cancer has been established.

The chapter by Dr. Eifel reviews trials of chemoradiation in cervical cancer, including the recent trials that established the value of this approach, and discusses several questions that remain to be resolved regarding this treatment, including the ideal dose and schedule and the effect of chemoradiation on compliance and complications.

One of the most exciting areas of combined modality therapy is the specific molecular targeted therapy in combination with radiation. Over the past decade there has been a quantum increase in the understanding of molecular mechanisms that underlie the process of tumor development, proliferation, invasion, and metastasis.

This has led to a growing awareness of mechanisms by which tumors and normal tissue are able to overcome damage from radiation injury. This knowledge has resulted in a vast amount of preclinical study of ways that these molecular abnormalities may be specifically targeted to result in clinical benefit, not only by potentially impacting on systemic disease, but by enhancing radiosensitivity. The last part of this book describes some of these agents and pathways.

Although we have made significant progress in our understanding of the role of combined modality therapy, much remains to be accomplished. Current and future research may provide exciting opportunities to improve response and survival for patients with tumors previously associated with a dismal prognosis.

ACKNOWLEDGMENT

I would like to thank my assistant, Laura Jewell Tyree, for her attention to detail and her many hours devoted to editing.

Hak Choy, *MD*

Contents

Contributors

Jaffer A. Ajani • *Department of Gastrointestinal Oncology, The University of Texas M. D. Anderson, Cancer Center, Houston, Texas*

Carlos L. Arteaga • *Department of Medicine and Cell Biology, Vanderbilt-Ingram Cancer Center, Nashville, TN*

Andrew Baxter • *Celltech Chiroscience, Great Abington, Cambridge, United Kingdom*

John Bird • *Celltech Chiroscience, Great Abington, Cambridge, United Kingdom*

William Blackstock • *Radiation Oncology and Cancer Biology, Wake Forest University Medical Center, Winston-Salem, NC*

Julie R. Brahmer • *The Sidney Kimmel Comprehensive Cancer Center at Johns Hopkins, Baltimore, MD*

Roger W. Byhardt • *Department of Radiation Oncology, Medical College of Wisconsin, Milwaukee, WI*

Bapsi Chak • *Department of Radiation Oncology, Vanderbilt University Medical Center, Nashville, TN*

Hak Choy • *Department of Radiation Oncology, Vanderbilt University Medical Center, Nashville, TN*

Walter J. Curran, Jr. • *Department of Radiation Oncology, Thomas Jefferson University Hospital, Philadelphia, PA*

Heather A. Curry • *Department of Radiation Oncology, Thomas Jefferson University Hospital, Philadelphia, PA*

Janet Dancey • *Investigational Drug Branch, Cancer Therapy Evaluation Program, National Cancer Institute, Bethesda, MD*

Robert B. Diasio • *Department of Pharmacology & Toxicology, University of Alabama at Birmingham (UAB) Comprehensive Cancer Center, Birmingham, AL*

Raymond N. DuBois • *Department of Gastroenterology, Vanderbilt University Medical Center, Nashville, TN*

Patricia J. Eifel • *The University of Texas M.D. Anderson Cancer Center, Houston, TX*

Cathy Eng • *The University of Texas M.D. Anderson Cancer Center, Houston, TX*

David S. Ettinger • *The Sidney Kimmel Comprehensive Cancer Center at Johns Hopkins, Baltimore, MD*

Arlene Forastiere • *The Sidney Kimmel Comprehensive Cancer Center at Johns Hopkins, Baltimore, MD*

Silvia C. Formenti • *Department of Radiation Oncology, New York University School of Medicine, New York, NY*

Elora Gupta • *Bristol-Myers Squibb, Wallingford, CT*

Dennis E. Hallahan • *Department of Radiation Oncology, Vanderbilt University Medical Center, Nashville, TN*

Jeffrey S. Humphrey • *Bristol-Myers Squibb, Wallingford, CT*

Larry Kleinberg • *The Sidney Kimmel Comprehensive Cancer Center at Johns Hopkins, Baltimore, MD*

Jerome Landry • *Department of Radiation Oncology, Emory University School of Medicine, Atlanta, Georgia*
Jason H. Lee • *Hudner Oncology Center, St. Anne's Hospital, Fall River, MA*
Robert M. MacRae • *Ottawa Regional Cancer Centre, Ottawa, Ontario*
Stacy L. Moulder • *Department of Hematology-Oncology, Vanderbilt Medical Center, Nashville, TN*
Joseph Naglich • *Bristol-Myers Squibb, Wallingford, CT*
Alexandria Phan • *Department of Gastrointestinal Oncology, The University of Texas M. D. Anderson Cancer Center, Houston, TX*
Karen Price • *Bristol-Myers Squibb, Wallingford, CT*
Hong Pyo • *Yonsei University College of Medicine, Seodaemun-KU, Seoul, Korea*
Tyvin A. Rich • *Department of Radiation Oncology, The University of Virginia Health System, Charlottesville, VA*
Bruce J. Roth • *The Paul V. Hamilton, M. D. and Virginia E. Howd Professor of Medicine and Urologic Oncology, Vanderbilt-Ingram Cancer Center, Nashville, TN*
Jack A. Roth • *Department of Thoracic and Cardiovascular Surgery, The University of Texas M. D. Anderson Cancer Center, Houston, TX*
Muhammad Wasif Saif • *Division of Hematology/Oncology, University of Alabama at Birmingham (UAB), Comprehensive Cancer Center, Birmingham, AL*
Scott Saxman • *Clinical Investigations Branch, Cancer Therapy Evaluation Program, National Cancer Institute, Bethesda, MD*
Daryl Sonnichsen • *Bristol-Myers Squibb, Wallingford, CT*
Don Stacy • *Department of Radiation Oncology, Vanderbilt University Medical Center, Nashville, TN*
Stephen G. Swisher • *Department of Thoracic and Cardiovascular Surgery, The University of Texas M. D. Anderson Cancer Center, Houston, TX*
Beverly A. Teicher • *Genzyme Corporation, Framingham, MA*
Everett E. Vokes • *Section of Hematology/Oncology, University of Chicago, Chicago, IL*
Matthew Volm • *Department of Medicine (Medical Oncology), New York University School of Medicine, New York, NY*
Christopher G. Willett • *Department of Radiation Oncology, Massachusetts General Hospital, Boston, MA*
Gary Yang • *Division of Radiation Oncology, The Johns Hopkins Oncology Center, Baltimore, MD*

I

General/Background

1 Chemoradiation

Biological Principles and Perspectives

Hak Choy, MD *and Robert M. MacRae,* MD

Contents

1. INTRODUCTION

The medical uses of ionizing radiation have expanded dramatically since Wilhelm Roentgen first discovered it at the end of the last century. In particular, it has proven to be an effective agent in the ongoing battle against cancer. It is presumed that the essential target for radiation is cellular DNA where it acts through the formation of free radicals to directly or indirectly cause double-stranded breaks. It is these double-stranded breaks in the DNA that are felt to be the lethal lesion that malignant cells sustain from therapeutic radiation.

It was in the period of World War II that it was possible to induce lasting remissions and potential cures of hematological malignancies with nitrogen mustard *(1)*, which was really the first chemotherapeutic agent put to widespread use in the treatment of malignant disease. Since that time, a multitude of other drugs have come and gone in the search for a cure. A few drugs appear to have found a more lasting place in the therapeutic armamentarium, including doxorubicin, cisplatinum, cyclophosphamide, and 5-fluorouracil. A new generation of drugs with varied mechanisms of action has appeared in the last decade and also has the potential to remain as key in the treatment of cancers.

From: *Chemoradiation in Cancer Therapy*
Edited by: H. Choy © Humana Press Inc., Totowa, NJ

These agents include paclitaxel, docetaxel, gemcitabine, irinotecan, and vinorelbine. Although oncologists and researchers have often tried to cure cancers with radiation alone or with various chemotherapeutic strategies, in general these have been met with limited success for any number of reasons, which will be outlined below. The strategy of integrating different treatment modalities into a more comprehensive approach to both local control and the treatment of micrometastatic disease, often referred to as combined modality therapy, has been met with some success. Although the delivery of neoadjuvant and adjuvant chemotherapy may contribute to improved local control, it is less clearly demonstrable than with concurrent therapy. This chapter will focus on combined modality therapy with an emphasis on concurrent chemoradiation. It will attempt to set the background with an examination of the rationale and the difficulties that are inherent with concurrent therapy from the point of view of both the delivery of radiation and of chemotherapy. Beyond this it will illustrate some of the gains achieved in therapy using a concurrent treatment approach. Finally it will focus on the potential for the future that lies in an increased understanding of the molecular players in neoplastic processes as well as the response of malignant cells to therapy with radiation and chemotherapy. The integration of new agents that are aimed against more specific cellular targets than either radiation or traditional cytotoxic chemotherapy may significantly influence the success of combined modality therapy in the future.

2. TREATMENT PARADIGMS

Surgical therapy as a sole modality often fails because micrometastatic disease is already present at the time of surgery or because malignant cells are present beyond the surgical margins of the resection. Radiation therapy is sometimes added before or after surgical resection to decrease the possibility of local recurrence when it is felt that there is a high enough probability of residual malignant cells being present after surgery. However, radiation therapy as both a sole modality of treatment or as an adjuvant or adjunctive therapy may fail to sterilize tumors because of micrometastases or because the dose of radiation that can be safely delivered is limited by the tolerance of the surrounding normal tissues. Certainly the explosion of new technology in the current computer age has improved our ability to deliver further radiation in a more conformal fashion. However, in those malignancies that have a high propensity for distant spread of disease, delivery of higher doses of conformal radiation may not prove to be a satisfactory approach to the problem. Unfortunately chemotherapy rarely proves to have a curative role on its own in the treatment of solid tumors.

3. BIOLOGY COMPLICATES THE DELIVERY OF RADIATION

The delivery of therapeutic radiation is limited by the tolerance of the surrounding normal tissues. Data have been compiled over many years that suggest which structures are able to tolerate certain doses with acceptable amounts of toxicity *(2)*. This model for thinking about how to plan the delivery of radiation has changed considerably with the advent of new computer- and automation-driven technologies that allow for the more conformal delivery of dose to the gross tumor and to the clinical target volume. New analytical tools called dose volume histograms, which allow for a definition of the dose delivered to a percentage of an organ, have begun to replace more traditional concepts of normal tissue tolerance (*see* Fig. 1). Although these technology-related advances allow

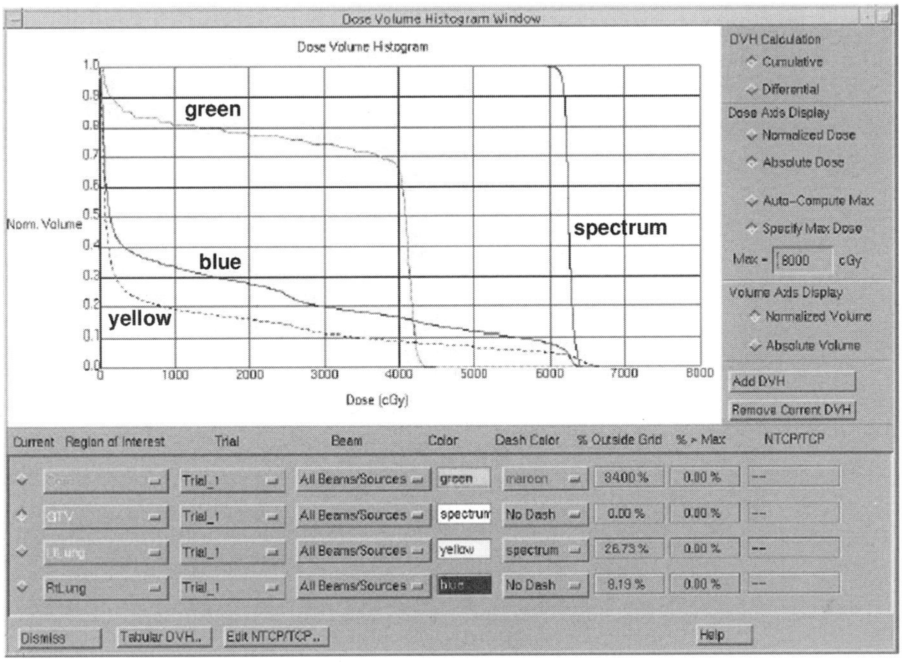

Fig. 1. This example of a cumulative dose volume histogram (DVH) exemplifies the manner in which three dimensional treatment planning allows the radiation oncologist to ensure that the tumor receives the planned dose while limiting the dose of radiation received by the normal structures. In this example 100% of the gross tumor volume (GTV) receives 70 Gy whereas the dose received by any length of the spinal cord is less than 45 Gy.

for the delivery of higher doses of radiation, this may only be an effective strategy in those tumors whose biology makes them amenable to a local therapy as the sole modality of treatment. Those tumors that have a predilection for the early dissemination of micrometastases cannot be effectively treated by a local therapy alone. However, those tumors that tend to remain localized for longer periods of time may have several biologic reasons that underlie their resistance to radiation.

3.1. Accelerated Repopulation

This is a hypothetical mechanism to explain the decrease in local control that is seen in some types of malignancy when the overall radiation treatment time becomes prolonged *(3)*. Actual tumor growth occurs at a rate that is significantly slower than the potential doubling time of the tumor cells, and this is related to what is called the *cell loss factor* (Φ). The cell loss factor in most human squamous cell cancers is felt to be in the range of 0.9, which is to say that cell production rates are approx 10 times faster than tumor growth rates *(4)*. It is felt that the acceleration of repopulation that occurs in squamous cell cancers during therapy leads to an effective tumor cell production rate approaching the potential tumor-doubling rate and that this occurs because of a decrease in the cell loss factor. This is supported by work from both Fowler and Dorr suggesting that this repopulation cannot be accounted for by a simple increase in the rate of the proliferation of surviving tumor cells alone but rather it requires a profound decrease in the cell loss factor as well *(5,6)*. Although some have hypothesized that increased tumor oxygenation seen during therapy is related to the increase in cellular repopulation that occurs, it may in fact be related to cellular density changes. Investigators who have looked at the squamous epithelium of the skin as a model for repopulation have seen that as the cellular density changes there are profound modifications in the expression of connexin 43, the major component of gap junctions, that in turn regulates cell-to-cell communication *(7)*.

Radiation treatment schemes that *accelerate* the dose delivery, i.e., attempt to deliver it in a shorter overall time, endeavor to compensate for any accelerated repopulation of the tumor that may be occurring. These schemes are often accompanied by increased morbidity. Ultimately a better understanding of the molecular and cellular events involved may give rise to measures that will allow us to compensate for accelerated repopulation in tumors or to induce repopulation in normal tissues earlier in a course of therapy in order to minimize treatment related morbidity.

3.2. Repair of Radiation-Induced DNA Damage

Traditional radiation survival curves from single dose experiments exhibit a shoulder that is thought to be indicative of the innate capacity of cells to repair radiation damage *(8)*. If the dose is fractionated into multiple treatments with sufficient time between treatments, all repairable damage may be corrected leading to an increase in the surviving fraction of malignant cells. There is, however, a probable limit to the effective reduction of the slope of the survival curve that is felt to represent unrepairable damage caused by radiation. This difference in the slopes of the radiation survival curve between a single dose experiment and fractionated radiation is felt to represent *sublethal damage repair* (SLDR) *(9)*.

Normal tissues are usually divided into early and late responding according to their responses to radiation. It is well known that late responding tissues, like the spinal cord, are better able to repair damage caused by radiation than malignant cells with conventional fractionation schemes using daily doses of 180–200 cGy compared with larger fraction sizes *(10)* and as such these fraction sizes are used to exploit this difference in the repair capacity for a therapeutic gain. The major rationale for the use of *hyperfractionated radiotherapy* wherein more than one fraction is delivered each day but the total treatment time remains the same as with conventional treatment, is to exploit this difference in repair capacity between tumors and normal tissues. Normally an increase of 20–30% in the total dose is needed to account for repair at the lower dose per fraction administered in a hyperfractionated scheme *(11)*. However, hyperfractionated radiation treatment schemes normally must reach a fine balance between the risk of allowing for accelerated repopulation and causing undo acute morbidity.

Another treatment strategy to deal with the interrelated phenomena of accelerated repopulation and repair has been to both accelerate and hyperfractionate therapy. Limiting acute morbidity most often complicates this strategy and in many cases the overall tumor control and late morbidity remain undefined. A more sophisticated understanding of repair mechanisms at a molecular level and their relation to treatment times may allow for increased clarity in understanding the utility of altered fractionation schemes to treat cancer.

3.3. Tumor Hypoxia

The equally intriguing phenomenon of tumor hypoxia has been documented to occur in a number of tumor types including cancers of the uterine cervix *(12,13)*, head and neck *(14,15)*, bladder *(16)* as well as in soft tissue sarcomas *(17)*. This is the result of inadequate blood supply to tissues that leads to the compromise of biological function and in the case of cancers this is usually related to abnormal or inadequate blood vessels, anemia, or the formation of methemoglobin or carboxyhemoglobin that will reduce the oxygen carrying capacity of the blood in smokers. There have been several observations collected over the last few decades that suggest that tumor hypoxia plays a key role in outcome. These observations are as follows: tumors often have lower median partial pressures of oxygen than their tissues of origin *(18)*; the presence of tumor hypoxia cannot necessarily be reliably predicted by factors like stage, size, histology, or grade; tumor-to-tumor oxygen variability is often greater than intratumor oxygenation differences *(19)*, and recurrent tumors often are more poorly oxygenated than their corresponding primary tumor *(20)*.

While the controversy about the exact role that anemia plays in determining outcome from radiation therapy is age old, i.e., big tumors bleed more and are more likely to spread vs tumors in anemic patients tend to be more hypoxic and hence more resistant to therapy, evidence is accumulating to suggest that reality is firmly rooted between both views. Radiosensitivity is known to be significantly limited when the partial pressure of oxygen is less than 25–30 mmHg *(21)*. It has been known for years that molecular oxygen will increase radiation-induced DNA damage through the formation of oxygen free radicals that act to inflict "indirect" damage beyond the "direct" effects of radiation on DNA *(22)*. There is also substantial evidence obtained over the last few years that tumor hypoxia induces genomic changes with subsequent upregulation of genes that are linked to radiation resistance *(23)*. Equally compelling are the experiments that have revealed that presence of tumor hypoxia is linked to an increased incidence of metastatic disease *(24)*. The microenvironmental signals in a hypoxic tumor environment are such that there is greater genomic instability and selection pressure to maintain those cells with increased angiogenic potential and decreased apoptotic potential. Improved understanding of this interesting phenomenon will ultimately lead to improved potential for therapeutic targeting of tumors.

4. BIOLOGY ALSO COMPLICATES THE DELIVERY OF CHEMOTHERAPY

The limitations of systemic chemotherapy are equally important to recognize prior to examining its integration with radiation. Although chemotherapy has earned a spot in the armamentarium against solid tumors, it is not often curative. Its use in the palliative setting is to reduce symptoms while decreasing the tumor burden and, though often effective, it is limited by its side effects as well as the emergence of resistance to the therapeutic effects of the drugs.

There are multiple factors that are felt to be relevant to a discussion of the emergence of resistance to chemotherapy. This list includes the current proliferative state of tumor cells, aspects of the tumor environment including vascular supply and volume of distribution of individual drugs, and the intrinsic sensitivity of tumor cells to various cytotoxic drugs. Common strategies to combat these problems include the combination of drugs with nonoverlapping toxicities *(25)* and differing mechanisms of action and possibly the rapid alteration of drugs to prevent the emergence of resistant cell populations as suggested by Coldman and Goldie *(26)*. A fundamental understanding at the

Table 1
Mechanisms Associated with Chemotherapy Related Resistance

Mechanism	*Drugs*
Decreased uptake	Methotrexate, melphalan, nitrogen mustards, cisplatin
Increased drug efflux	Taxanes, etoposide, anthracyclines
Decreased activation	Antimetabolites
Increased catabolism	Antimetabolites
Enzyme induction and/or alteration	Topoisomerase inhibitors, methotrexate
Drug deactivation by intracellular thiol compounds	Alkylators, cisplatin, anthracyclines
Increased DNA repair	Alkylators, cisplatin, anthracyclines
Decreased apoptotic rate	Alkylators, cisplatin, anthracyclines

Adapted from Tannock IF, Hill RP, eds. *The Basic Science of Oncology. Third edition.* Montreal: McGraw-Hill; 1998. Tannock and Hill. Chapter 17

molecular level of the mechanisms through which cells acquire resistance to chemotherapy is important in order to develop strategies to potentially circumvent this resistance. It is equally important to note that this resistance can function at multiple levels within a cell. Table 1 illustrates some of the basic mechanisms of resistance to the cytotoxic effects of chemotherapy.

5. PRINCIPLES GUIDING THE INTEGRATION OF CHEMORADIATION

Although the delivery of radiation and chemotherapy as sole modalities is definitely more complex than outlined above, there needs to be guiding principles that will allow for their successful integration in combined modality therapy. Peckham and Steele introduced several key concepts that govern the interactions of both radiation and chemotherapy when they are administered together in an attempt to improve the therapeutic effect of their separate administrations *(27)*.

Spatial cooperation is a term coined to describe a situation when disease in one particular anatomic site is missed by one modality but is treated adequately by another. The essence of this is that radiation is a local therapy that will not impact on metastatic disease beyond the planned field borders. Systemic cytotoxic chemotherapy is traditionally used to address the potential distant spread of cancer. In the original description of this mechanism there is no assumption of an interaction between the drugs and radiation with the idea being that the "best radiation" and "best chemotherapy" be administered independently of toxicities. The classic example used in several textbooks to illustrate this is the treatment of childhood leukemia with systemic chemotherapy, while their central nervous system, a potential sanctuary site where disease is not treated adequately by chemotherapy, is treated by radiation *(28)*. The reality of the interaction between radiation and chemotherapy is that the dose and timing of radiation are adjusted accordingly to minimize their impact on the neural tissues.

Toxicity independence definitely emerges as a real concern in the planning of combined modality therapy. As originally outlined, if two partially effective agents can be combined without having to alter their levels substantially, an improved therapeutic

Table 2
Nature of Radiation Enhancement

Enhancement	*Example*
Synergism	2 + 1 = 4
Additive	2 + 1 = 3
Subadditive	2 + 1 = 2.5
Interference	2 + 1 = 1.5
Antagonism	2 + 1 = 0.5

Adapted from Phillips TL. Chemical modification of radiation effects. *Cancer* 1977; Feb;39(2 Suppl):987–998.

result can be anticipated. Certainly this principle has been used widely in the justification of combination chemotherapies, however, when combining cytotoxic agents with radiation, one needs to choose agents that do not significantly enhance radiation-induced normal tissue damage. Examples of this principle are seen with the concurrent use of adriamycin and radiation in breast cancer *(29)* and actinomycin D and radiation in pediatric malignancies like Wilms' tumor *(30)*.

Protection of normal tissues is also a possible result of the interaction of radiation and systemic therapy. Peckham and Steele outlined this as "the combination of a chemotherapeutic agent with radiation allowing a greater dose of radiation to be given than would be tolerated otherwise" *(27)*. Although this area of combined therapy is relatively young, there are emerging examples of possible agents that may be administered concurrently with radiation to improve the tolerability of therapy, including amifostine *(31)*, granulocyte colony stimulation factor *(32)*, and keratinocyte growth factor *(33)*.

Enhancement of tumor response is of course the main topic of this chapter and this book. Enhancement is often used as a term to imply an increase in response and in the general sense is defined by a situation in which the administration of one agent increases the effectiveness of another or when the effect of the combination is greater than expected *(27)*. Interaction of different agents makes it difficult to characterize the exact nature of their interrelations especially in the in vivo situation. Table 2 points out the complexity involved in how exactly chemotherapies act to enhance the effects of ionizing radiation *(34)*. Beyond what the figure suggests is the fact that chemotherapies may be able to shrink disease such that smaller radiation fields and, consequently, higher radiation doses, may be used to treat tumors.

6. "IDEAL RADIOSENSITIZER"

Keeping the above principles in mind, Herscher et al. gives an excellent overview of the characteristics of an idealized radiation modifier *(35)*. In the case of the radiation protector more dose can be delivered to the tumor and in the case of a sensitizer more "effective" dose can be delivered. In theory the ideal radiation enhancer will have selective systemic activity against malignant but not against nonmalignant cells, will reach the tumor in adequate concentrations to affect radiation, and will have been studied such that the ideal timing with relation to radiation treatment delivery will be defined. Such a compound will increase the effects of radiation in one of several ways (*see* Fig. 2):

1. Increased initial damage: Agents that act to increase the initial DNA damage caused by ionizing radiation would be expected to augment the cytotoxicity caused by radiation

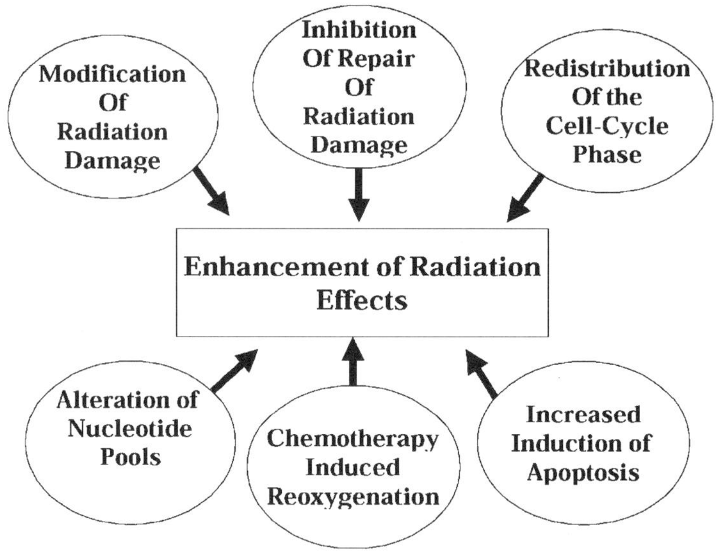

Fig. 2. Traditional ways of thinking about radiosensitization.

especially if they are able to saturate the repair systems. Good examples of agents that are felt to work in this manner include the halogenated pyrimidines *(36,37)*.

2. Repair inhibition: Agents that are able to impact the ability of a cell to repair DNA damage sustained from ionizing radiation are able to increase cytotoxicity. This is seen through a broadening of the shoulder in the traditional radiation survival curves. In practical terms there often remains a concern about the selectivity of cytotoxic agents for malignant tissues and the potential to increase normal tissue toxicity in this setting. Classical examples of drugs that are felt to act in this manner include cisplatin and the new oral platinum analogs *(38,39)*.
3. Redistribution: There are results of classical experiments that show that cells respond differently to radiation depending on which part of the cell cycle they are in when radiation is delivered. For human cancer cells the G_2M boundary appears to be the position in the cell cycle associated with the greatest sensitivity. It is likely that a drug that is able to block cell cycle progression in a radiosensitive phase will be associated with significant radiosensitization. The taxanes are an example of such a compound *(40)*.

Of course other methods of radiation enhancement may take place with reoxygenation of hypoxic tumor cells that may be increased with the use of chemotherapies like paclitaxel or gemcitabine *(41,42)*, improved drug access to the tumor cells after radiotherapy, or a lowering of the threshold for radiation-induced apoptosis as has been described with the use of gemcitabine *(43)*.

7. PRECLINICAL STUDIES

Before novel treatment strategies are attempted in the field of chemoradiation, there needs to be adequate preclinical data that establish whether the addition of drug X to radiation is likely to be of clinical benefit. Basic knowledge that needs to be sorted out in a laboratory setting includes: Is there a synergistic effect between the drug and radiation, is the timing between the drug administration and radiation important in achieving synergism, does this effect seen in an in vitro system translate into an animal model, and is this interaction likely to be clinically relevant such that human trials are warranted?

Terms like synergism and enhancement are often seen in the literature. It is important to remember a relevant definition of their true meaning in the setting of combined modality therapy. In general, enhancement is felt to describe any increase in effect greater than that observed with either radiation or chemotherapy alone, either on the tumor or the normal tissues *(44)*. Synergism, or supraadditivity as it is sometimes more clearly referred to, represents a subset of those enhancing interactions describing those situations when the combined response exceeds the range of additive responses even when corrected for the nonlinearity of survival curves *(44)*. Table 2, adapted from Phillips, provides a mathematical illustration of important relevant terminology.

7.1. The Isobologram

Although it is difficult to determine the exact nature of the chemoradiation interaction in animal and human systems unless biopsy and determination of surviving fractions is feasible, it is more straightforward to examine in an in vitro model. Dose-response curves are, in general, nonlinear. However, consideration of the calculation of supraadditivity, additivity, and subadditivity are more easily understood if a linear relationship is assumed for log survival. In this case when the dose of drug A vs dose of drug B is plotted for a given level of survival, it will produce a straight line. The line itself will represent true additivity. The region above the line will represent subadditivity and below the line supraadditivity *(27)*.

When dose-response curves are nonlinear as is usually the case, the process becomes more complex and an envelope of additivity is calculated to define the area in which the interaction of the two agents could be additive depending on how the two agents interact. The method described by Peckham and Steele *(27)* is explained as follows with the assumption that the dose response does not vary that much beyond a linear response. In their analysis, drugs A and D were assumed to yield linear responses and B and C yielded nonlinear responses.

In a mode I calculation which assumes that the agent response to agent A and B starts at zero cell kill, doses of agent A and agent B are chosen to give a total cell kill to level S (a selected level of cell kill for each analysis). The isoeffect curves that this analysis yields will bulge upward when one of the agents has a shoulder-type survival curve and downward when one survival curve bends upward. Mode II analysis uses the assumption that the incremental dose to yield the desired fractional survival is taken from the part of the curve that gives the greatest difference from mode I. In the case of the survival curve with a shoulder (curve B) it is taken from the steepest part, and in the case of the survival curve (curve C) that bends upward it is taken from the shallowest part. Calculation in these two modes will define the envelope of additivity, which accounts for the range of interaction between agents from no effect to the first dose of the second agent acting like a second dose of the other treatment *(44)*. *See* Fig. 3 adapted from Peckham and Steele.

8. IMPROVED THERAPEUTIC RATIO

Although the focus of this entire book is on chemoradiation, there are several notable areas where the use of concurrent chemoradiation has managed to change patterns of practice and had significant impact on treatment outcomes and overall quality of life.

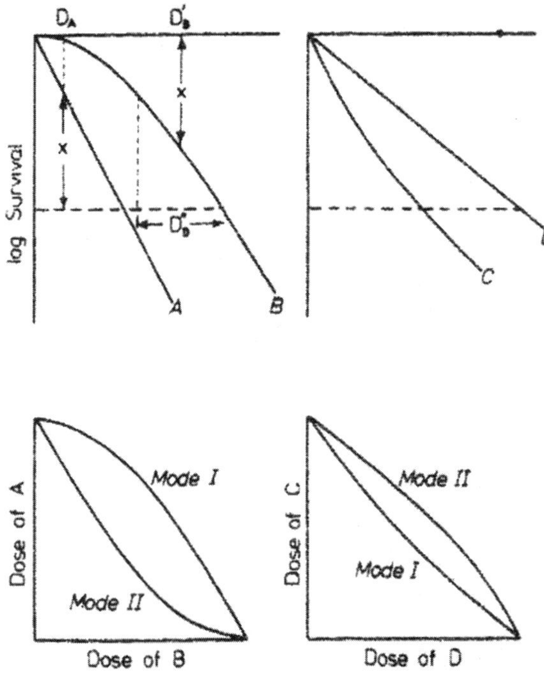

Fig. 3. The way in which an envelope of additivity may be calculated for two pairs of cytotoxic agents (A + B and C + D) where one of each pair gives a non-linear dose-response curve (isobologram analysis from Peckham and Steele ref. *27*).

The concept of the therapeutic ratio is key here as it implies that the effect of the combination therapy is greater in the tumor than in the relevant normal tissues within the treated radiation volume. The therapeutic ratio is often described in a mathematical formulation as the ratio of dose enhancement factors in the tumor divided by that in the normal tissues. The following are clear examples of clinical situations where the use of concurrent therapy has been found to be associated with an improvement in the therapeutic ratio.

8.1. Carcinoma of the Anal Canal

In this instance the early experience of Nigro et al. *(45)* suggested that there may not be a need to perform surgery as part of the initial therapy of this cancer and that it could be kept in reserve for local recurrence. Three patients treated with preoperative radiation, 5-fluorouracil, and mitomycin C were found to have complete pathologic responses at the time of their surgery. This work has been expanded upon by Cummings et al. *(46)* in their series of patients who were treated by various concurrent regimens over time and by several large intergroup studies *(47–49)* that have demonstrated the value of concurrent chemoradiation in this disease (*see* Table 3). The current standard practice for this disease in North America involves the use of concurrent chemoradiation.

8.2. Carcinoma of the Cervix

The National Cancer Institute in the United States issued a clinical alert when it became apparent that the addition of cisplatin-containing chemotherapy delivered with

Table 3
Randomized Trials of Concurrent Chemoradiation in Carcinoma of the Anus

Trial	*Number of patients*	*Therapy*	*Local control (%)*	*Overall survival 3/5 yr (%)*
UKCCCR	585	Radiation alone	39	58/–
		vs radiation with 5FU	61	65/–
		and MMC	$p = 0.0001$	
EORTC	110	Radiation alone	39	65/–
		vs radiation with 5FU	58	72/–
		and MMC	$p = 0.02$	
RTOG/ECOG	310	Radiation with 5FU	59	65
		vs radiation with 5FU	71	67
		and MMC	$p = 0.014$[a]	

[a]Four-year colostomy free survival; MMC = Mitomycin C; 5FU = 5-fluorouracil.

Table 4
Randomized Trials Illustrating the Benefit of Cisplatin-Based Concurrent Chemoradiation in Carcinoma of the Uterine Cervix

Trial	*Eligibility*	*Therapy*	*Number of patients*	*Local control (%)*	*Relative risk of death (%)*
RTOG 90-10	IB-IVA	RT(EF)	193	78[a]	
		RT + C+ 5FU	193	91[a]	0.48
SWOG 87-97	IB-IIA	RT	116	65	
		RT + C + 5FU	127	81	0.50
GOG 123	IB2	RT + TAH	183	76	
		RT + C + TAH	186	89	0.51
GOG 120	IIB-IVA	RT + HU	177		
		RT + C	176		0.57
		RT + C + HU + 5FU	173		0.55
GOG 85	IIB-IVA	RT + HU	191	70	
		RT + 5FU + C	177	75	0.79

RT = radiation, EF = extended fields, C = cisplatin, 5FU = 5 fluorouracil, TAH = extrafascial hysterectomy, HU = hydroxyurea.

[a]From local failure as site of first progression data.

concurrent radiation was found to increase the survival of patients with squamous cell carcinoma of the cervix. Table 4 shows the results of five randomized trials *(50–54)* that have now been published that lead to the clinical alert. The best schedule of delivery of cisplatin or any other chemotherapy has yet to be determined.

8.3. Small-Cell Lung Carcinoma

While the natural history of this malignancy involves early seeding of distant metastases, those patients who have localized or limited-stage small-cell carcinoma of the lung have potentially curable tumors where combined chemoradiation is important.

Meta-analyses that examined the value of thoracic radiation in the limited stage of this disease performed by both Pignon *(55)* and Warde *(56)* showed improvement in 2–3 yr survivals of 5%. Warde's analysis showed that thoracic radiation improved local control by 25%. A relatively recently published randomized trial has examined the benefit of delivering hyperfractionated radiation with the first cycle of chemotherapy and found that the 2- and 5-yr survivals with the hyperfractionated regimen were 47% and 26%, while they were only 41% and 16% with the once daily regimen *(57)*. On further analysis it was found that not only was the local control improved in the group that received hyperfractionated radiation but they also had decreased incidence of simultaneous local and distant failure, suggesting that improved local control may lead to improved survival even in this malignancy that tends to disseminate systemically. The principle of spatial cooperation enters the treatment realm again in this disease wherein the value of prophylactic cranial radiation is associated with a decrease in the incidence of brain metastases. This decreased incidence of brain metastases is associated with an increased survival in patients with limited-stage disease who have had a complete response to therapy *(58,59)*. As such, prophylactic cranial radiation forms a part of standard practice in many areas of the world in this patient population.

8.4. Wilms' Tumor

This pediatric cancer stands as an example of how cooperative group studies (NWTS and SIOP) have been able to integrate both chemotherapy and radiation into standard therapy while minimizing side-effects and dramatically improving cure rates as seen in the improvement of the 5-yr relative survival rates from 74% in 1974–1976 to 93% in 1989–1996 *(60)*. The fifth NWTS trial began in 1995 and is expected to continue until 2003 (*see* Table 5) *(60)*. This study will search for biological prognostic factors and examine the rates of cancer and birth defects in children born to survivors of Wilms' tumor.

9. WHAT IS HAPPENING AT THE MOLECULAR LEVEL?

The challenge for the future is to begin to better integrate the information that is rapidly accumulating from the revolution in the field in molecular biology to the chemoradiation armamentarium. Currently the accumulating data in a variety of research areas in oncology needs to become incorporated into the clinic, where no doubt it will make important contributions to disease outcome and patient care. Several examples of this are as follows.

9.1. Apoptosis

Programmed cell death is the definition of apoptosis, and there is increasing evidence that this is an important process in the determination of the radiation response to therapy *(61)*. The impact of this process on treatment needs to be accounted for in terms of both cancer cells and normal tissues like the salivary gland cells of the parotid that are often irreversibly damaged with treatment. Issues including the effects of the heterogeneity of tumors to undergo apoptosis and how fractionation schemes impact the apoptotic rate may be important. Of course, if apoptosis-prone tumor cells are more sensitive to radiation than those cells in which the apoptotic pathways are inhibited, then it may make sense to manipulate the gene expression of Bcl-2 or *p53* *(61)*.

Table 5
Guidelines for Therapy of Wilms' Tumor from NWTS-V

Stage	*Other factors*	*Therapy*	*Additional comments*
I	FH, <2 yr old, tumor <550 g	Nephrectomy only	Followed q 3 mo with CXR and abdominal ultrasound
	FH, >2 yr old or tumor >550 g	Pulse intensive VCR + ACD (for 18 wk)	No radiotherapy
	Any anaplasia		
II	FH		
III/IV	FH	VCR + ACD + DOX (for 24 wk) 10.8 Gy	Radiotherapy according to abdominal stage +/- whole lung radiation
II-IV	Focal anaplasia		
I-IV	CCSK	ACD + VCR + DOX + CYC + ET (for 24 wk) 10.8 Gy	Radiotherapy for all
II-IV	Diffuse anaplasia		
I-IV	Rhabdoid	Cb + ET + CYC (for 24 wk) 10.8 Gy	Radiotherapy for all

Cb = carboplatin, ET = etoposide, CYC = cyclophosphamide, DOX = doxorubicin, VCR = vincristine, ACD = actinomycin D.

9.2. Mechanisms of DNA Repair

Eukaryotic systems have four separate systems that repair double-stranded DNA breaks induced by radiation *(62)*:

1. Homologous recombinational repair (HRR).
2. Nonhomologous endjoining (NHEJ).
3. Single-strand annealing (SSA).
4. Break-induced replication (BIR).

All of these mechanisms appear to lead to the loss of genetic integrity with the exception of HRR. Because the loss of the Ku protein that is essential for NHEJ leads to extreme radiosensitivity, this was felt to be the major mammalian mechanism for DNA repair *(63)*. However, newer evidence suggests that HRR is also important *(64)*. Whether or not cells have the ability to decide which type of repair happens in transcribed regions of the DNA compared to the nontranscribed regions is not clear. Current preclinical strategies that may become more relevant to therapy in the future include the use of triplex-forming oligotrinucleotides with bound reactive chemicals that may be able to induce lesions in critical repair genes to increase the efficacy of radiation and/or chemotherapy.

9.3. Targeting Tumor Hypoxia

The evidence presented earlier, on the effects of combined modality therapy in carcinoma of the anal canal, may exploit to some extent the properties of mitomycin C as a hypoxic cell cytotoxin. This strategy remains valid, as many human tumors are less well oxygenated than the tissues from which they arose. The literature suggests that not only are these hypoxic tumors more difficult to control locally with therapy but that they may possess a more malignant phenotype with a higher propensity for distant spread. Tirapazamine is a drug developed and introduced into the clinic for its ability to target hypoxic cells *(65)*. It may be that this will lead to a therapeutic advantage as it will target hypoxic cells, not normal tissues, and second, it may be able to selectively target that cell population that is most resistant to current treatment and thus be able to improve combined modality therapy significantly.

10. NEW GENERATION OF MOLECULARLY TARGETED AGENTS

We are currently on the cusp of a new era in the treatment of cancers whereby we will learn to incorporate new drugs that are likely not cytotoxic on their own but when used in combination with standard chemotherapy and radiation hold the promise of superior tumor responses that will hopefully translate into improved local control and improved survival. At the same time it is reasonable to expect an increased selectivity for malignant cells compared to normal tissues given that many of these targets are either not altered in normal cells or their expression is not usually increased in normal tissues. This leads to the anticipation of no increase in normal tissue toxicities when these novel targeted agents are used to treat patients.

10.1. p53

p53 is a well-characterized tumor suppressor gene that has altered expression in a number of cancers. Its function is often characterized as the "guardian of the genome" and is involved in the balance of the processes of apoptosis and cell cycle regulation that are required for normal ongoing cellular and organ function *(66)*. When mammalian DNA is damaged, cells normally arrest in G_1 phase in order to repair the damage or if the damage is too extensive, programmed cell death is initiated; *p53* is intimately involved in the regulation of this decision-making step by cells as the protein becomes stabilized and its DNA binding activity increases in response to a number of stressors including UV damage, hypoxia, nucleotide depletion, DNA damaging agents, and hypoglycemia. p53 expression is known to impact a number of downstream genes *(66)* at a transcriptional level, including *Bcl-2*, *Bax*, *Fas/APO1*, and *Mdm2,* whereas its expression can be induced by any number of inappropriate proliferative signals in transformed cells *(67)* (*c-myc*, *E2F-1*, *ras*, and *E1A*). It becomes clear that changes in *p53* expression will have a profound impact on the cellular machinery's decision to pursue a pathway of inappropriately regulated proliferation.

Ample preclinical evidence that gene replacement therapy with *p53* was able to inhibit tumor growth in in vitro and in vivo scenarios has lead investigators to consider this strategy in humans. There are however a number of potential barriers to this therapy, including the efficiency of transduction, that may prove to be limiting. Recently conducted phase I and II *(68–70)* trials suggest that although the current technology allows for the transduction to occur, it may not have a significant impact on outcome. Further refinements in this strategy and larger trials are needed.

10.2. Cyclo-oxygenase2 (cox-2)

There is intriguing evidence that shows that nonsteroidal anti-inflammatory drugs have anticancer activity that could potentially lead to the use of these drugs or the newer generation of selective cox-2 inhibitors for their anticancer activity. Chapter 22 by Pyo et al. will expand upon this and address the impact of the interesting observation that a combination of the selective cox-2 inhibitor, SC-236, and radiation was found to cause a dose enhancement factor of at least 1.4 at a surviving fraction of 0.1 *(71)*.

10.3. Epidermal Growth Factor Receptor (EGFR)

The EGFR family members are perhaps the best studied of the receptor protein kinases, especially the two receptors encoded for by C-erbB1/EGFR and C-erbB2/HER2/neu. It is generally accepted that dysregulated expression of EGFR or its ligands is causative in the development and/or progression of tumorigenesis *(72)*. Abundant evidence exists that many human cancers express either EGFR or one of its common ligands, epidermal growth factor (EGF) or transforming growth factor-α (TGF-α) *(72)*. The literature also suggests that these ligands may promote angiogenesis, produce stromal proliferation, cause extracellular matrix deposition, and induce the release of cytokines *(73)*. All these actions may impact on a local tumor environment.

Upon binding of a ligand to the EGFR receptor, dimerization also occurs with activation of the intracellular kinase region of the protein. Autophosphorylation occurs, which creates a docking site for several signal-transducing proteins whose role it is to transmit the proliferative signal from the receptor to its downstream effectors. The precise signaling proteins activated and the signal delivered depend on the type of cell surface receptor that has been activated. There appears to be one of three ways *(74)* in which dysregulated expression of the EGFR receptor will lead to malignant transformation: the normal EGFR is overexpressed, a mutant receptor that is constitutively active without ligand binding, and autocrine activation of normal receptors through malignant cells producing activating ligands.

Although numerous strategies have been developed to target this cell surface receptor and its downstream effects, much of the current data that look at integrating this tactic with current radiation-based therapies have used monoclonal antibodies directed at the extracellular portion of the receptor (e.g., C225) *(75)* which are small molecules that competitively inhibit the intracellular kinase activity by binding to the adenosine triphosphate (ATP) binding site *(76)* (e.g., CI-1033). Both of these compounds show impressive preclinical results that suggest that this approach to therapy may prove very worthwhile. Chapter 18 by Moulder and Arteaga expands upon the potential role of EGFR inhibitors in the targeting of cancers.

10.4. Vascular Endothelial Growth Factor (VEGF)

The establishment of a blood supply to tumors is an important process in the growth of tumors. Certainly VEGF and its receptors on endothelial cells are pivotal in situations of tumor-related neovascularization. It has been found in situations of both benign and malignant neovascularization that the expression of both VEGF receptors, flt-1 and KDR, are strongly upregulated *(77)*. Models that provided supplemental VEGF after radiation to treated tumor cells lead to an enhancement of endothelial cell proliferation and survival *(78)*. Other models that use small molecular inhibitors of the VEGF receptor are able to demonstrate a reversion of radiation-resistant tumor phenotypes to radiation-sensitive phenotypes when used in combination therapy *(79)*. Numerous approaches are under development to attempt to target human tumor endothelial cells as a strategy to improve tumor control. Interesting preclinical results would seem to suggest that integrating these agents into radiation-based treatments would be beneficial.

10.5. Protein Kinase C (PKC)

The multigene family of protein kinase C, which functions downstream of receptor protein kinases, is involved in the transduction of signals that regulate normal develop-

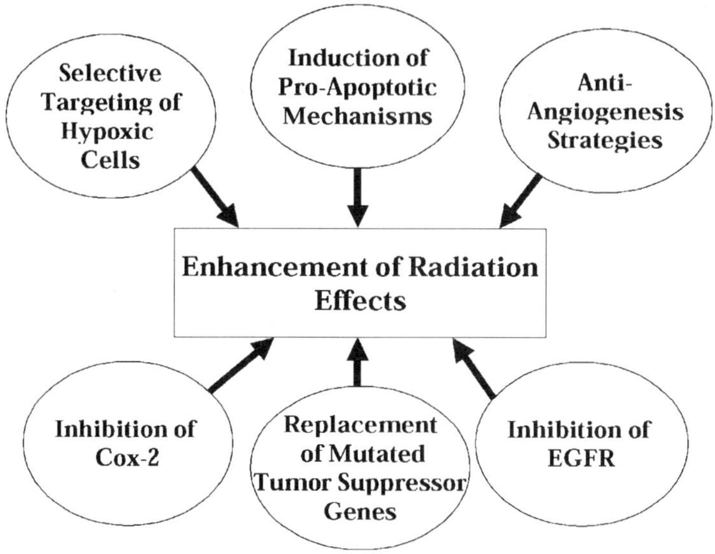

Fig. 4. Several biological mechanisms that have potential to alter sensitization strategies.

ment and cellular proliferation *(80)*. High PKC levels have been identified in certain tumor types including carcinoma of the breast, brain, and colon *(81–83)*. Manipulation of cellular PKC levels through transfection and antisense oligonucleotide strategies have indicated a role in carcinogenesis and cellular differentiation. Preclinical studies, which have examined the activity of a reversible inhibitor (PKC412) of certain PKCs including cdk1/cyclin B1, have found that it has substantial antitumor activity in a variety of murine xenografts on its own *(84)*. Furthermore, studies looking at the administration of this drug in combination with radiation have shown unique mechanisms for induced tumor growth delay depending on the *p53* status of the tumors. Those tumors that are +/+ for *p53* show a drastically increased rate of apoptotic-induced cell death for combination therapy whereas those that are –/– experienced an increased G_2 cell cycle distribution, which is the most radiosensitive part of the cell cycle *(85)*. While early clinical trials of this drug have shown that it can be safely administered on a chronic timetable, it is hopeful that in combined therapy this could significantly improve responses and survival.

There are numerous other new, targeted agents that hold the promise of improving outcomes from therapy not discussed above. They will aim to specifically block the action of numerous specific targets including cyclin-dependent kinases, mitogen-activated protein kinase, farnesyl transferases, mitogen-activated protein kinase kinase, PI 3'-kinase, matrix metalloproteinases, and Bcl-2. Figure 4 is illustrative of possible newer ways to think about radiosensitization as these novel agents are incorporated into the therapeutic armamentarium.

11. CONCLUSION

The accumulated experience over the past half-century has revealed that the delivery of chemotherapy and radiation as sole treatment modalities is complicated by multiple biologic phenomena. However, we have been able to successfully combine these modalities to improve the treatment of many solid tumors. In those tumors where significant cure rates have been achieved, efforts to decrease the overall amount of therapy to reduce both acute and chronic side effects are ongoing. However, in the majority of solid tumors the cure rates, especially those seen with locally advanced tumors, remain poor despite the integration of chemotherapy and radiation. It is the hope that by building on the revolution in molecular biology that new targeted therapies can be incorporated to improve existing treatment paradigms and allow for more patients to be cured of their malignancies.

REFERENCES

1. Gilman A. The initial clinical trial of nitrogen mustard. *Am J Surg* 1963; 105:574–578.
2. Emami B, Lyman J, Brown A, et al. Tolerance of normal tissue to therapeutic irradiation. *Int J Radiat Oncol Biol Phys* 1991; 21(1):109–122.
3. Trott KR, Kummermehr J. What is known about tumour proliferation rates to choose between accelerated fractionation or hyperfractionation? *Radiother Oncol* 1985; 3(1):1–9.
4. Trott KR. The mechanisms of acceleration of repopulation in squamous epithelia during daily irradiation. *Acta Oncol* 1999; 38(2):153–157.
5. Fowler JF. Rapid repopulation in radiotherapy: a debate on mechanism. The phantom of tumor treatment—continually rapid proliferation unmasked. *Radiother Oncol* 1991; 22(3):156–158.
6. Dorr W, Kummermehr J. Accelerated repopulation of mouse tongue epithelium during fractionated irradiations or following single doses. *Radiother Oncol* 1990; 17(3):249–259.
7. Liu K, Kasper M, Bierhaus A, et al. Connexin 43 expression in normal and irradiated mouse skin. *Radiat Res* 1997; 147(4):437–441.
8. Bristow RG, Hill RP. Molecular and cellular basis of radiotherapy. In Tannock IF, Hill RP, eds. The Basic Science of Oncology. Third edition. Montreal: McGraw-Hill; 1998. pp. 295–321.
9. Hall EJ. Radiobiology for the Radiologist. Fourth Edition. Philadelphia: JB Lippincott; 1994. pp 133–152.
10. Rosen EM, Fan S, Goldberg ID, et al. Biological basis of radiation sensitivity. Part 1: Factors governing radiation tolerance. *Oncology (Huntingt)* 2000; 14(4):543–550.
11. Saunders MI. Head and neck cancer: altered fractionation schedules. *Oncologist* 1999; 4(1):11–16.
12. Grogan M, Thomas GM, Melamed I, et al. The importance of hemoglobin lvels during radiotherapy for carcinoma of the cervix. *Cancer* 1999; 86(8):1528–1536.
13. Kapp DS, Fischer D, Gutierrez E, et al. Pretreatment prognostic factors in carcinoma of the uterine cervix: a multivariate analysis of the effect of age, stage, histology and blood counts on survival. *Int J Rad Onc Biol Phys* 1983; 9:44–53.
14. Warde P, O'Sullivan B, Bristow R, et al. T1/T2 glottic cancer managed by external beam radiotherapy: the influence of pretreatment hemoglobin on local control. *Int J Rad Onc Biol Phys* 1998; 41(2):347–353.
15. Lee WR, Berkley B, Marcial V, et al. Anemia is associated with decreased survival and increased locoregional failure in patients with locally advanced head and neck carcinoma: a secondary analysis of RTOG 85-27. *Int J Rad Onc Biol Phys* 1998; 42(5):1069–1075.
16. Pollack A, Zagars GK, Dinney CP, et al. Preoperative radiotherapy for muscle-invasive bladder carcinoma. Long term follow-up and prognostic factors for 338 patients. *Cancer* 1994; 74(10):2819–2827.
17. Brizel DM, Scully SP, Harrelson JM et al. Radiation therapy and hyperthermia improve the oxygenation of human soft tissue sarcomas. *Cancer Res* 1996; 56(23):5347–5350.
18. Becker A, Hansgen G, Bloching M, et al. Oxygenation of squamous cell carcinoma of the head and neck: comparison of primary tumors, neck node metastases, and normal tissue. *Int J Rad Onc Biol Phys* 1998; 42(1):35–41.
19. Brizel DM, Rosner GL, Prosnitz LR, et al. Patterns and variability of tumor oxygenation in human soft tissue sarcomas, cervical carcinomas, and lymph node metastases. *Int J Radiat Oncol Biol Phys* 1995 Jul 15; 32(4):1121–1125.
20. Hockel M, Schlenger K, Hockel S, et al. Tumor hypoxia in pelvic recurrences of cervical cancer. *Int J Cancer* 1998 Aug 21; 79(4):365–369.
21. Hockel M, Vaupel P. Tumor hypoxia: definitions and current clinical, biologic, and molecular aspects. *J Natl Cancer Inst* 2001 Feb 21; 93(4):266–276.
22. Breen AP, Murphy JA. Reactions of oxyl radicals with DNA. *Free Radic Biol Med* 1995; 18(6):1033–1077.

23. Sutherland RM. Tumor hypoxia and gene expression—implications for malignant progression and therapy. *Acta Oncol* 1998; 37(6):567–574.
24. Dachs GU, Tozer GM. Hypoxia modulated gene expression: angiogenesis, metastasis and therapeutic exploitation. *Eur J Cancer* 2000; 36(13 Spec No):1649–1660.
25. De Vita VT, Hellman S, Rosenberg SA. Cancer. Principles and Practice of Oncology, 5th edition. Lippincott-Raven. 1997. pp. 858–910.
26. Goldie JH, Coldman AJ, Gudauskas GA. Rationale for the use of alternating non-cross-resistant chemotherapy. *Cancer Treat Rep* 1982; 66(3):439–449.
27. Steel GG, Peckham MJ. Exploitable mechanisms in combined radiotherapy-chemotherapy: the concept of additivity. *Int J Radiat Oncol Biol Phys* 1979 Jan; 5(1):85–91.
28. Laver JH, Barredo JC, Amylon M, et al. Effects of cranial radiation in children with high risk T cell acute lymphoblastic leukemia: a Pediatric Oncology Group report. *Leukemia* 2000; 14(3):369–373.
29. Dubey AK, Recht A, Come S, et al. Why and how to combine chemotherapy and radiation therapy in breast cancer patients. *Recent Results Cancer Res* 1998; 152:247–254.
30. Wolff JA, Newton WA Jr, Krivit W, et al. Single versus multiple dose dactinomycin therapy of Wilms's tumor. A controlled co-operative study conducted by the Children's Cancer Study Group A (formerly Acute Leukemia Co-operative Chemotherapy Group A). *N Engl J Med* 1968; 279(6):290–294.
31. Lindegaard J C, Grau C. Has the outlook improved for amifostine as a clinical radioprotector? *Radiother Oncol* 2000; 57(2):113–118.
32. Vokes EE, Haraf DJ, Drinkard LC, et al. A phase I trial of concomitant chemoradiotherapy with cisplatin dose intensification and granulocyte-colony stimulating factor support for advanced malignancies of the chest. *Cancer Chemother Pharmacol* 1995; 35(4):304–312.
33. Danilenko DM. Preclinical and early clinical development of keratinocyte growth factor, an epithelial-specific tissue growth factor. *Toxicol Pathol* 1999; 27(1):64–71.
34. Phillips TL. Chemical modification of radiation effects. *Cancer* 1977 Feb; 39(2 Suppl):987–998.
35. Herscher LL, Cook JA, Pacelli R, et al. Principles of chemoradiation: theoretical and practical considerations. *Oncology (Huntingt)* 1999 Oct; 13(10 Suppl 5):11–22.
36. Franken NA, Van Bree CV, Kipp JB, et al. Modification of potentially lethal damage in irradiated Chinese hamster V79 cells after incorporation of halogenated pyrimidines. *Int J Radiat Biol* 1997; 72(1):101–109.
37. Kinsella TJ, Dobson PP, Mitchell JB, et al. Enhancement of X ray induced DNA damage by pre-treatment with halogenated pyrimidine analogs. *Int J Radiat Oncol Biol Phys* 1987; 13(5):733–739.
38. Dolling JA, Boreham DR, Brown DL, et al. Modulation of radiation-induced strand break repair by cisplatin in mammalian cells. *Int J Radiat Biol* 1998; 74(1):61–69.
39. Amorino GP, Freeman ML, Carbone DP, et al. Radiopotentiation by the oral platinum agent, JM216: role of repair inhibition. *Int J Radiat Oncol Biol Phys* 1999; 44(2):399–405.
40. Milas L, Milas MM, Mason KA. Combination of taxanes with radiation: preclinical studies. *Semin Radiat Oncol* 1999; 9(2 Suppl 1):12–26.
41. Milas L, Hunter NR, Mason KA et al. Role of reoxygenation in induction of enhancement of tumor radioresponse by paclitaxel. *Cancer Res* 1995; 55(16):3564–3568.
42. Mason KA, Milas L, Hunter NR, et al. Maximizing therapeutic gain with gemcitabine and fractionated radiation. *Int J Radiat Oncol Biol Phys* 1999; 44(5):1125–1135.
43. Lawrence TS, Eisbruch A, McGinn CJ, et al. Radiosensitization by gemcitabine. *Oncology (Huntingt)* 1999; 13(10 Suppl 5):55–60.
44. Phillips T. Biochemical Modifiers: Drug-Radiation Interactions. In Mauch PM, Loeffler JS, eds. Radiation Oncology: Technology and Biology. Philadelphia: WB Saunders Company; 1994. pp. 113–152.
45. Nigro ND, Vaitkevicius VK, Considine B Jr. Combined therapy for cancer of the anal canal: a preliminary report. *Dis Colon Rectum* 1974; 17(3):354–356.
46. Cummings BJ, Keane TJ, O'Sullivan B, et al. Epidermoid anal cancer: treatment by radiation alone or by radiation and 5-fluorouracil with and without mitomycin C. *Int J Rad Onc Biol Phys* 1991; 21(5):115–125.
47. Bartelink H, Roelofsen F, Eschwege F, et al. Concomitant radiotherapy and chemotherapy is superior to radiotherapy alone in the treatment of locally advanced anal cancer: results of a phase III randomized trial of the European Organization for Research and Treatment of Cancer Radiotherapy and Gastrointestinal Cooperative Groups. *J Clin Oncol* 1997; 15:2040–2049.
48. Flam M, John M, Pajak TF, et al. Role of mitomycin in combination with fluorouracil and radiotherapy, and of salvage chemoradiation in the definitive nonsurgical treatment of epidermoidcarcinoma of the anal canal: results of a phase III randomized intergroup study. *J Clin Oncol* 1996; 14:2527–2539.

49. UKCCCR: Epidermoid anal cancer: results from the UKCCCR randomised trial of radiotherapy alone versus radiotherapy, 5-fluorouracil, and mitomycin. UKCCCR Anal Cancer Trial Working Party. UK Coordinating Committee on Cancer Research. *Lancet* 1996; 348:1049–1054.
50. Whitney CW, Sause W, Bundy BN, et al. Randomized comparison of fluorouracil plus cisplatin versus hydroxyurea as an adjunct to radiation therapy in stage IIB-IVA carcinoma of the cervix with negative para-aortic lymph nodes: a Gynecologic Oncology Group and Southwest Oncology Group study. *J Clin Oncol* 1999; 17(5):1339–1348.
51. Rose PG, Bundy BN, Watkins EB, et al. Concurrent cisplatin-based radiotherapy and chemotherapy for locally advanced cervical cancer. *N Engl J Med* 1999; 340(15):1144–1153.
52. Keys HM, Bundy BN, Stehman FB, et al. Cisplatin, radiation, and adjuvant hysterectomy compared with radiation and adjuvant hysterectomy for bulky stage IB cervical carcinoma. *N Engl J Med* 1999; 340(15):1154–1161.
53. Morris M, Eifel PJ, Lu J, et al. Pelvic radiation with concurrent chemotherapy compared with pelvic and para-aortic radiation for high-risk cervical cancer. *N Engl J Med* 1999; 340(15):1137–1143.
54. Peters WA 3rd, Liu PY, Barrett RJ 2nd, et al. Concurrent chemotherapy and pelvic radiation therapy compared with pelvic radiation therapy alone as adjuvant therapy after radical surgery in high-risk early-stage cancer of the cervix. *J Clin Oncol* 2000; 18(8):1606–1613.
55. Pignon JP, Arriagada R, Ihde DC, et al. A meta-analysis of thoracic radiotherapy for small-cell lung cancer. *N Engl J Med* 1992 Dec 3; 327(23):1618–1624.
56. Warde P, Payne D. Does thoracic irradiation improve survival and local control in limited-stage small-cell carcinoma of the lung? A meta-analysis. *J Clin Oncol* 1992; 10(6):890–895.
57. Turrisi AT 3rd, Kim K, Blum R, et al. Twice-daily compared with once-daily thoracic radiotherapy in limited small-cell lung cancer treated concurrently with cisplatin and etoposide. *N Engl J Med* 1999; 340(4):265–271.
58. Kotalik J, Yu E, Markman BR, et al. Practice guideline on prophylactic cranial irradiation in small-cell lung cancer. *Int J Radiat Oncol Biol Phys* 2001; 50(2):309–316.
59. Auperin A, Arriagada R, Pignon JP, et al. Prophylactic cranial irradiation for patients with small-cell lung cancer in complete remission. Prophylactic Cranial Irradiation Overview Collaborative Group. *N Engl J Med* 1999; 341(7):476–484.
60. Neville HL, Ritchey ML. Wilms' tumor. Overview of National Wilms' Tumor Study Group results. *Urol Clin North Am* 2000; 27(3):435–442.
61. Meyn RE. Apoptosis and response to radiation: implications for radiation therapy. *Oncology (Huntingt)* 1997; 11(3):349–356.
62. Li L, Story M, Legerski RJ. Cellular responses to ionizing radiation damage. *Int J Radiat Oncol Biol Phys* 2001; 49(4):1157–1162.
63. Boubnov NV, Hall KT, Wills Z, et al. Complementation of the ionizing radiation sensitivity, DNA end binding, and V(D)J recombination defects of double-strand break repair mutants by the p86 Ku autoantigen. *Proc Natl Acad Sci USA* 1995; 92(3):890–894.
64. Johnson RD, Liu N, Jasin M. Mammalian XRCC2 promotes the repair of DNA double stranded breaks by homologous recombination. *Nature* 1999; 401:397–399.
65. Brown JM. Exploiting the hypoxic cancer cell: mechanisms and therapeutic strategies. *Mol Med Today* 2000; 6(4):157–162.
66. Roth JA, Grammer SF, Swisher SG, et al. Gene replacement strategies for treating non-small cell lung cancer. *Semin Radiat Oncol* 2000; 10(4):333–342.
67. Bristow RG, Benchimol S, Hill RP. The p53 gene as a modifier of intrinsic radiosensitivity: implications for radiotherapy. *Radiother Oncol* 1996; 40(3):197–223.
68. Swisher SG, Roth JA, Nemunaitis J, et al. Adenovirus-mediated p53 gene transfer in advanced non-small-cell lung cancer. *J Natl Cancer Inst* 1999; 91(9):763–771.
69. Schuler M, Rochlitz C, Horowitz JA, et al. A phase I study of adenovirus-mediated wild-type p53 gene transfer in patients with advanced non-small cell lung cancer. *Hum Gene Ther* 1998; 9(14):2075–2082.
70. Schuler M, Herrmann R, De Greve JL, et al. Adenovirus-mediated wild-type p53 gene transfer in patients receiving chemotherapy for advanced non-small-cell lung cancer: results of a multicenter phase II study. *J Clin Oncol* 2001; 19(6):1750–1758.
71. Petersen C, Petersen S, Milas L, et al. Enhancement of intrinsic tumor cell radiosensitivity induced by a selective cyclooxygenase-2 inhibitor. *Clin Cancer Res* 2000; 6(6):2513–2520.
72. Raymond E, Faivre S, Armand JP. Epidermal growth factor receptor tyrosine kinase as a target for anticancer therapy. *Drugs* 2000; 60 Suppl 1:15–23.

73. Baselga J. New therapeutic agents targeting the epidermal growth factor receptor. *J Clin Oncol* 2000; 18(21 Suppl):54S–9S.
74. Sartor CI. Biological modifiers as potential radiosensitizers: targeting the epidermal growth factor receptor family. *Semin Oncol* 2000; 27(6 Suppl 11):15–20.
75. Milas L, Mason K, Hunter N, et al. In vivo enhancement of tumor radioresponse by C225 antiepidermal growth factor receptor antibody. *Clin Cancer Res* 2000; 6(2):701–708.
76. Rao GS, Murray S, Ethier SP. Radiosensitization of human breast cancer cells by a novel ErbB family receptor tyrosine kinase inhibitor. *Int J Radiat Oncol Biol Phys* 2000; 48(5):1519–1528.
77. Gasparini G, Toi M, Gion M, et al. Prognostic significance of vascular endothelial growth factor protein in node-negative breast carcinoma. *J Natl Cancer Inst* 1997; 89(2):139–147.
78. Katoh O, Tauchi H, Kawaishi K, et al. Expression of the vascular endothelial growth factor (VEGF) receptor gene, KDR, in hematopoietic cells and inhibitory effect of VEGF on apoptotic cell death caused by ionizing radiation. *Cancer Res* 1995; 55(23):5687–5692.
79. Geng L, Donnelly E, McMahon G, et al. Inhibition of vascular endothelial growth factor receptor signaling leads to reversal of tumor resistance to radiotherapy. *Cancer Res* 2001; 61(6):2413–2419.
80. Schenk PW, Snaar-Jagalska BE. Signal perception and transduction: the role of protein kinases. *Biochim Biophys Acta* 1999; 1449(1):1–24.
81. O'Brian C, Vogel VG, Singletary SE, et al. Elevated protein kinase C expression in human breast tumor biopsies relative to normal breast tissue. *Cancer Res* 1989; 49(12):3215–3217.
82. Benzil DL, Finkelstein SD, Epstein MH, et al. Expression pattern of alpha-protein kinase C in human astrocytomas indicates a role in malignant progression. *Cancer Res* 1992; 52(10):2951–2956.
83. Kopp R, Noelke B, Sauter G, et al. Altered protein kinase C activity in biopsies of human colonic adenomas and carcinomas. *Cancer Res* 1991; 51(1):205–210.
84. Fabbro D, Ruetz S, Bodis S, et al. PKC412—a protein kinase inhibitor with a broad therapeutic potential. *Anticancer Drug Des* 2000; 15(1):17–28.
85. Zaugg K, Rocha S, Resch H, et al. Differential p53-dependent mechanism of radiosensitization in vitro and in vivo by the protein kinase C-specific inhibitor PKC412. *Cancer Res* 2001; 61(2):732–738.

2 Fluoropyrimidines as Radiation Sensitizers

Muhammad Wasif Saif, MD
and Robert B. Diasio, MD

CONTENTS

1. INTRODUCTION

Radiation sensitization with concurrent chemotherapy with an aim to improve radioresponse has long been a focus of investigation. As a result of these efforts, the concomitant use of cytostatic drugs and radiation has become the standard approach for many tumors including head and neck, rectal, anal, esophageal, pancreatic, and gastric cancers. The combined chemoradiation offers many potential advantages vs single modality treatment, such as reduction in local failure rates, eradication of micrometastases to enhance distant control, preservation of organ function, and decrease in tumor bulk prior to surgery to make complete resection possible and improve survival.

From: *Chemoradiation in Cancer Therapy*
Edited by: H. Choy © Humana Press Inc., Totowa, NJ

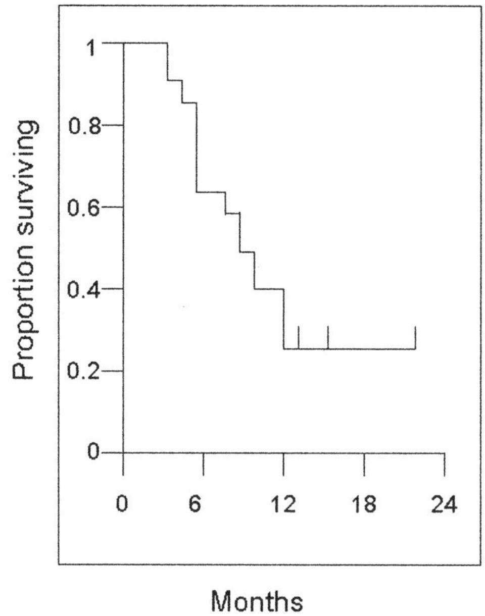

Fig. 1. Floxuridine radiosensitization—long-term freedom from liver progression for patients with nondiffuse primary hepatobiliary cancer treated with combined radiation therapy and hepatic artery infusion of floxuridine.

An ideal radiosensitizer would be the one that can maximize radiation therapy benefit, can be easily administered, can be optimally sequenced with radiation therapy for best effects, and have no overlapping toxicities with radiation. Although falling short in certain of these characteristics, 5-fluorouracil (5-FU) has become the most promising clinical radiosensitizer in combined chemoradiotherapy regimens.

Randomized trials have demonstrated that a combination of fluorouracil (5-FU)-based chemotherapy and radiotherapy significantly improves the survival of patients with both pancreatic *(1)* and rectal cancers *(2,3)* when compared with the administration of radiation alone. Furthermore, the improved response rates with use of biomodulators of 5-FU, such as lecovorin (LV) in colorectal cancers, led to the use of this biomodulator also in the combined chemoradiotherapy regimens involving 5-FU *(4)*. FdUrd is a related nucleoside, which has also been used with radiation. FdUrd is actively metabolized by the liver, and results in high regional drug concentrations with minimal systemic toxicity when administered via hepatic artery infusion *(5)*. FdUrd has also been tested with concurrent whole-liver radiation for colon carcinoma metastatic to the liver *(6,7)* (Fig. 1).

5-FU is an analog of uracil in which the hydrogen in the 5 position is replaced by fluorine, whereas FdUrd is an analog of deoxyuridine (Fig. 2). Its cytotoxicity is achieved through several mechanisms. In vitro studies have demonstrated enhanced cytotoxicity of radiation by fluorouracil. The combined effects of radiation and fluorouracil in controlling tumor growth are better than the additive effects of the two modalities given independently. The radiosensitizing efficacy of 5-FU depends on continuous exposure of tumor cells to 5-FU for 8 h or more following radiation *(8)*. Because of the short half-life of 5-FU, the drug must be administered as a continuous infusion (CI) to achieve prolonged tumor cell exposure to effective levels of 5-FU. This schedule of administration

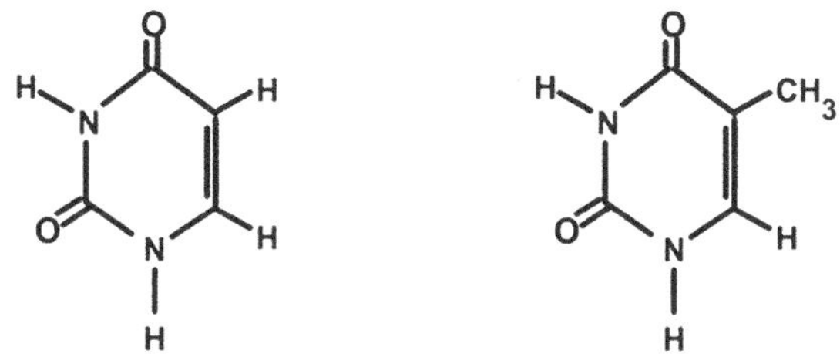

Uracil Thymine

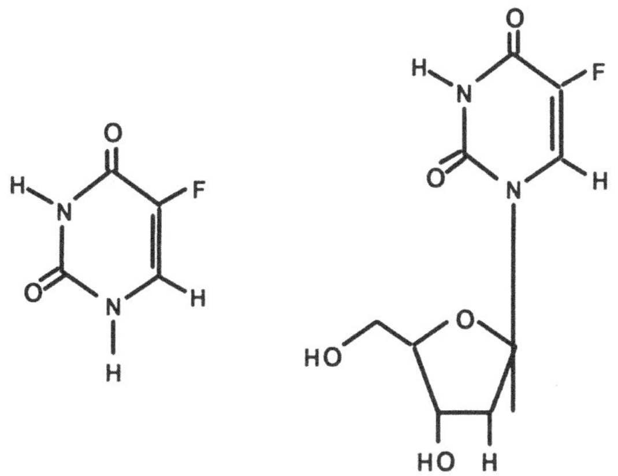

5-Fluorouracil (5-FU) 5-Fluoro-2'-deoxyuridine (FdUrd)

Fig. 2. Structure of fluorouracil (5-FU) and floxuridine (5-fluoro-2'-deoxyuridine, FdUrd).

is also associated with less myelotoxicity. Use of CI 5-FU infusion regimens, however, has been limited by the need for an indwelling venous catheter and a portable infusion pump. These catheters are associated with development of complications including thrombosis and infection *(9)*.

The recent availability of oral formulations of 5-FU, may provide not only an improvement in the ease of administration and the efficacy of fluoropyrimidine therapy, but also alleviate complications related to the catheters. Such agents include uracil:tegafur (UFT) and capecitabine (Xeloda).

The mechanisms of interaction between fluorouracil and radiation are not clearly understood. Different hypotheses have been postulated to explain the synergistic or potentiated effect of 5-FU with radiation including redistribution of cells to a more radiosensitive cell cycle phase, deranged pyrimidine pools with reduced capacity for repair of DNA damage, and activation of apoptosis. The effect of 5-FU on radiation damage also appears to vary in different cell lines, thus complicating the extrapolation of laboratory results into clinical practice.

2. PHARMACOLOGY OF FLUOROPYRIMIDINES

The fluoropyrimidines as a group can affect the synthesis and function of both deoxyribonucleic acid (DNA) and ribonucleic acid (RNA), and both of these two mechanisms

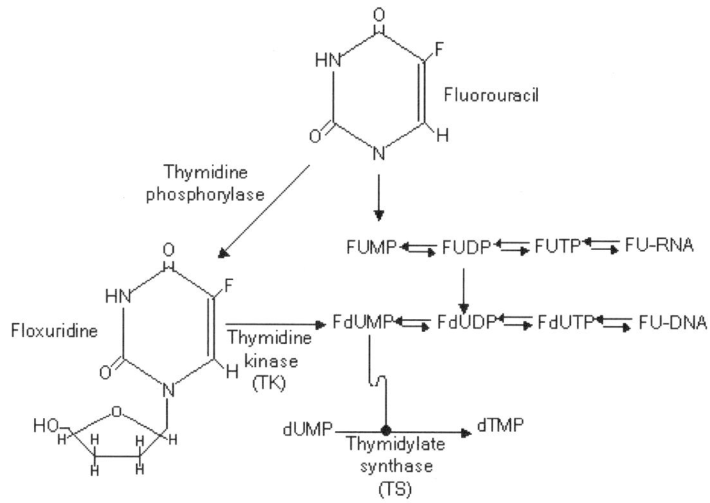

Fig. 3. Metabolism of the fluoropyrimidines: dTMP = deoxythymidine monophosphate, dUMP = deoxyuridine monophosphate, FdUDP = fluorodeoxyuridine diphosphate, FdUMP - fluorodeoxyuridine monophosphate, FdUTP = fluorodeoxyuridine triphosphate, FU-DNA= fluorouracil-deoxyribonucleic acid, FUDP = fluorouracil diphosphate, FUMP = fluorouracil monophosphate, FU-RNA = fluorouracil-ribonucleic acid, FUTP = fluorouracil triphosphate.

have lead to different consequences. Some cell lines are more sensitive to 5-FU's DNA-directed pathways, whereas RNA-medicated cytotoxicity predominates in other cell lines *(10,11)*.

2.1. DNA-Directed Effects of Fluropyrimidines

5-FU can be metabolized to form fluorodeoxyuridine monophosphate (FdUMP), which finally affects DNA. FdUrd is phosphorylated to FdUMP is (via thymidine kinase). For 5-FU to be converted into FdUMP, it involves at least two steps (Fig. 3). FdUMP is a potent inhibitor of the enzyme thymidylate synthase (TS), which is responsible for converting deoxyuridine monophosphate (dUMP) to deoxythymidine monophosphate (dTMP). TS inhibition leads to depletion of thymidine nucleotides and accumulation of deoxyurindine nucleotides, which leads to several events, including perturbations in other nucleotide pools, arrest in S phase of the cell cycle (growth arrest), and, ultimately, to DNA fragmentation and loss of clonogenicity *(12,13)*. In addition to inhibition of TS activity, FdUMP can be converted to fluorodeoxyuridine triphosphate (FdUTP) and become incorporated into DNA. The relative importance of TS inhibition and FdUTP incorporation into DNA on FdUrd-mediated DNA damage is not yet clear *(14,15)*.

2.2. RNA-Directed Effects of Fluropyrimidines

Although FdUrd produces only DNA-medicated cyotoxicity, 5-FU can also be metabolized to fluorouracil monophosphate (FUMP) and ultimately to fluorouracil triphosphate (FUTP), which can be incorporated into RNA in place of uridine triphosphate (UTP). In other words, incorporation of 5-FU into RNA mimics uracil *de novo* synthesis and affects the production of ribosomal RNAs (rRNAs) *(16,17)*. 5-FU also affects several aspects of messenger RNA (mRNA) function, including transcription *(18)*, translation *(19)*, and slicing *(20)*.

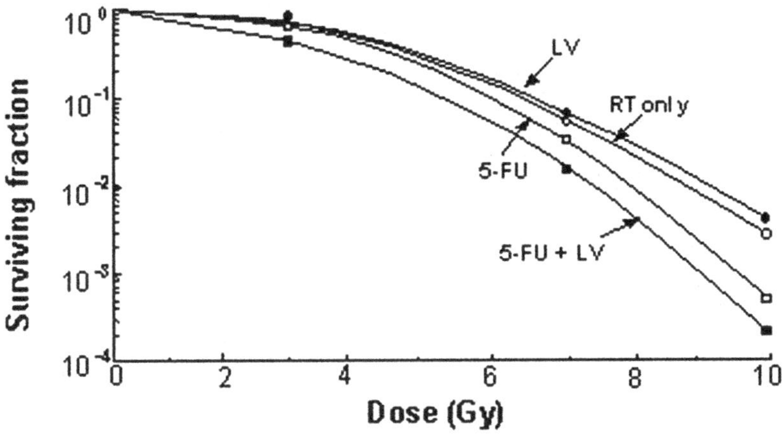

Fig. 4. 5-FU-induced radiosensitization of HT29 human colon cells is potentiated by LV. HT29 cells were exposed for 14 h to: median alone (○), 10 umol/L LV (●), 1 umol/L 5-FU (■). Cells were assessed and data are expressed as described in Fig. 4.

3. BIOMODULATION

The DNA-mediated effects of fluropyrimidines can be modulated by a number of agents, such as leucovorin (LV), levamisole, and interferon-alpha (IFN-alpha). LV prolongs TS inhibition by increasing the availability of the reduced folate cofactor necessary for formation of the inactive TS–FdUMP complex *(21)* (Fig. 4). Studies show alpha-interferon can potentiate 5-FU-mediated cyotoxicity, but the mechanisms are not yet defined *(22,23)*. Another approach to modulate the activity of fluoropyrimidines is the use of the nucleoside transport inhibitor dipyridamole. Dipyridamole probably permits 5-FU to enter the cell, and may trap intracellular nucleoside metabolites, hence increasing cytotoxicity *(24,25)*, but the exact mechanism underlying the selective cytotoxicity against tumor cells compared with normal tissues still needs to be determined.

4. FLUOROPYRIMIDINE-RADIATION INTERACTIONS

Fluoropyrimidine-radiation interactions can best be understood in terms of the fundamental mechanisms by which fluoropyrimidines lead to DNA damage and ultimately cell death. Two such mechanisms have been described as:

1. Futile repair.
2. Endonuclease activation.

4.1. Futile-Repair Hypothesis

The futile-repair hypothesis is based on the concept that "FdUrd treatment lethally deranges normal mechanisms of the cells for removing low levels of dUTP that become misincorporated in DNA." dUTP is a good substrate for DNA polymerases (alpha and beta). A high dUTP/thymidine triphosphate (dTTP) ratio occurs after treatment with sufficient concentrations of FdUrd, which subsequently leads to misincorporation of dUTP into DNA. Uracil-*N*-glycosylase, an enzyme that recognizes uracil misincorporation and cleaves the glycosidic bond, producing an apyrimidinic site. This site is recognized by an apurinic/apyrimidinic nuclease, producing a DNA break. The cell has several mechanisms for repairing DNA single-strand breaks *(26)*. One such repair mechanism under normal conditions is as follows: neighboring nucleotides are cleaved, DNA polymerase fills in the gap, and DNA ligase seals the new, correct bases (including dTTP) into place. On the other hand, in the case of a high dUTP/dTTP ratio, such as following administration of FdUrd, dUTP will still be favored over dTTP, and this futile cycle of excision and repair would repeat itself. As mentioned earlier, FdUTP can also be incorporated into DNA in place of dTTP, which would be expected to produce a similar futile cycle to that produced by dUTP incorporation. It has been hypothesized that larger gaps would occur over time that would be sensitive to other cellular nucleases, resulting in a potentially lethal DNA double-strand break and DNA fragmentation *(27)*. This is called "futile-repair hypothesis."

4.2. Endonuclease Activation

Hirota et al. *(28)* observed that treatment of FM3A murine mammary carcinoma cells with FdUrd produced cytotoxicity that was accompanied by the generation of DNA fragments having an unusually discrete size distribution (ranging from 50 to 200 kb). The lack of incorporated uracil in these cells and the finding that this damage could also be caused by agents that did not cause dUTP elevation and dTTP depletion argued against the futile repair hypothesis *(28)*. It was found that the fragment size range noted in these cells is similar to the estimated size of an individual replication unit, and it was proposed that the observed pattern of damage resulted from selective digestion of actively replicating DNA by an induced endonuclease activity. This hypothesis was further supported by findings that lysates prepared from FdUrd-treated FM3A cells contained an endonuclease activity that was absent from control cells, and that the appearance of this endonuclease activity could be prevented by inhibiting protein synthesis with cyclohexamide treatment *(29)*.

In brief, it is postulated that futile repair and endonuclease activation may both lead to DNA fragmentation after FdUrd treatment, with the dominant process depending on a cell-line-specific factor. Neither of the two observed fragmentation patterns resembles the random damage produced by ionizing radiation.

5. MECHANISMS OF RADIOSENSITIZATION BY FLUOROPYRIMIDINES

There are four hypotheses that underline the combined effect of chemoradiation therapy employing fluoropyrimidines:

1. Fluoropyrimidines cause changes in nucleotide pools that alone increase the cytotoxicity of radiation (i.e., by depleting substrates used in the repair of radiation-induced DNA damage).
2. Fluoropyrimidines do radiosensitize by causing redistribution of cells into a relatively sensitive phase of the cell cycle (early S).
3. Radiosensitization depends on the incorporation of FdUTP into DNA.
4. Radiation as a potentiation for fluoropyrimidine-mediated cytotoxicity.

5.1. Nucleotide Pool Perturbations

One hypothesis for fluoropyrimidine-induced radiosensitization is that fluoropyrimidines induce changes in nucleotide pools including the ability of polymerases to

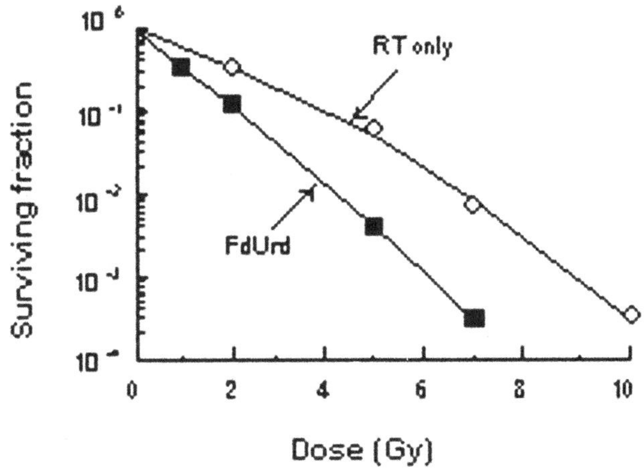

Fig. 5. HuTu80 human colon cancer cells are radiosensitized by FddUrd. HuTu80 cells were irradiated under control conditions (O) or after a 14-h exposure to 100 nmol L FdUrd (■). They were then assessed doe survival using a clonogenic assay. Data are expresses as the mean (point) ± SE (bar), which is within the symbol unless indicated.

find the correct base required for DNA repair. This alteration leads to either misrepaired or unrepaired DNA double-strand breaks, which is consistent with the decrease in sublethal damage repair and DNA double-strand break repair. Studies have indicated that both 5-FU *(30)* and FdUrd *(12)* deplete dTTP pools in human colorectal cancer cells within 1–2 h of drug exposure, whereas radiosensitization takes many hours to ensue. This suggests that nucleotide pool perturbations may result in radiosensitization under some circumstances, but pool changes alone do not seem to be the sole mechanism responsible to fluropyrimidine-induced radiosensitization.

5.2. Cell Cycle Redistribution

Another proposal is that radiosensitization embarks from 5-FU-induced cell cycle redistribution. Both 5-FU and FdUrd result in arrest of S phase cells and block cells that are not in S phase at the G1/S interface. Studies in rodent *(31)* and HeLa cells *(32)* have revealed that early S phase is a relatively sensitive phase of the cell cycle, thereby suggesting that fluoropyrimidine-mediated radiosensitization may result from redistribution into a more radiosensitization phase of the cell cycle. Investigators also tried to evaluate dependence on the timing of exposure to fluoropyrimidines in relation to radiation on the resultant radiosensitization, such as to correlate the enhancement ratio with the fraction of cells in early S phase *(12)* (Fig. 5).

Cell cycle redistribution may not be the sole factor if cells are irradiated before drug exposure, but it has been shown that 5-FU can sensitize even when cells are irradiated before drug exposure. Byfield et al. found that 5-FU radiosensitizes HeLa cells only when the drug exposure followed radiation (the cells were treated with 5-FU, either before or after radiation, for up to 8 d). A similar finding was observed on HT29 human colon cancer cells, except that in these experiments cells were exposed to 5-FU for a maximum of only 30 min before radiation *(33)*. These observations demonstrate that radiosensitization can be produced in the absence of cell cycle redistribution.

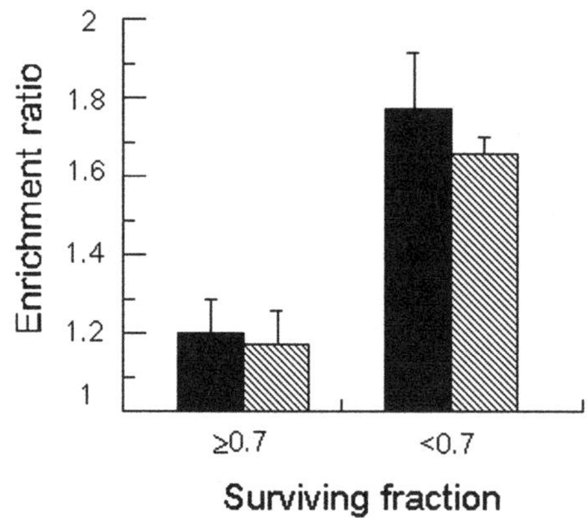

Fig. 6. FdUrd-induced radiosensitization is greater under treatment conditions that produce cytotoxicity. Data from Miller and Kinsella et al. and the data from Bruso et al. and Lawrence et al., the average radiation enhancement ratio is shown for a variety of FdUrd treatment conditions.

Investigations were also focused to assess cell cycle redistribution when cells are exposed to fluoropyrimidines before radiation. Lawrence et al. used a mechanical technique called centrifugal elutriation to obtain populations enriched in various phases of the cell cycle and found large differences in radiation sensitivity during different phases of the cell cycle, HT29 cells evidenced no significant differences in radiation sensitivity during different phases of cell cycle *(34,35)*. These findings suggest that although cell cycle redistribution accompanies fluoropyrimidine treatment, it does not appear to cause the increase in radiation sensitivity observed.

5.3. Incorporation of FdUTP into DNA

CB3717 is a TS inhibitor and does not incorporate into DNA. CB3717 is also a potent radiosensitizer of HT29 cells (under the same conditions as FdUrd) *(35)*. This finding reflects that incorporation of FdUTP into DNA may not be a prerequisite for radiosensitization.

5.4. Radiation as a Potentiation for Fluoropyrimidine-Mediated Cytotoxicity

It has been postulated that radiation may act as a potentiator of fluoropyrimidine-medicated cytotoxicity. This possibility is borne out of the observation that fluoropyrimidine-induced radiosensitization of human colon cancer cells tends to occur under conditions that produce at least some cytotoxicity by the drug alone *(15,33,36,37)*. This hypothesis is further supported by the data employing FdUrd treatment in HT29 cells, which showed that enhancement ratio was significantly greater when surviving fraction was <0.7 than when the surviving fraction was ≥0.7 ($p < 0.05$ by *t* test) (Fig. 6).

6. PHARMACOLOGICAL AND SCHEDULING REQUIREMENTS FOR OBTAINING EFFECTIVE RADIOSENSITIZATION WITH FLUOROPYRIMIDINES

6.1. Effect of Pharmacology of 5-FU on Radiosensitization

5-FU has a short half-life (10–15 min). Bolus doses of 5-FU disappear from the blood stream rapidly because of hepatic degradation of drug. Since radiosensitization requires constant drug exposure, bolus drug dosing cannot achieve effective radiosensitization *(38)*. Pharmacologic studies have also shown that 5-FU has nonlinear pharmacokinetics, which is another pharmacologic factor as with its radiosensitizing effect *(39,40)*. Nonlinear pharmacokinetics may occur due to the presence of two mechanisms competing for drug removal: removal of drug by proliferating body tissues, largely through incorporation into RNA, and hepatic degradation *(40)*. It is postulated that these two mechanisms are antagonistic because hepatic degradation eliminates the drug whereas incoporation of the drug into RNA is one of the mechanisms of action responsible for the cytoxicity of 5-FU *(41)*. Clinically, these two phenomena interact and result in essentially no drug demonstrable when 5-FU is infused at doses below 15 mg/kg/24 h. The investigators hypothesized that under such conditions, 5-FU "clearance" equals the cardiac output, i.e., the drug is totally cleared during a single passage (subject to minor differences in tissue bed uptake). However, at dosages higher than about 15mg/kg/24 h, a linear relationship between infusion dose and mean plasma level have been noted (>15–65 mg/kg/24 h). The plasma 5-FU levels obtained during continuous infusions between dose levels of 15 and 65 mg/kg/d provide the concentrations necessary to cause significant cytotoxicity in human tumor cells in tissue culture and to induce radiosensitization. This observation suggested a quantitative relationship between tissue culture data and 5-FU levels required for in vivo cytotoxic radiosensitization of tumor cells *(42)*.

6.2. Effect of Scheduling of 5-FU on Radiosensitization

The studies have also suggested the "scheduling" requirements for obtaining radiosensitization induced by 5-FU, and that 5-FU must be present for at least 24 h after each (and every) radiation fraction to achieve maximum radiosensitization. Investigators also tried to determine the optimum duration of the infusion. Moertel et al. studied CI up to 24 h in duration and found no significant difference in toxicity vs bolus therapy *(43)*. On the other hand, Seifert et al. showed that 5-FU infusions for 5 d resulted in a marked shift in limiting toxicity *(44)*. Byfield et al. examined 72-h infusions of 5-FU and found central nervous system (CNS) toxicity, previously not seen with shorter infusions (where marrow suppression is the main toxicity) *(40)*. Lokich et al. studied "protracted" infusions in which 5-FU is essentially infused constantly until toxicity, tumor progression, or mechanical complications affected the therapy *(45)*. The studies proposed that infusion between 96 h and infinite hours (PI: protracted infusion) can be used for radiosensitizing regimens provided the drug is infused to limiting toxicity. In almost all patients this toxicity will involve some components of each patient's squamous cell renewal system.

6.3. Integration of 5-FU and Radiation

Byfield proposed certain principles that may govern the development of radiosensitization produced by 5-FU *(23,46,47)*.

6.3.1. Duration of Schedule

The infusion should be at least 96 h and preferably be protracted infusion. The schedule is based on the degree of radiosensitization as a function of primary 5-FU cytotoxicity. Although radiosensitization can be achieved with infusions shorter than 96 h, neurological side-effects become a limiting toxicity *(40)*. Therefore, probably 96 h is the "shortest" infusion that is both safe and effective in inducing radiosensitization (Figs. 7 and 8).

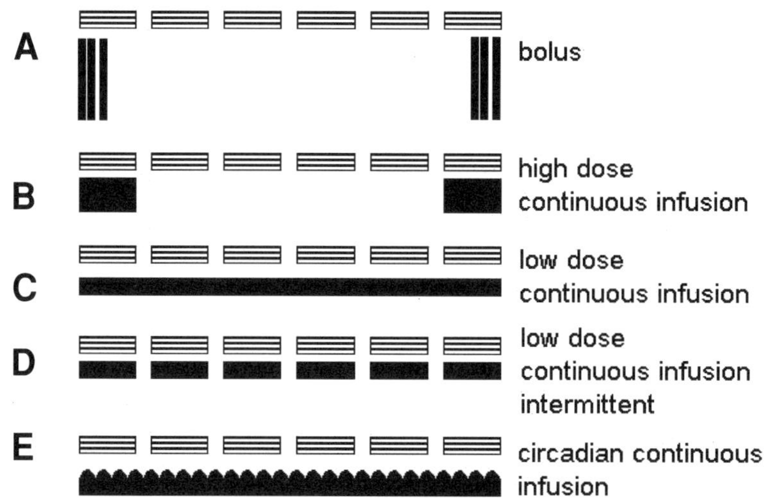

Fig. 7. A schematic representation of treatment of 5-FU and external irradiation. The stippled rectangles represent weekly irradiation (9 Gy total/wk, given in five doses of 1.8 Gy). Concurrent 5-FU is represented by the solid bars beneath the irradiation, and the height of the bars represents the peak level of radiosensitizing chemotherapy. By using protracted infusional schedules of 5-FU, radiosensitizing chemotherapy can be given with each daily dose of irradiation (from 5 to 35 d). Newer schedules using continuous intermittent and circadian schedules have achieved high tumor activity with acceptable toxicity in recent trials.

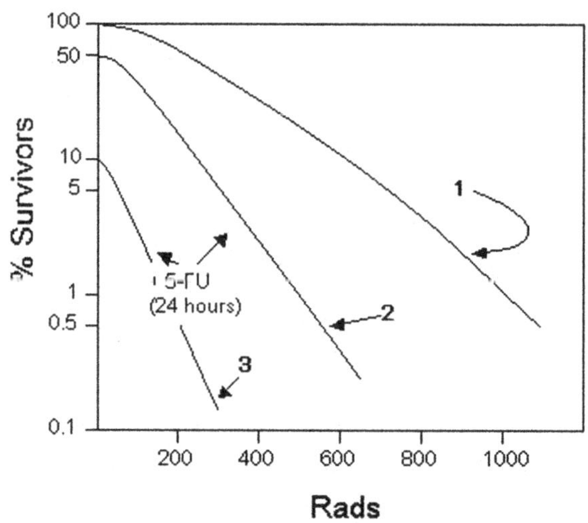

Fig. 8. Diagram of 5-FU radiosensitization. Curve 1: Radiation survival curve for cells not treated with 5-FU. Curve 2: Radiation survival curve for cells treated postradiation with sufficient 5-FU to kill 50% of the cells without radiation (partial response equivalent). Curve 3: Radiation survival curve with 5-FU killing to 10% (typical of cell system very sensitive to 5-FU).

Table 1
Cancers Sensitive to 5-FU Radiosensitization

Cancers
Esophagus
Anus
Larynx
Vulva
Penis
Bladder
Rectum
Head and neck
Pancreas
Gastric

6.3.2. Fractionation Scheme of Radiation

Investigators have employed all schemes inducing conventional fractionation (180–200 rad/d), hyperfractionation, and hypofractionation. There is no convincing evidence that infused 5-FU affects the late effects of radiation, which are a function, primarily, of the daily treatment fraction size. However, the capacity to combine radiosensitizing infused 5-FU with hyperfractionated radiation should be considered, especially in patients requiring retreatment where tolerance is an issue and can be increased by hyperfractionation.

6.3.3. Cyclicity of Administration of 5-FU

Cyclicity of administration is vital in the use of 5-FU as a radiosensitizer. The concept of cyclical treatment has been well established in cancer chemotherapy and alien to classical radiation therapy (where it is termed "split-course" therapy). 5-FU radiosensitizes tumor tissue as well as normal cells. However, this normal tissue radiosensitization is limited to the irradiated field. Suitable fractionation (i.e., cyclical therapy) can permit rapid normal tissue recovery *(23)*. The results of infused 5-FU and radiation in head and neck cancer supports the principle that cyclical treatment with 5-FU does not suffer from the limitations apparent in split-course radiation treatments.

The above described "principles" imply that optimal therapy should include tumors that are 5-FU-sensitive or, in other words, are derived from normal tissues sensitive to infused 5-FU. Tumors insensitive to 5-FU cannot be radiosensitized using this approach *(42)*.

Practically speaking, 5-FU infused at 25–30 mg/kg/d continuously for 5 d will radiosensitize virtually all 5-FU-sensitive tumors listed in Table 1. Although the "optimal" regimen has yet to be established, the 5-d schedule of 5-FU currently appears close to an ideal regimen.

7. ROLE OF *p53* IN 5-FU-INDUCED RADIOSENSITIZATION

The role of *p53* in flouropyrimidine-radiation interaction remains controversial. Some investigators have suggested that cells which are *p53* mutated are more resistant to radiation *(48)*, whereas others have found that *p53* status is unrelated to radiation sensitization *(49–51)*. Studies on SW620 cells (which are not sensitized) and HT29 cells (which are sensitized) that have the identical *p53* mutations, revealed that *p53* status does not play an independent role in fluoropyrimidine-mediated radiosensitization *(52)*. It has also been found that RKO cells, which are mutant, wild-type (wt), or effectively null (through E6 transfection) in *p53*, are equally radiosensitized by FdUrd. Interestingly enough, fluoropyrimidines lead to elevation of *p53* levels in cells with wt *p53 (53)*. It is also known that *p53* elevation produced by TS inhibition occurs when cells enter S (i.e., after having passed through the G_1 checkpoint) *(54)*. This all leads to a model in which fluoropyrimidine-treated cells progress through the classic G_1 checkpoint and into S phase for several hours before arresting or progressing (slowly); the latter condition is associated with radiosensitization.

8. ROLE OF 5-FU RADIOSENSITIZATION IN GENE THERAPY

Although it is beyond the scope of this chapter to delve deeply into gene therapy, it is worth mentioning that 5-FU could have a potential role as a radiosensitizer in this complex area as well. It has been revealed that the bacterial enzyme cytosine deaminase (CD) can be introduced into cells, so that they become capable of converting 5-flucytosine (nontoxic antifungal agent) into 5-FU *(55)*. 5-FU produced from 5-flucytosine in cells containing CD can also radiosensitize *(56)*. Another possibility is that the activation of this agent under the control of a carcinoembryonic antigen (CEA) promoter could allow nonspecificity of the introduction of the CD gene, relying on the presence of CEA for the tumor specificity. However, only a fraction of cells are transduced in vivo and these cells must be capable of killing the rest of the tumor (the bystander effect), thereby disqualifying this concept. In the case of intracellular CD, high levels of intracellular 5-FU are generated from 5-flucytosine, which tends to kill the "factory" before the bystander *(57)*. It underlines the basis to develop gene therapy strategies for both direct cytotoxicity and radiosensitization that maximize the bystander effect.

9. ORAL FORMS OF 5-FU

The recent availability of oral formulations of 5-FU involving the ability to modulate the anabolic and catabolic metabolism of 5-FU with LV and dihydropyrimidine dehydrogenase (DPD) inhibitors has provided a substantial improvement in the ease of administration and may probably improve the efficacy of fluoropyrimidine-induced radiosensitization. Such oral fluoropyrimidines include UFT (uracil:tegafur) plus oral LV (Orzel™), an oral DPD-inhibitory fluoropyrimidine (DIF), and capecitabine (Xeloda; Roche).

With daily administration, Orzel results in similar concentrations of 5-FU as those achieved with CI 5-FU, without the necessity for indwelling catheters and infusion pumps. The predominant toxicity of Orzel is gastrointestinal and myelosuppression *(58)*. Capecitabine is an oral prodrug of 5-FU. Capecitabine is an approved agent (by FDA) that offers potential for simulating an intermittent continuous infusion of 5-FU without the inconvenience and morbidity associated with indwelling catheters. Clinical data suggest a favorable safety profile when given alone. Another compelling reason to evaluate capecitabine in combination with radiotherapy is that some tumors have high levels of thymidine phosphorylase (dThdPase). In the clinical studies, high tumor levels of this enzyme correlated with low likelihood of benefit to 5-FU. In contrast, high intratumoral dThdPase levels in preclinical models are associated with enhanced sensitivity to capecitabine. Moreover, combining capecitabine with radiotherapy may mimic the radiosensitizing effect of 5-FU when given intravenously *(59)*.

9.1. Orzel in Combination with Radiation Therapy

The regimes combining Orzel and capecitabine with radiation therapy have become the focus of increasing interest in the management of patients' various malignancies including rectal, anal, locally advanced head and neck, esophageal, and pancreatic cancers.

9.2. Head and Neck Cancer

Takahashi et al. *(60)* found that UFT with concurrent radiotherapy was both effective and well tolerated, with a response rate approaching 94%. Fujii et al. *(61)* performed a phase I study and reported that UFT 300 mg/m^2 daily and carboplatin AUC: 5.0 d 1 every 8 wk was well tolerated with local radiation and recommended this dose schedule for phase II evaluation. Rivera et al. *(62)* in a phase II study in patients with stage III and IV squamous cell cancer of the head and neck involving UFT (6 mg/kg on d 1–21), vinorelbine (25 mg/m^2 on d 1 and 8) and CDDP (100 mg/m^2 on d 1), the combination being repeated every 21 d for four cycles followed by UFT (5 mg/kg/d) and carboplatin (100 mg/m^2/wk) administered concurrently with radiation found encouraging results. Gonzalez-Larriba et al. *(63)* performed a phase III study comparing UFT (300 mg/m^2 d 2 to 20) and CDDP (100 mg/m^2 d 1) with CI 5-FU (100 mg/m^2 d 2–6) and CDDP (100 mg/m^2 d 1) (both regimens repeated every 21 d for four cycles) as neoadjuvant therapy prior to radiation therapy (50–70 Gy) in patients with stage III and IV head and neck cancer. The overall response rates of the two arms were 79% vs 73%, overall survival of 37 vs 15 wk, and time to progression of 14.5 and 8.5 wk, respectively. However, the trend in each efficacy parameter favored the UFT/CDDP arm.

9.3. Nonsmall-Cell Lung Cancer

Takeda et al. *(64)* performed a phase I/II study consisting of low-dose CDDP (6–10 mg/m^2/d) and UFT (600 mg/d) combined with radiotherapy (50 Gy/25 fractions) as postoperative adjuvant therapy following curative resection for patients with nonsmall-cell lung cancer (NSCLC). The combined therapy was well tolerated and resulted in a disease-free survival rate of 78% at 2 yr. Another study in a small number of patients with unresectable stage III nonsmall-cell lung cancer, UFT (400 mg/m^2 on d 1–52) and CDDP (80 mg/m^2 on d 8, 29, and 50) were administered with radiation therapy (total dose of 60.8 Gy in 38 fractions on d 1–52). Among 17 evaluable patients, 94% (16 patients) achieved partial responses with median time to tumor progression of 30 wk, and the 1-yr survival rate of 80% *(65)*.

9.4. Gastric Cancer

UFT was studied in combination with radiation therapy in patients with locally advanced, inoperable gastric carcinoma. Tsukiyama et al. *(66)* evaluated combined modality therapy (CMT) consisting of UFT and mitomycin-C administered together with radiation therapy, and reported local control in 70% of patients with advanced inoperable gastric cancer.

9.5. Pancreatic Cancer

Robert et al. *(67)* conducted a phase I trial in patients with pancreatic cancer, consisting of UFT/LV (starting dose of UFT was 150 mg/m^2/d, escalated in increments of 50 mg/m^2/d with three patients per cohort to a current level of 300 mg/m^2/d), LV 90 mg/d, both in three divided doses for 35 d starting on d 1 of radiation, and concurrent radiation therapy (45 Gy; 1.8 Gy/d). The preliminary results revealed minimal hematologic toxicity (except for one episode of grade 4 neutropenia on d 38) and infrequent and reversible nonhematologic toxicity, median survival of 12.5 mo (range 4–19 mo) and the median time to progression of 9 mo. Patient accrual was stopped because an MTD had not been reached at the 300 mg/m^2/d dose of UFT. A second phase of the study is planned incorporating changes in patient selection criteria and in treatment schedule.

9.6. Rectal Cancer

Hoff et al. *(68)* performed a phase I study in patients with clinical stage II and III rectal carcinoma involving preoperative chemoradiotherapy consisting of UFT starting at 250 mg/m^2/d (escalated by 50 mg/m^2/d for subsequent levels) plus LV (90 mg/d) combined with radiotherapy (45.0 Gy) followed later by surgery. Then postoperatively, patients received adjuvant UFT/LV (UFT 300 mg/m^2/d and LV 90 mg/d) in a 28-d schedule every 35 d for four cycles. The recommended dose level of UFT with radiation was 350 mg/m^2/d with 90 mg/d of LV. de la Torre et al. *(69)* conducted a phase II study of UFT/LV (300 mg/m^2/d UFT and 30 mg/d LV on days 8–35) administered with concurrent pelvic radiation (total dose of 35 Gy) in patients with unresectable or recurrent rectal cancer, and found that 13% of patients had a complete response, 69% a partial response, and complete pathologic response was observed in 9%. Studies aiming at postoperative UFT/LV plus radiotherapy are ongoing at present.

10. CAPECITABINE (XELODA) IN COMBINATION WITH RADIATION THERAPY

Xeloda mimics continuous FU infusion with a more convenient administration schedule. In addition, it has been demonstrated in experimental models that radiation upregulated dThdPase activity in tumor tissue. It has also been demonstrated that Xeloda given in combination with radiation therapy was associated with superior activity when compared to either given alone, whereas FU and XRT in combination did not show clear evidence of an additive effect *(70)*.

A phase I study of Xeloda in combination with XRT in rectal cancer is in the adjuvant, neoadjuvant, and palliative settings *(71–73)*. The DLT of the combination is hand-foot syndrome and mild to moderate leukopenia, diarrhea, and local skin reaction *(71–73)*. The recommended dose for phase 2 studies is Xeloda 825 mg/m^2 twice daily without interruption in combination with standard dose of radiation. Promising activity has been demonstrated in neoadjuvant therapy with six objective responses in seven evaluable patients including one pathological confirmed CR.

11. CLINICAL INDICATIONS OF FLOUROPYRIMIDINE-INDUCED RADIOSENSITIZATION

The use of 5-FU in combination with radiotherapy has shown improved survival in various malignancies including unresectable pancreatic cancer, resectable pancreatic cancer, Dukes B2 and C rectal cancer, esophageal cancer, and hepatobiliary cancer (Table 2). Similarly, 5-FU with concurrent radiation has also been used for organ preservation in different tumors involving bladder cancer, anal cancer, and laryngeal cancer (Table 3).

Table 2
Malignancies in which Fluoropyrimidines and Radiation Therapy Appear to Improve Survival

Ref.	*Disease*	*Group*	*Treatment*	*Survival*
1	Unresectable pancreatic cancer	GITSG	Radiation (40 Gy) + 5-FU	42.2 wk[a]
			Radiation alone (60 Gy)	22.9 wk[a]
78	Resectable pancreatic cancer	GITSG	Radiation alone (40 Gy) + 5-FU	21.0 mo[a]
			No adjustment treatment	10.9 mo[a]
2	Dukes B2 and C rectal cancer	GITSG	No adjuvant therapy	35%[b]
			Radiation (40–44 Gy + 5-FU + semustine	55%[b]
3	Dukes B2 and C rectal cancer	NCCTG	Radiation (45-50.4 Gy) alone	35%[c]
			Radiation (45–50.4 Gy)+ 5-FU +/- semustine	55%[c]
80	Dukes B2 and C rectal cancer	NCCTG	Radiation (54 Gy) + bolus 5-FU +/- semustine	60%[d]
			Radiation (54 Gy) + infusion 5-FU +/- semustine	70%[d]
76	Esophageal cancer	RTOG	Radiation (64 Gy) alone	8.9 mo[a]
			Radiation (50 Gy)+5-FU + cisplatin	12.5 mo[a]
85	Primary hepatobiliary cancer	University of Michigan	Radiation + hepatic arterial floxuridine	16 mo

[a]Median survival.
[b]5-yr survival.
[c]7-yr survival.
[d]4-yr survival.
[e]Phase I/II study.

Table 3
Malignancies in which 5-FU and Radiation Therapy Have Been Used for Organ Preservation

Ref.	*Disease*	*Treatment*	*Number of patients*	*Percentage of organ sparing*
86	Bladder cancer	Radiation (60 Gy) + 5-FU	34	70%
87		Radiation (60–65 Gy)	19	89%
81	Anal cancer	Radiation (30 Gy) + 5-FU + mitomycin	45	76%
82		Radiation (30–45 Gy) + 5-FU + mitomycin	22	100%
88	Laryngeal cancer	5-FU + cisplatin + radiation (66–76 Gy)[a]	332	64%

[a]Sequential delivery of chemotherapy and radiation.

11.1. Esophageal Cancer

The feasibility of concomitant chemoradiotherapy has been evaluated in numerous studies in esophageal cancer, given either as preoperative treatment or as primary therapy. In most of these studies, fluorouracil was an integral part of the chemotherapy regimen. Byfield et al. *(74)* evaluated the efficacy of 5-FU infusion (for 5 d) and 10 Gy of radiation (in four fractions given every 2 wk) for a total of six cycles. Five of six patients achieved complete responses and were alive at the time of the report (range: 1–22 mo). Coia et al. *(75)* reported the results of 57 patients with stage I or II esophageal cancer who received fluorouracil infusion (for 4 d × two cycles, starting on d 2 and 29), and CMT (on d 2) with radiation (60 Gy in 30 fractions). The 3- and 5-yr actuarial survivals were 29% and 18%, respectively. The disease-specific survival was 41% and 30% at 3 and 5 yr, respectively. In a randomized intergroup trial, 121 patients with localized esophageal cancer were administered either 64 Gy of radiation alone or four cycles of fluorouracil and cisplatin plus 50 Gy of radiation. The results showed 24-mo survival of 38% in the chemoradiotherapy arm vs 10% in the radiation-alone arm ($p = 0.001$). An additional follow-up revealed a 3-yr survival of 31% in the chemoradiotherapy arm vs no 3-yr survival in the radiation-only arm *(77)*. The local failure rate was 44% in the combined-modality arm vs 65% in the radiation-only arm ($p < 0.01$). Within 12 mo, the rate of distant metastasis was 22% in the combined-modality arm vs 38% in the radiation-only arm ($p = 0.005$), and more toxicity was associated with the combined-modality treatment. In addition, 44% of patients in the combined-modality arm had severe side effects and 20% had life-threatening side effects vs 25% and 3%, respectively, in the radiation-alone arm.

The results of the intergroup trial compound the concept of radiosensitization, since a lower dose of radiation in the combined-modality group improved local control compared with the radiation-alone group. The chemotherapy also decreased the risk of micrometastasis. Despite the better outcome with chemoradiotherapy, the overall prognosis of these patients remains poor. No randomized trials comparing chemoradiotherapy with esophagectomy have been performed; it seems that chemoradiotherapy provides a reasonable alternative to esophagectomy in selected patients.

11.2. Pancreatic Cancer

In a Gastrointestinal Tumor Study Group (GITSG) trial *(78)*, patients were randomized to adjuvant chemoradiotherapy or to observation alone after complete resection. Radiation was administered in two courses of 20 Gy each, separated by an interval of 2 wk, for a total dose of 40 Gy. Fluorouracil was given for three consecutive days at the beginning of each radiation course and was then continued once weekly for 2 yr. Although only a small number of patients were evaluated, the study suggested a significant survival benefit for the combined treatment arm vs the control arm (median survival: 20 mo vs 11 mo, respectively). However, 71% of the treatment arm and 86% of the control arm developed recurrent disease.

The GITSG then randomized 194 patients with locally advanced, unresectable pancreatic cancer to receive 60 Gy of radiation alone, 40 Gy of radiation plus fluorouracil, or 60 Gy radiation plus fluorouracil *(1)*. The median time to progression was 12.6 wk for the radiation group vs 30–34 wk for the combined-modality groups. The median survival for radiation-alone group was 5.5 mo vs 10 mo for the combined-modality group. Although the median survival of patients receiving 60 Gy was slightly better than those who received 40 Gy, the difference was not significant.

In another GITSG study, patients with locally unresectable pancreatic cancer were randomized to multidrug chemotherapy (streptozocin, CMT, and fluorouracil) or to 54 Gy of radiation plus fluorouracil followed by the same three-drug chemotherapy regimen. Overall survival for the combined chemoradiotherapy group was superior, i.e., 41% at one year vs 19% for the chemotherapy group *(79)*.

11.3. Rectal Cancer

The GITSG randomized patients with resected Dukes B2 or C rectal cancer to one of four arms: no adjuvant therapy, postoperative radiotherapy of 40–48 Gy, postoperative chemotherapy with fluorouracil (500 mg/m^2 on the first 3 d and the last 3 d of radiotherapy) and semustine, or combined chemotherapy and radiotherapy *(2)*. Two hundred and two evaluable patients of the original 227 patients showed at 7 yr, the survival of 56% for the combined treatment group compared with 32% for the control group ($p = 0.005$). Both locoregional and distant recurrence decreased, but the main advantage was improved locoregional control. The chemotherapy alone or radiotherapy alone groups did not improve local control or survival significantly.

The Mayo Clinic/North Central Cancer Treatment Group (NCCTG) randomized patients with resected rectal cancer and tumor penetration through the rectal wall or with metastatically involved lymph nodes were assigned to postoperative radiation alone (45–50.4 Gy) or to two courses of chemotherapy with fluorouracil and semustine followed by concomitant fluorouracil and radiotherapy and two additional courses of chemotherapy *(3)*. At 5 yr, the recurrence-free survival was 37% for the radiation group vs 58% for the combined-modality group ($p = 0.0016$). The overall survival was 44% for the radiation group vs 57% for the combined-modality group ($p = 0.025$). The incidence of severe late complications was similar between the two treatment groups. An intergroup trial demonstrated the benefit of protracted fluorouracil infusion when given concomitantly with radiation as indicated by a significant decrease in recurrence (from 47% to 37%) and distant metastasis (from 40% to 31%) compared with those who received bolus fluorouracil *(80)*. Survival was better in patients treated with protracted venous infusion of fluorouracil. Patients in the protracted fluorouracil group had a higher incidence of severe diarrhea, whereas the bolus fluorouracil group had more severe myelosuppression.

11.4. Anal Cancer

The Wayne State regimen consisted of two cycles of fluorouracil infusion (1000 mg/m^2/d d 1–4 and on d 29–32), and CMT (15 mg/m^2 on d 1) with radiation (total dose of 30 Gy) *(81)*. The results revealed overall 5-yr survival rates of 70–90% and preservation of anal sphincter function in more than two-thirds of the patients. The main toxicities of CMT may include severe, life-threatening hematologic and pulmonary toxicity, and hemolytic uremic syndrome. Cummings et al. *(82)* evaluated its contribution to the efficacy of the combined modality therapy in a series of nonrandomized protocols in which patients were treated with radiation plus fluorouracil and CMT, radiation plus fluorouracil, or radiation only. The local control and cause-specific survival for patients receiving radiation and fluorouracil plus CMT were significantly superior compared with those receiving radiation and fluorouracil or radiation alone. In a randomized trial by the Radiation Therapy Oncology Group (Study 87-04), patients were treated with 45 Gy of radiation and two courses of fluorouracil (1000 mg/m^2/d for 4 d on wk 1 and 4) *(82)*. They were randomized to receive or not receive CMT (10 mg/m^2 on d 1 and 29). Preliminary results suggested significant improvements in the four-year locoregional control (82% vs 64%, respectively), colostomy-free survival (71% vs 59%, respectively), and survival without evidence of disease (73% vs 51%, respectively) for patients who received both fluorouracil and CMT vs those who received fluorouracil alone. The difference in overall survival was not statistically significant (76% vs 67%, respectively). Patients receiving fluorouracil and CMT were also noted to have a higher incidence of severe toxicities than those receiving fluorouracil alone. This study confirmed that CMT constitutes an important component of the combined chemoradiotherapy modality at the cost of increased toxicity. In a study that included 20 patients with locally recurrent and/or metastatic anal cancer, fluorouracil and cisplatin achieved a 55% response rate *(83)*. The preliminary result of a phase II trial by the Eastern Cooperative Oncology Group (ECOG) using fluorouracil, cisplatin, and 59.4 Gy of radiation showed an overall response rate of 92% and a complete response rate of 74% *(84)*. An intergroup randomized study is underway to determine whether a high dose (59.4 Gy) is more effective than a moderate dose (45 Gy) of radiation and whether fluorouracil plus cisplatin is a more effective chemotherapy regimen than fluorouracil plus CMT.

12. SUMMARY

The pharmacologic studies indicated that intrinsic pharmacokinetics of 5-FU hinder their ability to reproduce the conditions required for radiosensitization. Indeed, the short half-life of the drug (from hepatic removal) preclude anything other than addictive effects when bolus drug is added to any variety of radiation fractionation scheme. These two sets of requirements together demonstrated that a continuous infusion (in which drug is made present for at least 24 h after each radiation fraction) would be optimal. In summary, 5-FU is a potent radiosensitizer under the following defined circumstances.

1. 5-FU has to be present for at least 24 h after each radiation exposure in order to establish the radiosensitive state. Prior exposure to the drug (with its removal after X-ray exposure) has no effect on radiation survival.
2. In order for 5-FU to render cells sensitive to radiation, a demonstrable degree of cell killing by 5-FU has to occur. In other words, some effectiveness of drug alone must be seen (equivalent quantitatively to killing slightly short of a clinical partial response).
3. 5-FU-insensitive human cancers probably cannot be radiosensitized by 5-FU.

Although, there are theoretical advantages of combining chemotherapy and radiotherapy to enhance cytotoxicity, 5-FU combined with concurrent radiation has been shown to improve treatment outcome in several malignancies, in particular, gastrointestinal cancers. Despite this progress, further efforts are required to improve the current results by well-designed randomized clinical trials, especially involving newer/oral agents. Basic laboratory research is also indicated to elucidate the underlying mechanisms of interaction between 5-FU and radiation, to facilitate the development of more effective drugs, and to provide the framework for future clinical trials.

REFERENCES

1. Moertel CG, Frytak S, Hahn RG, et al. Therapy of locally unresectable pancreatic carcinoma: A randomized comparison of high dose (6000 rads) radiation alone, moderate dose radiation (4000 rads + 5-fluorouracil), and high dose radiation +5-fluorouracil. *Cancer* 1981; 48:1705–1710.
2. Gastrointestinal Tumor Study Group. Prolongation of the disease-free interval in surgically treated rectal carcinoma. *N Eng J Med* 1985; 312:1465–1472.
3. Krook JE, Moertel CG, Gunderson LL, et al. Effective surgical adjuvant therapy for high-risk rectal carcinoma. *N Eng J Med* 1991; 324:709–715.
4. Minsky BD, Cohen AM, Kemeny N, et al. Enhancement of radiation-induced downstaging of rectal cancer by fluorouracil and high-dose leucovorin chemotherapy. *J Clin Oncol* 1992; 10:79–84.

5. Ensminger WD, Rosowsky A, Raso V, et al. A clinical pharmacological evaluation of hepatic arterial infusions of 5-fluoro-2'-deoxyuridine and 5-fluorouracil. *Cancer Res* 1978; 38:3784–3792.
6. Byfield JE, Barone RM, Frankel SS, et al. Treatment with combined intra-arterial 5-FUdR infusion and whole-liver radiation for colon carcinoma metastatic to the liver. *Am J Clin Oncol* 1984; 7:319–325.
7. Raju PI, Maruyama Y, DeSimone P, et al. Treatment of liver metastases with a combination of chemotherapy and hyperfractionated external radiation therapy. *Am J Clin Oncol* 1987; 10:41–43.
8. Lawrence TS, Tepper JE, Blackstock AW. Flouropyrimidine-radiation interaction in cells and tumors. *Semin Radiat Oncol* 1997; 7:260–266.
9. Monreal M, Davant E. Thrombotic complications of central venous catheters in cancer patients. *Acta Haematol* 2001; 106(1–2):69–72.
10. Daher GC, Harris BE, Diasio RB. Metabolism of pyrimidine analogues and their nucleosides. *Pharmacol Ther* 1990; 48:189–222.
11. Parker WB, Cheg YC. Metabolism and mechanism of action of 5-fluorouracil. *Pharmacol Ther* 1990; 48:381–395.
12. Miller EM, Kinsella TJ. Radiosensitization by fluorodeoxyuridine: Effects of thymidylate synthase inhibition and cell synchronization. *Cancer Res* 1992; 52:1687–1694.
13. Heimburger DK, Shewach DS, Lawrence TS. The effect of fluorodeoxyuridine on sublethal damage repair in human colon cancer cells. *Int J Radiat Oncol Biol Phys* 1991; 21:983–987.
14. Kufe DW, Scott P, Fram R, et al. Biologic effect of 5-fluoro-2'-deoxyuridine incorporation in L1210 deoxyribonucleic acid. *Biochem Pharmcol* 1983; 32:1337–1340.
15. Danenberg PV, Heidelberger C, Mulkins MA, et al. The incorporation of 5-fluoro-2'-deoxyuridine into DNA of mammalian tumor cells. *Biochem Biophys Res Commun* 1981; 102:654–658.
16. Goel R, Cleary SM, Horton C, et al. Selective intraperitoneal biochemical modulation of methotrexate by dipyridamole. *J Clin Oncol* 1989; 7:262–269.
17. Wilkinson DS, Pitot HC. Inhibition of ribosomal ribonucleic acid maturation in Novikoff hepatoma cells by 5-fluorouracil and 5-fluorouridine. *J Biol Chem* 1973; 248:63–68.
18. Greenhalgh DA, Parish JH. Effect of 5-fluorouracil combination therapy on RNA processing in human colonic carcinoma cells. *Br J Cancer* 1990; 61:415–419.
19. Iwata T, Watanabe T, Kufe DW. Effects of 5-fluorouracil on globin mRNA synthesis in murine erythroleukemia cells. *Biochemistry* 1986; 25:2703–2707.
20. Dolnick BJ, Pink JJ. Effects of 5-fluorouracil in dihydrofolate reductase and dihydrofolate reductase mRNA from methotrexate-resistant KB cells. *J Biol Chem* 1985; 260:3006–3014.
21. Houghton JA, Houghton P, Wooten RS. Mechanism of induction of gastrointestinal toxicity in the mouse by 5-fluorouracil, 5-fluorourdine, and 5-fluoro-2'-deoxyuridine. *Cancer Res* 1979; 39:2406–2413.
22. Chu E, Zinn S. Boarman D, et al. Interaction of gamma interferon and 5-fluorouracil in the H630 human colon carinoma cell line. *Cancer Res* 1990; 50:5834–5840.
23. Wadler S, Wersto R, Weinberg V, et al. Interaction of fluorouracil and interferon in human colon cancer cell lines: Cytotoxic and cytokinetic effects. *Cancer Res* 1990; 50:5735–5739.
24. Grem, JL, Mulcahy T, Miller EM, et al. Interaction of deoxyuridine with fluorouracil and dipyridamole in a human colon cancer cell line. *Biochem Pharmacol* 1989; 38:51–59.
25. Curtin NJ, Harris AL, Aherne GW. Mechanism of cell death following thymidylate synthase inhibition: 2-deoxyuridine-5-triphosphate accumulation, DNA damage, and growth inhibition following exposure to CB3717 and dipyridamole. *Cancer Res* 1991; 51:2346–2352.
26. Friedberg EC, Hanawalt PC (eds). DNA Repair, New York; Marcel Dekker, 1988.
27. Ingraham H. Dickey L, Goulian M. DNA fragmentation and cytotoxicity from increased cellular deoxyuridylate. *Biochemistry* 1986; 25:3225–3230.
28. Hirota Y, Yoshioka A, Tanaka S, et al. Imbalance of deoxyribonucleoside triphosphates, DNA double-strand breaks and cell death caused by 2-chlorodeoxyadenosine in mouse FM3A cells. *Cancer Res* 1989; 49:915–919.
29. Yoshioka A. Tanaka S, Hiraoka O, et al. Deoxyribonucleoside triphosphate imbalance. 5-fluorodeoxyuridine-induced DNA double strand breaks in mouse FM3A cells and the mechanism of cell death. *J Biol Chem* 1987; 262:8235–8241.
30. Berger SH, Hakala MT. Relationship of dUMP and free FdUMP pools to inhibition of thymidylate synthase by 5-fluorouracil. *Mol Pharmacol* 1984; 25:303–309.
31. Sinclair WK. Cyclic X-ray responses in mammalian cells in vitro. *Radiat Res* 1968; 33:620–643.
32. Terasima T, Tolmach LJ. Variation in several responses of Hela cells to x-irradiation during the division cycle. *Biophys J* 1963; 3:11–33.

33. Byfield JE, Sharp TR, Tang S, et al. Phase I and II trial of cyclical 5-day infused 5-fluorouracil and coincident radiation in advanced cancer of the head of neck. *J Clin Oncol* 1983; 2:406–413.
34. Smalley SR, Kimler BF, Evans RG. 5-fluorouracil modulation of radiosensitivity in cultured human carcinoma cells. *Int J Radiat Oncol Biol Phys* 1991; 20:207–211.
35. Lawrence TS, Davis M, Tang HY, et al. Fluorodeoxyuridine-mediated radiosensitization of human colon cancer cells is not caused by cell cycle redistribution. *Proc AACR* 1992; 33:502, (abstr 3002).
36. Bruso CE, Shewach DS, Lawrence TS. Fluorodeoxyuridine-induced radiosensitization and inhibition of DNA double strand break repair in human colon cancer cells. *Int J Radiat Oncol Biol Phys* 1990; 19:1411–1417.
37. Lawrence TS, Davis MA, Maybaum J, et al. The potential superiority of bromodeoxyuridine to iododeoxyuridine as a radiation sensitizer in the treatment of colorectal cancer. *Cancer Res* 1992; 52:3698–3704.
38. Chadwick M, Chang C. Comparative physiologic dispositions of 5-fluoro-2'-deoxyuridine and 5-fluorouracil in mice bearing solid L1210 lymphocytic leukemia. *Cancer Treat Rep* 1976; 60(7): 845–855.
39. Myers CE. The pharmacology of the fluoropyrimidines. *Pharmacol Rev* 1981; 33:1–15.
40. Byfield JE, Sharp TR, Frankel SS, et al. Phase I and pharmacologic study of 72-hour infused 5-fluorouracil in man. *Amer J Clin Oncol* 1985; 8:429–440.
41. Valerote F, Santelli G. 5-fluorouracil (FUra). *Pharmacol Ther* 1984; 24:107–132.
42. Byfield JE. 5-FU radiation sensitization. *Invest New Drugs* 1989; 7:111–116.
43. Moertel CG, Schutt AJ, Reitemeier RJ, et al. A comparison of 5-fluorouracil administered by slow infusion and rapid injection. *Cancer Res* 1972; 32:2717–2719.
44. Seifert P, Baker LH, Reed ML, et al. A comparison of 5-fluorouracil administered by slow infusion and rapid injection. *Cancer Res* 1972; 32:2717–2719.
45. Lokich J. Bothe A, Fine N, et al. Phase I study of protracted venous infusion of 5-fluorouracil. *Cancer* 1981; 48:2565–2568.
46. Byfield JE. Theoretical basis and clinical applications of 5-fluorouracil used as a radiosensitizer. In: Rosenthal CJ, Rothman M (eds) Clinical Applications of Continuous Infusion Chemotherapy and Concomitant Radiation Therapy, Plenum Publishing Corp. New York, 1986, pp. 113–125.
47. Byfield JE. The clinical use of 5-fluorouracil and other halopyrimidines as radiosensitizers in man. In: Lokich J (ed) Cancer Chemotherapy by Infusion. Precept Press, Chicago, 1987, pp. 479–501.
48. Lowe SW, Schmitt EM, Smith SW, et al. p53 is required for radiation-inducted apoptosis in mouse thymocytes. *Nature* 1993; 362:847–849.
49. Brachman DG, Beckett M, Graves D, et al. p53 mutation does not correlate with radiosensitivity n 24 head and neck cancer cell lines. *Cancer Res* 1993; 53:3667–3669.
50. Slichenmyer WJ, Nelson WG, Slebos RJ, et al. Loss of p53-associated G1 checkpoint does not decrease cell survival following DNA damage. *Cancer Res* 1993; 53:4164–4168.
51. Zellars R, Naida J, Davis MA, et al. The effect of p53 overexpression on radiation sensitivity of human colon cancer cells. *Radiat Oncol Investing* 1997; 5:43–49.
52. Rodrigues NR, Rowan A, Smith MEF, et al. p53 mutations in colorectal cancer. *Proc Natl Acad Sci USA* 1990; 87:7555–7559.
53. Tishler RB, Calderwood SK, Coleman CN, et al. Increases in sequence specific DNA binding by p53 following treatment with chemotherapeutic and DNA damaging agents. *Cancer Res* 1993; 53:2212–2216, (suppl).
54. Matsui S, Arrendondo A, Wrzosek C, et al. DNA damage and p53 induction do not cause ZD1694 induced cell cycle arrest in human colon carcinoma cells. *Cancer Res* 1996; 56:4715–4723.
55. Huber BE, Austin EA, Richards CA, et al. Metabolism of 5-fluorocytosine to 5-fluorouracil in human colorectal tumor cells transduced with the cytosine deaminase gene: Significant antitumor effects when only a small percentage of tumor cells express cytosine deaminase. *Proc Natl Acad Sci USA* 1994; 91:8302–8306.
56. Khil MS, Kim JH, Mullen CA, et al. Radiosensitization by 5-fluorocytosine of human colorectal carcinoma cells in culture transduced with cytosine deaminase gene. *Clin Cancer Res* 1996; 2:53–57.
57. Ng EY, Rehemtulla A, Laurence TS, et al. Preferential cytotoxicity of cells transduced with cytosine deaminase compared to bystander cells after treatment with 5-flucytosine. *Radiat Res Soc Proc* 1977.
58. Hoff PM, Pazdur R, Benner SE, Canetta R. UFT and leucovorin: a review of its clinical development and therapeutic potential in the oral treatment of cancer. *Anticancer Drugs* 1998; 9:479–490.
59. Budman DR, Meropol NJ, Reigner B, et al. Preliminary studies of a novel oral fluoropyrimidine carbamate: capecitabine. *J Clin Oncol* 1998; 16:1795–1802.

60. Takahashi H, Yao K, Sawaki S, Kubota A, Tsukuda M, Miyake H, Horiuchi M, Takeyama I, Kikuchihara M, Kubota T, et al. Investigation of UFT and radiation combination therapy of head and neck cancer mainly in laryngeal cancer. *Gan To Kagaku Ryoho* 1990; 17:2037–2042.
61. Fujii M, Nameki H, Kawaura M, et al. A dose finding study of carboplatin (CBDCA) + UFT in head and neck cancer. *Proc Am Soc Clin Oncol* 1998; 18:406a (abstr 1564).
62. Rivera F, Lopez-Brea M, Lopez-Vega J, Pascual C, Rubio A, et al. High activity of UFT vinorelbine and cisplatin (UFTVP) as induction chemotherapy for locally advanced squamous cell head and neck carcinoma (SCHNC). *Proc Am Soc Clin Oncol* 1997; 16:386a (abstr 1376).
63. Gonzalez-Larriba J, Garcia Carbonero I, Sastre Valera J, Perez Segura P, Diaz-Rubino E. Neoadjuvant therapy with cisplatin/fluorouracil vs cisplatin/UFT in locally advanced squamous cell head and neck cancer. *Oncology (Huntingt)* 1997; 11(9 Suppl 10): 90–97.
64. Ito H, Takeda Y, Uno T, et al. A Phase I/II trial of UFT and low-dose cisplatin plus concurrent thoracic radiotherapy (TRT) for resected P-N2 non-small cell lung cancer. *Proc Am Soc Clin Oncol* 1999; 18:510a (abstr 1966).
65. Ichinose Y, Yano T, Asoh H, et al. UFT plus cisplatin with concurrent radiotherapy for locally advanced non-small-cell lung cancer. *Oncology (Huntingt)* 1999; 13(7 Suppl 3): 98–101.
66. Tsukiyama I, Akine Y, Kajiura Y, et al. Radiation therapy for advanced gastric cancer. *Int J Radiat Oncol Biol Phys* 1988; 15:123–127.
67. Robert F, Raben D, Spencer S. UFT/oral calcium folinate plus radiation in pancreatic cancer. *Oncology (Huntingt)* 1999; 13(7 Suppl 3):127–128.
68. Hoff PM, Janjan N, Saad Ed, et al. Phase I study of preoperative oral uracil and tegafur plus leucovorin and radiation therapy in rectal cancer. *J Clin Oncol* 2000; 18:3529–3534.
69. de la Torre A, Ramos S, Valcarcel FJ, et al. Phase II study of radiochemotherapy with UFT and low-dose oral leucovorin in patients with unresectable rectal cancer. *Int J Radiat Oncol Biol Phys* 1999; 45:629–634.
70. Sawada N, Ishikawa T, Sekiguchi F, Tanaka Y, Ishitsuka H. X-ray irradiation induces thymidine phosphorylase and enhances the efficacy of capecitabine in human xenografts. *Clin Cancer Res* 1999; 5(10):2948–2953.
71. Dunst J, Reese T, Frings S. Phase I Study of Capecitabine Combined with Simultaneous Radiotherapy Rectal Cancer. ASCO 2001, 149a.
72. Yoon W-H, Choi J-H, Kim J-R, et al. Enhanced Tumoricidal Effect of Preoperative Chemoradiation Using Capecitabine for Locally Advanced Rectal Cancer. ASCO 2001, 104b.
73. Ben-Josef E, Vaishampayan UN, Vaitkevicius VK, et al. A Single Institution Experience with Concurrent Capecitabine and Radiation Therapy in Gastrointestinal Malignancies. ASCO 2001, 1436.
74. Byfield JE, Barone R, Mendelsohn J, et al. Infusional 5-fluorouracil and X-ray therapy for non-resectable esophageal cancer. *Cancer* 1980; 45:703–708.
75. Coia LR, Engstrom PF, Paul AR, et al. Long-term results of infusional 5-FU, mitomycin-C, and radiation as primary management of esophageal carcinoma. *Int J Radiat Oncol Biol Phys* 1991; 20:29–36.
76. Herskovic A, Martz K, al-Sarraf M, et al. Combined chemotherapy and radiotherapy compared with radiotherapy alone in patients with cancer of the esophagus. *N Engl J Med* 1992; 326:1593–1598.
77. Al-Sarraf M, Pajak T, Herskovic A, et al. Progress report of combined chemo-radiotherapy (CT-RT) vs radiotherapy (RT) alone in patients with esophageal cancer. An intergroup study. *Proc Annu Meet Am Soc Clin Oncol* 1993; 12:197.
78. Kalser MH, Ellenberg SS. Pancreatic cancer: adjuvant combined radiation and chemotherapy following curative resection. *Arch Surg* 1985; 120:899–903.
79. Gastrointestinal Tumor Study Group. Treatment of locally unresectable carcinoma of the pancreas: comparison of combined-modality therapy (chemotherapy plus radiotherapy) to chemotherapy alone. *J Natl Cancer Inst* 1988; 80:751–755.
80. O'Connell MJ, Martenson JA, Wieand HS, et al. Improving adjuvant therapy for rectal cancer by combining protracted-infusion fluorouracil with radiation therapy after curative surgery. *N Engl J Med* 1994; 331:502–507.
81. Nigro ND, Vaitkevicius VK, Considine B. Combined therapy for cancer of the anal canal: a preliminary report. *Dis Colon Rectum* 1974; 17:354–356.
82. Flam MS, John JM, Pajak T, et al. Radiation (RT) and 5-fluorouracil (5-FU) vs radiation, 5-FU, mitomycin-C (MMC) in the treatment of anal carcinoma: results of a phase III randomized RTOG/ ECOG intergroup trial. *Proc Annu Meet Am Soc Clin Oncol* 1995; 14:191. Abstract A443.

83. Mahjoubi M, Sadek H, Francois E, et al. Epidermoid anal canal carcinoma (EACC): activity of cisplatin and continuous 5-fluorouracil in metastatic and/or local recurrent disease. *Proc Annu Meet Am Soc Clin Oncol* 1990; 9:114.
84. Martenson JA, Lipitz S, Wagner H, et al. Phase II trial of radiation therapy, 5-fluorouracil and cisplatin in patients with anal cancer. *Int J Radiat Oncol Biol Phys* 1995; 32(suppl 1):158.
85. Robertson JM, Lawrence TS, Walker S. The treatment of colorectal liver metastases with conformal radiation therapy and regional chemotherapy. *Int J Rad Oncol Biol Phys* 1995; 32:445–450.
86. Russel KJ, Bioleau MA, Higano C. Combined 5-FU and irradiation for transitional cell carcinoma of the urinary bladder. *Int J Rad Oncol Biol Phys* 1990; 19:693–699.
87. Rotman M, Macchia R, Silverstein M. Treatment of advanced bladder carcinoma with irradiation and concomitant 5-FU infusion. *Cancer* 1987; 59:710–714.
88. Induction chemotherapy plus radiation compared with surgery plus radiation in patients with advanced laryngeal cancer: The Department of Veterans Affairs Laryngeal Cancer Study Group. *N Eng J Med* 1991; 324:1685–1690.

II

Mechanisms of Interaction of Specific Chemotherapeutic Agents with Radiation

3 The Role of Platinum Complexes in Combined Modality Therapy

Beverly A. Teicher, PhD

CONTENTS

1. CHEMISTRY AND BIOCHEMISTRY

Platinum complexes are one of the most important classes of antitumor agents to enter the clinic in the last 30 yr. Cisplatin (*cis*-diamminedichloroplatinum II), the first of a group of antitumor platinum complexes, was shown by Rosenberg et al. *(1)* to possess antibiotic activity and in subsequent studies *(2)* to have antitumor activity in murine tumor models. In 1972 the National Cancer Institute introduced cisplatin into clinical trials. Cisplatin is a water-soluble inorganic square planar coordination complex containing a central platinum atom surrounded by two chlorine atoms and two ammonia moieties (Fig. 1). Platinum complexes are characterized by slow rates of ligand substitution reactions compared with other metal complexes *(3–5)*. Because of the slow reactions involved in platinum drugs binding to DNA, other intracellular nucleophiles such as glutathione may compete with DNA for reaction *(6)*. Platinum complexes may also bind to metallothioneins, cytosolic proteins of molecular weight 6000–7000 that contain 20 cysteine residues *(7)*. The primary mechanism of inhibition of tumor growth by cisplatin appears to be inhibition of DNA synthesis *(8,9)*. The *cis* configuration of the chloride leaving groups of cisplatin favors the formation of intrastrand crosslinks in DNA *(10–14)*. Recently, the crystal structure of a double-stranded DNA decamer containing a single interstrand crosslink of cisplatin formed between opposite guanine residues in the 5'-GC sequence was solved *(15)*. In another study using short oligodeoxyribonucleotides duplexes (10 and 20 base pairs) containing a central sequence AGCGA/TCGCT,

From: *Chemoradiation in Cancer Therapy*
Edited by: H. Choy © Humana Press Inc., Totowa, NJ

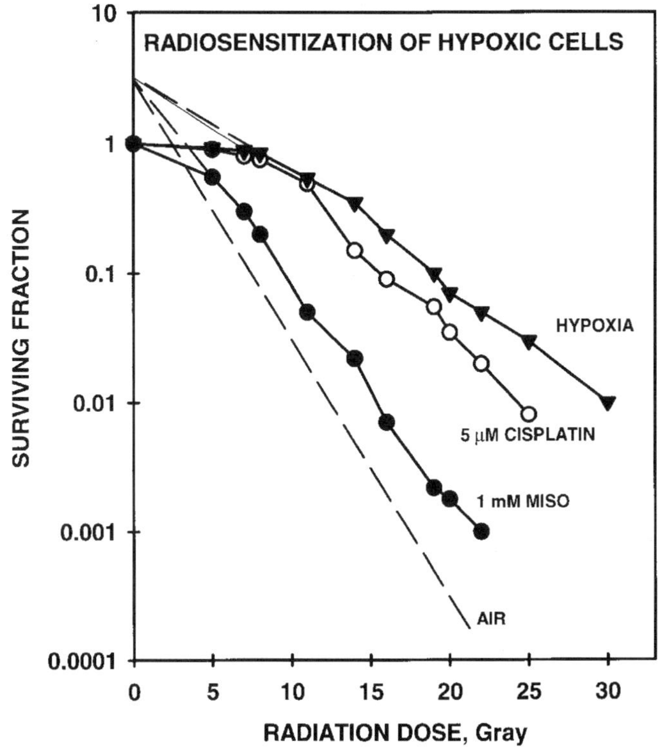

Fig. 1. Radiosensitization of hypoxic V79 cells by 5 µ*M* cisplatin compared to 1 m*M* misonidazole. The enhancement ratio for the cisplatin (5 µ*M*) in this experiment was 1.15. Adapted from Stratford et al. *(153)*.

the interstrand crosslink formed by cisplatin between guanine residues in the opposite strands in the 5'-GC sequence was labile at 37°C and rearranged into an intrastrand crosslink *(16)*. Thus, the frequency of specific cisplatin adducts could be locally and transiently altered in DNA in the cell nucleus during some phase (or phases) of the cell cycle and could be different from those in DNA modified in cell-free media *(17)*. DNA interstrand crosslinks of cisplatin inhibit transcription elongation by both prokaryotic and eukaryotic RNA polymerases *(18)* and thus may be more lethal than the more frequent intrastrand crosslinks *(17)*.

The carrier ligands, that is, the chemical moieties bound to platinum that are not the leaving groups and become part of the lesion on DNA, of the platinum antitumor agents appear to play an important role in determining efficacy against tumors with both intrinsic and acquired resistance to cisplatin *(19)*. Both cisplatin and carboplatin have *cis*-diammine carrier ligands, therefore there is a high level of cross-resistance between cell lines and tumors for these compounds. Oxaliplatin, JM216, and ZDO473 each have different carrier ligands. Major mechanisms of platinum resistance include decreased accumulation of the compound in cells, increased inactivation by glutathione, increased efflux of the platinum compound, increased nucleotide excision repair, and decreased mismatch repair *(20–22)*. In addition, increased tolerance of platinum–DNA adducts, that is, an increase in the number of platinum adducts required to inhibit cell growth, play an important role in resistance to these drugs *(23–26)*. Increased tolerance of platinum–

DNA adducts most likely reflects increased DNA repair such as nucleotide excision repair and postreplication repair including translesion synthesis, gap filling, and template switching during replication *(27,28)*.

Since the first reports of accumulation defects in cells with acquired resistance to cisplatin *(29,30)*, research effort has been directed toward defining the mechanism(s) by which cisplatin enters and leaves cells *(31–34)*. A clear case for carrier-mediated transport for cisplatin cannot be made because accumulation of cisplatin is not saturable or inhibitable with structural analogs *(35–39)*. Cisplatin has never been shown to be a substrate for the MDR-1 gene product, the multidrug resistance P-glycoprotein, or for the multiple resistance protein (MRP-1) *(40)*. However, cells expressing high levels of canalicular multispecific organic anion transporter (cMOAT, MRP-2) are resistant to cisplatin *(41–43)*. The mechanism by which cMOAT, which is expressed primarily in liver, confers resistance to cisplatin is not clear. The expression of MRP-3, MRP-4, or MRP-5 does not confer resistance to cisplatin *(44,45)*.

DNA mismatch repair (MMR) plays an important role in maintaining the integrity of the genome and in repairing mispaired bases in DNA *(46)*. The loss of DNA mismatch repair has been correlated with a decrease in the tendency of certain tumor cells to undergo drug-induced apoptosis after DNA damage, thus loss of DNA mismatch repair correlates with increased tumor cell survival and drug resistance *(47,48)*. The loss of DNA mismatch repair correlates with acquisition of resistance to cisplatin as well as resistance to a wide variety of DNA damaging agents *(47)*. Durant et al. *(49)* showed that *Saccharomyces cerevisiae* acquired resistance to cisplatin and carboplatin when DNA mismatch repair genes were inactivated.

2. RADIOSENSITIZATION

The greatest research effort on radiation sensitizers has focused on organic compounds; however, platinum complexes conform to the hypotheses for radiation sensitizers since they are electron affinic and react preferentially with the hydrated electron in aqueous solution. Early studies of cisplatin in combination with radiation therapy suggested a synergistic effect in antitumor activity *(50,51)*. Much of the initial data were obtained using cells in tissue culture *(52)*, these data indicated that the potential of cisplatin to inhibit repair of radiation-induced damage to DNA could be an important contributor to the enhanced tumor cell killing seen in vivo by the combination of these two modes of treatment.

Cisplatin was first characterized as a radiation sensitizer using hypoxic *Bacillus megaterium* spores *(53)*. Radiation sensitization by cisplatin was confirmed in vegetative *Escherichia coli* with a maximum sensitizer enhancement ratio of 1.77 in anoxic bacteria at a cisplatin concentration of 50 μM *(54)*. Zimbrick et al. *(55)* extended these studies to other platinum complexes. The earliest studies in mammalian cells used hypoxic V-79 Chinese hamster cells and showed a small radiation sensitization with 8 μM of cisplatin *(56)*. Nias and Szumiel *(57)* first reported that pretreatment of Chinese hamster ovary (CHO) cells with a platinum complex could sensitize well-oxygenated cells to radiation. Wodinsky et al. *(58)* showed that cisplatin potentiated the effect of whole-body radiation therapy in mice inoculated intraperitoneally with P388 leukemia compared with either modality alone. Therapeutic potentiation was found in MTG-B subcutaneous tumors and intracerebral RBT when the animals were treated with cisplatin and radiation *(59)*.

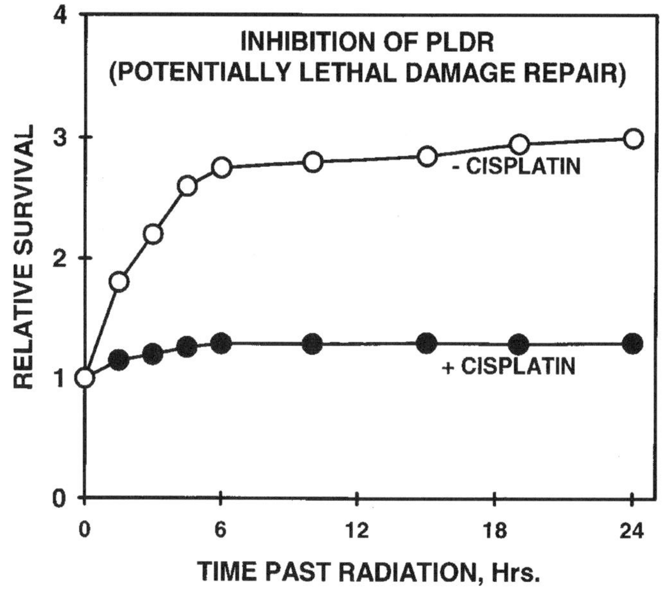

Fig. 2. Potentiation of rat H4 hepatoma by 2.5 μ*M* cisplatin present during the postirradiation incubation prior to assay for viability demonstrating inhibition of PLD recovery. Relative survival of plateau phase cells irradiated with 7.5 Gy after incubation for different time periods or in the presence of cisplatin. Results have been corrected for drug toxicity. Adapted from Carde and Laval *(154)*.

These studies were followed by others that demonstrated the potential for therapeutic enhancement by combined cisplatin–radiation treatments with primary murine bladder cancer *(60)*, EMT-6 mammary tumors and KHT and RIF-1 sarcomas *(61)*, and Lewis lung carcinoma *(62)*.

Preclinical studies identified two potential mechanisms for the increased tumor cell killing observed with the combination of cisplatin with radiation therapy *(63,64)*. The first mechanism, radiosensitization of hypoxic cells, was characterized by the increase in the final slope of the radiation dose response curve for hypoxic cells (Fig. 1). The degree of radiosensitization was cisplatin concentration dependent and resulted in enhancement ratios of 1.0–1.3 after correction for the direct cell killing by the cisplatin. The second effect was observed as the inhibition of the repair of potentially lethal damage (PLD) (Fig. 2). When stationary phase cell cultures are irradiated, there is an increase in survival over time if the cultures stand unperturbed; there is a reduction in this survival when platinum complexes are added immediately following irradiation. Thus, cisplatin inhibits PLD repair. In some cell lines an abrogation of the shoulder of the radiation cell survival curve was observed. This reduction of the shoulder has been attributed to an inhibition of sublethal damage repair (SLDR) by cisplatin. Cisplatin free-radical-mediated sensitization may involve the ability to scavenge free electrons formed by the interaction between radiation and DNA. This reduction of the platinum moiety from Pt(II) to Pt(I) may stabilize otherwise reparable damage to DNA *(64)*.

Although cisplatin rose to a compound of major interest through its performance in laboratory studies, carboplatin emerged as promising as a second-generation platinum complex on the basis of promising early clinical trial data *(65–68)*. Carboplatin was

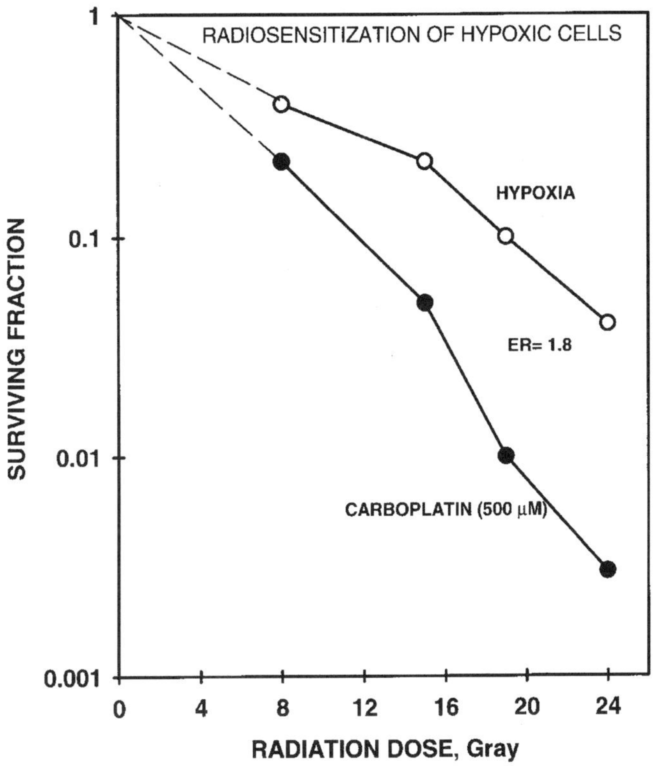

Fig. 3. Radiosensitization of hypoxic V79 cells by 500 μ*M* carboplatin compared to hypoxia without drug. The carboplatin data are corrected for cytotoxicity from the drug. Cells were exposed to carboplatin for 1 h at 37°C before irradiation. Adapted from Douple et al. *(63)*.

reported to be a radiation sensitizer of hypoxic V79 cells and CHO cells when the cells were exposed to 100–200 μ*M* of carboplatin *(69)*. Douple et al. *(63)* found an enhancement ratio (ER) of approx 1.8 when V79 cells were exposed to 500 μ*M* of carboplatin for 1 h prior to and during irradiation. At a concentration of 500 μ*M*, the surviving fraction from the carboplatin alone was 0.55 (Fig. 3).

A supraadditive effect of cisplatin and radiation in murine tumors was first reported by Lelieveld et al. *(70)* using a mouse mammary tumor latency assay. The decrease in tumor cell survival with cisplatin administered 5 h prior to radiation therapy was approximately two logs larger than expected for additive effects of the single agents. The effect was only obtained when the tumor was irradiated under hypoxic conditions (blood supply clamped off) and at high radiation doses. In some tumor models greater-than-additive effects were obtained with the combination of cisplatin and radiation therapy under normal conditions (unclamped) after correction for the drug activity effects; in other tumors supraadditivity of the combination treatment was less apparent *(60,70,71)*. In most cases, the greatest effects were obtained when the cisplatin was present in the tumor at the time of radiation delivery. In general, greater-than-additive tumor cell killing in vivo has been most reliably obtained when cisplatin has been administered along with fractionated radiation therapy *(64)*. Analyses of preclinical data along with probability of interactions between cisplatin and radiation in the presence of DNA allowed predictions to be made of optimizing the scheduling of these treatments *(73)*.

3. CLINICAL STUDIES: HEAD AND NECK CANCER

Early clinical studies clearly demonstrated that cisplatin could be administered safely and concurrently with radiation therapy *(73–75)*. Early clinical trials that demonstrated the promise of the combination of cisplatin and radiation therapy included the treatment of brain tumors *(76,77)*, head and neck tumors *(78)*, malignant melanoma *(79)*, and bladder cancer *(80)*. Early clinical trial integrating carboplatin administration with radiation therapy was carried out in patients with locally advanced nonsmall cell lung cancer (NSCLC) *(81)*. A hypothesis put forth by Coughlin and colleagues *(81)* was that the best clinical outcomes would be achieved with the combination of cisplatin and radiation therapy in tumors that were responsive to cisplatin.

As a biomarker or surrogate marker, several groups developed methodology for measuring platinum–DNA adduct levels in clinical samples *(82,83)*. These methods included ELISA assay *(84)*, HPLC assay *(85)*, and atomic absorption spectroscopy *(82,86)*. Most platinum–DNA adduct determinations were made in nucleated peripheral blood cells but some were made in tumor biopsy material. Platinum–DNA adduct levels in peripheral blood cells correlated with disease response in advanced stage ovarian cancer, testicular cancer, and breast cancer *(87–90)*. In a blinded Phase I study of the combination of cisplatin and carboplatin, a cohort of 49 patients including 24 different tumor types was assessed for platinum–DNA adduct level using atomic absorption spectroscopy *(91,92)*. It was found that platinum–DNA adduct level after the first dose of chemotherapy was directly related to disease response, regardless of tumor type. Similarly, Schellens et al. *(93)* in a study of 45 patients who received cisplatin-based therapy, found that platinum–DNA adduct area under the curve (AUC) was directly related to a favorable clinical response regardless of tumor type. It is well recognized that cellular resistance to cisplatin is multifactorial; however, low levels of resistance have most frequently been associated with efficient DNA repair *(92,94)*.

The initial combination modality clinical studies with cisplatin and fractionated radiation therapy was carried out in head and neck cancer with weekly cisplatin (120–160 mg/m^2) and conventional single daily fraction radiation *(95)*. In a follow-up intergroup study, patients were randomized to radiation therapy alone or to radiation therapy plus 20 mg/m^2/wk cisplatin *(96)*. Both studies showed no major increase in normal tissue toxicity in the radiation field and showed an increase in response rate. There was no increase in complete response rate or in survival. Bachaud et al. *(97)* carried out a randomized study comparing radiation therapy alone with concurrent cisplatin (50 mg/m^2) and radiation therapy in postoperative patients. This trial produced a significant reduction in local recurrence and improved disease-free survival with 59% of the patients receiving the full planned dose of cisplatin.

A study of 124 patients with unresectable head and neck cancer receiving cisplatin (100 mg/m^2) every three weeks for three courses along with fractionated radiation therapy (66 to 73.8 Gy) was carried out by the Radiation Therapy Oncology Group (RTOG) *(98)*. Although only 61% of the patients received the full planned dose of cisplatin, comparison of patient survival with historical controls from the RTOG database of patients suggested improved survival with the combination regimen for all patients and particularly for patients with nasopharyngeal cancer *(99)*.

Wheeler et al. *(100,101)* took another tack and treated patients with unresectable head and neck cancer with cisplatin (40 mg/m^2) daily for 5 d per course for three cycles along with radiation therapy (200 cGy/d) to a dose of 70 Gy. The first cycle of cisplatin was started on treatment d 1. Several studies evaluated cisplatin and 5-fluorouracil along with radiation therapy in head and neck cancer *(102–106)*. In general, these clinical trials found increased local toxicity and significant numbers of patients did not complete the chemotherapy; however, there were higher response rates, greater frequency of histologic clearing of tumor, reduced locoregional recurrence rate, and decrease in deaths due to cancer.

Later trials built on the early findings. Jeremie et al. *(107)* demonstrated improved survival and lower recurrence rates with the use of cisplatin and radiation therapy compared with radiation therapy alone in patients with stage III and IV disease. Similarly, Bachaud et al. *(108)* employed postoperative concurrent cisplatin and radiation therapy vs radiation therapy alone in a phase III study of stage III and IV disease. The 2- and 5-yr survival rates were 72% and 36% for the combination therapy and 46% and 13% for radiation therapy alone. In another phase III study of stage III and IV resectable disease, patients were treated with cisplatin and 5-fluorouracil and radiation therapy (1.8–2.0 Gy/d to a total of 68 to 72 Gy) or radiation therapy alone *(109)*. The complete response rates were 76% for the chemoradiation combination and 50% for radiation therapy only. Brizel et al. *(110)* utilized hyperfractionated radiation therapy with or without concomitant cisplatin and 5-fluorouracil for locally advanced disease. The hyperfractionated schedule for the radiation alone patients was 125 cGy two times per day to a total of 75 Gy, while the patients on the combination therapy arm received 125 cGy to a total of 70 Gy. After 3 yr of follow-up the patients in the chemoradiation therapy group had better overall survival (55% vs 34%), relapse-free survival (61% vs 41%), and control of local disease (70% vs 44%). Al-Sarraf et al. *(111)* studying advanced nasopharyngeal cancer patients compared radiation therapy alone with radiation therapy and concomitant cisplatin and adjuvant cisplatin and 5-fluorouracil, found 3-yr survival rates of 47% for radiation therapy alone and 78% for the combination treatment regimen. Robbins et al. *(112)* have reported their trial with intra-arterial supradoses of cisplatin (150 mg/m^2 weekly × 4) with radiation (66–74 Gy) in mainly stage IV disease and using sodium thiosulfate to neutralize the cisplatin. A complete response rate at local regional sites was 75% and an impressive 5-yr disease-free survival and an overall survival of 58% and 40%, respectively *(113)*. Several phase III trials to find optimal dosing and delivery of cisplatin and radiation therapy are on-going *(114,115)*. Recently, there have been two reports of improved outcome with concurrent chemoradiotherapy for advanced carcinoma of the nasopharynx, these are Cooper et al. *(116,117)* and Cheng et al. *(118)*. Cheng et al. *(118)* studied 107 patients with stage II, III, and IV nasopharyngeal carcinoma with 70 Gy administered in 35 fractions (five fractions per week) along with two courses of chemotherapy consisting of cisplatin and 5-fluorouracil during treatment weeks 1 and 6 and for two additional monthly courses after completion of the radiation therapy. With a median follow-up of 44 mo, the 5-yr survival rate overall was 84%, the disease-free survival was 74%, and the locoregional control rate was 90%. The overall 3-yr survivals were 100% for stage II patients, 93% for stage III patients, and 69% for stage IV patients. The disease-free 3-yr survival was 97% for stage II patients, 88% for stage III patients, and 52% for stage IV patients.

4. CLINICAL STUDIES: LUNG CANCER

A number of studies have evaluated treatment regimens including concurrent chemotherapy and radiation therapy in patients with advanced local stage III nonsmall-cell lung cancer *(119)*. There were early nonsurgical trials that examined combinations of cisplatin or carboplatin with thoracic radiation *(120)*. There have been several phase II trials evaluating concurrent platinum chemotherapy and radiation therapy as preoperative treatment *(121–125)*. Thoracic irradiation was compared with cisplatin and concurrent radiation therapy in at least four randomized trials in stage III nonsmall-cell lung cancer by the early 1990s *(126–129)*. Although the cisplatin regimens and radiation regimens varied, none of these clinical trials showed a significant survival benefit for the combined modality treatment vs radiation therapy alone. Schaake-Koning et al. *(126)*, in a phase II study in patients with inoperable lung cancer, showed that the best improvement in survival occurred when cisplatin was administered daily with radiation therapy rather than weekly with radiation therapy (Fig. 4).

The Southwest Oncology Group (SWOG) conducted a phase II trial with continuous thoracic radiation to a total dose of 61 Gy and simultaneous daily cisplatin (5 mg/m^2) and found acceptable toxicity *(130)*. Another trial utilized a split-course of thoracic radiation therapy to a total dose of 50 Gy and simultaneous daily continuous infusion cisplatin (5 mg/m^2) and found a 35% 2-yr survival rate with relatively mild toxicity *(131)*. Weekly doses of carboplatin were administered with continuous thoracic irradiation to a total dose of 60 Gy in a phase II trial that resulted in a 45% response rate *(132)*.

The earliest combination chemotherapy and radiation trials in nonsmall-cell lung cancer included cisplatin and 5-fluorouracil and concurrent radiation therapy and found survival results comparable to those for sequential chemotherapy and radiation or to daily cisplatin and radiation therapy without surgery *(119,121)*. Phase II studies of stage IIIa and IIIb nonsmall-cell lung cancer patients treated with the combination of cisplatin with etoposide and 5-fluorouracil and either single daily radiation fractionation or twice daily radiation fractionation prior to surgery produced similar clinical results *(119,121)*. Complete surgical resection was accomplished in 70% of the patients, the median survival was 22 mo and the 2-yr survival rate was 45%.

5. CLINICAL STUDIES: CERVICAL AND OTHER CANCERS

Early studies of radiation sensitization involved comparisons of cisplatin and 5-fluorouracil and radiation therapy with hydroxyurea and radiation therapy carried out by the Gynecologic Oncology Group (GOG) for treatment of stages IIB to IVA disease *(133,134)*. There have been several clinical trials testing cisplatin or cisplatin-based regimens with radiation therapy in locally advanced cervix cancer *(135)*. A phase II trial of more than 70 patients with stage IB (bulky) to IVA cervix cancer received radiation therapy (external beam plus low-dose-rate brachytherapy) along with cisplatin to provide radiosensitization and optimize the dose intensity of the cisplatin *(136–138)*. The cisplatin dose was 20 mg/m^2/d × 5 every 3 wk to a total dose of 400 mg/m^2. Radiation therapy was designed to deliver 80 Gy to point A and 55 Gy to point B. In the initial follow-up report 91% of patients had complete responses. At 4 yr, more than 75% of stage IB to IIB patients were alive; however, only 25% of patients with stage III disease were alive with no plateau seen on the curve. Amifostine has been studied as a normal tissue protector with cisplatin and radiation therapy for treatment of locally advanced cervical cancer *(135)*. The results of three phase II clinical trials have recently been reported showing an improvement in local control and survival in cervical cancer patients after concomitant cisplatin and radiotherapy *(139–141)*. Santin et al. *(142)* examined the

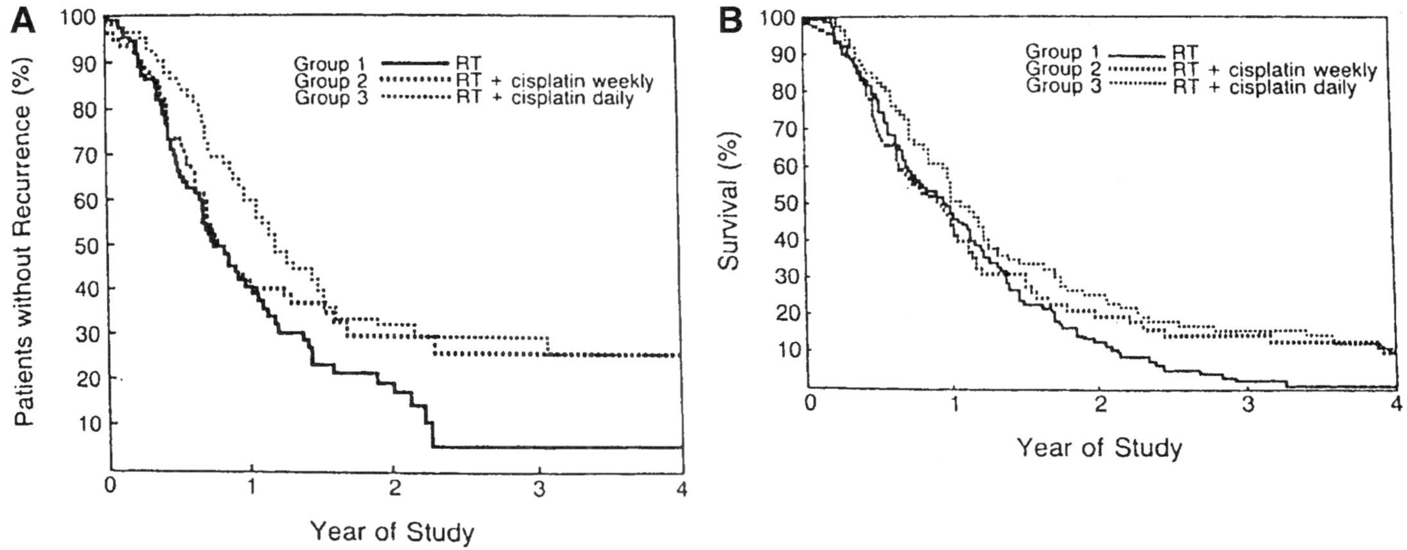

Fig. 4. Local control and survival in inoperable lung cancer patients treated with RT alone, weekly cisplatin or daily cisplatin *(155)*.

effect of therapy on the immune system of cervical cancer patients undergoing external irradiation and intracavity brachytherapy with or without concurrent cisplatin and found that administration of concurrent cisplatinum with radiation therapy may have synergistically increased cytotoxic effects of radiation on tumor cells but did not alter the magnitude or characteristics of the radiation-induced immunosuppression. The role of concurrent radiation therapy and chemotherapy consisting of 5-fluorouracil and cisplatin was explored in the treatment of local–regionally advanced vulvar cancer and results appeared positive *(143)*. The combination of cisplatin or carboplatin and radiation therapy has been discussed for locally advanced prostate cancer *(144)*. Kaufman et al. *(145)* conducted a study of 34 patients to assess the safety, tolerance, and efficacy of transurethral surgery plus concomitant cisplatin, 5-fluorouracil, and radiation therapy in conjunction with selective bladder preservation in patients with muscle-invading bladder cancer. This protocol included high-dose hypofractionated radiation therapy and had a 67% complete response rate to induction therapy and a 66% three-year survival rate with an intact bladder.

6. CARBOPLATIN AND OXALIPLATIN

Carboplatin, introduced in 1981, as an alternative to cisplatin has a similar activity profile but a very different toxicity profile to the original platinum complex *(146–148)*. Carboplatin and cisplatin have been compared in numerous studies and, in general, the carboplatin-containing regimens were essentially equivalent to and less toxic than the cisplatin-containing regimens *(146,147)*. Belani et al. *(149)* performed a study of concurrent carboplatin and radiotherapy in patients with inoperable stage III nonsmall-cell lung cancer and achieved a response rate of 33%. Carboplatin with concomitant radiotherapy has been evaluated in head and neck tumors *(150)*. In this study 103 patients with advanced head and neck carcinoma treated with radiation therapy plus carboplatin (60–70 mg/m^2/d, d 1–5 and 29–33) had 1-yr and 2-yr survival rates of 77% and 53%, respectively.

Oxaliplatin (trans-L-diaminocyclohexane oxalate platinum II) was selected for development based on preclinical antitumor activity in murine leukemia lines and in colon cancer models *(151,152)*. The clinical development of oxaliplatin has been primarily in colorectal cancer alone and in combination with 5-fluorouracil.

7. CONCLUSIONS

Platinum complexes came to be anticancer agents through the serendipitious observation and intellectual pursuit of that observation by Dr. Barnett Rosenberg. The preclinical data needed to support the passage of cisplatin and then carboplatin, oxaliplatin, and others into clinical trial was generated by the cancer research community very quickly. The preclinical support of the notion that platinum complexes could interact with ionizing radiation in a manner that produced greater-than-additive cytotoxicity within the field of radiation exposure also moved quickly from the laboratory bench to clinical trial. Over the past 12–15 yr, the combination of a platinum complex and radiation therapy administered concomitantly as a valuable therapeutic regimen has been well established in head and neck cancer and supported to lesser degrees in nonsmall-cell lung cancer, cervical cancer, and others. The future will likely bring combinations including growth factor inhibitors and antiangiogenic agents along with a platinum and radiation. These combination regimens may broaden the applicability of platinum/radiation combinations.

REFERENCES

1. Rosenberg B, VanCamp L, Krigas T. Inhibition of cell division in *Escherichia coli* by electrolysis products from platinum electrode. *Nature* 1965; 205:698–699.
2. Rosenberg B, VanCamp L, Trosko J, Mansour VH. Platinum compounds: a new class of potent antitumour agent. *Nature* 1969; 222:385–386.
3. Lippard SJ. New chemistry of an old molecule: cis-[Pt(NH3)2Cl2]. *Science* 1982; 218:1075–1082.
4. Lippard SJ (ed) Platinum, Gold and Other Metal Chemotherapeutic Agents, ACS Symposium Series No. 209. 1983; America Chemical Society: Washington, DC.
5. Pinto AL, Lippard SJ. Binding of the antitumor drug cis-diamminedichloro-platinum(II) (cisplatin) to DNA. *Biochem Biophys Acta* 1985; 780:167–180.
6. Dedon PC, Borch RF. Characterization of the reactions of platinum antitumor agents with biologic and nonbiologic sulfur-containing nucleophiles. *Biochem Pharmacol* 1987; 36:1955–1964.
7. Kelley SL, Basu A, Teicher BA, Hacker MP, Hamer DH, Lazo JS. Overexpression of metallothionein confers resistance to anticancer drugs. *Science* 1988; 241:1813–1815.
8. Howle JA. Gale GR. Cis-dichlorodiammineplatinum (II). Persistent and selective inhibition of deoxyribonucleic acid synthesis in vivo. *Biochem Pharmacol* 1970; 19(10):2757–2762.
9. Taylor DM, Tew KD, Jones JD. Effects of cis-dichlorodiammine platinum (II) on DNA synthesis in kidney and other tissues of normal and tumour-bearing rats. *Eur J Cancer (Oxford)* 1976; 12(4):249–254.
10. Roberts JJ. IN: Platinum Coordination Complexes in Cancer Chemotherapy. Springer-Verlag: Heidelberg, 1974; pp. 79–97.
11. Roberts JJ, Pascoe JM. In: Advances in Antimicrobial and Antineoplastic Chemotherapy Vol. II. 1972; University Park Press: Baltimore, pp. 249–252.
12. Rosenberg B. Platinum coordination complexes in cancer chemotherapy. *Naturwissenschaften* 1973; 60:399–406.
13. Roos IA, Arnold M. Interaction of an anti-tumour active platinum complex with DNA. J Clin Hematol Oncol 1977; 7:374–390.
14. Thomson AJ, Mansy S. In: Advances in Antimicrobial and Antineoplastic Chemotherapy Vol. III. 1972; Baltimore University Press: Baltimore, pp. 199–203.
15. Coste F, Malinge J-M, Serre L, Shepard W, Roth M, Leng M, Zelwer C. Crystal structure of a double-stranded DNA containing a cisplatin interstrand crosslink at 1.63°A resolution: hydration at the platinated site. *Nucleic Acids Res* 1999; 27:1837–1184.
16. Perez C, Leng M, Malinge JM. Rearrangement of interstrand crosslinks into intrastrand crosslinks in cis-diamminedichloroplatinum(II)-modified DNA. *Nucleic Acids Res* 1997; 25:896–903.
17. Brabec V. Chemistry and structural biology of 1,2-interstrand adducts of cisplatin. In: (Kelland LR, Farrell N, eds) Platinum-Based Drugs in Cancer Therapy 2000; Humana Press Inc.: Totowa, NJ; pp. 37–61.
18. Corda Y, Job C, Anin MF, Leng M, Job D. Transcription by eukaryotic and prokaryotic RNA ploymerases of DNA modified at a d(GG) or a d(AG) site by the antitumor drug cis-diamminedichloroplatinum(II). *Biochemistry* 1991; 30:222–230.
19. Chaney SG, Vaisman A. DNA adduct tolerance and bypass. In: (Kelland LR, Farrell N, eds) Platinum-Based Drugs in Cancer Therapy 2000; Humana Press Inc.: Totowa, NJ; pp. 129–148.
20. Eastman A, Richon VM. Mechanisms of cellular resistance to platinum coordination complexes. In: (McBrien DCH, Slater TF, eds) Biochemical Mechanisms of Platinum Anticancer Drugs 1986; IRL: Oxford, UK; pp. 91–119.
21. Johnson SW, Ozols RF, Hamilton TC. Mechanisms of drug resistance in ovarian cancer. *Cancer* 1993; 71:644–649.
22. Hill BT. Drug resistance: an overview of the current state of the art. *Int J Oncol* 1996; 9:197–203.
23. Lanzi C, Perego P, Supino R, et al. Decreased drug accumulation and increased tolerance to DNA damage in tumor cells with a low level of cisplatin resistance. *Biochem Pharmacol* 1998; 55:1247–1254.
24. Johnson SW, Shen DW, Pastan I, Gottesman MM, Hamilton TC. Cross-resistance, cisplatin accumulation and platinum-DNA adduct formation and removal in cisplatin-sensitive and –resistant human hepatoma cell lines. *Exp Cell Res* 1996; 226:133–139.
25. Shellard SA, Fichtinger-Schepman AMJ, Lazo JS, Hill BT. Evidence of differential cisplatin DNA adduct formation, removal and tolerance of DNA damage in three human lung carcinoma cell lines. *Anti-Cancer Drugs* 1993; 4:491–500.

26. Schmidt W, Chaney SG. Role of carrier ligand in platinum resistance of human carcinoma cell lines. *Cancer Res* 1993; 53:799–805.
27. Naegeli H. Roadblocks and detours during DNA replication: mechanisms of mutagenesis in mammalian cells. *Bioessays* 1994; 16:557–564.
28. Kaufmann WK. Pathways of human cell post-replication repair. *Carcinogenesis* 1989; 10:1–11.
29. Andrews PA, Howell SB. Cellular pharmacology of cisplatin: perspective on mechanisms of acquired resistance. *Cancer Cells* 1990; 2:35–43.
30. Andrews PA. Cisplatin Accumulation. In: (Kelland LR, Farrell N, eds) Platinum-Based Drugs in Cancer Therapy 2000; Humana Press Inc.: Totowa, NJ; pp. 89–113.
31. Andrews PA. Mechanisms of acquired resistance to cisplatin. *Cancer Treat Res* 1994; 73:217–248.
32. Teicher BA, Holden SA, Herman TS, et al. Characteristics of five human tumor cell lines and sublines resistant to cis-diamminedichloroplatinum(II). *Int J Cancer* 1991; 47:252–260.
33. Katabami M, Fijita H, Haneda H, et al. Reduced drug accumulation in a newly established human lung squamous-carcinoma cell line resistant to cis-diamminedichloroplatinum(II). *Biochem Pharmacol* 1992; 44:394–397.
34. Loh SY, Mistry P, Kelland LR, Abel G, Harrap KR. Reduced drug accumulation as a major mechanism of acquired resistance to cisplatin in a human ovarian carcinoma cell line: circumvention studies using novel platinum (II) and (IV) ammine/amine complexes. *Br J Cancer* 1992; 66:1109–1115.
35. Andrews PA, Velury S, Mann SC, Howell SB. Cis-Diamminedichloroplatinum(II) accumulation in sensitive and resistant human ovarian carcinoma cells. *Cancer Res* 1988; 48:68–73.
36. Mann SC, Andrews PA, Howell SB. Short-term cis-diamminedichloroplatinum(II) accumulation in sensitive and resistant human ovarian carcinoma cells. *Cancer Chemotherap Pharmacol* 1990; 25:236–240.
37. Scanlon KJ, Safirsten RL, Thies H, Gross RB, Waxman S, Guttenplan JB. Inhibition of amino acid transport by cis-diamminedichloroplatinum(II) derivatives in L1210 murine leukemia cells. *Cancer Res* 1983; 43:4211–4215.
38. Hromas RA, North JA, Burns CP. Decreased cisplatin uptake by resistant L1210 leukemia cells. *Cancer Lett* 1987; 36:197–201.
39. Kelland LR, Mistry P, Abel G, et al. Mechanism-related circumvention of acquired cis-diamminedichloroplatinum(II) resistance using two pairs of human ovarian carcinoma cell lines by ammine/amine platinum(IV) dicarboxylates. *Cancer Res* 1992; 52:3857–3864.
40. Lautier D, Canitrot Y, Deeley RG, Cole SPC. Multidrug resistance mediated by the multidrug resistance protein (MRP) gene. *Biochem Pharmacol* 1996; 52:967–977.
41. Ishikawa T, Bao J, Yamane Y, Akimaru K, Frindrich K, Wright CD, et al. Coordinated induction of MRP/GS-X pump and gamma-glutamylcysteine synthetase by heavy metals in human leukemia cells. *J Biol Chem* 19967; 271:14,981–14,988.
42. Akimaru K, Kuo MT, Furuta K, Suzuki M, Noyori R, Ishikawa T. Induction of MRP/GS-X pump and cellular resistance to anticancer prostaglandins. *Cytotechnology* 1996; 19:221–227.
43. Fujii R, Mutoh M, Sumizawa T, Chen Z, Yoshimura A, Akiyama S. Adenosine triphosphate-dependent transport of leukotriene C4 by membrane vesicles prepared from cisplatin-resistant human epidermoid carcinoma tumor cells. *J Natl Cancer Inst* 1994; 86:1781–1784.
44. Kool M, de Haas M, Scheffer GL, Scheper RJ, van Eijik MJT, Julia A-M, et al. Analysis of expression of cMOAT (MRP2), MRP3, MRP4 and MRP5, homologues of the multidrug resistance-associated protein gene (MRP1), in human cancer cell lines. *Cancer Res* 1997; 57:5902–5910.
45. Borst P, Kool M, Evers R. Do cMOAT (MRP2), other MRP homologues and LRP play a role in MDR? *Cancer Biol* 1997; 8:205–213.
46. Modrich P. Strand-specific mismatch repair in mammalian cells. *J Biol Chem* 1997; 272:24,727–24,730.
47. Anthoney DA, McIlwrath AJ, Gallagher WM, Edlin ARM, Brown R. Microsatellite instability, apoptosis and loss of p53 function in drug resistant tumor cells. *Cancer Res* 1996; 56:1374–1381.
48. Brown R. Cisplatin resistance in ovarian cancer. In: (Kelland LR, Farrell N, eds) Platinum-Based Drugs in Cancer Therapy 2000; Humana Press Inc.: Totowa, NJ; pp. 115–128.
49. Durant ST, Morris MM, Illand M, et al. Dependence on RAD52 and RAD1 for anticancer drug resistance mediated by inactivation of mismatch repair genes. *Current Biology* 1999; 9:51–54.
50. Douple EB, Richmond RC, Logan ME. Therapeutic potentiation in a muse mammary tumor and an intracerebral rat brain tumor by combined treatment with cis-dichlorodiammineplatinum (II) and radiation. *J Clin Hematol Oncol* 1977; 7:585–603.

51. Soloway MS, Gehrki G. Radiation therapy of experimental murine bladder cancer. *Surgical Forum* 1977; 28:559–561.
52. Douple EB, Richmond RC. Platinum complexes as radiosensitizers of hypoxic mammalian cells. *Br J Cancer* 1978; 37(Suppl III):98–102.
53. Richmond RC, Powers EL. Radiation sensitization of bacterial spores by cis-dichlorodiammine-platinum (II). *Radiat Res* 1976; 68:251.
54. Richmond RC, Zimbrick JD, Hykes DL. Radiation-induced DNA damage and lethality in e-coli as modified by the antitumor agent cis-dichlorodiammineplatinum (II). *Radiat Res* 1977; 71:447.
55. Zimbrick JD, Aruni S, Richmond RC. Studies on radiosensitization of Escherichia coli cells by cis-platinum complexes. *Int J Radiat Oncol Biol Phys* 1979; 5:1351–1354.
56. Bertrand M, Deen DF. Factors influencing the recovery from potentially lethal damage (PLD) in mammalian cells in vitro and in vivo. *Cancer Treat Rev* 1980; 7:1–15.
57. Szumiel I, Niah AHW. The effect of combined treatment with a platinum complex and ionizing radiation on Chinese hamster ovary cells in vitro. *Br J Cancer* 1976; 33:450.
58. Wodinsky I, Swiniarski J, Kensler CJ, Venditti JM. Combination radiotherapy and chemotherapy for P388 lymphocytic leukemia in vivo. *Cancer Treat Rep* 1974; 4:73.
59. Douple EB, Richmond RC, Logan ME. Therapeutic potentiation in a mouse mammary tumour and an intracerebral rat brain tumour by combined treatment with cis-dichlorodiammineplatinum (II) and radiation. *J Clin Hematol Oncol* 1977; 7:585–603.
60. Soloway MS, Morris CR, Sudderth B. Radiation therapy and cis-diamminedichloroplatinum(II) in transplantable and primary murine bladder cancer. *Int J Radiat Oncol Biol Phys* 1979; 5:1355–1360.
61. Twentyman PR, Kallman RF, Brown JM. The effect of time between x-irradiation and chemotherapy on the growth of three solid mouse tumors. III. Cis-Diamminedichloro-platinum. *Int J Radiat Oncol Biol Phys* 1979; 5:1365–1367.
62. Kovacs CJ, Schenken LL, Burholt DR. Therapeutic potentiation of combined cis-dichlorodi-ammineplatinum (11) and irradiation by ICRF-159. *Int J Radiat Oncol Biol Phys* 1979; 5:1361–1364.
63. Douple EB, Richmond RC, O'Hara JA, Coughlin CT. Carboplatin as a potentiator of radiation therapy. *Cancer Treat Revs* 1985; 12(Suppl A):111–124.
64. Dewit L. Combined treatment of radiation and cis-diamminedichloroplatinum (II): A review of experimental and clinical data. *Int J Radiat Oncol Biol Phys* 1987; 13:403–426.
65. Calvert AH, Harland SJ, Newell DR, Siddik ZH, Jones AC, McElwain TJ, Raju S, Wiltshaw E, Smith IE, Baker JW, Peckham MJ, Harrap KR. Early clinical studies with cis-diammine-1,1-cyclobutane dicarboxylate platinum II. *Cancer Chemotherap Pharmacol* 1982; 9:140–147.
66. Calvert AH, Harland SJ, Harrap KR, Wiltshaw E, Smith IE. JM8 development and clinical projects. In: (Hacker MP, Douple EB, Krakoff IH, eds), Platinum Coordination Complexes in Cancer Chemotherapy 1984; Martinus-Nijhoff: Boston, pp. 240–252.
67. Van Echo DA, Egorin MJ, Whitacre MY, Olman EA, Aisner J. Phase I clinical and pharmacologic trial of carboplatin daily for 5 days. *Cancer Treat Rep* 1984; 68:1103–1114.
68. Curt GA, Grygiel JJ, Corden BJ, Ozols RF, Weiss RB, Tell DT, Myers CE, Collins JM. A phase I and pharmacokinetic study of diamminecyclobutane-dicarboxylatoplatinum (NSC241240). *Cancer Res* 1983; 43:4470–4473.
69. Chibber R. Radiosensitizing and cytotoxic action of some Rh(II) carboxylates in vitro: a comparison with Pt(II) complexes. Ph.D. Dissertation 1984; Department of Chemistry, Hatfield Polytechnic, Hatfield, Hertfordshire, England.
70. Lelieveld P, Scoles MA, Brown JM, Kallmann RF. The effect of treatment in fractionated schedules with the combination of x-irradiation and six cytostatic drugs on the RIF-1 tumor and normal mouse skin. *Int J Radiat Oncol Biol Phys* 1985; 11:111–121.
71. Bartelink H, Kallmann RF, Rapacchietta D, Hart AAM. Therapeutic enhancement in mice by clinically relevant dose and fractionation schedules of cis-diamminedichloroplatinum(II) and irradiation. *Radiotherap Oncol* 1986; 6:61–74.
72. Begg AC. Cisplatin and radiation: interaction probabilities and therapeutic possibilities. *Int J Radiat Oncol Biol Phys* 1990; 19:1183–1189.
73. Haselow RE, Adams GS, Oken MM, Goudsmit A, Lerner HJ, Marsh JC. Simultaneous cis-platinum (DDP) and radiation therapy (RT) for locally advanced unressectable head and neck cancer. *Int J Radiat Oncol Biol Phys* 1982; 8:201.
74. Keizer HJ, Karim ABMF, Njo KH, et al. Feasibility study on daily administration of cis-diammine-dichloroplatinum(II) in combination with radiotherapy. *Radiotherap Oncol* 1984; 1:227–234.

75. Leipzig B, Wetmore SJ, Putzeys R, Suen JY, Snyderman NL. Cisplatin potentiation of radiotherapy-long term follow-up. *Arch Otolaryngol* 1985; 111:114–118.
76. Stewart DJ, Leavens M, Maor M, et al. Human central nervous system distribution of cis-diamminedichloroplatinum and use as a radiosensitizer in malignant brain tumors. *Cancer Res* 1982; 42:2474–2479.
77. Stewart DJ, Wallace S, Feun L, et al. A phase I study of intracarotid artery infusion of cis-diammine dichloroplatinum(II) in patients with recurrent malignant intracerebral tumors. *Cancer Res* 1982; 42:2059–2062.
78. Leipzig B. Cisplatin sensitization to radiotherapy of squamous cell carcinoma of the head and neck. *Amer J Surg* 1983; 146:462–465.
79. Reimer RR, Gahbauer R, Bukowski RM, et al. Simultaneous treatment with cisplatin and radiation therapy for advanced solid tumors: a pilot study. *Cancer Treat Rep* 1981; 65:219–222.
80. Herr HW, Yagoda A, Batata M, Sogani PC, Whitmore WF. Planned preoperative cisplatin and radiation therapy for locally advanced bladder Cancer. *Cancer* 1983; 52:2205–2208.
81. Coughlin CT, Richmond RC. Biologic and clinical developments of cisplatin combined with radiation: concepts, utility, projections for new trials and the emergence of carboplatin. *Semin Oncol* 1989; 16(Suppl 6):31–43.
82. Reed E, Sauerhoff S, Piorier MC. Quantitation of platinum-DNA binding in human tissues following therapeutic levels of drug exposure—a novel use of graphite furnace spectrometry. *Atomic Spectroscopy* 1988; 9:93–95.
83. Dabholkar M, Reed E. Cisplatin. In: (Pinedo HM, Longo DL, Chabner BA, eds), Cancer Chemotherapy and Biological Response Modifiers Annual 16, Elsevier Sciences B.V., 1996, pp. 88–110.
84. Poirier MC, Lippard SJ, Zwelling LA, et al. Antibodies elicited against cis-diamminedichloroplatinum(II)-DNA adducts formed in vivo and in vitro. *Proc Natl Acad Sci USA* 1982; 79:6443–6447.
85. Fichtinger-Schepman AMJ, Dijt FJ, De Jong WH, van Oosterom AR, Berends F. In vivo cis-diamminedichloroplatinum(II)-DNA adduct formation and removal as measured with immunochemical techniques. In: (Nicolini M, ed), Platinum and Other Metal Coordination Compounds in Cancer Chemotherapy 1988; Martinus Nijhoff Publishing: Boston, pp. 32–46.
86. Perera R, Tang D, Reed E, et al. Multiple biologic markers in testicular cancer patients treated with platinum-based chemotherapy. *Cancer Res* 1992; 52:3558–3565.
87. Reed FP, Yuspa SH, Zwelling LA, Ozols RF, Poirier MC. Quantitation of cisplatin-DNA intrastrand adducts in testicular and ovarian cancer patients receiving cisplatin chemotherapy. *J Clin Invest* 1986; 77:545–550.
88. Reed E, Ozols RF, Tarone R, Yuspa SH, Poirier MC. Platinum-DNA adducts in leukocyte DNA correlate with disease response in ovarian cancer patients receiving platinum-based chemotherapy. *Proc Natl Acad Sci USA* 1987; 84:5024–5028.
89. Reed E, Ozols RF, Tarone R, Yuspa SH, Piorier MC. The measurement of cisplatin-DNA adduct levels in testicular cancer patients. *Carcinogenesis* 1988; 9:1909–1911.
90. Gupta-Burt S, Shamkhani H, Reed E, et al. Correlation between patient response in ovarian, breast, and colon cancer and platinum drug-DNA adduct formation. *Cancer Epidem, Biomarkers Preven* 1993; 2:229–234.
91. Parker RJ, Gill I, Tarone R, et al. Platinum-DNA damage in leukocyte DNA of patients receiving carboplatin and cisplatin chemotherapy measured by atomic absorption spectrometry. *Carcinogenesis* 1991; 12:1253–1258.
92. Reed E, Parker RJ, Gill I, et al. Platinum-DNA adduct in leukocyte DNA of a cohort of 49 patients with 24 different types of malignancy. *Cancer Res* 1993; 53:3694–3699.
93. Schellens JH, Ma J, Planting AS, et al. Relationship between the exposure to cisplatin, DNA-adduct formation in leukocytes and tumor response in patients with solid tumors. *Br J Cancer* 1996; 73:1569–1575.
94. Eastman A, Schulte N, Sheibani N, Sorenson CM. Mechanisms of resistance to platinum drugs. In: (Nicolini M, ed), Platinum and Other Metal Coordination Compounds in Cancer Chemotherapy 1988; Martinus Nijhoff Publishing: Boston, pp. 178–196.
95. Haselow RE, Adams GL, Oken MM, Goudsmit A, Lerner HJ, Marsh JC. Cisplatinum with radiation therapy for locally advanced unresectable head and neck cancer. *Proc Amer Soc Clin Oncol* 1983; 2:160.
96. Haselow RE, Warshaw MG, Okin MM, et al. Radiation alone versus radiation plus weekly low-dose cisplatinum in unresectable cancer of the head and neck. In: (Fee WE Jr, Geopfert H, Johns ME, Strong EW, Ward PH, eds). Head and Neck Cancer 1990; Decker BC: Toronto, pp. 279–281.

97. Bachaud J-M, David J-M, Boussin G, Daly N. Combined radiotherapy and weekly cisplatin infusion for advanced squamous cell carcinoma of the head and neck: preliminary report of a randomized trial. *Int J Radiat Oncol Biol Phys* 1991; 20:243–246.
98. Marcial VA, Pajak TF, Mohuiddin M, et al. ConComitant cisplatin chemotherapy and radiotherapy in advanced mucosal squamous cell carcinoma of the head and neck. *Cancer* 1990; 66:1861–1868.
99. Al-Sarraf M, Pajak TF, Cooper JS, Mohuiddin M, Herskovic A, Ager PJ. Chemo-radiotherapy in patients with locally advanced nasopharyngeal carcinoma: a Radiation Therapy Oncology Group study. *J Clin Oncol* 1990; 8:1342–1351.
100. Wheeler R, Salter M, Stephens S, et al. Simultaneous high dose cisplatin and radiation therapy for unresectable squamous cancer of the head and neck: a phase I/II study. *Monogr Natl Cancer Inst* 1988; 6:339–341.
101. Wheeler RH, Spencer S. Cisplatin plus radiation therapy. *J Infusional Chemo* 1995; 5:61–66.
102. Marcial VA, Hanley JA, Hendrickson F, Ortiz H. Split course radiation therapy of carcinoma of the base of the tongue: results of a prospective national collaborative clinical trial conducted by the Radiation Therapy Oncology Group. *Int J Radiat Oncol Biol Phys* 1983; 9:437–443.
103. Overgaard J, Hjelm-Hansen M, Johansen LV, Anderson AP. Comparison of conventional and split course radiotherapy as primary treatment in carcinoma of the larynx. *Acta Oncol* 1988; 27:147–152.
104. Withers HR, et al. The hazard of accelerated tumor clonogen repopulation during radiation therapy. *Acta Oncol* 1988; 27:131–146.
105. Taylor SG, Murthy AK, Caldarelli DD, et al. Combined simultaneous cisplatin/5-FU infusion chemotherapy and split course radiation in head and neck cancer. *J Clin Oncol* 1989; 7:846–856.
106. Adelstein DJ, Sharan VM, Earle AS, et al. Long-term results after chemoradiotherapy for locally confined squamous-cell head and neck cancer. *Amer J Clin Oncol* 1990; 13:440–447.
107. Jeremie B, Shibamoto Y, Stanisavljevic B, Milojevic L, Milicic B, Nikolie N. Radiation therapy alone or with concurrent low-dose either cisplatin or carboplatin in locally advanced unresectable squamous cell carcinoma of the head and neck: a prospective randomized trial. *Radiotherap Oncol* 1997; 43:29–37.
108. Bachaud JM, Cohen-Jonathan E, Alzieu C, David JM, Serrano E, Daly-Schveitzer N. Combined postoperative radiotherapy and weekly cisplatin infusion for locally advanced head and neck carcinoma: final report of a randomized trial. *Int J Radiat Oncol Biol Phys* 1996; 36:999–1004.
109. Adelstein DJ, Saxton JP, Lavertu P, et al. A phase III trial comparing concurrent chemotherapy and radiotherapy with radiotherapy alone in resectable stage III and IV squamous cell head and neck cancer: preliminary results. *Head Neck* 1997; 19:567–573.
110. Brizel DM, Alberx MF, Fisher SR, et al. Hyperfractionated irradiation with or without concurrent chemotherapy for locally advanced head and neck cancer. *N Engl J Med* 1998; 338:1798–1804.
111. Al-Sarraf M, LeBlanc M, Giri PGS, et al. Chemoradiotherapy versus radiotherapy in patients with advanced nasopharyngeal cancer: phase III randomized intergroup study 0099. *J Clin Oncol* 1998; 16:1310–1317.
112. Robbins KT, Kumar P, Regine WF, et al. Efficacy of targeted supradose cisplatin and concomitant radiation therapy for advanced head and neck cancer: the Memphis experience. *Int J Radiat Oncol Biol Phys* 1997; 38:263–271.
113. Robbins KT, Kumar P, et al. Efficacy of targeted supradose cisplatin and concomitant radiation therapy for advanced head and neck cancer: the Memphis experience. *Int J Radiat Oncol Biol Phys* 1996; 38:263–271.
114. Sharma VM, Wilson WR. Radiosensitization of advanced squamous cell carcinoma of the head and neck with cisplatin during concomitant radiation therapy. *Eur Arch Otorhinolaryngol* 1999; 256:462–465.
115. Bartelink H, Begg AC, Martin JC, et al. Translational research offers individually tailored treatments for cancer patients. *The Cancer J* 2000; 6:2–10.
116. Cooper JS, Lee H, Torrey M, et al. Improved outcome secondary to concurrent chemoradiotherapy for advanced carcinoma of the nasopharynx: Preliminary corroboration of the Intergroup experience. *Int J Radiat Oncol Biol Phys* 2000; 47:861–866.
117. Cooper JS. Concurrent chemotherapy and radiation therapy for advanced stage carcinoma of the nasopharynx. *Int J Radiat Oncol Biol Phys* 2000; 48:1277–1279.
118. Cheng SH, Jian J J-M, Tsai SYC, et al. Long-term survival of nasopharyngeal carcinoma following concomitant radiotherapy and chemotherapy. *Int J Radiat Oncol Biol Phys* 2000; 48:1323–1330.
119. Bonomi P. Treatment of stage III non-small cell lung cancer with thoracic radiation therapy and simultaneous platinum chemotherapy. *Semin Oncol* 1994; 21(Suppl 6):101–108.

120. Robinow JS, Shaw EG, Eagan RT, et al. Results of combination chemotherapy and thoracic irradiation therapy for unresectable non-small cell carcinoma of the lung. *Int J Radiat Oncol Biol Phys* 1989; 17:1203–1210.
121. Bonomi P, Faber LP. Neoadjuvant chemoradiation therapy in non-small cell lung cancer: The RusUniversity experience. *Lung Cancer* 1993; 9:383–390.
122. Weiden PL, Piantodosi S. Preoperative chemotherapy cisplatin and fluorouracil and radiation therapy in stage III non-small cell lung cancer: A phase II study of the Lung Cancer Study Group. *J Natl Cancer Onst* 1991; 83:266–272.
123. Strauss GM, Herndon JE, Sherman DD, et al. Neoadjuvant chemotherapy and radiotherapy followed by surgery in stage IIIa non-small cell carcinoma of the lung: report of a Cancer and Leukemia Group B phase II study. *J Clin Oncol* 1992; 10:1237–1244.
124. Weirberg A, Yashar J, Posner M, et al. Combined modality therapy for stage IIIa non-small cell carcinoma of the lung. *Proc Amer Soc Clin Oncol* 1992; 11:293.
125. Rusch VW, Albain KS, Crowley JJ, et al. Surgical resection of stage IIIa and stage IIIb non-small cell lung cancer after concurrent induction chemoradiotherapy. *J Thoracic Cardiovasc Surg* 1993; 105:97–106.
126. Schaake-Koning C, Vanden Bogaert W, Dalesio O, et al. Effects of concomitant cisplatin and radiotherapy on inoperable non-small cell lung cancer. *N Engl J Med* 1992; 326:524–530.
127. Trovo MG, Minotel E, Fravelun G, et al. Radiotherapy versus radiotherapy enhanced by cisplatin in stage III non-small cell lung cancer. *Int J Radiat Oncol Biol Phys* 1992; 24:11–16.
128. Soresi E, Clerici M, Grilli R, et al. A randomized clinical trial comparing radiation therapy versus radiation therapy plus cis-dichlorodiammine platinum in the treatment of locally advanced non-small cell lung cancer. *Semin Oncol* 1988; 15:20–25.
129. Ansari R, Tokara R, Fisher W, et al. A phase III study of thoracic irradiation with and without concomitant cisplatin in locally advanced unresectable non-small cell lung cancer, a Hoosier Oncology Group study. *Proc Amer Soc Clin Oncol* 1991; 10:242.
130. Hazuka M, Crowley J, Bunn P, et al. Concurrent daily low-dose cisplatin combined with chest irradiation in locally advanced non-small cell lung cancer. Preliminary results of a Southwest Oncology Group study. *Proc Amer Soc Clin Oncol* 1992; 11:295.
131. Ravasl G, Bodini AV, Milani F, et al. Continuous infusion of cisplatin and concurrent radiotherapy in non-resectable stage III lung cancer. *Lung Cancer* 1991; 7:164.
132. Belani CP, Slawson R, Van Echo D, et al. Concurrent carboplatin and radiotherapy for unresectable stage III non-small cell lung cancer. *Lung Cancer* 1991; 7:159.
133. Stehman FB. Experience with hydroxyurea as a radiosensitizer in carcinoma of the cervix. *Semin Oncol* 1992; 19:48–52.
134. Muggia FM, Muderpach. Platinum compounds and endometrial cancers: focus on carboplatin. *Semin Oncol* 1994; 21(Suppl 2):35–41.
135. Wadler S, Goldberg G, Fields A, et al. The potential role of amifostine in conjunction with cisplatin in the treatment of locally advanced carcinoma of the cervix. *Semin Oncol* 1996; 23(Suppl 8):64–68.
136. Runowicz CD, Wadler S, Rodriguez-Roddriguez L, et al. Concomitant cisplatin and radiotherapy in locally advanced cervical carcinoma. *Gynecol Oncol* 1989; 34:395–401.
137. Runowicz CD, Smith HO, Goldbert G. Multimodality therapy in locally advanced cervical cancer. *Curr Opin Obstet Gynecol* 1993; 5:92–98.
138. Fields A, Anderson P, Goldbert GL, et al. Mature results of a phase II trial of concomitant cisplatin/pelvic radiotherapy for locally advanced squamous cell carcinoma of the cervix. *Gynecol Oncol* 1996; 61:416–422.
139. Keys HM, Bundy BN, Stehman FB, et al. Cisplatin, radiation and adjuvant hysterectomy compared with radiation and adjuvant hysterectomy for bulky stage Ib cervical carcinoma. *N Engl J Med* 1999; 340:1154–1161.
140. Morris M, Eifel PJ, Jiandong L, et al. Pelvic radiation with concurrent chemotherapy compared with pelvic and para-aortic radiation for high-risk cervical cancer. *N Engl J Med* 1999; 340:1137–1143.
141. Rose PG, Bundy BN, Watkins EB, et al. Concurrent cisplatin-based radiotherapy and chemotherapy for locally advanced cervical cancer. *N Engl J Med* 1999; 340:1144–1153
142. Santin AD, Hermonat PL, Ravaggi A, et al. Effects of concurrent cisplatinum administration during radiotherapy vs radiotherapy alone on the immune function of patients with cancer of the uterine cervix. *Int J Radiat Oncol Biol Phys* 2000; 48:997–1006.

143. Koh W-J, Wallace J, Greer BE, et al. Combined radiotherapy and chemotherapy in the management of local-regionally advanced vulvar cancer. *Int J Radiat Oncol Biol Phys* 1993; 26:809–816.
144. Coughlin CT, Richmond RC, Page RL. Platinum drug delivery and radiation for locally advance prostate cancer. *Int J Radiat Oncol Biol Phys* 1994; 28:1029–1038.
145. Kaufman DS, Winter KA, Shipley WU, et al. The initial results in muscle-invading bladder cancer of RTOG 95-06: phase I/II trial of transurethral surgery plus radiation therapy with concurrent cisplatin and 5-fluorouracil followed by selective bladder preservation or cystectomy depending on the initial response. *The Oncologist* 2000; 5:471–476.
146. Ruckdeschel JC. The future role of carboplatin. *Semin Oncol* 1994; 21(Suppl 12):114–118.
147. Lokich J, Anderson N. Carboplatin versus cisplatin in solid tumors: an analysis of the literature. *Ann Oncol* 1998; 9:13–21.
148. Highley MS, Calvert AH. Clinical experience with cisplatin and carboplatin. In: (Kelland LR, Farrell N, eds) Platinum-Based Drugs in Cancer Therapy 2000; Humana Press Inc.: Totowa, NJ; pp. 171–194.
149. Belani CP, Aisner J. Combined chemotherapy and radiation in locally advanced non-small cell lung cancer. *Semin Oncol* 1994; 21(Suppl 12):79–90.
150. Zamboglou N, Schnabel T, Kolotas C, et al. Carboplatin and radiotherapy in the treatment of head and neck cancer: six years' experience. *Semin Oncol* 1994; 21(Suppl 12):45–53.
151. Lebwohl D, Canetta R. Clinical development of platinum complexes in cancer therapy: an historical perspective and an update. *Eur J Cancer* 1998; 34:1522–1534.
152. O'Dwyer PJ, Stevenson JP, Johnson SW. Clinical experience:DACH-based platinum drugs. In: (Kelland LR, Farrell N, eds) Platinum-Based Drugs in Cancer Therapy 2000; Humana Press Inc.: Totowa, NJ; pp. 231–249.
153. Stratford IJ, Williamson C, Adams GE. Combination studies with misonidazole and a cis-platinum complex: cytotoxicity and radiosensitization in vitro. *Br J Cancer* 1980; 41:517–522.
154. Carde P, Laval F. Effect of cis-dichlorodiammine platinum II and x-rays on mammalian cell survival. *Int J Radiat Oncol Biol Phys* 1981; 7:929–933.
155. Bartelink H, Begg AC, Martin JC, et al. Translational research offers individually tailored treatments for cancer patients. *Cancer J Scientific American* 2000; 6(1):2–10.

4 Taxanes in Combined Modality Therapy

Robert M. MacRae, MD and Hak Choy, MD

CONTENTS

1. INTRODUCTION

The taxanes are a relatively new group of plant-derived chemotherapeutic agents that have been studied quite extensively in both preclinical studies and in clinical trials. This group of drugs, which includes paclitaxel (Taxol) and docetaxel (Taxotere), act as mitotic spindle inhibitors through their promotion of microtubule assembly and retardation of disaggregation. Paclitaxel is a natural product derived from the bark of the Pacific yew (*Taxus brevifolia*) whereas taxotere is a semisynthetic analog prepared from the needles of the European yew (*Taxus baccata*) *(1)*. The taxanes as a group have had significant success in the treatment of solid tumors in the setting of both metastatic disease and adjuvant therapy as well as in locally advanced disease where they are combined with radiation in either a sequential or concurrent fashion. There are also several newer taxanes/ microtubule inhibitors that are under development that appear to have promising activities in the completed preclinical studies. They include taxoltere metro *(2)*, the epothilones *(3)*, and the BMS compounds 184476 and 188797 *(4)*. This chapter will provide an

From: *Chemoradiation in Cancer Therapy*
Edited by: H. Choy © Humana Press Inc., Totowa, NJ

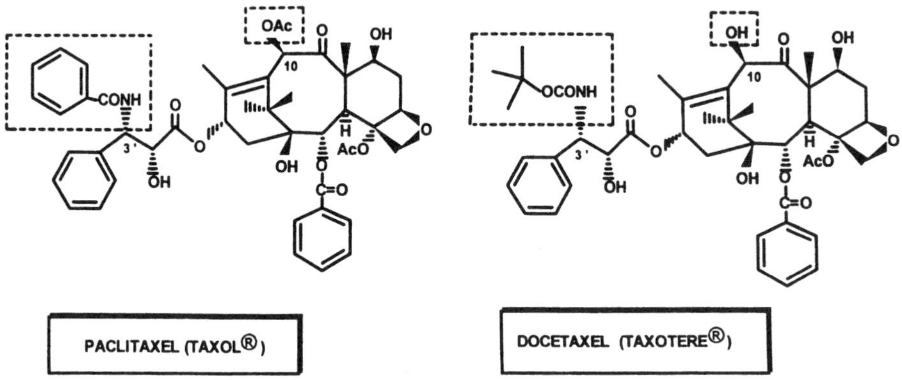

Fig. 1. Chemical structure of the taxanes. The chemical structures of docetaxel and paclitaxel. From ref. *5*.

overview of the current status of the taxanes and their combination with radiation in the treatment of human malignancy through a review of the preclinical literature on the subject. It will then focus on the status of clinical practice with a look into the future and the place of taxanes at the start of the new millennium.

Paclitaxel, which is the prototypic drug in this group, was originally found through a screening program at the National Cancer Institute where thousands of plant extracts were screened for activity *(1)*. Both paclitaxel and docetaxel consist of a complex taxane ring structure with a four-member oxetan ring attached at C-4 and C-5 and a bulky ester side chain at C-13 *(5)* (*see* Fig. 1). The taxanes bind to the N-terminal 31 amino acid sequence of the beta-tubulin subunit of the tubulin polymers *(6)* at a site distinct from that of the vinca alkaloids, guanosine 5'-triphosphate (GTP), colchicines, and podophyllotoxin *(1)*. Its binding leads to the stabilization of tubulin polymers by shifting the dynamic equilibrium between tubulin dimers and the microtubules in favor of the polymerized state *(7)*. Docetaxel has a significantly increased affinity for this binding site in comparison to paclitaxel *(8)* and will also form polymers at a faster rate relative to paclitaxel. Although there is also in vitro suggestion that docetaxel more cytotoxic to cells in culture *(9)*, this does not necessarily translate into greater clinical efficacy because this increased activity may also portend increased toxicity as well.

Although taxanes bind to β-tubulin promoting microtubule polymerization and stabilization of the spindle complex, they serve to cause a sustained mitotic block at the metaphase/anaphase boundary. This block will occur at a lower concentration than that which is required to increase the microtubule mass *(10)*. However, it is not completely clear how this interaction with microtubules translates into cell death. Morphologic features and the characteristic DNA fragmentation patterns seen in the setting of apoptosis have been documented in tumor cells after therapy with taxanes *(10)*. These observations are accompanied by the phosphorylation of Bcl-2, an anti-apoptotic protein, changing the cellular balance between Bax and Bcl-2 to a status that favors apoptosis *(11)*.

Evidence has also come to light that suggests that cells containing p53 mutations are more sensitive to paclitaxel's cytotoxic effects than those with wild-type copies of the gene *(12–14)*. Wang et al. outline how the *p53* status may impact on paclitaxel sensitivity in their review of paclitaxel induced cell death *(15)*. They suggest that:

1. The loss of *p53*-dependent G_1 arrest promotes the progression of cells to G_2/M phase where they are the target of mitotic arrest.
2. With loss of *p53* function, $p21^{WAF1/CIP1}$ is no longer upregulated and is unable to help cells escape from their state of mitotic arrest.
3. Wild-type *p53* will downregulate the levels of microtubule associated protein 4 (MAP-4) so that, when *p53* function is absent, the high levels of MAP-4 will stabilize microtubules and sensitize cells to paclitaxel therapy.

The concentration of paclitaxel appears to be important in determining the exact apoptotic mechanism at work. When cells are treated with lower concentrations of the drug (10–100 n*M*), the mitotic spindle may be the only microtubule formation significantly affected, as it is more sensitive than other microtubule structures *(16)*. This altered spindle may lead to the triggering of mitotic spindle checkpoint genes that cause apoptosis *(17,18)*. The use of high concentrations of paclitaxel (>200 n*M*) may lead to the induction of apoptosis independent from mitotic arrest, which may be an advantage in that this would allow for the targeting of growth-arrested tumor cells *(15)*.

The literature is also starting to show a significant volume of papers that concentrate on the possible mechanisms of paclitaxel resistance seen in tumors *(15)*. These include:

1. Mutations in the amino acid sequence of β-tubulin that abolish the paclitaxel binding site *(19)*.
2. Upregulation of anti-apoptotic genes like Bcl-2 *(20)* and Bcl-X_L *(21)* or the downregulation of Bax *(22)*.
3. Increased drug efflux resulting from the increased production of mdr-1 *(23)* or other membrane pumps.
4. Differential expression of tubulin isotypes *(24)*.
5. Capase mutations *(25)* in malignant cells.

Ultimately it is increased understanding of the mechanisms that underlie taxane-mediated cell death that will allow for the development of improved therapies for malignancies.

2. PHARMACOLOGY

Both docetaxel and paclitaxel share several common pharmacological properties including large volumes of distribution (except for the central nervous system), long elimination half lives, rapid tissue uptake, and considerable hepatic metabolism involving the cytochrome P-450 system *(26)*. Docetaxel has linear pharmacokinetic behavior at clinically relevant doses *(26)* with avid serum protein binding and extensive tissue binding. Fecal excretion accounts for approx 80% of drug deposition and less than 10% is excreted renally *(1)*. Although many of the characteristics of paclitaxel are similar to docetaxel, a notable difference exists at the pharmacokinetic level with nonlinear or saturable clearance. This has profound implications as increasing doses of the drug will disproportionately increase drug exposure.

Both drugs are highly lipid soluble and as such are prepared and administered in dilutants (paclitaxel in Cremophor EL and docetaxel in polysorbate 80). Both medications are normally administered with dexamethasone, H_1 and H_2 antagonists as premedications to decrease the incidence of the acute hypersensitivity reaction (HSR) (dyspnea with bronchospasm, urticaria, and hypotension) that has been observed to occur *(1,27)*. It is uncertain as to whether or not these vehicles may contribute to the incidence of the HSR. Myelosuppression is the limiting toxicity of both taxanes. Clinical studies with paclitaxel have shown that the severity of neutropenia correlates with the duration that the plasma levels are above 50–100 nmol/L *(28)*.

These drugs produce other notable toxicities including a peripheral neuropathy characterized by numbness, paresthesia, and a symmetric distal loss of sensation including proprioception, vibration, pinprick, and temperature effects in a "glove and stocking" distribution *(1)*. Myalgias and malaise are also common peritreatment complaints. Paclitaxel has also been associated with cardiac rhythm disturbances, myocardial ischemia, and reversible alopecia. Docetaxel has been associated with skin toxicity in the form of a puritic maculopapular rash on the forearms and hands as well as alopecia, nail changes, and stomatitis that is seen more frequently than with paclitaxel. Docetaxel has also been found to cause a unique fluid retention syndrome characterized by edema and third spacing of fluids including pleural effusions and ascites. The use of prophylactic steroid therapy and lower single doses appears to have decreased the incidence and severity of this side-effect *(1)*.

Both of the taxanes have become integral to the treatment of several malignancies including: breast cancer *(29–31)*, ovarian cancer *(29,32)*, nonsmall-cell lung cancer (NSCLC) *(29,33)*, and bladder cancer *(34)*. The combination of paclitaxel and carboplatin was the preferred first-line regimen for all stages of NSCLC by the majority of medical oncologists (55%) in a recent survey undertaken by investigators from Vanderbilt University *(35)*. The recent approval of taxotere as second-line therapy for NSCLC *(36)* is also tribute to the impact of these drugs in the most common malignancy encountered in the developed world. The substantial impact that these drugs have had in advanced malignancies in combination with their unique radiosensitizing properties has lead to the interest that exists in the exploration of their concurrent use with radiation in locally advanced disease.

3. RADIOSENSITIZING ABILITIES OF THE TAXANES

The taxanes act to cause cells to arrest their progression through the cell cycle at the G2-M phase. This is of significant interest because this is exactly the point in the cell cycle where cells are more sensitive to the lethal effects of ionizing radiation *(37)*. Taxanes also act to induce programmed cell death. Milas et al. have looked at the relationship among mitotic arrest, apoptosis, and the antineoplastic activity of paclitaxel in 16 murine tumors *(38)*. Using a single dose of paclitaxel of 40 mg/kg, mitotic arrest was induced in all tumors in varying degrees, however, apoptosis was induced in only 50% of tumors. The antitumor efficacy of paclitaxel correlated best with mitotic arrest as quantitated by absolute growth delay. This study also showed that the pretreatment levels of apoptosis correlated with both paclitaxel-induced apoptosis and tumor growth delay. Therefore both pretreatment apoptotic rate and paclitaxel apoptotic rate could potentially act as predictors of the response to paclitaxel.

The major rationale for combining a taxane with radiation relates to the induction of a cell cycle block at the G_2/M point where cells are more sensitive to the damaging effects of radiation. Tishler reported an enhancement factor of 1.8 when human astrocytomas cells were incubated with paclitaxel for 24 h prior to receiving radiation *(39)*. Choy et al. have reported on paclitaxel's sensitizing effects in a human lung cancer cell line, HL-60, finding a slightly lower enhancement ratio, 1.48 *(40)*, using a 1-h exposure of paclitaxel at a concentration of only 3.0×10^{-8} (*see* Fig. 2). It is important to note that in all studies

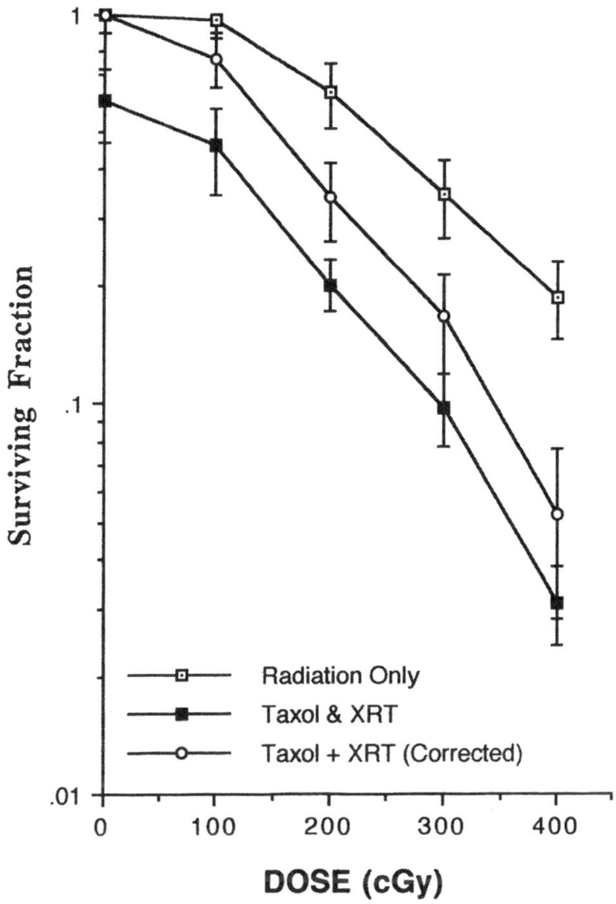

Fig. 2. The radiation sensitizing effects of paclitaxel and concurrent ionizing radiation in a human lung cancer cell line, HL-60. From ref. *40*.

performed examining the radiosensitizing abilities of paclitaxel a range of interactions have been demonstrated, from supraadditivity to additivity to as little as sub-additive results *(38)*. These results have also demonstrated that not all tumor cell lines are sensitized to the effects of ionizing X-ray therapy (XRT) by taxanes and the exposure time to the drug is likely equally, if not more important than the concentration of the drug in achieving radiosensitization.

In most studies where a supraadditive interaction was seen, cells were incubated with the drug prior to irradiation *(38)*. In general the use of moderate concentrations (5–100 nmol/L) of paclitaxel in the culture medium for over 24 h lead to maximum sensitization. Most studies used actively proliferating cells in order to conduct their experiments and most investigators reached the conclusion that maximal radiosensitization occurred when cells were arrested in G_2 and M, as this part of the cell cycle is the most sensitive to radiation damage. This assumption does, however, presuppose that the majority of the G_2/M arrested cells will not die unless they are exposed to ionizing XRT. Plateau phase, i.e., nonproliferating, cells were found to be sensitized to radiation by paclitaxel albeit to a lesser extent than actively proliferating cells, so other mechanisms must also be involved *(38)*.

Other suggested mechanisms for the increased radiosensitization seen with both paclitaxel and docetaxel include an increased alpha component of DNA damage and the fact that docetaxel is toxic for S-phase cells that are maximally radiation resistant *(41,42)*.

Certain other conditions are associated with only an additive or even a subadditive response when taxol is combined with radiation *(38)*. These conditions include:

1. Paclitaxel-mediated G_1 arrest, which creates a more resistant subpopulation of cells that counteracts the effects of a G_2/M block.
2. Paclitaxel-induced cell cycle effects like G_2/M block in cells destined to die before irradiation.
3. Incubation conditions, timing of the addition of drug or drug concentrations that are insufficient to exert cellular effects.

Although there is less literature on the effects of docetaxel in combination with radiation, it also appears to be a powerful radiosensitizer. Among the reports is data from Amorino et al. *(43)* who looked at the enhancement of radiation effects by the combination of docetaxel and carboplatin in vitro. H460 large cell lung carcinoma cells were incubated with docetaxel and paclitaxel with or without carboplatin and were then irradiated. The most impressive results were found with the combination of docetaxel (25 n*M*) and carboplatin (100 μ*M*), which gave a dose enhancement ratio of 1.55. The dose enhancement ratio for the combination of paclitaxel and carboplatin (100 μ*M*) was in the same range at 1.50. Creane et al. *(44)* looked at the effect of docetaxel on radiation response in three different cell lines that have widely different responses to radiation alone. Their experiments indicated that docetaxel had the greatest cytotoxic and radiosensitizing effect on the SW48 (*p53*^{WT}) cell line. The degree of radiosensitization was not improved by increasing the drug concentration despite the fact that higher doses of drug were more cytotoxic. Both of the other cell lines (HT 29 and SW48), which carry mutant *p53*, were less sensitive to the effects of docetaxel even though their malignant potential is different. The authors conclude that a functional *p53* gene product is essential for sensitizing effects of docetaxel to be seen and that its increased lethality is likely related to increased apoptotic potential in more sensitive cell lines.

Milas et al. *(45)* have published data looking at the efficacy of docetaxel on the therapeutic ratio of fractionated radiotherapy in vivo using MCa-4 mammary adenocarcinoma (prototype docetaxel-sensitive tumor) and SCC-VII squamous cell carcinoma (prototype docetaxel-resistant tumor) xenografts. In this set of experiments the investigators looked at two different delivery schemes for the docetaxel with radiotherapy: a single bolus (33 mg/kg) 24 h before 5 d of fractionated radiotherapy and daily delivery of docetaxel (8 mg/kg) with radiation delivered at the peak of mitotic arrest (9 h for MCa-4 cells and 6 h for SCC-VII tumors). They found that the best schedule for the two cell lines was different; the MCa-4 tumors responded better with a single dose of the drug, while the SCC-VII responded better to daily drug administration. Enhancement factors were 2.04 and 2.0 for each tumor type respectively. The authors also reported that the final therapeutic gain of the daily docetaxel was reduced because of increased normal tissue effects using normal mouse jejunal cells as a model. It was suggested that the enhancement seen in the docetaxel-sensitive tumor was related to an additional increase in reoxygenation of hypoxic tumor cells with each fraction beyond what reoxygenation was caused by the direct cytotoxic effects of the drug on its own. They felt that a similar phenomenon might be taking place in their docetaxel-resistant tumor model, only that the reoxygenation effect was greater with daily administration of the drug. Their conclusions were that there is room for greater individualization of therapy in the future and this should be based on correlates including pretreatment levels of apoptosis in a tumor, assessment of its oncogene status including *p53*, Bax, and Bcl-2, or changes seen in these parameters seen within 1–2 d after treatment with the drug.

In an excellent review of the literature on the interaction between radiation and the taxanes, especially looking at the effects of paclitaxel, Milas et al. *(38)* outline how they came to realize that reoxygenation played such a substantial role in the potentiation of tumor radioresponse. It has been well established for years that tumors contain areas of hypoxic cells that are normally 2.5 to 3 times less sensitive to radiation than normal cells *(37)*. Both radiation and chemotherapies can cause reoxygenation through their preferential killing of those oxygenated cells that are located close to blood vessels. Milas et al. summarized observations that showed:

1. Massive loss of tumor cells though the apoptotic pathway was restricted to the perivascular region.
2. Radioenhancement occurring during this period of cell loss became even more impressive when apoptotic cells were removed from the tumor *(38)*.

Experiments in which tumor xenografts were treated with paclitaxel and radiation in hypoxic and noroxic conditions were pursued *(46)*. It was found that the creation of hypoxic conditions greatly reduced the efficacy of paclitaxel in its enhancement of radioresponse. Measurements of tumor oxygenation using Eppendorf histographs confirmed that the median tumor PO_2 increased from the control value of 6.8 mmHg to 10.5 mmHg at 24 h to 31.2 mmHg at 48 h after paclitaxel treatment. In the same vane, Milas et al. *(46)* documented that the percentage of hypoxic cells was decreased from 32% in untreated tumors to 4%, 2%, and 1% at 9, 24, and 48 h after drug administration. In combination with reoxygenation, the induction of apoptosis and the induction of mitotic arrest in G_2-M phase leads to the radiosensitization that is associated with concurrent use of the taxanes.

Importantly, an agent that attempts to enhance the therapeutic ratio must be able to selectively enhance the effect on tumors more compared to the enhancement that occurs in normal tissues. Like most chemotherapy agents those tissues at greatest risk are those with a rapid turnover time, such as the normal gastrointestinal mucosa and the skin. When looking at jejunal crypt cells it was seen that at the peak of mitotic arrest there was a slight enhancement of radiation effect with a relative enhancement ratio of 1.07 at the 10-surviving cell isoeffective dose, however, by the time that 24–96 h had passed, there was a slight radioprotection that occurred with paclitaxel administration in concert with radiation *(47)*. Similar results are seen with the concurrent administration of docetaxel *(45)*. The authors suggest that the radioprotection seen is related to the rapid regeneration of epithelial cells after their initial depletion by the taxanes because of a shortening of their cell cycle or a recruitment of noncycling cells.

4. APPLICATION IN THE CLINIC

These preclinical works with the taxanes have now lead to the clinic where experience has shown that concurrent radiation and paclitaxel or docetaxel leads to impressive response rates in several solid tumor types *(48–50)*. The large bulk of experience has been acquired with locally advanced nonsmall-cell lung cancer and advanced head and neck primary cancers where protocols have integrated both taxanes with concurrent radiation to improve responses and outcomes. Ongoing research continues in order to refine the administration, sequencing, and integration of these agents with other chemotherapies, new biological response modifiers and radiation therapy.

5. NONSMALL-CELL LUNG CANCER

5.1. Paclitaxel

There have been several different phase I trials that have examined the concurrent administration of radiation with taxol-based chemotherapy. Interestingly, the timing of administration of taxol has been fairly extensively explored in the phase I setting with: a 7-wk continuous infusion of taxol *(51)*, daily dosing *(52)*, twice weekly dosing *(53)*, weekly dosing *(54,55)*, dosing every 2 wk *(56)*, dosing with three weekly cycles *(57)*, and a 120-h (5-d) continuous infusion repeated every 3 wk during the course of radiation therapy *(58)*.

In a series of trials conducted during the mid to late 1990s Choy et al. examined the activity of taxol and radiation delivered in a concurrent fashion to patients with locally advanced NSCLC *(54,59–61)*. In the initial phase I experience, paclitaxel was administered as a 3-h intravenous (iv) infusion, repeated every week for 6 wk with concurrent thoracic radiation to a total dose of 60 Gy *(54)*. The starting dose of paclitaxel was 10 mg/m^2 with escalation in 10-mg/m^2 increments until the maximum tolerated dose (MTD) of 60 mg/m^2/wk was reached. The major acute toxicity was found to be reversible esophagitis. In a subsequent phase II trial (LUN-27) *(59)* 33 previously untreated patients with unresectable stage III A or B NSCLC received 60 mg/m^2 weekly for 6 wk with concurrent thoracic radiation. Of the 27 evaluable patients there was a 76% overall response rate (3 CRs and 22 PRs) and the 1-, 2-, and 3-yr survivals were 61%, 33%, and 18%. Reversible esophagitis was once again the major acute toxicity, however, it was felt to be manageable.

Choy et al. have published two further phase II trials of concurrent paclitaxel and carboplatin. In both trials the two drugs were administered weekly with paclitaxel at a dose of 50 mg/m^2 and carboplatin at a dose of 2 AUC. The first of these trials, LUN-56 *(60)*, combined these two drugs with once daily radiation to a dose of 66 Gy and the second trial, LUN-63 *(61)*, used hyperfractionated radiation to a total dose of 69.6 Gy directed at the primary tumor. They have shown similar promising results in patient populations where 70% have stage IIIB disease. LUN-56, which enrolled 40 patients, showed a 76% response rate and 1-, 2-, and 3-yr median survivals of 54, 46, and 32%; 43 patients were enrolled on LUN-63. In this trial there was a 79% response rate and a median survival of 14.3 mo. Encouraging 1- and 2-yr survivals of 61% and 35% were seen.

Certainly these three phase II trials performed at Brown and Vanderbilt Universities have shown promising results in terms of response rate, median survival, and 1- and 2-yr survivals (Table 1). Esophagitis has been the major acute toxicity seen in these trials. When using RTOG criteria, the rate of grade 3/4 esophagitis in the three phase II trials was 17%, 25%, and 26%, respectively *(63)*. While these rates of esophagitis are significant and certainly higher than the rate seen when treating with radiation alone, the symptoms are manageable and they appear to be restricted to the acute setting. On multivariate

Table 1
Outcomes in Three Phase II Trials
of Paclitaxel-Based Chemoradiotherapy for Locally Advanced NSCLC

	Choy (59) LUN-27	*Choy (60) LUN-56*	*Choy (61) LUN-63*
Evaluable patients	33	39	43
Response rate (%)	76	76	79
Median survival (months)	20	20.5	14.3
2-yr survival (%)	36	46	35
Local recurrence only (%)	—	29	35
Local and distant recurrence (%)	—	21	10
Distant recurrence only (%)	—	50	55
Brain only recurrence (%)	—	71	45

Patterns of failure data is not available for LUN-27.

analysis there was no significant correlation between esophageal toxicity and gender, histology, length of esophagus in the primary or boost fields, and disease stage. Perhaps more interesting are the data collected from the LUN-56 and -63 trials on the patterns of failure. Local recurrence is the site of first failure in approx 30–35% of cases. Of those with distant metastatic disease with no apparent local recurrence, 55% are failing in the brain. This result correlates with the results of other studies and certainly raises the prospect of prophylactic cranial radiation to decrease this rate of distant relapse further.

Lau et al. have reported on their experience of administering radiation with taxol dosed twice a week for locally advanced nonsmall-cell lung cancer *(53)*. Their phase II trial was conducted combining low-dose radiosensitizing chemotherapy with concurrent radiation followed by consolidation chemotherapy *(62)*. The induction chemoradiation consisted of paclitaxel, 30 mg/m^2 iv over 1 h, twice weekly for 6 wk; carboplatin, AUC of 1.5, weekly for 6 wk; and concurrent daily thoracic radiation for a total of 61 Gy. The consolidation chemotherapy consisted of two 21-d cycles of paclitaxel 200 mg/m^2 over 3 h and carboplatin AUC = 6. With the last report of their data, 34 patients had been enrolled. The overall response rate was 71%. With a median follow-up of 20 mo, the median survival was 20 mo and 2-yr actuarial survival was 40% (95% CI: 20% to 65%). The authors have concluded that this regimen is quite promising and as such it will be compared with a standard cisplatin/etoposide/radiation regimen for stage III NSCLC in a SWOG phase III trial.

Socinski et al. have reported on their phase I/II experience with dose-escalated thoracic radiation in the setting of a combined modality approach to locally advanced NSCLC *(55,64)*. Two cycles of carboplatin and paclitaxel (AUC 6 and 225 mg/m^2/3h q21d) were followed on d 43 by weekly carboplatin and paclitaxel (AUC 2 and 45 mg/m^2/3h × 6) and thoracic radiotherapy (TRT), 50 Gy was delivered to the prechemotherapy tumor volume and areas of suspected microscopic spread in the mediastinum with a 1.0–2.0 cm margin. Boost volumes included the primary tumor volume and all radiographically positive nodes with a 1.0 cm margin. The total dose of radiation was escalated through four cohorts of patients 60, 66, 70, 74 Gy without reaching any of the planned toxicity endpoints. The overall response to the therapy was 50% (3% CR, 47%

PR) and median survival was 26 mo. The 3-yr survival probability is 0.47 *(64)*. Because dose escalation was limited to 74 Gy without reaching a maximally tolerated dose, a further trial is underway to find the true MTD of dose-escalated thoracic radiation with concurrent carboplatin–paclitaxel-based chemotherapy.

The CALGB has reported on a randomized phase II trial of induction chemotherapy followed by concurrent thoracic radiation and platinum-based chemotherapy *(65)* with the purpose of examining the activity of three of the newer chemotherapeutic agents—gemcitabine, paclitaxel, and vinorelbine—in the setting of locally advanced NSCLC. Patients in arm 2 received concurrent cisplatin and paclitaxel and thoracic radiation after two induction cycles of chemotherapy with the same drugs. The paclitaxel–cisplatin arm had a response rate of 64% and a median survival of 14.7 mo. While this trial may not have delivered paclitaxel in an optimal fashion to achieve maximal radiosensitization, it does reveal that the use of paclitaxel in this patient population is a very reasonable treatment strategy. Further ongoing phase II and III trials should prove helpful in evaluating paclitaxel's efficacy in this treatment setting.

5.2. Docetaxel

There is certainly less data available on the role of concurrent docetaxel with radiation in the treatment of locally advanced nonsmall-cell lung cancer. Koukourakis et al. *(66)* have reported on their phase I/II experience of administering radiation concurrently with docetaxel for stage IIIB NSCLC. In the phase II portion of their study, 30 mg/m^2 of docetaxel was given weekly with concurrent 64 Gy of thoracic radiation. Esophagitis was the main side effect of the regimen wherein 17% of patients needed a two-week treatment delay and another 31% of patients required minor delays (3–7 d). Thirty-five patients were enrolled and evaluable, and the overall response rate was 80% (34% CR). The median survival was 12 mo, and 1-yr survival rate was reported as being 48%.

Aamdal et al. *(67)* investigated the role of docetaxel in concurrent chemoradiotherapy in locally advanced NSCLC in another phase I/II study. The maximally tolerated dose of docetaxel delivered with chest radiation was 40 mg/m^2. In the phase II study, 33 patients were treated with weekly docetaxel (30 mg/m^2/d) concurrent with only 50 Gy of thoracic radiation. With 24 evaluable patients, the overall response rate was 62.5%. With 9 mo follow-up, the median survival time was 13.6 mo, and the 1-yr survival rate was 59.4%. Choy et al. *(68)* and Murakami et al. *(69)* have performed phase I studies as well. The major difference here was that these investigators chose to examine the role of weekly docetaxel/carboplatin delivered concurrently with radiation in stage III NSCLC. Using 20–40 mg/m^2 of docetaxel and 1–2 AUC of carboplatin weekly, they achieved overall response rates of 62% and 92%, respectively. Similarly, Segawa et al. *(70)* have reported on their phase I-II experience with concurrent docetaxel plus cisplatin with thoracic radiation. Using their recommended weekly dose of 40 mg/m^2 docetaxel and 40 mg/m^2 cisplatin, 33 patients were enrolled to yield an overall response rate of 70%. Their two-year survival was quite respectable at 41%. Nyman et al. *(71)* conducted a phase II trial in stage III NSCLC where docetaxel and cisplatin were also delivered concomitantly with thoracic radiation. Patients received an initial two courses of induction systemic docetaxel (75 mg/m^2) and cisplatin (75 mg/m^2), and the third course was given concomitantly with radiotherapy. With 24 evaluable patients, an overall response rate of 79% was achieved as was a 2 yr overall survival of 43%.

The oncology community in the United States appears to have embraced the use of paclitaxel in combination with concurrent thoracic radiation in the treatment of NSCLC. Investigators from Vanderbilt University recently reported the results of an American practice pattern survey for nonsmall-cell lung carcinoma for the year 1997 *(35)*. They found that in the setting of nonmetastatic disease, 45% of respondents preferred paclitaxel–carboplatin chemotherapy as the drugs of choice with concurrent or sequential radiotherapy. This certainly reveals that a large number of physicians are choosing paclitaxel-based therapies for locally advanced NSCLC based on its toxicity profile and phase II evidence. However, it is unlikely that either a paclitaxel- or docetaxel-containing regimen will perform significantly better than the other in the combined modality treatment of unresectable stage III NSCLC. As many of the large cooperative oncology groups are incorporating paclitaxel-based regimens into their new trials it would seem that taxane-based therapy has come to stay.

6. SMALL-CELL LUNG CANCER

The concept of delivering concurrent chemoradiation has long since been established in the therapy of limited-stage small-cell lung cancer. It has been shown to contribute to both local control and survival in two meta-analyses *(72,73)*. Standard therapy includes the concurrent delivery of thoracic radiation with either the first or second cycle cisplatin–etoposide chemotherapy *(74,75)*. With the advent of a newer generation of chemotherapeutic agents, investigators have hoped that their incorporation into treatment regimens may allow the cure rates to be pushed beyond their current 20–25% range for limited stage disease.

6.1. Paclitaxel

At present there is no published data looking at the addition of docetaxel to regimens that attempt to treat limited-stage disease. However, there are some early data that are now available looking at the contribution of paclitaxel administered in a concurrent fashion in this disease *(76)*. In one of the only publications on the subject, Levitan et al. *(77)* outline their experience with a multi-institutional phase I/II trial of paclitaxel, cisplatin, and etoposide with concurrent radiation for limited-stage small-cell lung carcinoma. In this treatment schema the radiation was delivered concurrently with the first two cycles of chemotherapy (where the paclitaxel escalation occurred) for a total dose of 45 Gy (1.8 Gy/fraction for 5 wk) and then a further two cycles of chemotherapy of fixed dose were delivered. The maximally tolerated dose of paclitaxel was found to be 135 mg/m^2 in the concurrent phase. If one includes patients treated on both the phase I and II sections of the trial, the overall response rate was 96% (complete responses, 39%; partial responses, 57%). After a median follow-up period of 23 mo (range, 9–40 mo), the median survival time was 22.3 mo. Hainsworth et al. *(78)* also reported on patients treated with two different doses of paclitaxel, carboplatin, and etoposide for small-cell lung cancer. Those patients who had limited-stage disease also received thoracic radiation therapy (1.8 Gy/d; total dose, 45 Gy) administered concurrently with courses three and four of chemotherapy. The overall response rate was 98%, with 71% complete responses and the median survival time had not been reached at 16 mo of follow-up. In general this was well-tolerated therapy with the predictable levels of grade 3–4 toxicities including myelosuppression, esophagitis, and febrile neutropenia. Finally Bremnes et al. *(79)* have also looked at the addition of paclitaxel to cisplatin/

etoposide chemoradiation therapy. They have seen a 95% response rate (80% CR, 15% PR) in a population of 20 patients in the results that have been reported. This trial is ongoing. The results of phase II trials done by the RTOG and ECOG looking at the addition of paclitaxel to platinum, etoposide, and thoracic-radiation-based protocols are awaited.

7. BRAIN TUMORS

Early on it was felt that the addition of a taxane to current radiation-based treatment regimens could potentially have significant bearing on the outcome of therapy for malignant gliomas, which are associated with a discouraging local control rate and poor long-term survival. This early enthusiasm was based in part on its demonstrated activity in a wide variety of solid tumors including in vitro and in vivo evidence of enhancement of radiation effects in primary brain tumors *(48,49,80)*.

7.1. Paclitaxel

Glantz et al. from Brown University undertook a phase I dose-escalation study of weekly administration of paclitaxel with concurrent radiotherapy in patients with newly diagnosed glioblastoma multiforme (GBM), anaplastic astrocytomas, and astrocytomas *(81,82)*. Their trial revealed the surprising result of a dose escalation from 20 mg/m^2/wk to 275 mg/m^2/wk. The authors found that the MTD was 250 mg/m^2/wk with a limiting peripheral sensory neuropathy and recommended that 225 mg/m^2/wk be used in phase II trials. While 60 patients received at least one dose of the drug, 56 received all the planned doses. On analysis of patient outcome it was seen that survival varied according to histology as would be predicted, however, within the GBM group only, the performance status and patient age were predictors of outcome in a proportional hazards analysis. Also tempering this early enthusiasm for combination therapy in this tumor site was analysis of the cerebrospinal fluid (CSF) concentrations in patients receiving concurrent treatment *(83)*. Investigators found that in human subjects the CSF concentrations never went above about 8% of the plasma concentrations, and although this appeared disappointing, they also presented data that no quantifiable amount of paclitaxel could be found in either normal rat brain, or in malignant tumors in the brains of four rats studied. The authors did caution that doses of paclitaxel lower than that detectable by HPLC were able to give rise to sensitization of some tumor cell lines and therefore they could not rule out a real effect of the paclitaxel on the tumor.

Lederman's *(84,85)* results from his retrospective analysis of patients with recurrent GBMs treated with fractionated stereotactic radiation and weekly paclitaxel are encouraging. The reported median survival of 14.2 mo is significantly better than historical controls treated with single fraction radiosurgery alone. This result, while encouraging, is fraught with selection bias. Table 2 shows the results of several phase II series of primary brain tumors treated with concurrent paclitaxel and radiation, none of which are very encouraging for their outcome improvements. Follow-up on Glantz et al.'s original experience has reported on 12 patients who underwent a second surgery due to symptoms and an enlarging mass on MRI *(86)*. Pathological examination of these patients' surgical specimens revealed evidence of radionecrosis many weeks earlier than would have otherwise been anticipated. While the radionecrosis stands as proof of principle that paclitaxel was causing some radiosensitization in the brain, its

Table 2
Concurrent Paclitaxel and Radiation for Primary Malignant Brain Tumors

Study	*Design*	*Number of patients*	*Toxicities*	*Response*
RTOG *(87)*	Phase II (225 mg/m^2 weekly)	62 enrolled with 91% receiving Rx	4 hypersensitivity 4 late sensory neuropathy	23% CR/PR 9.7 mo median survival
Julka *(88)*	Phase II (60 mg/m^2 weekly)	18 enrolled	Neuropathy	1 yr survival of 70%
Fountzilas *(89)*	Phase II (100 mg/m^2 weekly)	33 enrolled	Alopecia Hematological	36% CR/PR 10.7 mo median survival

lack of specificity between tumor and normal tissue illustrates that its potential in providing a long-term curative option that allowed for a good quality of life is limited.

7.2. Docetaxel

The experience with docetaxel in the setting of concurrent treatment of primary brain neoplasms is restricted. There were no responses noted in 18 patients with recurrent malignant gliomas treated with 75–100 mg/m^2 of docetaxel alone *(90)*. A case report of no effect in an individual with leptomeningeal disease is also discouraging *(91)*. A solitary study from Greece has shown that nine patients with GBMs treated with hyperfractionated radiation and concurrent twice-weekly docetaxel (up to 23 mg/m^2 with each dose) did not yield a response better than historical controls *(92)*. Overall the literature would suggest that the benefit from a combination of radiation and a taxane for the treatment of a malignant brain tumor appears to be trivial at best.

8. GENITOURINARY CANCERS

Traditionally carcinoma of the bladder has been treated by radical cystectomy in the United States. There is, however, an emerging interest in organ preservation as seen in other disease sites *(93)*. Certainly the experience from trials including a phase III trial that was not powered to detect a survival difference, is that combined chemoradiation usually using a cisplatin-based chemotherapy regimen and concurrent radiation leads to increased levels of local control *(94)*.

8.1. Docetaxel

Vaverais and the group from Greece *(95)* have looked at the administration of primary chemoradiation following maximal transurethral resection of bladder tumors within 4 wk by weekly cisplatin (30 mg/m^2) and docetaxel (40 mg/m^2) and total 65.2–74 Gy. A total of 37 of 42 enrolled patients received treatment and with a median follow-up of over 2 yr the survival was 78% and the pelvic control rate was 75%. During the trial the significant rate of myelotoxicities seen lead to a dose reduction in the docetaxel to 20 mg/m^2. Chronic toxicities included low-grade cystitis and four of the treated patients were later identified to have contracted bladders although the severity of the condition and the need for surgery is not reported.

8.2. Paclitaxel

A similar small phase II trial from Germany has reported on seven patients receiving concurrent chemoradiation for transitional cell carcinoma of the bladder with cisplatin and paclitaxel *(96)*. The authors conclude that this combination is at least feasible given an acceptable acute toxicity profile and reasonable efficacy. Another small series is reported by Nichols et al. *(97)* where eight patients received radiation with concurrent paclitaxel and carboplatin in an attempt at bladder preservation. Three of the patients remain free of distant metastases, and local recurrence has occurred in three.

The lack of data reinforces the need to conduct randomized trials in the area of carcinoma of the bladder, and given the radiosensitizing action of the taxanes, they are worthy of consideration in these protocols. The RTOG phase I/II trial looking at concurrent cisplatin, paclitaxel, and hyperfractionated radiation with selective bladder preservation and adjuvant chemotherapy is ongoing and it may serve as the basis for future randomized trials in the area *(98)*.

9. GYNECOLOGICAL CANCERS

The experience with either of the taxanes in the combined modality setting with any of the gynecological tumors is limited. With the relatively recent publication of several landmark trials showing that concurrent cisplatin based chemotherapy improves survival in cervical cancer *(99–101)*, the door would appear to be open to try and improve upon those results with the addition of paclitaxel or possibly by decreasing the side-effects of concurrent treatment by reducing or replacing the cisplatin. The current literature contains information on three trials looking at the role of paclitaxel in combined modality treatment; there is no data looking at the addition of docetaxel to radiation in a setting of cervical cancer or any other gynecological malignancy for that matter. Chen et al. from the University of Minnesota *(102)* looked at the addition of weekly paclitaxel to concurrent cisplatin (30 mg/m^2) and pelvic radiation in a phase I trial. They escalated the dose to 50 mg/m^2 and found that the combination was well tolerated with a 93% response rate in 16 patients. Toxicity was minimal with only one case of grade III neutropenia and nausea, vomiting, and diarrhea requiring rehydration in two patients. Two Italian trials have also added paclitaxel to concurrent radiation in the treatment of cervix cancer. Bruzzone et al. *(103)* gave 50 mg/m^2 every 15 d for four cycles with 50 Gy of external beam radiation and an external or intracavitary boost to eight patients. Overall they concluded that the treatment is well tolerated and are planning to pursue this with more aggressive chemotherapy to follow combined paclitaxel/radiation. De Palo et al. *(104)* gave concurrent weekly paclitaxel (40 mg/m^2) with radiation to 14 patients with *de novo* or recurrent disease. There have been responses in 9 of 14 patients with very acceptable toxicities. Currently, the Gynecologic Oncology Group has two ongoing phase I/II trials *(105,106)* looking at the addition of paclitaxel to concurrent cisplatin and radiation in patients with cervix cancer and the second trial more specifically addresses the addition of paclitaxel to cisplatin and extended field radiation in those patients with proven paraortic micrometastases *(106)*. These regimens may form the basis for future randomized trials in cervical cancer if they do not trigger excessive morbidity.

There is also a single study looking at the addition of paclitaxel to adjuvant radiation for patients with high-risk early stage carcinoma of the endometrium *(107)*. Essentially they have shown that post total abdominal hysterectomy, bilateral salingo-oopherectomy, and surgical staging that 13 patients were able to tolerate weekly paclitaxel (60 mg/m^2) with 50.4 Gy of adjuvant pelvic radiation with a tolerable amount of side-effects in a broad mix of tumor stages. They acknowledge that larger prospective trials are warranted to show that this approach to therapy has an impact on local control and/or long term-survival in this disease.

10. BREAST

Given the well-known systemic activity of the taxanes against breast cancer coupled with their radiosensitizing abilities, it would seem logical to combine them in the therapy of locally advanced breast cancer *(108)*. Skinner et al. *(109)* reported updated results of a trial looking at the concurrent delivery of paclitaxel and radiation in locally advanced breast cancer. Originally the trial was designed to give 60 mg/m^2 weekly during radiation with a total dose of 50 Gy in 25 fractions, however, the first two patients developed unexpected significant skin toxicity, so the doses were amended to give 30 mg/m^2 twice weekly during 45 Gy of radiation. Of 29 patients enrolled, 28 were assessable for clinical response and toxicity, and 27 were assessable for pathological response. An objective clinical response was achieved in 89% and at the time of surgery, 33% had no or minimal microscopic residual disease. Chemoradiation-related acute toxicity was limited; however, surgical complications occurred in 41% of patients. This encouraging result needs further long-term follow-up to assess both the local control rates of these locally advanced tumors as well as the cosmetic results. Bellon et al. *(110)* have also reported on their series of 44 patients who received either concurrent paclitaxel or docetaxel with their adjuvant radiation during breast cancer therapy. It would seem that the skin toxicity in their series was high with 38% of patients requiring a break in treatment, which lasted an average of 8 d. They report that the rate of Grade 3 skin toxicity with concurrent docetaxel was significantly higher than with paclitaxel. It would seem that there is a significant increased skin morbidity to the delivery of concurrent taxanes and breast/chest wall irradiation. Further investigation of an optimal sequencing/dosing schedule needs to be done.

11. GASTROINTESTINAL

Within the multiple subsites of this tumor grouping, most work has been done in esophageal cancer. The large majority of these patients have been treated with paclitaxel in combination with radiation (Table 3). The experience with docetaxel is essentially limited to patients treated on phase I trials for thoracic malignancies that used radiation in combination with docetaxel *(68,111)*. The situation is much the same for both pancreatic and gastric cancers as well. The rationale for looking at combination therapy that incorporates paclitaxel is much the same as in other disease sites, i.e., its activity in systemic disease *(112)*, its potent preclinical radiosensitizing properties *(38)*, and evidence from randomized trials that there is a benefit to combined modality therapy that includes at least radiation and chemotherapy *(113–116)*.

11.1. Paclitaxel

Wright et al. from the Massachusetts General Hospital reported interesting results from their intensive trial of preoperative paclitaxel, cisplatin, and 5-fluorouracil with hyperfractionated radiation (total tumor dose of 58.5 Gy and 45 Gy to the mediastinum)

Table 3
Paclitaxel in Preoperative Therapy for Carcinoma of the Esophagus

Study	*Design*	*Number of patients*	*Response*	*2 yr survival*
Wright	Phase I/II concurrent pre-op Cisplatin 20 mg/m^2 d 1–5, 29–33 5-Fluorouracil 800 mg/m^2/d d 1–5, 29–33 Paclitaxel 75–125 mg/m^2 d 1, 29 58.5 Gy to primary hyperfractionated	42 entered 40 eligible for resection 36 resected	14/36 pCR	61%
Safran	Phase II-concurrent pre-op/definitive Paclitaxel 60 mg/m^2 weekly Cisplatin 25 mg/m^2 d 1, 8, 15, 22 39.6 Gy in 1.8 Gy fractions if inoperable to 50.4 Gy total	41 entered	12 pCR	42%
Meluch	Phase II-concurrent pre-op Paclitaxel 200 mg/m^2 d 1, 22 Carboplatin AUC = 6 d 1, 22 5-Fluorouracil 225 mg/m^2/d 1–42 45 Gy in 1.8 Gy daily fractions	50 entered 40 eligible for resection 34 resected	17/34 pCR 17/34 pPR	54%
Adelstein	Phase II-concurrent pre-op Cisplatin 20 mg/m^2/d 1–4, 22–25 Paclitaxel 175 mg/m^2 d 1, 29 45 Gy	40 entered 40 eligible for resection 37 resected	9/40 pCR 15/40 pPR	30%*
Schnirer	Phase II pre-op 5-Fluorouracil 300 mg/m^2/d 1–42 Paclitaxel 45 mg/m^2 weekly 45–50.4 Gy in 1.8 Gy fractions	10 entered 6 eligible for resection 5 resected	1/5 pCR 2/5 had >90% necrosis	Not reported

pCR = pathologic complete response, pPR = pathologic partial response, *3 yr survival.

(117). The phase I portion of this trial determined that the safe scheduling to move into the phase II portion was 100 mg/m^2 every 4 wk during radiation. Unfortunately, this protocol ended up being rather toxic requiring on average 7 d of hospital stay to deal with side effects of therapy. Interestingly, 36 of 40 patients were able to undergo resection and of those who had surgery, there were 14 (39%) pathologic complete responses. These investigators report that they hope that decreasing the intensity of the thoracic radiation will increase the tolerability of the regimen without compromising the response seen. Safran et al. from Brown University, where much of the initial work with paclitaxel and radiation was done, have reported on their experience with paclitaxel, cisplatin, and radiation in esophageal cancer *(118)*. They found that when paclitaxel was administered at 60 mg/m^2 with cisplatin 25 mg/m^2 weekly on d 1, 8, 15, and 22 and radiation to a total dose of 39.60 Gy, in 1.80 Gy fractions, for 22 treatments that 2-yr progression-free rates were 40%. Patients with medical or surgical contraindications to esophagectomy received an additional 2 wk of paclitaxel with a radiation boost to 50.4 Gy. Other trials confirming

similar rates of response and survival have also been reported with similar regimens *(119,120)*. In contrast Adelstein et al. claim in their nonrandomized comparison with historical controls that were treated with 5-fluorouracil based therapy that there was no survival related benefit seen to the addition of paclitaxel *(121)*. Perhaps at this point in time, the statement "paclitaxel-based treatments must be carefully and prospectively studied before their incorporation into the standard management of esophageal cancer" *(122)* is the best language to summarize the state of contemporary preoperative combined modality therapy in esophageal cancer.

The combined modality studies that have attempted to address the role of paclitaxel in stomach and pancreatic cancers have also originated from Brown University. These investigators acknowledge that while the benefit of combined modality therapy in this patient population is limited by toxicities, the lack of truly effective agents leaves opportunity to examine the effect of a known radiosensitizer like paclitaxel *(123)*. In their phase I study of both locally advanced gastric and pancreatic adenocarcinomas, the dose-limiting toxicities of abdominal pain, nausea, and anorexia were seen when 60 mg/m^2 paclitaxel was administered with 50 Gy of radiation. There was a substantial response rate with 11 of 23 patients (48%) having radiological-objective responses *(124)*. In their phase II experience treating patients with locally advanced pancreatic tumors using 50.4 Gy of radiation in 28 treatments with weekly paclitaxel (50 mg/m^2), Safran et al. report a 26% response rate, a median survival of 8 mo and a 1-yr survival of 30% *(125)*. They also state that survival was heavily influenced by systemic relapse with only 2 of 44 patients experiencing local recurrence at site of first progression. They also suggest that the results of the recently completed RTOG phase II trial will yield more insight into the utility of paclitaxel-based regimens. Likewise their protocol in locally advanced gastric cancer shows that the delivery of paclitaxel–radiation is feasible to treat these tumors and that it affords reasonable local control *(126)*. However, further studies need to be done to better define the overall role of this therapy as a strategy to treat gastric cancers.

12. HEAD AND NECK

The combination of chemotherapy with radiation therapy is a rational effort to reduce both the rate of locoregional failure and the frequency of distant metastasis in patients with squamous cell carcinoma of the head and neck. Its role, however, remains controversial to some extent despite evidence from several meta-analyses that the use of chemotherapy in an adjuvant or adjunctive fashion is associated with an improvement in local control as well as overall survival *(127–129)*. Certainly the meta-analysis from El-Sayed and Nelson *(128)* suggests that concurrent treatment leads to an absolute 8% decrease in the mortality rate. This relatively small benefit does come at the expense of increased toxicity. Investigators looking at the use of concurrent taxanes, whether it be paclitaxel or docetaxel, have hoped that their addition might improve outcome without further increasing toxicity. Given the lack of randomized data from trials that have incorporated these drugs it is really too early to say what their true impact will be.

12.1. Paclitaxel

Investigators have taken several different approaches to the integration of paclitaxel into radical therapy in head and neck cancer. Rosenthal et al. undertook a multicenter phase I study where 7-wk continuous infusion of paclitaxel was administered during radical radiation *(130)*. They enrolled 27 patients and 19 of them who received greater than 70 Gy were also assessed for response. At 17 mg/m^2/d skin toxicity required a 2-wk break in radiation for all three patients. As such the recommended dose for phase II trials was 10.5 mg/m^2/d. Initial locoregional control was achieved in 58% of patients and it persisted in 38%. Two other groups *(131,132)* decided to explore the influence of a 120-h continuous infusion of chemotherapy every 3 or 4 wk during curative radiation therapy. Machtay *(132)* found that the MTD was 100 mg/m^2/ 96 h when delivered on a 4-wk time schedule. Dose-limiting toxicities were as expected—mucositis and dermatitis. Sunwoo *(131)* reported that in 33 untreated patients using a 3-wk 96-h infusion of paclitaxel during radiation that at 3 mo postcompletion of therapy a 76% complete response at the primary site was possible and at 36 mo posttherapy locoregional control was maintained in 55.7% with overall survival of 57.8%. Treated patients experienced many of the same toxicities as in other reported trials. Steinberg and the group at Case Western University have also reported on a 24-h infusion of paclitaxel during radiotherapy in a phase I setting *(133)*. Toxicities included febrile neutropenia as well as significant mucositis requiring enteral feeding tubes in most patients. Pharmacokinetic studies here showed that at least 75 mg/m^2 achieved near steady-state mean plasma concentrations that greatly exceeded established in vitro thresholds for the induction of mitotic arrest and altered microtubule function.

The common link with many clinical studies of chemoradiation in head and neck cancers is the significant mucositis that patients experience during therapy. Acrein has reported on a trial that attempts to deliver Ethyol as a protective agent to lessen the side effects of weekly paclitaxel *(134)*.

The use of weekly paclitaxel (45 mg/m^2) and carboplatin (100 mg/m^2) has been reported *(135,136)*. This combination as used to treat 62 patients with stage III and IV squamous cell carcinoma of the head and neck concurrently with radical radiotherapy lead to a clinical complete response rate of 75% both at the primary and in the neck with a median survival of 33 mo *(135)*. The authors report a retrospective comparison to similar patients treated with concurrent carboplatin alone or concurrent carboplatin and bleomycin and show on multivariate analysis that complete response and treatment with paclitaxel were predictive for survival *(136)*. This result while encouraging is retrospective in nature and is subject to potential bias.

Eckardt et al. have reported on a strategy with concurrent paclitaxel and carboplatin delivered in a neoadjuvant fashion with 40 Gy in resectable cases of head and neck cancer *(137,138)*. In their latest report of the 28 patients available for reporting of pathological response postsurgery, 53% or 15 patients achieved a complete response and 13 or 47% achieved a partial response to induction therapy. The high pathological response rates will in fact lead to further study within the DOSAK Cooperative Study Group.

More aggressive chemoradiation that is paclitaxel-containing has also been investigated. Kies et al. have reported on 64 patients with stage IV cancers treated with 120-h infusion of paclitaxel (20 mg/m^2/d) and fluorouracil (600 mg/m^2/d) for five 2-wk cycles with weekly dosing of oral hydroxyurea and hyperfractionated radiation to a total dose of 65–75 Gy. The 3-yr overall survival was 60%, however, the 3-yr locoregional control has been reported as 86%. Of concern are the complaints of compromised swallowing posttherapy in 47% of patients and the 84% rate of grade 3–4 mucositis seen during therapy.

12.2. Docetaxel

A few different strategies have been pursued attempting to integrate docetaxel into treatment regimens for locally advanced head and neck cancers. These include a dose-escalation strategy with single-agent chemotherapy *(140)* where weekly docetaxel was administered with 70 Gy of fractionated radiation starting at a dose of 15 mg/m^2. Despite enrolling six patients in this entry level, the trial was closed because of unacceptable toxicity including grade 4 skin and pulmonary complications and also a treatment-related death. Other schemes have been tried as well. Koukourakis et al. *(141)* have investigated the escalation of novel concurrent therapy that includes both docetaxel and irinotecan with 66–70 Gy of conventionally fractionated radiation. They found an impressive 75% radiological complete response rate and a 25% partial response rate; however, the incidence of grade 3–4 mucositis was dose-limiting. They suggest that 20 mg/m^2 of taxotere and 40 mg/m^2 of irinotecan is the maximally tolerated dose for weekly administration of these drugs.

The group from the Dana Farber Cancer Institute has also explored the addition of docetaxel to therapy. First they have published results of a phase I/II study that adds docetaxel to cisplatin-, fluorouracil-, and leucovorin-based induction therapy for patients with stage III or IV squamous cell carcinoma of the head and neck *(142)*. Twenty-three patients in total were treated with this regimen and the MTD of docetaxel at 60 mg/m^2 iv on the first day of each cycle was found for induction therapy. This was followed by definitive hyperfractionated radiation to at least 72 Gy to the primary and 66 Gy to lymph nodes greater than two centimeters. The overall response rate to the induction chemotherapy was 100%, which is certainly impressive; however, the toxicities were also remarkable. This strategy has progressed to examining concurrent docetaxel post-induction chemotherapy *(143)*. The reported results of this study showed that the MTD of weekly docetaxel was 25 mg/m^2 with mucositis halting escalation. The clinical outcome was also acceptable. As mentioned before the additional benefit of taxane-based chemoradiation in head and neck cancers has yet to be established in randomized trials despite reported responses and acceptable toxicities.

13. METASTATIC DISEASE

Concurrent therapy for the treatment of more than three brain metastases using paclitaxel and radiation has been explored in a phase III trial *(144)*. The hypothesis here being that high-dose paclitaxel in combination with cranial radiation should improve local control while providing systemically active amounts of chemotherapy. Unfortunately, there was no statically significant improvement in survival seen. There is certainly a place to further explore the benefits and toxicities experienced with concurrent taxane-based therapy with radiation in metastatic disease. The role of the taxanes in concurrent chemoradiotherapy with sarcomas and pediatric tumors has not been explored at this time.

14. NOVEL TAXANES

The success of taxane-based therapy in cancer treatment has stimulated interest in further improving its efficacy profile and in identifying new tubulin-active agents. Two taxane analogs, BMS-184476 and BMS-188797, demonstrate greater activity than paclitaxel or docetaxel in a number of human tumor cell lines as well as in rodent solid tumors and human xenografts *(4,145)*. BMS-184476 was discovered to be more potent than paclitaxel in cells expressing mutated tubulin or a high level of the multidrug resistance protein. However, it showed no superiority in those cells that contain wild-type tubulin or in those that do not overexpress the multidrug resistance protein. The improved cytotoxic effects of BMS-184476 in cell lines containing paclitaxel-specific resistance may contribute to its observed in vivo superiority *(146)*. Both of these newer taxanes are presently in phase I trials evaluating different schedules of administration *(147–150)*.

Properties of water solubility and oral bioavailability have important potential implications including reduced hypersensitivity reactions and reduced toxicities that may be associated with diluants currently used with paclitaxel and docetaxel, cremophor, and Tween-80. The reduced attendant cost of administering oral chemotherapies in protracted treatment regimens is also an important consideration. The orally administered taxane analogs, BMS-185660 and BMS-275183, demonstrate comparable levels of activity with intravenously administered paclitaxel in preclinical testing and are currently completing phase I testing *(151,152)*. Other novel taxane agents that may soon be entering clinical testing include IND5109 *(153,154,156)*, SB-T-1213 *(155)*, SB-T-1250 *(155)*, SB-T-101187 *(155)*, IND 5390 *(157)*, TXD258 *(158)*. Although these compounds are beginning to undergo clinical testing in advanced disease, there is really little data on the interaction of novel taxanes with radiation. One report of a novel taxane, taxolteremetro, suggests that it was able to enhance the radiation cell kill in some of the cell lines tested compared to paclitaxel under euoxic conditions *(2)*. The real test for the future will be to see if these compounds are able to improve the therapeutic index when used in combination with radiation either by increasing the tumor cell kill or by more selectively targeting tumor cells compared to normal tissues.

15. CONCLUSION

The initial experience with the taxanes and especially with paclitaxel in the realm of combined modality therapy has had a substantial impact on the treatment of cancers both in the United States and worldwide. Paclitaxel delivered in concert with radiation provides a classical model of the development of clinically applicable treatment strategies from laboratory-based studies. The initial in vitro works of Tishler *(39)* and Choy *(40)* have translated in a very tangible way into approaches that are clinically applicable and in the next generation of randomized clinical trials their efficacy will be compared to more traditional chemotherapies in the combined modality setting. While the experience to date with both paclitaxel and docetaxel has been largely positive, the mortality rates in many of the solid tumor types remind us that much more needs to be done.

REFERENCES

1. Rowinsky EK. The development and clinical utility of the taxane class of antimicrotubule chemotherapy agents. *Annu Rev Med* 1997; 48:353–374.
2. Yang LX, Wang HJ, Holton RA. In vitro efficacy of a novel chemoradiopotentiator—taxoltere metro. *Int J Radiat Oncol Biol Phys* 2000; 46(1):159–163.
3. Altmann KH, Wartmann M, O'Reilly T. Epothilones and related structures—a new class of microtubule inhibitors with potent in vivo antitumor activity. *Biochim Biophys Acta* 2000; 1470(3):M79–91.
4. Rose WC, Fairchild C, Lee FY. Preclinical antitumor activity of two novel taxanes. *Cancer Chemother Pharmacol* 2001; 47(2):97–105.
5. Vaishampayan U, Parchment RE, Jasti BR, Hussain M. Taxanes: an overview of the pharmacokinetics and pharmacodynamics. *Urology* 1999; 54(6A Suppl):22–29.
6. Rao S, Krauss NE, Heerding JM, et al. 3'-(p-azidobenzamido)taxol photolabels the N-terminal 31 amino acids of beta-tubulin. *J Biol Chem* 1994; 269(5):3132–3134.

7. Manfredi JJ, Horwitz SB. Taxol: an antimitotic agent with a new mechanism of action. *Pharmacol Ther* 1984; 25(1):83–125.
8. Diaz JF, Andreu JM. Assembly of purified GDP-tubulin into microtubules induced by taxol and taxotere: reversibility, ligand stoichiometry, and competition. *Biochemistry* 1993; 32(11):2747–2755.
9. Ringel I, Horwitz SB. Studies with RP 56976 (taxotere): a semisynthetic analogue of taxol. *J Natl Cancer Inst* 1991; 83(4):288–291.
10. Jordan MA, Wendell K, Gardiner S, Derry WB, Copp H, Wilson L. Mitotic block induced in HeLa cells by low concentrations of paclitaxel (Taxol) results in abnormal mitotic exit and apoptotic cell death. *Cancer Res* 1996; 56(4):816–825.
11. Haldar S, Chintapalli J, Croce CM. Taxol induces Bcl-2 phosphorylation and death of prostate cancer cells. *Cancer Res* 1996; 56(6):1253–1255.
12. Wahl AF, Donaldson KL, Fairchild C, et al. Loss of normal p53 function confers sensitization to Taxol by increasing G2/M arrest and apoptosis. *Nat Med* 1996; 2(1):72–79.
13. Vikhanskaya F, Vignati S, Beccaglia P, et al. Inactivation of p53 in a human ovarian cancer cell line increases the sensitivity to paclitaxel by inducing G2/M arrest and apoptosis. *Exp Cell Res* 1998; 241(1):96–101.
14. Zaffaroni N, Silvestrini R, Orlandi L, Bearzatto A, Gornati D, Villa R. Induction of apoptosis by taxol and cisplatin and effect on cell cycle-related proteins in cisplatin-sensitive and -resistant human ovarian cells. *Br J Cancer* 1998; 77(9):1378–1385.
15. Wang TH, Wang HS, Soong YK. Paclitaxel-induced cell death: where the cell cycle and apoptosis come together. *Cancer* 2000; 88(11):2619–2628.
16. Jordan MA, Wendell K, Gardiner S, Derry WB, Copp H, Wilson L. Mitotic block induced in HeLa cells by low concentrations of paclitaxel (Taxol) results in abnormal mitotic exit and apoptotic cell death. *Cancer Res* 1996; 56(4):816–825.
17. Taylor SS, McKeon F. Kinetochore localization of murine Bub1 is required for normal mitotic timing and checkpoint response to spindle damage. *Cell* 1997; 89(5):727–735.
18. Taylor SS, Ha E, McKeon F. The human homologue of Bub3 is required for kinetochore localization of Bub1 and a Mad3/Bub1-related protein kinase. *J Cell Biol* 1998; 142(1):1–11.
19. Giannakakou P, Sackett DL, Kang YK, et al. Paclitaxel-resistant human ovarian cancer cells have mutant beta-tubulins that exhibit impaired paclitaxel-driven polymerization. *J Biol Chem* 1997; 272(27):17,118–17,125.
20. Gazitt Y, Rothenberg ML, Hilsenbeck SG, Fey V, Thomas C, Montegomrey W. Bcl-2 overexpression is associated with resistance to paclitaxel, but not gemcitabine, in multiple myeloma cells. *Int J Oncol* 1998; 13(4):839–848.
21. Liu JR, Fletcher B, Page C, Hu C, Nunez G, Baker V. Bcl-xL is expressed in ovarian carcinoma and modulates chemotherapy-induced apoptosis. *Gynecol Oncol* 1998; 70(3):398–403.
22. Huang Y, Ray S, Reed JC, et al. Estrogen increases intracellular p26Bcl-2 to p21Bax ratios and inhibits taxol-induced apoptosis of human breast cancer MCF-7 cells. *Breast Cancer Res Treat* 1997; 42(1):73–81.
23. Huang Y, Ibrado AM, Reed JC, et al. Co-expression of several molecular mechanisms of multidrug resistance and their significance for paclitaxel cytotoxicity in human AML HL-60 cells. *Leukemia* 1997; 11(2):253–257.
24. Kavallaris M, Kuo DY, Burkhart CA, et al. Taxol-resistant epithelial ovarian tumors are associated with altered expression of specific beta-tubulin isotypes. *J Clin Invest* 1997; 100(5):1282–1293.
25. Panvichian R, Orth K, Day ML, Day KC, Pilat MJ, Pienta KJ. Paclitaxel-associated multimininucleation is permitted by the inhibition of caspase activation: a potential early step in drug resistance. *Cancer Res* 1998; 58(20):4667–4672.
26. Rowinsky EK. The taxanes: dosing and scheduling considerations. *Oncology (Huntingt)* 1997; 11(3 Suppl 2):7–19.
27. Weiss RB, Donehower RC, Wiernik PH, et al. Hypersensitivity reactions from taxol. *J Clin Oncol* 1990; 8(7):1263–1268.
28. Huizing MT, Keung AC, Rosing H, et al. Pharmacokinetics of paclitaxel and metabolites in a randomized comparative study in platinum-pretreated ovarian cancer patients. *J Clin Oncol* 1993; 11(11):2127–2135.
29. Crown J, O'Leary M. The taxanes: an update. *Lancet* 2000 Apr 1; 355(9210):1176–1178.
30. Nabholtz JM, North S, Smylie M, et al. Docetaxel (Taxotere) in combination with anthracyclines in the treatment of breast cancer. *Semin Oncol* 2000; 27(2 Suppl 3):11–18.

31. Kaufman PA. Paclitaxel and anthracycline combination chemotherapy for metastatic breast cancer. *Semin Oncol* 1999; 26(3 Suppl 8):39–46.
32. Piccart MJ, Bertelsen K, James K, et al. Randomized intergroup trial of cisplatin-paclitaxel versus cisplatin-cyclophosphamide in women with advanced epithelial ovarian cancer: three-year results. *J Natl Cancer Inst* 2000; 92(9):699–708.
33. Schiller JH, Harrington D, Sandler A, et al. A Randomized Phase III Trial of Four Chemotherapy Regimens in Advanced Non-Small Cell Lung Cancer (NSCLC) (abstract 2). 2000. *Pro Am Soc Clin Oncol* 19:1a.
34. Bellmunt J, Guillem V, Paz-Ares L, et al. Gemcitabine/paclitaxel-based three-drug regimens in advanced urothelial cancer. *Eur J Cancer* 2000; 36 Suppl 2:17–25.
35. Choy H, Shyr Y, Cmelak AJ, Mohr PJ, Johnson DH. Patterns of practice survey for nonsmall-cell lung carcinoma in the U.S. *Cancer* 2000; 88(6):1336–1346.
36. Shepherd FA, Dancey J, Ramlau R, et al. Prospective randomized trial of docetaxel versus best supportive care in patients with non-small-cell lung cancer previously treated with platinum-based chemotherapy. *J Clin Oncol* 2000; 18(10):2095–2103.
37. Hall EJ. *Radiobiology for the Radiobiologist Fourth Edition.* J.B. Lippincott Company. Philadelphia. 1994.
38. Milas L, Milas MM, Mason KA. Combination of taxanes with radiation: preclinical studies. *Semin Radiat Oncol* 1999; 9(2 Suppl 1):12–26.
39. Tishler RB, Geard CR, Hall EJ, Schiff PB. Taxol sensitizes human astrocytoma cells to radiation. *Cancer Res* 1992; 52(12):3495–3497.
40. Choy H, Rodriguez FF, Koester S, Hilsenbeck S, Von Hoff DD. Investigation of taxol as a potential radiation sensitizer. *Cancer* 1993; 71(11):3774–3778.
41. Hennequin C, Giocanti N, Favaudon V. S-phase specificity of cell killing by docetaxel (Taxotere) in synchronised HeLa cells. *Br J Cancer* 1995; 71(6):1194–1198.
42. Hennequin C, Giocanti N, Favaudon V. Interaction of ionizing radiation with paclitaxel (Taxol) and docetaxel (Taxotere) in HeLa and SQ20B cells. *Cancer Res* 1996; 56(8):1842–1850.
43. Amorino GP, Hamilton VM, Choy H. Enhancement of radiation effects by combined docetaxel and carboplatin treatment in vitro. *Radiat Oncol Investig* 1999; 7(6):343–352.
44. Creane M, Seymour CB, Colucci S, Mothersill C. Radiobiological effects of docetaxel (Taxotere): a potential radiation sensitizer. *Int J Radiat Biol* 1999; 75(6):731–737.
45. Mason KA, Kishi K, Hunter N, et al. Effect of docetaxel on the therapeutic ratio of fractionated radiotherapy in vivo. *Clin Cancer Res* 1999; 5(12):4191–4198.
46. Milas L, Hunter NR, Mason KA, Milross CG, Saito Y, Peters LJ. Role of reoxygenation in induction of enhancement of tumor radioresponse by paclitaxel. *Cancer Res* 1995; 55(16):3564–3568.
47. Mason KA, Milas L, Peters LJ. Effect of paclitaxel (taxol) alone and in combination with radiation on the gastrointestinal mucosa. *Int J Radiat Oncol Biol Phys* 1995; 32(5):1381–1389.
48. Choy H. Taxanes in combined modality therapy for solid tumors. *Crit Rev Oncol Hematol* 2001; 37(3):237–247.
49. Choy H. Combining taxanes with radiation for solid tumors. *Int J Cancer* 2000; 90(3):113–127.
50. Choy H. Taxanes in combined-modality therapy for solid tumors. *Oncology (Huntingt)* 1999; 13(10 Suppl 5):23–38.
51. Dowell JE, Sinard R, Yardley DA, et al. Seven-week continuous-infusion paclitaxel concurrent with radiation therapy for locally advanced non-small cell lung and head and neck cancers. *Semin Radiat Oncol* 1999; 9(2 Suppl 1):97–101.
52. Rathmann J, Leopold KA, Rigas JR, et al. Daily paclitaxel and thoracic radiation therapy for non-small cell lung cancer: preliminary results. *Semin Radiat Oncol* 1999; 9(2 Suppl 1):130–135.
53. Lau D, Ryu J, Gandara D, et al. Concurrent twice-weekly paclitaxel and thoracic irradiation for stage III non-small cell lung cancer. *Semin Radiat Oncol* 1999; 9(2 Suppl 1):117–120.
54. Choy H, Akerley W, Safran H, et al. Phase I trial of outpatient weekly paclitaxel and concurrent radiation therapy for advanced non-small-cell lung cancer. *J Clin Oncol* 1994; 12(12):2682–2686.
55. Socinski MA, Rosenman JG, Schell MJ, et al. Induction carboplatin/paclitaxel followed by concurrent carboplatin/paclitaxel and dose-escalating conformal thoracic radiation therapy in unresectable stage IIIA/B nonsmall cell lung carcinoma: a modified Phase I trial. *Cancer* 2000; 89(3):534–542.
56. Kirkbride P, Gelmon K, Eisenhauer E, et al. Paclitaxel and concurrent radiotherapy in locally advanced non-small cell lung cancer: the Canadian experience. *Semin Radiat Oncol* 1999; 9(2 Suppl 1): 102–107.

57. Langer CJ. Concurrent chemoradiation using paclitaxel and carboplatin in locally advanced non-small cell lung cancer. *Semin Radiat Oncol* 1999; 9(2 Suppl 1):108–116.
58. Herscher LL, Hahn SM, Kroog G, et al. Phase I study of paclitaxel as a radiation sensitizer in the treatment of mesothelioma and non-small-cell lung cancer. *J Clin Oncol* 1998; 16(2):635–641.
59. Choy H, Safran H, Akerley W, et al. Phase II trial of weekly paclitaxel and concurrent radiation therapy for locally advanced non-small cell lung cancer. *Clin Cancer Res* 1998; 4(8):1931–1936.
60. Choy H, Akerley W, Safran H, et al. Multiinstitutional phase II trial of paclitaxel, carboplatin, and concurrent radiation therapy for locally advanced non-small-cell lung cancer. *J Clin Oncol* 1998; 16(10):3316–3322.
61. Choy H, Devore RF 3rd, Hande KR, et al. A phase II study of paclitaxel, carboplatin, and hyperfractionated radiation therapy for locally advanced inoperable non-small-cell lung cancer (a Vanderbilt Cancer Center Affiliate Network Study). *Int J Radiat Oncol Biol Phys* 2000; 47(4):931–937.
62. Lau D, Leigh B, Gandara D, Edelman M, Morgan R, Israel V, Lara P, Wilder R, Ryu J, Doroshow J. Twice-weekly paclitaxel and weekly carboplatin with concurrent thoracic radiation followed by carboplatin/paclitaxel consolidation for stage III non-small-cell lung cancer: a California Cancer Consortium phase II trial. *J Clin Oncol* 2001; 19(2):442–447.
63. Choy H, LaPorte K, Knill-Selby E, et al. Esophagitis in combined modality therapy for locally advanced non-small cell lung cancer. *Semin Radiat Oncol* 1999; 9(2 Suppl 1):90–96.
64. Socinski MA, Halle J, Schell MJ, et al. Induction (I) and Concurrent (C) Carboplatin/Paclitaxel (C/P) with Dose-Escalated Thoracic Conformal Radiotherapy (TCRT) in Stage IIIA/B Non-Small Cell Lung Cancer (NSCLC): A Phase I/II Trial. *Proc Am Soc Clin Oncol* 2000; 19: Abstract 1940.
65. Vokes EE, Leopold KA, Herndon JE, et al. CALGB Study 9431: A randomized phase study of cisplatin with gemcitabine or paclitaxel or vinorelbine as induction chemotherapy and concomitant chemoradiotherapy for unresectable stage III non-small cell lung cancer. *Lung Cancer* 2000; 29(S1):49(Abstract 158).
66. Koukourakis MI, Bahlitzanakis N, Froudarakis M, et al. Concurrent conventionally fractionated radiotherapy and weekly docetaxel in the treatment of stage IIIB non-small cell lung carcinoma. *Br J Cancer* 1999; 80:1792–1796.
67. Aamdal S, Lauvvang G, Owre K, et al. A phase I/II study of docetaxel (Taxotere) combined with concurrent radiation therapy in locally advanced non-small cell lung cancer (NSCLC). *Lung Cancer* 2000; 29(Suppl 1):100 (abstract 327).
68. Choy H, DeVore RF, Porter LL, et al. Phase I trial of outpatient weekly docetaxel (DTX) Carboplatin (CBDCA) and concurrent thoracic radiation therapy (TRT) for stage III unresectable non-small-cell lung cancer: A Vanderbilt Cancer Center Affiliate Network (VCCAN) Trial. *Pro Am Soc Clin Oncol* 1999; 18:475a (abstract 1833).
69. Murakami H, Kubota K, Ohe Y, et al. Phase I study of weekly docetaxel (DTX) and carboplatin (CBDCA) with concurrent thoracic radiotherapy (TRT) for stage III non-small cell lung cancer (NSCLC). *Lung Cancer* 2000; 29(Suppl 1):111 (abstract 367).
70. Segawa Y, Ueoka H, Kiura K, et al. A phase I/II study of docetaxel (TXT) and cisplatin (CDDP) with concurrent thoracic radiotherapy (TRT) for locally advanced non-small-cell lung cancer (LA-NSCLC). *Proc Am Soc Clin Oncol* 2000; 19:508a.
71. Nyman J, Mercke C. Accelerated radiotherapy with docetaxel and cisplatin as induction and concomitant chemotherapy for stage III non-small cell lung cancer. *Lung Cancer* 2000; 29(Suppl 1):98.
72. Warde P, Payne D. Does thoracic irradiation improve survival and local control in limited-stage small-cell carcinoma of the lung? A meta-analysis. *J Clin Oncol* 1992; 10(6):890–895.
73. Pignon JP, Arriagada R, Ihde DC, et al. A meta-analysis of thoracic radiotherapy for small-cell lung cancer. *N Engl J Med* 1992; 327(23):1618–1624.
74. Turrisi AT 3rd, Kim K, Blum R, Sause WT, Livingston RB, Komaki R, Wagner H, Aisner S, Johnson DH. Twice-daily compared with once-daily thoracic radiotherapy in limited small-cell lung cancer treated concurrently with cisplatin and etoposide. *N Engl J Med* 1999; 340(4):265–271.
75. Murray N, Coy P, Pater JL, et al. Importance of timing for thoracic irradiation in the combined modality treatment of limited-stage small-cell lung cancer. The National Cancer Institute of Canada Clinical Trials Group. *J Clin Oncol* 1993; 11(2):336–344.
76. Ettinger DS. Concurrent paclitaxel-containing regimens and thoracic radiation therapy for limited-disease small cell lung cancer. *Semin Radiat Oncol* 1999; 9(2 Suppl 1):148–150.

77. Levitan N, Dowlati A, Shina D, et al. Multi-institutional phase I/II trial of paclitaxel, cisplatin, and etoposide with concurrent radiation for limited-stage small-cell lung carcinoma. J Clin Oncol 2000; 18(5):1102–1109.
78. Hainsworth JD, Gray JR, Stroup SL, Kalman LA, Patten JE, Hopkins LG, Thomas M, Greco FA. Paclitaxel, carboplatin, and extended-schedule etoposide in the treatment of small-cell lung cancer: comparison of sequential phase II trials using different dose-intensities. J Clin Oncol 1997; 15(12):3464–3470.
79. Bremnes RM, Sundstrom S, Aasebo U, Vilsvik J. Paclitaxel in combination with cisplatin, etoposide and thoracic radiotherapy for limited stage small cell lung cancer (SCLC): a phase II study (abstract 1826). *Pro Am Soc Clin Oncol* 1998; 17:475a.
80. Glantz MJ, Chamberlain MC, Chang SM, Prados MD, Cole BF. The role of paclitaxel in the treatment of primary and metastatic brain tumors. *Semin Radiat Oncol* 1999; 9(2 Suppl 1):27–33.
81. Glantz MJ, Choy H, Kearns CM, Akerley W, Egorin MJ. Weekly, outpatient paclitaxel and concurrent cranial irradiation in adults with brain tumors: preliminary results and promising directions. *Semin Oncol* 1995; 22(5 Suppl 12):26–32.
82. Glantz MJ, Choy H, Kearns CM, et al. Phase I study of weekly outpatient paclitaxel and concurrent cranial irradiation in adults astrocytomas. *J Clin Oncol* 1996; 14(2):600–609.
83. Glantz MJ, Choy H, Kearns CM, et al. Paclitaxel disposition in plasma and central nervous systems of humans and rats with brain tumors. *J Natl Cancer Inst* 1995; 87(14):1077–1081.
84. Lederman G, Arbit E, Odaimi M, Wertheim S, Lombardi E. Recurrent glioblastoma multiforme: potential benefits using fractionated stereotactic radiotherapy and concurrent taxol. *Stereotact Funct Neurosurg* 1997; 69(1–4 Pt 2):162–174.
85. Lederman G, Arbit E, Odaimi M, Lombardi E, Wrzolek M, Wronski M. Fractionated stereotactic radiosurgery and concurrent taxol in recurrent glioblastoma multiforme: a preliminary report. *Int J Radiat Oncol Biol Phys* 1998; 40(3):661–666.
86. Wehbe T, Glantz M, Choy H, Glantz L, Cortez S, Akerley W 3rd, Mills P, Cole B. Histologic evidence of a radiosensitizing effect of Taxol in patients with astrocytomas. *J Neurooncol* 1998; 39(3):245–251.
87. Langer CJ, Paulus R, Ruffer J, Movsas B, Murray K, Rhodes H, Curran WJ. Pro Am Soc Clin Oncol. Phase II RTOG Trial of Weekly Paclitaxel (TAX) and Conventional External Beam Radiation Therapy for Supratentorial Glioblastoma Mutiforme (abstract 534) 1999. 18.
88. Julka PK, Awasthy BS, Rath GK, Agarwal S, Varna T, Mahapatra AK, Singh R. A study of concurrent radiochemotherapy with paclitaxel in glioblastoma multiforme. *Australas Radiol* 2000; 44(1):84–87.
89. Fountzilas G, Karavelis A, Capizzello A, Kalogera-Fountzila A, Karkavelas G, Zamboglou N, Selviaridis P, Foroglou G, Tourkantonis A. Radiation and concomitant weekly administration of paclitaxel in patients with glioblastoma multiforme. A phase II study. *J Neurooncol* 1999; 45(2):159–165.
90. Forsyth P, Cairncross G, Stewart D, Goodyear M, Wainman N, Eisenhauer E. Phase II trial of docetaxel in patients with recurrent malignant glioma: a study of the National Cancer Institute of Canada Clinical Trials Group. *Invest New Drugs* 1996; 14(2):203–206.
91. Herrington JD, Di Nunno L, Rinehart JJ. Lack of CNS penetration of docetaxel in a patient with leptomeningeal carcinomatosis. *Ann Pharmacother* 1998; 32(5):611–612.
92. Koukourakis MI, Giatromanolaki A, Schiza S, Kakolyris S, Georgoulias V. Concurrent twice-a-week docetaxel and radiotherapy: a dose escalation trial with immunological toxicity evaluation. Int *J Radiat Oncol Biol Phys* 1999; 43(1):107–114.
93. Kim HL, Steinberg GD. The current status of bladder preservation in the treatment of muscle invasive bladder cancer. *J Urol* 2000; 164(3 Pt 1):627–632.
94. Coppin CM, Gospodarowicz MK, James K, et al. Improved local control of invasive bladder cancer by concurrent cisplatin and preoperative or definitive radiation. The National Cancer Institute of Canada Clinical Trials Group. *J Clin Oncol* 1996; 14(11):2901–2907.
95. Varveris H, Delakas D, Anezinis P, et al. Concurrent platinum and docetaxel chemotherapy and external radical radiotherapy in patients with invasive transitional cell bladder carcinoma. A preliminary report of tolerance and local control. *Anticancer Res* 1997; 17(6D):4771–4780.
96. Dunst J, Weigel C, Heynemann H, Becker A. Preliminary results of simultaneous radiochemotherapy with paclitaxel for urinary bladder cancer. *Strahlenther Onkol* 1999; 175 Suppl 3:7–10.
97. Nichols RC Jr, Sweetser MG, Mahmood SK, Malamud FC, Dunn NP, Adams JP, Kyker JS, Lydick K. Radiation therapy and concomitant paclitaxel/carboplatin chemotherapy for muscle invasive transitional cell carcinoma of the bladder: a well-tolerated combination. *Int J Cancer* 2000; 90(5): 281–286.

98. RTOG 9906. A Phase I/II Trial in Patients with Muscle-Invading Bladder Cancer of Transurethral Surgery Plus Taxol, Cisplatin and BID Irradiation Followed by Either Selective Bladder Preservation or Radical Cystectomy and Adjuvant Chemotherapy. Study Protocol.
99. Peters WA 3rd, Liu PY, Barrett RJ 2nd, Stock RJ, Monk BJ, Berek JS, Souhami L, Grigsby P, Gordon W Jr, Alberts DS. Concurrent chemotherapy and pelvic radiation therapy compared with pelvic radiation therapy alone as adjuvant therapy after radical surgery in high-risk early-stage cancer of the cervix. *J Clin Oncol* 2000; 18(8):1606–1613.
100. Keys HM, Bundy BN, Stehman FB, et al. Cisplatin, radiation, and adjuvant hysterectomy compared with radiation and adjuvant hysterectomy for bulky stage IB cervical carcinoma. *N Engl J Med* 1999; 340(15):1154–1161.
101. Morris M, Eifel PJ, Lu J, et al. Pelvic radiation with concurrent chemotherapy compared with pelvic and para-aortic radiation for high-risk cervical cancer. *N Engl J Med* 1999; 340(15):1137–1143.
102. Chen MD, Paley PJ, Potish RA, Twiggs LB. Phase I trial of taxol as a radiation sensitizer with cisplatin in advanced cervical cancer. *Gynecol Oncol* 1997; 67(2):131–136.
103. Bruzzone M, Franzone P, Ghione G, et al. Combined Treatment with Paclitaxel (P) and Radiotherapy (RT) in Patients (Pts) with Advanced Cervical Cancer (ACC) (abstract 1592). *Pro Am Soc Clin Oncol* 2000; 19.
104. De Palo G, Cerrotta A, Gardani G, et al. Concurrent Radiotherapy and Taxol as Radiosensitizer in Locally Advanced or Recurrent Carcinoma of the Uterine Cervix (abstract 1404). *Pro Am Soc Clin Oncol* 1998; 17:364a.
105. GOG-9803 Phase I/II Study of Radiotherapy Combined With Paclitaxel and Cisplatin in Patients With Stage IB2, IIA, IIB, IIIB, or IVA Invasive Carcinoma of the Cervix.
106. GOG-9804 Phase I/II Study of Extended Field Radiation Therapy With Concurrent Paclitaxel and Cisplatin Chemotherapy in Patients With Previously Untreated Carcinoma of the Cervix Metastatic to the Para-aortic Lymph Nodes. Study Protocol. http://www.cancer.gov/search/clinical_trials
107. Frigerio L, Mangili G, Aletti G, Carnelli M, Garavaglia E, Beatrice S, Ferrari A. Concomitant radiotherapy and paclitaxel for high-risk endometrial cancer: first feasibility study. *Gynecol Oncol* 2001; 81(1):53–57.
108. Formenti SC, Symmans WF, Volm M, et al. Concurrent paclitaxel and radiation therapy for breast cancer. *Semin Radiat Oncol* 1999; 9(2 Suppl 1):34–42.
109. Skinner KA, Silberman H, Florentine B, et al. Preoperative paclitaxel and radiotherapy for locally advanced breast cancer: surgical aspects. *Ann Surg Oncol* 2000; 7(2):145–149.
110. Bellon JR, Lindsley KL, Ellis GK, Gralow JR, Livingston RB, Austin Seymour MM. Concurrent radiation therapy and paclitaxel or docetaxel chemotherapy in high-risk breast cancer. *Int J Radiat Oncol Biol Phys* 2000; 48(2):393–397.
111. Mauer AM, Masters GA, Haraf DJ, et al. Phase I study of docetaxel with concomitant thoracic radiation therapy. *J Clin Oncol* 1988; 16: 159–164.
112. Blanke CD, Choy H, Teng M, et al. Concurrent paclitaxel and thoracic irradiation for locally advanced esophageal cancer. *Semin Radiat Oncol* 1999; 9(2 Suppl 1):43–52.
113. Cooper JS, Guo MD, Herskovic A, et al. Chemoradiotherapy of locally advanced esophageal cancer: long-term follow-up of a prospective randomized trial (RTOG 85-01). Radiation Therapy Oncology Group. *JAMA* 1999; 281(17):1623–1627.
114. Kelsen DP, Ginsberg R, Pajak TF, et al. Chemotherapy followed by surgery compared with surgery alone for localized esophageal cancer. *N Engl J Med* 1998; 339(27):1979–1984.
115. Burmeister BH, Denham JW, O'Brien M, et al. Combined modality therapy for esophageal carcinoma: preliminary results from a large Australasian multicenter study. *Int J Radiat Oncol Biol Phys* 1995; 32(4):997–1006.
116. Walsh TN, Noonan N, Hollywood D, Kelly A, Keeling N, Hennessy TP. A comparison of multimodal therapy and surgery for esophageal adenocarcinoma. *N Engl J Med* 1996; 335(7):462–467.
117. Wright CD, Wain JC, Lynch TJ, et al. Induction therapy for esophageal cancer with paclitaxel and hyperfractionated radiotherapy: a phase I and II study. *J Thorac Cardiovasc Surg* 1997; 114(5):811–815.
118. Safran H, Gaissert H, Akerman P, et al. Paclitaxel, cisplatin, and concurrent radiation for esophageal cancer. *Cancer Invest* 2001; 19(1):1–7.
119. Meluch AA, Hainsworth JD, Gray JR, et al. Preoperative combined modality therapy with paclitaxel, carboplatin, prolonged infusion 5-fluorouracil, and radiation therapy in localized esophageal cancer: preliminary results of a Minnie Pearl Cancer Research Network phase II trial. *Cancer J Sci Am* 1999; 5(2):84–91.

120. Schnirer II, Komaki R, Yao JC, et al. Pilot study of concurrent 5-fluorouracil/paclitaxel plus radiotherapy in patients with carcinoma of the esophagus and gastroesophageal junction. *Am J Clin Oncol* 2001; 24(1):91–95.
121. Adelstein DJ, Rice TW, Rybicki LA, et al. Does paclitaxel improve the chemoradiotherapy of locoregionally advanced esophageal cancer? A nonrandomized comparison with fluorouracil-based therapy. *J Clin Oncol* 2000; 18(10):2032–2039.
122. Thirion P, Piedbois Y, Adelstein DJ. (2001). Preoperative Chemoradiotherapy Using Taxanes for Locally Advanced Esophageal Carcinoma. *J Clin Oncol* 2001; 19:1880–1882.
123. Safran H, Akerman P, Cioffi W, et al. Paclitaxel and concurrent radiation therapy for locally advanced adenocarcinomas of the pancreas, stomach, and gastroesophageal junction. *Semin Radiat Oncol* 1999; 9(2 Suppl 1):53–57.
124. Safran H, King TP, Choy H, et al. Paclitaxel and concurrent radiation for locally advanced pancreatic and gastric cancer: a phase I study. *J Clin Oncol* 1997; 15(3):901–907.
125. Safran H, Moore T, Iannitti D, et al. Paclitaxel and concurrent radiation for locally advanced pancreatic cancer. *Int J Radiat Oncol Biol Phys* 2001; 49(5):1275–1279.
126. Safran H, Wanebo HJ, Hesketh PJ, et al. Paclitaxel and concurrent radiation for gastric cancer. *Int J Radiat Oncol Biol Phys* 2000; 46(4):889–894.
127. Munro AJ. An overview of randomised controlled trials of adjuvant chemotherapy in head and neck cancer. *Br J Cancer* 1995; 71(1):83–91.
128. El-Sayed S, Nelson N. Adjuvant and adjunctive chemotherapy in the management of squamous cell carcinoma of the head and neck region. A meta-analysis of prospective and randomized trials. *J Clin Oncol* 1996; 14(3):838–847.
129. Pignon JP, Bourhis J, Domenge C, Designe L. Chemotherapy added to locoregional treatment for head and neck squamous-cell carcinoma: three meta-analyses of updated individual data. MACH-NC Collaborative Group. Meta-Analysis of Chemotherapy on Head and Neck Cancer. *Lancet* 2000; 355(9208):949–955.
130. Rosenthal DI, Lee JH, Sinard R, et al. Phase I study of paclitaxel given by seven-week continuous infusion concurrent with radiation therapy for locally advanced squamous cell carcinoma of the head and neck. *J Clin Oncol* 2001; 19(5):1363–1373.
131. Sunwoo JB, Herscher LL, Kroog GS, et al. Concurrent paclitaxel and radiation in the treatment of locally advanced head and neck cancer. *J Clin Oncol* 2001; 19(3):800–811.
132. Machtay M, Aviles V, Kligerman MM, et al. A phase I trial of 96-hour paclitaxel infusion plus accelerated radiotherapy of unresectable head and neck cancer. *Int J Radiat Oncol Biol Phys* 1999; 44(2):311–315.
133. Steinberg L, Hassan M, Olmsted L, et al. A phase I trial of radiotherapy and simultaneous 24-hour paclitaxel in patients with locally advanced head and neck squamous cell carcinoma. *Semin Oncol* 1997; 24(6 Suppl 19):S19-51–S19-56.
134. Amrein PC, McIntyre J, Colevas AD, Wang CC, Varvares M, Fabian. A phase I trial of concurrent taxol and Bid radiotherapy with and without ethyol in patients with advanced squamous cell carcinoma of the head and neck. (abstract 1651) *Pro Am Soc Clin Oncol* 2000; 19:418a.
135. Suntharalingam M, Haas ML, Conley BA, et al. The use of carboplatin and paclitaxel with daily radiotherapy in patients with locally advanced squamous cell carcinomas of the head and neck. *Int J Radiat Oncol Biol Phys* 2000; 47(1):49–56.
136. Suntharalingam M, Haas ML, Van Echo DA, et al. Predictors of response and survival after concurrent chemotherapy and radiation for locally advanced squamous cell carcinomas of the head and neck. *Cancer* 2001; 91(3):548–554.
137. Eckardt A, Wildfang I, Karstens JH. Simultaneous radiochemotherapy with taxol/carboplatin in advanced operable head-neck tumors. Preliminary results. *Strahlenther Onkol* 1999; 175 Suppl 3:11–13.
138. Eckardt A, Wildfang I, Rades D, et al. Mulicenter phase II study of preoperative concurrent paclitaxel, carboplatin and radiotherapy in stage III/IV resectable cancer of the oropharynx and oral cavity: an interim analysis (abstract 1658). *Pro Am Soc Clin Oncol* 2000; 19:420a.
139. Kies ME, Haraf D, Rosen F, Stenson K, List M, Brockstein B, Chung T, Mittal B, Pelzer H, Portugal L, Rademaker A, Weichselbaum R, Vokes EE. Concomitant Infusional Paclitaxel and Fluorouracil, Oral Hydroxyurea, and Hyperfractionated Radiation for Locally Advanced Squamous Head and Neck Cancer. *J Clin Oncol* 2001; 19:1961–1969.
140. Hesse K, Heinrich B, Zimmermann F, et al. Combined radiochemotherapy with docetaxel in patients with unresectable locally advanced head and neck tumors. *Strahlenther Onkol* 2000; 176(2):67–72.

141. Koukourakis MI, Bizakis JG, Skoulakis CE, et al. Combined irinotecan, docetaxel and conventionally fractionated radiotherapy in locally advanced head and neck cancer. A phase I dose escalation study. *Anticancer Res* 1999; 19(3B):2305–2309.
142. Colevas AD, Busse PM, Norris CM, et al. Induction chemotherapy with docetaxel, cisplatin, fluorouracil, and leucovorin for squamous cell carcinoma of the head and neck: a phase I/II trial. *J Clin Oncol* 1998; 16(4):1331–1339.
143. Tishler RB, Posner MR, Colevas AD, et al. Phase I study of concurrent taxotere/radiation after induction chemotherapy in patients with squamous cell cancer of the head and neck (abstract 1547). *Pro Am Soc Clin Oncol* 1999; 18:400a.
144. Glantz MJ, Choy H, Chakravarthy A, et al. A randomized phase III trial of concurrent paclitaxel and whole brain radiotherapy (WBRT/) vs. WBRT alone for brain metastases. *Pro Am Soc Clin Oncol* 1999; 19:140a.
145. Ferrante K, Winograd B, Canetta R. Promising new developments in cancer chemotherapy. *Cancer Chemother Pharmacol* 1999; 43(Suppl): S61–S68.
146. Menendez A, Laidlaw J, Raventos-Suarez C, et al. In vitro characterization of BMS-184476, a novel taxane with promising preclinical activity. *Proc Am Assoc Cancer Res* 2000; 41:554 (abstract 3529).
147. Highely M, Sessa C, Hughes A, et al. Phase I and pharmacokinetic (PK) study of BMS-184476, a new taxanes analog, given weekly in patients with advanced malignancies. *Proc Am Soc Clin Oncol* 1999; 18:168a (abstract 644).
148. Hidalgo M, Aylesworth C, Ferrante K, et al. Phase I and pharmacokinetic (PK) study of BMS-184476, a potent and soluble taxane analog, as a 1-hour infusion every 3 weeks. *Proc Am Soc Clin Oncol* 1999; 18:168a (abstract 645).
149. Stevenson JP, Gallagher M, Sun W, et al. Phase I clinical and pharmacokinetic study of the taxanes analog BMS-184476 administered as a 1-hour iv infusion in combination with carboplatin every 21 days. *Proc Am Assoc Cancer Res* 2000; 41:608 (abstract 3871).
150. Advani R, Fischer GA, Jambalos C, et al. Phase I study of BMS-188797, a new taxane analog administered weekly in patients with advanced malignancies (abstract 422). *Pro Am Soc Clin Oncol* 2001; 20:106a.
151. Rose WC, Lee FYF, Golik J, et al. Preclinical oral antitumor activity of BMS-185660, a paclitaxel derivative. *Cancer Chemother Pharmacol* 2000; 46:246–250.
152. Trump DL, Egorin M, Ramanathan R, et al. A novel oral taxane (BMS-275183): a phase I trial with evaluation of pharmacokinetics, pharmacodynamics and bioavailability.
153. Nicoletti MI, Colombo T, Rossi C, et al. IDN5109, a taxane with oral bioavailability and potent antitumor activity. *Cancer Res* 2000; 60(4):842–846.
154. Gallo D, Ferlini C, Distefano M, et al. Anti-tumour activity of a panel of taxanes toward a cellular model of human cervical cancer. *Cancer Chemother Pharmacol* 2000; 45(2):127–132.
155. Ferlini C, Distefano M, Pignatelli F, et al. Antitumour activity of novel taxanes that act at the same time as cytotoxic agents and P-glycoprotein inhibitors. *Br J Cancer* 2000; 83(12):1762–1768.
156. Tortora G, Caputo R, Damiano V, et al. Specific Inhibition of EGFR Tyrosine Kinase with ZD1839 ('Iressa') Combined with a Protein Kinase a Antisense and the Novel Taxane IDN5109 Causes Cooperative Inhibition of Tumour Growth and Angiogenesis. *Proceedings of the AACR*, Vol. 42, March 2001. abstract 4315.
157. Taraboletti G, Gatto C, Riva A, et al. Anti-Angiogenic and Anti-Metastatic Activity of IDN 5390, a New C-Seco Taxane Derivative. *Proceedings of the AACR*, Vol. 42, March 2001. abstract 3162.
158. Vrignaud P, Lejeune P, Bissery MC. TXD258, a New Taxoid, with Oral Antitumor Activity. *Proceedings of the AACR*, Vol. 42, March 2001. Abstract 1975.

5 Camptothecin Radiation Sensitization

Tyvin A. Rich, MD

CONTENTS

1. INTRODUCTION

The camptothecin analog CPT-11 has recently been approved for the treatment of 5-fluorouracil (5-FU)-resistant colorectal cancer *(1)*, thus opening a new chapter in chemotherapeutic radiation sensitization. The camptothecins (CPT) are potent radiation sensitizers and are in their infancy in clinical studies. The combination of CPT with irradiation builds onto successful radiation-sensitization trials with 5-FU *(2)*, because both classes of agents are cytotoxic for S-phase cells. They each have a defined role in the treatment of colorectal cancer, a site where radiation sensitization has improved local–regional control and overall survival (Table 1). Radiation sensitization with these agents is dose and schedule dependent and additional knowledge about this combination treatment, based on new laboratory data, may help optimize the use of the CPTs as radiosensitizers.

2. CAMPTOTHECINS AS ANTITUMOR AGENTS

Camptothecin is a plant alkaloid obtained from the *Camptotheca acuminata* tree. It was first evaluated clinically, as a sodium salt, in the 1960s and 1970s, but was abandoned because of severe and unpredictable hemorrhagic cystitis *(3,4)*. Irinotecan (CPT-11) and Rubetecan are semisynthetic, water-soluble derivatives of camptothecin possessing

From: *Chemoradiation in Cancer Therapy*
Edited by: H. Choy

Table 1
Factors Affecting 5-FU (5-fluorouracil) and CPT-11 (Irinotecan) Radiation Sensitization

Factor	*5-FU*	*CPT-11*
Metabolism	5-FU must be converted into a nucleotide precursor (5FdUMP or 5FdUTP to interfere with thymidylate synthase or RNA metabolism)	Yes, must be metabolized to SN-38 by carboxylesterase
Dose dependency	Yes	Yes
Time dependent cytotoxicity	Yes ($\ln SF = C \times t^k$)[a]	Probable
Sequence with irradiation	Post-XRT sensitization	Variable; needs to be present in some concentration at the time of XRT in some systems.
Preferred method of administration for radiation sensitization	Protracted venous infusion	Repeated administration; weekly schedules under investigation
Circadian dependent cytotoxicity	Yes, widened therapeutic window when administered in the rest phase	Yes, animal and initial clinical data indicate chronotolerance

[a]Survival fraction (SF) is proportional to the drug concentration (*C*) × time (*t*) product. The exponent k is a positive integer.

greater in vitro and in vivo activity and associated with less severe and more predictable toxicity than camptothecin *(5–7)*.

Both camptothecin and Irinotecan inhibit topoisomerase I (TOPO-1), a nuclear enzyme that plays a critical role in DNA replication and transcription *(6)*. The mechanism of action involves a primary lesion induced by camptothecin in conjunction with human DNA topoisomerase "cleavable" complexes *(8)*. The properties of these complexes from in vitro studies suggest that CPT binds at the interface between TOPO-1 and DNA and inhibits religation in the cleavage/religation reaction. This inhibition appears to be uncompetitive because CPT binds neither the enzyme nor the DNA substrate but interacts with the enzyme DNA complex to form a reversible nonproductive complex. Alternatively, a drug interpolation model has been suggested in which CPT interacts with the DNA by interpolation at the site of cleavage. An additional model suggests there are interactions between CPT and TOPO-1 via a flip-based model at the +1 position *(8)* although other evidence suggests there may be multiple mechanisms for trapping TOPO-1 cleavable complexes.

CPTs kill cells in S-phase by the mechanism involving the replication fork collision model. It is known that reversible TOPO-1 CPT DNA cleavable complexes are in themselves nonlethal and that collisions with an advancing replication fork cause cell death *(8)*. Several biochemical events follow collision with the replication fork: the formation of double-strand breaks, irreversible arrest of the replication fork, and the formation of TOPO-1-linked DNA break at the site of collision. These mechanisms account for the S-phase-specific cytotoxicity seen at relatively low doses of camptothecin.

At higher concentrations of CPT, non-S-phase cells can be killed by CPT, which appears to be mainly an apoptotic death mechanism *(8)*. In addition to the DNA replication fork collision model, TOPO-1–CPT–DNA cleavable complexes alter transcription machinery causing RNA synthesis arrest. Collisions between RNA polymerase complex and the CPT-cleavable complex on the template strand of transcription can arrest RNA transcription and can convert reversible TOPO-1-cleavable complexes into irreversible TOPO-1-linked single-strand breaks. Another mechanism of DNA damage is the involvement of transcription-coupled repair and the repair of TOPO-1-mediated DNA damage that has been suggested for studies of Cockayne syndrome cells. Recent studies show that repair of TOPO-1-mediated DNA damage may involve TOPO-1 degradation *(8)*. CPT-induced TOPO-1 degradation depends on E1 and 26S proteasomes, suggesting involvement of the ubiquitin/26S proteasome pathway. These collisions trigger ubiquitin/26S proteasome-dependent degradation of TOPO-1. There is also a potential role for tyrosyl/DNA phosphodiesterase, which is involved in the removal of residual peptides *(8)*. CPT can also induce rapid conjugation of SUMO-1 to TOPO-1 implicating the ubiquitination and SUMOylation of TOPO-1 pathways that share reaction characteristics *(9)*. Both appear to be dependent on the formation of TOPO-1-cleavable complexes and both are unaffected by treatment with replication inhibitor aphidicolin or the poly(ADP-ribose) polymerase inhibitor, 3-amino-benzamide. These two reaction pathways differ in several ways depending on transcription and phosphorylation status, and whether these occur in tumor or normal cells. These processes may thus be important in leveraging differences between cancer and normal cells. For example, clinical treatment involves the possibility of CPT-induced TOPO-1 downregulation, which may be defective in tumor cell lines. The molecular mechanism for altered regulation of TOPO-1 downregulation in tumor cells is not clear, however. This could impact treatment schedule, since TOPO-1 downregulation rebounds higher and quicker than normal tissue cells and thus intermittent treatment would be a less favorable model of scheduling than a protracted treatment schedule.

New TOPO-1 inhibitors are being developed as the limitations of the current generation of camptothecins are understood *(10,11)*. In general, the limitations of the camptothecins are the rapid reversibility of TOPO-1 DNA cleavage complexes, E ring opening resulting in an inactive carboxylate, poor solubility, and high binding to human serum albumin, thereby reducing clinical effectiveness. The development of new camptothecins is based on understanding of TOPO-1 isomerase protein expression and mutation, interactions between TOPO-1 and the DNA cleavable complex as well as DNA lesion fixation, lesion processing, and cell cycle effects with regard to cell cycle checkpoints and apoptosis controls. Pharmacologic factors are being reviewed with regard to structure activity relationships, distribution in tissues and cells, metabolic conversion, solubility, and formulation, and how these factors affect therapy *(12)*. Dosing schedules that choose a best-tolerated time model based on understanding increased cytotoxicity of this class of agents for S-phase or the rapidly populating normal tissue compartments may also impact treatment schedules *(1)*.

3. CLINICAL PHARMACOLOGY OF THE CPTS

This chapter will focus on Irinotecan because this is one of the most actively used agents in the clinic today *(13,14)*. Irinotecan is converted by carboxylesterases to its more active metabolite, SN-38. In vitro, SN-38 is 250- to 1000-fold more potent than CPT-11 as an inhibitor of TOPO-1 activity *(6)*. The enzymatic cleavage (hydrolysis) of the carbamate bond of CPT-11 to form the active species SN-38 has been shown to be mediated by hepatic microsomal and serum carboxyl-esterase in animals. These serine hydroxylases have been found in hepatic microsomes, kidney, lung, intestine, brain, and erythrocytes. The ability of various human tissues to produce SN-38 from CPT-11 has been compared *(6)*. Enzymatic hydrolysis was fastest in human liver (42.4 ng SN-38/mg protein/h), with the kidney showing the second highest activity at 24% of the liver value. Activity in normal spleen, lung, and pancreatic tissue ranged between 16% and 18% of the liver value. Liver tumors produced significant, but slightly lower, amounts of SN-38 than normal liver tissue *(15)*. Based on these results, human liver was proposed to be the major site of bioactivation of CPT-11, with extrahepatic metabolism in other normal and tumor tissues likely. Similar to camptothecin and its other analogs (e.g., topotecan, 9-AC), both CPT-11 and its more active metabolite, SN-38, are reversibly hydrolyzed from active lactone forms to hydroxy acid (carboxylate) forms. This hydrolysis is pH-dependent, with equilibrium favoring the hydroxy acid form at physiological pH. The closed lactone ring is a structural requirement for activity of the camptothecins, since studies have demonstrated that the open-ring hydroxy acid form is a less potent inhibitor of TOPO-1 and a much less potent antitumor agent *(6)*.

The mean terminal half-life of SN-38 in plasma is slightly longer than that for CPT-11: 11.5 ± 3.8 h vs 6.3 ± 2.2 h (lactone forms). Peak plasma concentrations for CPT-11 occur at the end of the infusion. The time to peak SN-38 concentration is highly interpatient dependent but generally occurs 30–90 min after the end of infusion *(16)*. Murine studies suggest that the liver may concentrate CPT-11, convert CPT-11 to SN-38, and eliminate via biliary excretion CPT-11, SN-38, and the glucuronide conjugate of SN-38 (SN-38G). In rats, 55% of radiolabeled CPT-11 was excreted unchanged in the bile within 24 h while 21.7% was transformed to SN-38. Overall, 73% of the radioactivity could be recovered from the feces of rats and 25% from the urine. It recently was demonstrated that plasma concentrations of SN-38 glucuronide occur 0.5–3 h after the SN-38 peak and that plasma levels generally exceeded those of SN-38 *(17)*. In one patient, bile concentrations of CPT-11 were 10- to 60-fold higher than plasma concentrations during the first 6 h following administration, whereas bile concentrations of SN-38 were two- to ninefold higher *(16)*.

A full characterization of the metabolic pathways of CPT-11 in human cancer patients has not been undertaken. The incomplete recovery of the irinotecan dose based on urine and bile determinations of irinotecan, SN-38, and SN-38 glucuronide suggests the presence of additional unidentified metabolites. Recently, a major metabolite, 7-ethyl-10-[4-*N*-(5-aminopenatoic acid)-1-piperidino]carbonyloxycamptothecin, has been identified in dogs and humans, suggesting the presence of an additional metabolic pathway *(18)*. Renal clearance has not been reported to be a major route of elimination for these compounds in humans.

4. INTERACTION WITH IRRADIATION

TOPO-1 active drugs like Irinotecan, Topotecan, and 9-AC cause synergistic killing when given with irradiation, even in cells from highly radioresistant tumors *(19–24)*. The cumulative data favor a mechanism of synergistic killing caused by altered DNA lesion modification and enhanced apoptosis. Alterations in cell cycle regulation may also play a role in the synergy between these two agents in some cancers. Some evidence exists for participation by nuclear factor kappa B (NF-κB), a known anti-apoptotic factor activated in various cancer cells by TOPO-1 drugs *(25)*. NF-κB activation is dependent on initial nuclear DNA damage and is dependent on cytoplasmic signaling events. The cytoplasmic signaling leading to NF-κB activation after TOPO-1 exposure is diminished in cells lacking nuclei and in CEM-C2 cells that express mutant TOPO-1 protein that cannot interact with TOPO on active drugs. The NF-κB activation was also intensified in S-phase and in cells blocked by aphidocolin suggesting that activation was a result of double-strand break formation due to TOPO-1 poisoning and DNA replication. These data suggest that the blocking of anti-apoptotic NF-κB responses may improve radiotherapy results.

In vivo, combination 9-aminocamptothecin (9-AC) and irradiation is more effective when fractionated compared to single doses *(26)*. We found a dose modifying factor (DMF) of only 1.12 after 4 mg/kg of 9-AC and 15 Gy compared to a DMF of 2.8 with an isoeffective radiation dose (28 Gy) plus an equitoxic total dose of fractionated 9-AC. Reasons for the superiority of fractionated treatments over single treatment may be related to the formation and equilibration of stabilized DNA–TOPO-1 cleavable complexes during repeated CPT administration *(27,28)*. Another possibility is that of a "synchronizing" effect of fractionated irradiation through the selective cytotoxicity in G2-M cells after irradiation enriches the fraction of S-phase cells that are sensitive to CPT treatment (a "chemosensitizing" effect). Regardless of the mechanism of action, *fractionated CPT* alone increases cytotoxicity compared to a large single CPT treatment in human xenografts and repeated clinical administration schedules are justified.

Another consideration for using CPTs in the clinic are acute diarrhea and myelosuppression that are the typical dose-limiting toxicities with this class of S-phase chemotherapeutic agents. Our laboratory results with chronomodulated CPT suggest that acute morbidity can be spared when the rapidly proliferating normal tissues are treated when they are least sensitive *(26)*. The circadian time dependence for acute toxicity in the gut and the bone marrow has been described for other S-phase agents including the CPTs in ICR mice *(29)*. The explanation for this effect appears to be related to circadian cytokinetics of the murine gastrointestinal tract because the peak incorporation of bromodeoxyuridine into S-phase cells occurs around 2 AM *(30)*. Another factor influencing circadian-dependent toxicity of these drugs may be the enzymatic activity of the intestinal flora such as B-glucuronidase or intestinal tissue carboxylesterase, which converts CPT-11 into active metabolites in the intestinal lumen. An understanding of the chronopharmacology of the CPTs could provide valuable answers that have clinical relevance. We thus hypothesize that administration of CPTs during the human rest phase may allow dose escalation and provide a basis for increased radiation sensitization compared to nonchronomodulated sensitizer administration. A recent report on the treatment of advanced colorectal cancer patients with chronomodulated CPT-11 showed that dose escalation was possible and supports this view *(1)*. These laboratory data suggest optimal scheduling of the CPTs with irradiation occurs with repeated dosing. They provide a rationale for using fractionated treatments in the clinic and treatment schedules now being piloted with irinotecan using daily and weekly dosing schedules. Comparisons of toxicity and efficacy of these differing schedules in humans are not yet available. There is also evidence for circadian-dependent cytotoxicity and radiation sensitization, and when used as radiation sensitizers a chronomodulated delivery schedule should also be evaluated in the clinic.

5. TOPOTECAN

Topotecan is a water-soluble TOPO-I inhibitor with cytotoxic activity in a variety of preclinical models. Topotecan exhibits schedule dependency in vivo, and has high cytotoxic activity with repeated dose schedules *(31)*. In murine systems, there is evidence that *reducing the dose intensity* (by prolonging the drug administration schedule) provides a therapeutic advantage because of reduced host toxicity and equal or superior tumor responses. In clinical studies with topotecan, a short plasma half-life also suggests that prolonged drug exposure by infusion could be effective. In a phase I trial with escalating low-dose topotecan infusion, an increased therapeutic ratio was found when compared to an intermittent dosing schedule *(32)*. Neutropenia is usually the dose-limiting toxicity for topotecan.

In phase II studies with topotecan alone, there is cytotoxic activity in lung cancer with intermittent dose schedules *(33)*, as well as in lung cancer patients with topoisomerase II refractory disease *(34)*. In advanced head and neck cancer topotecan is well-tolerated and has single-agent activity similar to that of cisplatin, 5-fluorouracil, and methotrexate *(35)*. Decreased production or mutation of TOPO-1 can cause resistance to the cytotoxic effects of topotecan and other CPTs; active efflux of TPT by P-glycoprotein-mediated transport might also contribute to resistance.

Topotecan has radiation-sensitizing properties demonstrated in log- and plateau-phase cell cultures *(23,36)* and in murine fibrosarcomas *(37,38)*. Trials have begun in patients with nonsmall-cell lung cancer (NSCLC) and in those with central nervous system (CNS) tumors.

Clinical evidence for radiation sensitization has been demonstrated in a dose-escalation trial for patients with locally advanced, inoperable nonsmall-cell lung cancer (NSCLC) *(39)*. Twelve patients received 60 Gy (2 Gy/d) plus topotecan delivered by bolus injection d 1–5, and again on d 22–26, beginning on the same day as irradiation. The initial dose level was 0.5 mg/m^2; dose levels of 0.75 mg/m^2 and 1.0 mg/m^2 were also tested. Doses higher that 0.5 mg/m^2 were associated with relatively high hematologic and gastrointestinal toxicity. The results of treatment showed 5 of 12 patients alive (2 without evident disease) and 7 dead of disease; late pulmonary toxicity was not reported. Topotecan has also been used with cranial irradiation for patients with glioblastoma multiforme and for children with intrinsic pontine gliomas. In both of these trials, topotecan is given daily as a 30 min infusion 30–120 min prior to irradiation.

6. IRINOTECAN

Irinotecan treatment schedules differ from 125 to 150 mg/m^2 once a week for 4 wk followed by a 2-wk drug free interval (United States), to 350 mg/m^2 once every 3 wk (Europe), or 100 mg/m^2/wk or 150 mg/m^2 every 2 wk (Japan). Differing intermittent treatment schedules using cytokine support for neutropenia, or intensive loperamide to counteract diarrhea, have also been reported *(14)*. These tolerable CPT-11 regimens have produced median durations of response that range from 5.6 to 10.6 mo in colorectal patients; disease stabilization occurs in 30 to 71% *(40)*. Response rates of 26% and 32% have been reported for previously untreated colorectal cancer patients; higher response rates have been reported for non-5-FU-refractory patients (only 7–21%). Symptoms of diarrhea, nausea, and vomiting are common toxicities; other side effects are asthenia, abdominal pain, leukopenia, and neutropenia. In the US trials at least one of these adverse events occurred in >50% of patients. Grade 3 or 4 toxicity occurs in about one-third of patients and the most common grade 3 or 4 event is severe late diarrhea.

CPT-11 has significant activity in nonsmall-cell lung cancer *(41)* and it has been combined with irradiation in phase I/II trials in Japan. CPT-11 is a prodrug that must be converted to an active form, SN-38, by carboxylesterase, which has been found in liver, in blood, and in lung cancer biopsies. Carboxylesterase was detected by immunostaining with an antihuman carboxylesterase polyclonal antibody and by indirect immunostaining in lung squamous cell carcinomas that had significantly higher levels than adenocarcinoma cells ($p < 0.05$). Other studies in 10 human lung cancers cell lines showed that SN-38 levels increased significantly over 24 h suggesting that human lung cancer cells efficiently convert CPT-11 to SN-38.

Radiation sensitization with irinotecan in two human lung cancer xenografts has been reported *(42)*. In these experiments, CPT-11 was administered in nontoxic doses 1 h prior to a single dose of irradiation. In other reports radiation sensitization with CPT occurred during or after irradiation *(43)*.

7. OTHER AGENTS: 9-AMINO-CAMPTOTHECIN, 9-NITRO-CAMPTOTHECIN

The rationale for combining 9-AC with irradiation was based on in vitro work with human colon and pancreatic cancer cell lines showing dose dependency for cytotoxicity and radiation sensitization and other reports that it is a potent radiation sensitizer in vivo *(21)*. Unfortunately, this agent is not very well tolerated in man and clinical studies have been abandoned *(12)*. Another agent is 9-nitro-camptothecin that is converted into 9-AC in vivo, which has also been shown to be active in vitro and in vivo *(44,45)*.

8. CLINICAL STUDIES: LUNG CANCER

In a clinical phase I trial using CPT-11 with concurrent irradiation (60 Gy in 30 fractions over 6 wk) for NSCLC, the maximum tolerated dose (MTD) was 60 mg/m^2 (by 90 min iv infusion) when given weekly for 6 wk *(46)*. A follow-up phase II trial was then performed in previously untreated patients with high performance status with a diagnosis of unresectable stage IIIA/B NSCLC *(47)*. In 24 patients with varied histologic diagnoses and a median age of 60 yr (range 44–72), six planned courses of CPT-11 were delivered in 71% and another 21% of these patients received five courses. External beam irradiation to the thorax was completed in 88% and three patients had a treatment delay because of fever or fatigue. The overall objective response rate was 79%. Acute toxicities were limited to one grade-3 leukocytopenia and two grade-3 neutropenias. Other toxicities included three grade-3 hypoxemia due to pneumonitis, two with temporary grade-3 esophagitis, and one with a grade-3 fever. Grade-3/4 diarrhea was not observed. These authors conclude that weekly CPT-11 and concurrent radiation therapy is an active combination treatment for locally advanced NSCLC. The high incidence of pneumonitis with this treatment combination needs further investigation.

Phase I trials are now underway using CPT-11 plus irradiation for patients with advanced or recurrent colorectal cancer. In one study, a single weekly dosage of 30 mg/kg of CPT-11 is given intravenously in combination with infusional 5-FU (300 mg/m^2/d) and concurrent pelvic radiotherapy (50 Gy). This approach builds onto an existing standard practice of infusional chemoradiation and uses a dose modification of the common drug-dosing scheme for CPT-11 used today in the United States. Phase I and II trials with CPT-11 have demonstrated clinical activity and radiation sensitization in NSCLC.

9. OTHER THORACIC MALIGNANCIES

A Phase I study has been underway at the M.D. Anderson Cancer Center for patients with advanced unresectable gastric, gastroesophageal, or esophageal cancer *(48)*. Patients must not have had previous treatment, and eligibility criteria regarding a baseline hematologic and liver function tests are standard. Previous treatment with irinotecan or topotecan (Hycamtin) or prior radiotherapy were exclusion criteria. The treatment plan consisted of a Phase I dose-escalation study beginning at 30 mg/m^2 and extending to a dose of 70 mg/m^2. A weekly dose of irinotecan was modified according to blood counts. Radiotherapy treatment consisted of 45–50 Gy in 1.8 Gy fractions for a total of 25–28 fractions delivered over 5 wk. The irinotecan was administered 1 h prior to administration of radiation therapy on d 1 of each week of radiotherapy. In 18 patients enrolled between January and November of 1998, there were 12 patients evaluable for toxicities and response. There was a male predominance of 16:2 and ages ranged from 30–76 with a median age of 59. Six patients had esophageal cancer, nine had lesions of the GE junction, and three had tumors in the stomach. The predominant histology was adenocarcinoma and three had signet ring cell carcinoma. There were 12 T-3 patients and 6 T-4 patients; 6 had N-0 disease, and 12 had what was considered N-1 disease. The dose-escalation study revealed that the MTD was 60 mg/m^2, and it was recommended that a dose for the Phase II study is 45 mg/m^2 administered weekly with radiotherapy. The toxicities involved in the Phase I study revealed major toxicities were hematologic. Neutropenia and neutropenic fever along with sepsis and chills were common. Two patients had hemorrhage and two patients had severe anemia. Regarding GI toxicities, there were two patients with nausea, four with vomiting, three with dehydration, three with anorexia, and one with constipation. No patient had severe pneumonitis. In the 12 evaluable patients, seven (58%) had a response, including two complete responses. There were four patients with no change, and one patient had progressive disease. The median time to progression was 27.5 wk and survival ranged from 1 to 15 mo with a median survival of 8 mo.

Although this trial is small, it fits with results from Japanese studies and those reported from Vanderbilt showing that a range of 30–40 mg/m^2 given weekly can be combined with daily irradiation.

10. RECTAL CANCER

The group at the Thomas Jefferson University Hospital, Philadelphia, PA have evaluated the use of weekly irinotecan in conjunction with 5-FU infusion in a Phase I study *(49)*. The trial attempted to combine a weekly dose of irinotecan with continuous infusion 5-FU in conjunction with 45 Gy given in 1.8 Gy fractions over 5 wk. The objective of this Phase I study was to determine the MTD of weekly irinotecan in previously untreated patients with primary recurrent clinical stage T-3, T-4 adenocarcinoma of the rectum. The trial began with escalating doses of irinotecan at 30–50 mg/m^2 given over 90 min on d 1, 8, 15, and 22. 5-Fluorouracil was initially given as a protracted intravenous infusion of 300 mg/m^2 per day, which was subsequently reduced to a dose of 225 mg/m^2 on d 1–5 with weekly irradiation. Surgery was performed 8–10 wk following completion of

Table 2
Radiation Therapy Oncology Group RTOG R-0012 Randomized Phase II Trial of Preoperative Combined Modality Chemoradiation for Distal Rectal Cancer

			Schema
S		R	
T	Clinical	A	Arm 1: CVI 5-FU (250 mg/m^2/d, 7 d/wk, until completion of RT)
			+ Pelvic RT 45.6 Gy (1.2 Gy/b.i.d., ≥ 6 h interval)
	Staging		
R	1. T3	N	+ Boost to tumor (9.6 Gy for T3 and 14.4 Gy for fixed T4)*
	2. T4		+ Surgery**4–10 wk after completion of RT.
A		D	
T		O	Arm 2: CVI 5-FU (225 mg/m^2/d, M-F, 120 h/weekly,
			until completion of RT) plus CPT-11 (50 mg/m^2, once weekly × 4)
I		M	+ Pelvic RT 45 Gy (1.8 Gy/d)
			+ Boost to tumor (5.4 Gy for T3 and 9 Gy for fixed T4)*
F		I	+ Surgery**4–10 wk after completion of RT.
Y		Z	
		E	

*Boost radiation may be delivered using conformal 3D techniques.

**IORT (optional) may be delivered to areas of tumor fixation at time of surgery. Maintenance chemotherapy is recommended for all patients post.

treatment. A total of 38 patients were enrolled in the trial and the finalized and recommended dose for the Phase II study is 50 mg/m^2 weekly, given with conventional protracted infusion 5-FU during a course of radiotherapy.

The RTOG trial R0102 is now open for patient accrual and will be a randomized Phase II comparison of 5-FU infusion plus irinotecan and conventionally fractionated radiotherapy to a dose of 50.4 Gy (Table 2). This will be compared to a hyperfractionated radiotherapy arm given in conjunction with protracted venous infusion of 5-FU. Readers interested in participating should contact the radiotherapy oncology group headquarters in Philadelphia, PA.

A different chemoradiation approach being used is based on Phase I data with daily low-dose CPT-11 *(50)*. The rationale here is that camptothecin-stabilized DNA–TOPO1 cleavable complexes are reversible and thus frequent CPT-11 dosing may favor production of these complexes. This is supported by the fact that the half-life of SN-38 is relatively long and daily bolus injections can result in a concentration x time product similar to a continuous infusion. CPT-11 was administered in a Phase I fashion for five consecutive days for 2 wk followed by a 1 wk rest. In 20 previously treated patients with advanced tumors (16 with colorectal cancer) acute toxicity over first two cycles (6 wk duration) was mild diarrhea and neutropenia. Two patients with colorectal cancer achieved a partial response and six others had stable disease. Grade 3 diarrhea and neutropenic fever were seen at the highest dose level (22 mg/m^2/d), and dose escalation was stopped. This treatment scheme delivers 88% of the amount of drug given on a more standard weekly × four schedule. The investigators feel that less heavily pretreated patients might tolerate higher doses. A Phase I chemoradiation study using this schedule with concurrent pelvic RT for locally advanced rectal cancer has been completed but there are no data available yet as to the efficacy or toxicity of treatment.

REFERENCES

1. Rich TA, Kirichenko AV. Camptothecin radiation sensitization: mechanisms, schedules, and timing. *Oncology (Huntingt)* 1998; 12(8 Suppl 6):114–120.
2. Rich TA. Irradiation Plus 5-Fluorouracil: Cellular Mechanisms of Action and Treatment Schedules. *Semin Radiat Oncol* 1997; 7(4):267–273.
3. Moertel CG, Schutt AJ, Reitemeier RJ, Hahn RG. Phase II study of camptothecin (NSC-100880) in the treatment of advanced gastrointestinal cancer. *Cancer Chemother Rep* 1972; 56(1):95–101.
4. Muggia FM, Creaven PJ, Hansen HH, Cohen MH, Selawry OS. Phase I clinical trial of weekly and daily treatment with camptothecin (NSC-100880): correlation with preclinical studies. *Cancer Chemother Rep* 1972; 56(4):515–521.
5. Kunimoto T, Nitta K, Tanaka T, et al. Antitumor activity of 7-ethyl-10-[4-(1-piperidino)-1-piperidino]carbonyloxy-camptothec in, a novel water-soluble derivative of camptothecin, against murine tumors. *Cancer Res* 1987; 47(22):5944–5947.
6. Kawato Y, Furuta T, Aonurna M, Yasuoka M, Yokokura T, Matsumoto K. Antitumor activity of a camptothecin derivative, CPT-11, against human tumor xenografts in nude mice. *Cancer Chemother Pharmacol* 1991; 28(3):192–198.
7. Rothenberg ML. Topoisomerase I inhibitors: review and update. *Ann Oncol* 1997; 8(9):837–855.
8. Liu LF, Desai SD, Li TK, Mao Y, Sun M, Sim SP. Mechanism of action of camptothecin. *Ann NY Acad Sci* 2000; 922:1–10.
9. Desai SD, Mao Y, Sun M, Li TK, Wu J, Liu LF. Ubiquitin, SUMO-1, and UCRP in camptothecin sensitivity and resistance. *Ann NY Acad Sci* 2000; 922:306–308.
10. Kohn KW, Pommier Y. Molecular and biological determinants of the cytotoxic actions of camptothecins. Perspective for the development of new topoisomerase I inhibitors. *Ann NY Acad Sci* 2000; 922:11–26.
11. Giovanella BC, Harris N, Mendoza J, Cao Z, Liehr J, Stehlin JS. Dependence of anticancer activity of camptothecins on maintaining their lactone function. *Ann NY Acad Sci* 2000; 922:27–35.
12. Takimoto CH. Why drugs fail: of mice and men revisited. *Clin Cancer Res* 2001; 7(2):229–230.
13. Rothenberg ML, Cox JV, DeVore RF, et al. A multicenter, phase II trial of weekly irinotecan (CPT-11) in patients with previously treated colorectal carcinoma. *Cancer* 1999; 85(4):786–795.
14. Rothenberg ML. The current status of irinotecan (CPT-11) in the United States. *Ann N Y Acad Sci* 1996; 803:272–281.
15. Hsiang YH, Hertzberg R, Hecht S, Liu LF. Camptothecin induces protein-linked DNA breaks via mammalian DNA topoisomerase I. *J Biol Chem* 1985; 260(27):14873–14878.
16. Drengler RL, Kuhn JG, Schaaf LJ, et al. Phase I and pharmacokinetic trial of oral irinotecan administered daily for 5 days every 3 weeks in patients with solid tumors. *J Clin Oncol* 1999; 17(2):685–696.
17. Gupta E, Lestingi TM, Mick R, Ramirez J, Vokes EE, Ratain MJ. Metabolic fate of irinotecan in humans: correlation of glucuronidation with diarrhea. *Cancer Res* 1994; 54(14):3723–3725.
18. Rivory LP, Riou JF, Haaz MC, et al. Identification and properties of a major plasma metabolite of irinotecan (CPT-11) isolated from the plasma of patients. *Cancer Res* 1996; 56(16):3689–3694.
19. Chastagner P, Merlin JL, Marchal C, et al. In vivo potentiation of radiation response by topotecan in human rhabdomyosarcoma xenografted into nude mice. *Clin Cancer Res* 2000; 6(8):3327–3333.
20. Hennequin C, Giocanti N, Balosso J, Favaudon V. Interaction of ionizing radiation with the topoisomerase I poison camptothecin in growing V-79 and HeLa cells. *Cancer Res* 1994; 54(7):1720–1728.
21. Kirichenko AV, Travis EL, Rich TA. Radiation enhancement by 9-aminocamptothecin. Evidence for improved therapeutic ratio with a multiple dose schedule. *Ann NY Acad Sci* 1996; 803:312–314.
22. Kirichenko AV, Rich TA, Newman RA, Travis EL. Potentiation of murine MCa-4 carcinoma radioresponse by 9-amino-20(S)-camptothecin. *Cancer Res* 1997; 57(10):1929–1933.
23. Mattern MR, Hofmann GA, McCabe FL, Johnson RK. Synergistic cell killing by ionizing radiation and topoisomerase I inhibitor topotecan (SK&F 104864). *Cancer Res* 1991; 51(21):5813–5816.
24. Zanier R, De Salvia R, Fiore M, Degrassi F. Topoisomerase I activity and cellular response to radiation in Chinese hamster cells. *Int J Radiat Biol* 1996; 70(3):251–259.
25. Huang TT, Wuerzberger-Davis SM, Seufzer BJ, et al. NF-kappaB activation by camptothecin. A linkage between nuclear DNA damage and cytoplasmic signaling events. *J Biol Chem* 2000; 275(13):9501–9509.
26. Kirichenko AV, Rich TA. Radiation enhancement by 9-aminocamptothecin: the effect of fractionation and timing of administration. *Int J Radiat Oncol Biol Phys* 1999; 44(3):659–664.

27. Furman WL, Stewart CF, Poquette CA, et al. Direct translation of a protracted irinotecan schedule from a xenograft model to a phase I trial in children. *J Clin Oncol* 1999; 17(6):1815–1824.
28. Rodriguez-Galindo C, Radomski K, Stewart CF, Furman W, Santana VM, Houghton PJ. Clinical use of topoisomerase I inhibitors in anticancer treatment. *Med Pediatr Oncol* 2000; 35(4):385–402.
29. Ohdo S, Makinosumi T, Ishizaki T, et al. Cell cycle-dependent chronotoxicity of irinotecan hydrochloride in mice. *J Pharmacol Exp Ther* 1997; 283(3):1383–1388.
30. Kirichenko AV, Mason K, Straume M, Teates CD, Rich TA. Nuclear scintigraphic assessment of intestinal dysfunction after combined treatment with 9-amino-20(S)-camptothecin (9-AC) and irradiation. *Int J Radiat Oncol Biol Phys* 2000; 47(4):1043–1049.
31. Slichenmyer WJ, Rowinsky EK, Donehower RC, Kaufmann SH. The current status of camptothecin analogues as antitumor agents. *J Natl Cancer Inst* 1993; 85(4):271–291.
32. O'Dwyer PJ, LaCreta FP, Haas NB, et al. Clinical, pharmacokinetic and biological studies of topotecan. *Cancer Chemother Pharmacol* 1994; 34 Suppl:S46–S52.
33. Perez-Soler R, Glisson BS, Lee JS, et al. Treatment of patients with small-cell lung cancer refractory to etoposide and cisplatin with the topoisomerase I poison topotecan. *J Clin Oncol* 1996; 14(10): 2785–2790.
34. Perez-Soler R, Fossella FV, Glisson BS, et al. Phase II study of topotecan in patients with advanced non-small-cell lung cancer previously untreated with chemotherapy. *J Clin Oncol* 1996; 14(2):503–513.
35. Robert F, Soong SJ, Wheeler RH. A phase II study of topotecan in patients with recurrent head and neck cancer. Identification of an active new agent. *Am J Clin Oncol* 1997; 20(3):298–302.
36. Lamond JP, Wang M, Kinsella TJ, Boothman DA. Concentration and timing dependence of lethality enhancement between topotecan, a topoisomerase I inhibitor, and ionizing radiation. *Int J Radiat Oncol Biol Phys* 1996; 36(2):361–368.
37. Kim JH, Kim SH, Kolozsvary A, Khil MS. Potentiation of radiation response in human carcinoma cells in vitro and murine fibrosarcoma in vivo by topotecan, an inhibitor of DNA topoisomerase I. *Int J Radiat Oncol Biol Phys* 1992; 22(3):515–518.
38. Boscia RE, Korbut T, Holden SA, Ara G, Teicher BA. Interaction of topoisomerase I inhibitors with radiation in cis- diamminedichloroplatinum(II)-sensitive and -resistant cells in vitro and in the FSAIIC fibrosarcoma in vivo. *Int J Cancer* 1993; 53(1):118–123.
39. Graham MV, Jahanzeb M, Dresler CM, Cooper JD, Emami B, Mortimer JE. Results of a trial with topotecan dose escalation and concurrent thoracic radiation therapy for locally advanced, inoperable nonsmall-cell lung cancer. *Int J Radiat Oncol Biol Phys* 1996; 36(5):1215–1220.
40. Rothenberg ML, Blanke CD. Topoisomerase I inhibitors in the treatment of colorectal cancer. *Semin Oncol* 1999; 26(6):632–639.
41. Takeda K, Negoro S, Kudoh S, et al. Phase I/II study of weekly irinotecan and concurrent radiation therapy for locally advanced non-small cell lung cancer. *Br J Cancer* 1999; 79(9-10):1462–1467.
42. Tamura K, Takada M, Kawase I, et al. Enhancement of tumor radio-response by irinotecan in human lung tumor xenografts. *Jpn J Cancer Res* 1997; 88(2):218–223.
43. Omura M, Torigoe S, Kubota N. SN-38, a metabolite of the camptothecin derivative CPT-11, potentiates the cytotoxic effect of radiation in human colon adenocarcinoma cells grown as spheroids. *Radiother Oncol* 1997; 43(2):197–201.
44. Pantazis P, Harris N, Mendoza J, Giovanella B. Conversion of 9-nitro-camptothecin to 9-amino-camptothecin by human blood cells in vitro. *Eur J Haematol* 1994; 53(4):246–248.
45. Bernacki RJ, Pera P, Gambacorta P, Brun Y, Greco WR. In vitro antitumor activity of 9-nitro-camptothecin as a single agent and in combination with other antitumor drugs. *Ann N Y Acad Sci* 2000; 922:293–297.
46. Kobayashi K, Shinbara A, Kamimura M, et al. Irinotecan (CPT-11) in combination with weekly administration of cisplatin (CDDP) for non-small-cell lung cancer. *Cancer Chemother Pharmacol* 1998; 42(1):53–58.
47. Fukuoka M, Masuda N, Kudoh S, Negoro S. Irinotecan in small-cell lung cancer—Japanese trials. *Oncology (Huntingt)* 2000; 14(7 Suppl 5):57–62.
48. Komaki R, Janjan NA, Ajani JA, et al. Phase I study of irinotecan and concurrent radiation therapy for upper GI tumors. *Oncology (Huntingt)* 2000; 14(12 Suppl 14):34–37.
49. Mitchell EP. Irinotecan in preoperative combined-modality therapy for locally advanced rectal cancer. *Oncology (Huntingt)* 2000; 14(12 Suppl 14):56–59.
50. Saltz LB. Clinical Use of Irinotecan: Current Status and Future Considerations. *Oncologist* 1997; 2(6):402–409.

6 The Role of Gemcitabine in Combined Modality Therapy

Jerome Landry, MD, *William Blackstock,* MD, *Robert M. MacRae,* MD, *Gary Yang,* MD, *and Hak Choy,* MD

CONTENTS

1. INTRODUCTION

Gemcitabine is a novel pyrimidine nucleoside analog with a broad spectrum of clinical antitumor activity. In addition to its initial approved indication in pancreatic carcinoma, gemcitabine has been licensed for the treatment of nonsmall-cell lung cancer (NSCLC) *(1)*. The focus of this chapter will be to examine the current preclinical and clinical evidence probing the efficacy of gemcitabine as a clinically useful radiosensitizing agent. It will begin by examining the mechanism of action of the drug itself at a cellular and molecular level.

2. PHARMACOLOGY

Gemcitabine is a relatively new chemotherapeutic agent that belongs to the nucleoside analog category (*see* Fig. 1). It is a synthetic analog of deoxycitidine wherein the two hydrogens of the two-carbon atom are replaced with two fluorine atoms *(2)*. Gemcitabine is believed to be actively transported across the cellular membrane where it is converted to its monophosphate form, 2', 2'-difluorodeoxycytidine monophosphate (dFdCMP), by deoxycytidine kinase *(3)*. It is thought that a base-specific (d)CMP kinase catalyzes the

From: *Chemoradiation in Cancer Therapy*
Edited by: H. Choy © Humana Press Inc., Totowa, NJ

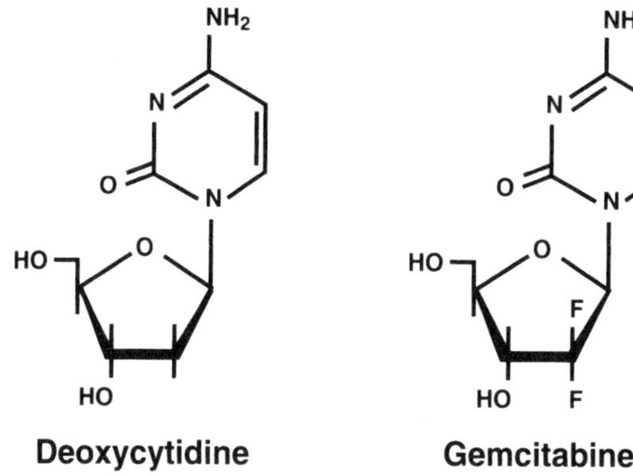

Fig. 1. Structure of gemcitabine.

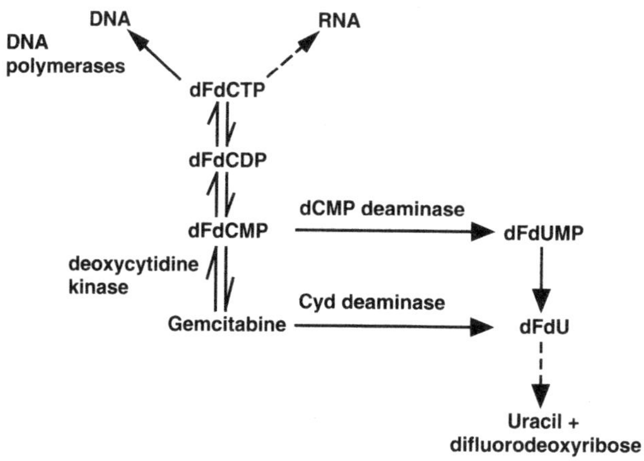

Fig. 2. Metabolism of gemcitabine.

conversion to the dFdCDP form *(2)* and the nonspecific nucleoside diphosphate kinase will lead the conversion to the triphosphate or dFdCTP form *(2)*. This process of conversion to a phosphorylated compound appears to be essential for the manifestation of the cytotoxic properties of the drug *(3)*. The drug itself also begins to act as a substrate inhibitor of deoxycytidine kinase at concentrations greater than 20 µmol/L *(4)*. This provides the rationale for clinical investigations that have attempted to maximize gemcitabine triphosphate accumulation in cells by limiting the rate of infusion of the drug *(5,6)*. Cytidine deaminase is the enzyme responsible for the rapid clearance of gemcitabine during its clinical use, and, fortunately, this deamination product appears to be biologically inactive *(7)*. There are other lesser pathways involved in the metabolism of gemcitabine whose significance is unknown (*see* Fig. 2).

The biologic action of gemcitabine on its own is due almost completely to its effects on DNA metabolism. Early studies of this drug in leukemic cell lines showed that notable decreases in cellular dNTPs occurred with the use of the drug *(8)*. These decreases were most impressive in terms of the levels of 2'-deoxycytidine 5'-triphosphate (dCTP), however, 2'-deoxyadenosine 5'-triphosphate (dATP) and 2'-deoxyguanosine 5'-triphosphate (dGTP) were also affected. It is felt that part of this is due to the inhibitory effects of gemcitabine diphosphate on ribonucleoside diphosphate reductase *(9)*. There is, however, a role for the direct incorporation of the drug into DNA as an additional mechanism underlying its cytotoxicity, as seen in experiments where DNA synthesis is not fully restored after the addition of missing deoxynucleosides into culture medium *(10)*. Overall, it is believed that S phase cells, which actively incorporate gemcitabine into DNA, are most susceptible to drug-induced apoptosis *(11,12)*, which is felt to be the major mode of action of the drug.

Important studies have shown that the triphosphate of gemcitabine can be incorporated into extending primer strands by both the α and ε forms of the human DNA polymerase on a competitive footing with dCTP *(10)*. Despite the fact that gemcitabine was incorporated into the elongating DNA strand at the 3' terminus, it was possible to incorporate one other base into the strand after gemcitabine *(2)* (termed "masked chain termination"), although it was difficult to add another dFdCTP. It is felt that the G:C richness of the particular sequence as well as the intracellular ratio of dCTP:dFdCTP are key determinants of strand elongation *(2)*. Equally interesting is the fact that the proofreading abilities of DNA polymerase operate at only a fraction of their potential efficiency when it comes to excising gemcitabine analogs *(10)*. The significance of the level of incorporation of gemcitabine into DNA and the induction of apoptosis appear to be linked.

A discussion of the methods underlying the "self-potentiation" of gemcitabine is also important when discussing its mechanisms of action. They are outlined below *(2)*:

1. dFdCDP acts as an inhibitory substrate for ribonucleotide reductase, which is the enzyme that produces deoxynucleotides needed for replication and repair.
2. dFdCTP competes directly with dCTP for incorporation into DNA.
3. Deoxycytidine kinase, which phosphorylates bases, is inhibited by deoxycytidine and dCTP, so, as their intracellular levels fall, more gemcitabine can be phosphorylated.
4. dCTP is also a cofactor for the activation of dCMP deaminase, which is the enzyme responsible for gemcitabine deactivation. Therefore, lower dCTP levels translate into less gemcitabine deactivation.
5. dFdCTP also inhibits dCMP deaminase, leading to less gemcitabine deactivation.
6. At high cellular concentrations dFdCTP inhibits CTP synthetase so that CTP and dCTP production is further down regulated.

All of these mechanisms are felt to be important in contributing to the cytotoxicity seen with gemcitabine as a sole agent. In fact, an understanding of these interactions will be important to fully appreciate the interaction of gemcitabine with ionizing radiation as well.

3. CLINICAL EFFICACY

This drug has clinical activity in a number of malignancies including pancreatic, lung, ovarian, bladder, and breast cancer *(13)*. In fact, it was initially approved for the treatment of metastatic pancreatic cancer based on studies showing that it improved overall quality of life *(14,15)*. Overall gemcitabine is well tolerated with its major dose limiting toxicity being myelosuppression as it is with the other antimetabolites. Nausea and vomiting are not uncommon; however, they are only severe in fewer than 15% of patients. Transient rashes that tend to be macular, erythematous, and puritic, flu-like symptoms, and alopecia may occur. Optimal systemic dosing of this drug is not necessarily defined and certainly the optimal dosing for combined therapy with radiation is undefined at this stage. Most regimens using the drug for its systemic effect administer between 800 and 1250 mg/m^2 iv once a week for 3 out of a 4-wk cycle *(13)*.

Table 1
Summary of the Available Preclinical Data on Gemcitabine's Radiosensitizing Potential

Cell type	*Relative enhancement ratio*	*Ref.*
Human colon carcinoma (HT29)	1.76	*(20)*
Human colon carcinoma (Widr)	1.08–1.57	*(21)*
Hela (human cervical carcinoma)	1.04–2.47	*(22)*
Squamous cell carcinoma #4197	1.03–1.67	*(22)*
Chinese hamster lung fibroblasts (V79)	1.05–1.45	*(21)*
SQD9 human head and neck squamous cell carcinoma	1.3	*(23)*
SCC61 human head and neck squamous cell carcinoma	1.5	*(23)*
Human pancreatic adenocarcinoma panc-1	1.68	*(19)*
Human pancreatic adenocarcinoma BxPC-3	1.74	*(19)*
Human breast cancer MDA-MB 231	1.47–1.58	*(24)*
Glioblastoma D54	Not sensitized	*(25)*
Glioblastoma U251	1.7	*(25)*

4. PRECLINICAL DATA OF GEMCITABINE AS A RADIOSENSITIZER

Although the exact mechanism by which gemcitabine serves to sensitize cells to damage from ionizing radiation is not well defined, there is burgeoning literature on the subject. Nucleoside analogs including fludarabine, cladrabine, and gemcitabine are felt to be attractive agents to combine with radiation for multiple reasons. First of all, these agents are S phase specific *(16)* and as such should be selectively toxic to proliferating cells. This may serve to decrease the cell proliferation that can occur during fractionated radiotherapy. Second, cell cycle redistribution induced by these agents can serve to improve cell kill by allowing more cells to be treated in the more sensitive parts of the cell cycle *(17)*. As DNA synthesis inhibitors these drugs may act to inhibit the repair of radiation-induced DNA damage *(18)*. Finally, as this class of drugs acts as DNA chain terminators, if incorporated into areas where DNA repair has occurred after radiation, they may cause the triggering of the apoptotic response *(19)*. This would serve to extend the cytotoxicity of these nucleoside analogs to non-S phase agents.

4.1. In Vitro

In addition to the above-outlined cytotoxic effects of gemcitabine, it also serves to act as a radiation sensitizer in many cell lines (*see* Table 1). Depending on the cell line tested, the drug concentration, the schedule of administration, and the cell proliferative status (e.g., plateau vs exponential growth), relative enhancement ratios (RERs) in the range of 1.1–2.5 have been reported. There is no evidence that preferential radiosensitization occurs in more radioresistant cell lines.

Initial experiments have shown that gemcitabine has a potent enhancing effect on the cellular effects of ionizing radiation; reports with rodent EMT6 *(26)* cells and with HT-29 human colon carcinoma cell lines *(27)* showed that noncytotoxic concentrations of the drug lead to significant enrichment of radiation-induced cell lethality (Fig. 3). In the latter study it was found that the noncytotoxic concentrations of the drug (10 n*M*

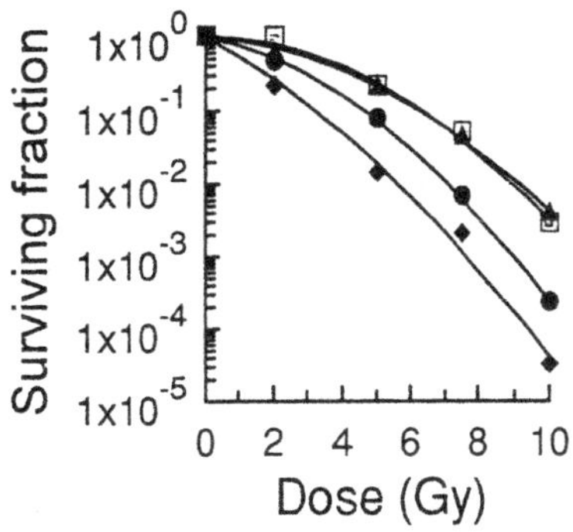

Fig. 3. Effect of gemcitabine on the sensitivity of HT-29 cells to radiation. Cells were incubated with no drug, 3 n*M*, 10 n*M*, and 30 n*M* gemcitabine for 24 h followed by radiation. Surviving fraction was corrected for cell survival in the absence of radiation. From Shewach et al. *Cancer Res* 1994; 54:3218-3223.

dFdCyd for 24 h or 30 n*M* dFdCyd for 16 h) yielded enhancement ratios of approx 2.0. These concentrations of the drug appear to only have effects on the pool of dATP; however, higher concentrations of the drug that impact the intracellular levels of dGTP and dCTP do not appear to correlate with further increases in radiosensitization. The authors concluded that dATP depletion is an important factor in the radiosensitizing nature of gemcitabine.

The group from the University of Michigan also looked at radio sensitization with this compound in the pancreatic cancer cell lines, Panc-1 and BxPC-3 *(19)*, which are known to differ in their endogenous nucleotide pools by a factor of 10. Although they found that the Panc-1 cell line was significantly more resistant to the cytotoxic effects of gemcitabine as a single agent, they did find that an equivalent degree of sensitization to radiation occurred using 10 n*M* in the BxPC-3 cells and 100 n*M* Panc-1 cells (these conditions did not lead to appreciable drug-alone-related cytotoxicity). This sensitization lead to enhancement ratios of 1.7–1.8 and was significant after 16 h of treatment. The authors reported that, while the Panc-1 cells accumulated significantly higher levels of dFdCTP, there was no increased sensitization to radiation seen. They felt confident in concluding that dFdCTP levels were not the primary determinant of radiation sensitivity in this interaction. They went on to look at the effects of gemcitabine on intracellular nucleotide pools and found that under conditions where significant radiosensitization occurred the levels of 2'-deoxythymidine 5'-triphosphate (dTTP), dCTP, and dGTP were minimally affected; however, there was a profound decrease in dATP levels to even less than 1% of control values (Fig. 4). When lower concentrations of the drug that did not evoke significant radiosensitization were tested, there was not such a marked effect on dATP levels and the authors went on to suggest that the intracellular decrease in dATP levels is intimately linked to the RERs seen when gemcitabine is used in combination with radiation. They went on further to suggest that this gemcitabine effect on intracellular nucleotide levels is seen with other radiosensitizing nucleoside analogs including: fluorodeoxyuridine *(16)*, which deceases sublethal damage repair and depletes dTTP and increase dATP pools, and bromodeoxyuridine *(16)*, which decreases repair of radiation-induced DNA damage and also decreases dCTP and dTTP pools.

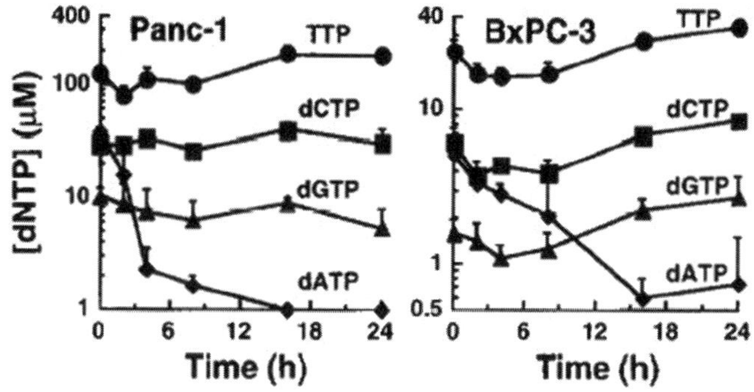

Fig. 4. The effect of gemcitabine on dNTP pools in human pancreas cells. Panc-1 and BxPC-3 cells were exposed for 2–24 h to 100 or 10 n*M*, respectively. Cells were then assessed for intracellular dNTP pools. From ref. *21*.

The degree of sensitization achieved also appears to be profoundly affected by the cell-cycle phase. It is well established that cells in S phase are much more radioresistant than cells in other phases of the cell cycle *(28)*. Interesting results from Latz et al. show quite clearly that cells that are pretreated with gemcitabine no longer show a progressive increase in radioresistance as they move toward DNA replication and therefore sensitization appears to be greatest in S phase *(21)*.

Gemcitabine's radiosensitizing abilities also appear to be rooted in its ability to lower the threshold for radiation-induced apoptosis to occur *(1)*. Apoptosis, or programmed cell death, is distinguished by specific cytologic features. There is also evidence that gemcitabine treatment of RKO-P but not RKO-E6 cells leads to increased production of both Bax and *p53 (29)*, which are both pro-apoptotic proteins. Certainly this mechanism is seen with other cytotoxic drugs and radiation including paclitaxel *(30)*, which when given prior to a single treatment with radiation will increase the level of radiation-induced apoptosis that occurs, with the effect being dependent on the interval between the drug administration and radiation delivery. In vivo investigations discussed below show support for the role of apoptosis in the radiosensitization that occurs with gemcitabine. Supportive results suggest that one of the primary modes of action for gemcitabine's radiosensitizing abilities, its lowering of the apoptotic threshold, come from Belgium where Grégoire et al. have demonstrated that radiosensitization with either gemcitabine or fludarabine is not mediated by increased induction or repair inhibition of DNA double-stranded breaks *(18)*. In essence the current evidence supports the notion that gemcitabine mediated radiosensitization occurs through a combination of mechanisms that appear to include nucleotide pool perturbations, cell cycle redistribution, and reduction of the apoptotic threshold.

4.2. In Vivo

Although the body of preclinical literature examining the radiation–gemcitabine interaction is growing, there are a few in vivo studies that have built on the work done in cell culture. Joschko et al. from Australia published the first set of experiments looking at gemcitabine and radiation with a human tumor xenograft model using Balb C athymic nude mice and xenografts created from the injection of FaDu cells isolated from a human hypopharyngeal tumor *(31)*. They looked at various schedules of the delivery of gemcitabine with 40 Gy in 2 Gy fractions delivered twice daily on d 1–5 and

8–12 and assessed the efficacy of the various strategies using growth-delay studies as well as assessing apoptosis scores at specified time points. There was no significant enhancement of tumor regrowth seen with the daily dose schedule used by the investigators. They found that when gemcitabine was delivered once weekly at the maximum tolerated dose (MTD) (430 mg/kg/injection for the drug alone) with radiation that there was a regrowth delay enhancement seen. When the drug was delivered in a twice-weekly fashion at the MTD of 160 mg/kg, there was significant enhancement of radiation sensitivity as the regrowth enhancement ratio increased to 3.3 ± 0.5; however, there were 60% toxic deaths within the first three weeks. Significant enhancement was seen even when the twice-weekly dose was decreased to 100 and 50 mg/kg; however, there were still 33% and 22% toxic deaths, respectively. While tumors treated with both radiation and gemcitabine showed greater number of apoptotic cells than those treated with radiation alone, there was no enhancement of apoptosis over the level seen with the drug alone. The authors advise that while the twice-weekly schedule lead to radiosensitization of tumors, the toxicity seen even with drug levels significantly lower than the MTD of the drug on its own should cause investigators to proceed cautiously in their development of human dose schedules.

An interesting report of in vivo work looking at different scheduling schemes was also recently published wherein the authors have two major conclusions *(32)*. First of all they saw that for equal gemcitabine induced toxicity with once-weekly and twice-weekly drug regimens, the twice-weekly regimen produced significantly more radiation-induced mucosal sensitization when radiation was added to the drug delivery. From this observation they suggest that proper dose-finding studies likely need to be done with each particular drug–radiation combination before embarking on phase II trials. Their second observation was that the twice-weekly dosing schedule produced a higher therapeutic index with a greater antitumor effect than once-weekly dosing.

In a similar in vivo experiment performed in an attempt to find optimal scheduling of drug delivery in combination with radiation, Milas et al. *(33)* found the largest enhancement of growth delay when the drug was delivered 24–60 h before irradiation in mice bearing SA-NH (murine sarcoma model) tumors. Interestingly, the use of gemcitabine in combination with radiation also decreased the rate of developing lung metastases in those mice that attained durable local control from 73% in those treated with radiation alone to 40% in the combined modality group. This observation has been confirmed in a second study with a larger number of mice *(34)*. This preclinical work is supportive of the principles of combined modality therapy in that gemcitabine helped in minimizing the primary tumor burden and this translated into decreased systemic spread of tumor cells in a significant percentage of study animals.

These same authors also report a dose-dependent increase in the apoptotic rate after the administration of gemcitabine *(33)*, which they believe correlates with the elimination of the more radioresistant S phase population of cells and redistribution of the remaining cells into more radiosensitive compartments of the cell cycle. They also report in another study that reoxygenation of the resistant hypoxic fraction of tumor cells is also a mechanism for the action of gemcitabine *(34)*. Therefore, elimination of these S phase tumor cells may aid the radiation response by not only causing cell cycle synchronization but also by leading to reoxygenation of hypoxic cells.

The early clinical experience, which is described in greater detail in a later section of this chapter, lead clinical investigators to realize that gemcitabine, while able to significantly impact on tumor response, also appeared to lower the clinical threshold for the induction of pneumonitis. As such, Grégoire et al. undertook experiments to look at the lung tolerance *(35)* using a LD_{50} scheme where the dose of thoracic radiation, treating mice with radiation alone was compared to gemcitabine administration 3 and 48 h prior to irradiation. They found that the combined treatment with gemcitabine and radiation lead to a slight enhancement of the pulmonary effects of radiation with a dose modifying factor of approx 1.10. They suggest that the earlier death of mice treated with gemcitabine 3 h prior to irradiation might be due to an increase in esophagitis in this group although they did not have data to support this. They conclude that at least with single dose irradiation that gemcitabine minimally enhanced lung sensitivity to radiation, and they suggested that in order to avoid unexpected toxicities proper phase I/II trials be performed. Mason and the group from the MD Anderson Cancer Center *(34)* looked at the enhancement of the radiation effect in the normal jejunum and found there was a significant schedule-dependent increase in the effect of radiation with enhancement ratios of up to 1.46. They also caution that proper dose-finding studies need to be done prior to forging ahead with larger-scale clinical trials.

Overall the preclinical data derived from both in vitro and in vivo studies suggest that gemcitabine holds the potential to be a very potent and useful complementary treatment to be used with ionizing radiation. These studies as a whole suggest that it acts through several mechanisms including nucleotide pool perturbation, reduction of the apoptosis threshold, cell cycle redistribution, and possibly by the reduction of tumor cell hypoxia to increase the effectiveness of ionizing radiation at controlling malignant neoplasms.

5. EARLY CLINICAL EXPERIENCE

As the preclinical data have suggested, gemcitabine is indeed a potent radiosensitizer. There are notable case reports in the literature of normal tissue toxicities occurring in patients that are felt to be related either to the drug alone (e.g., acute interstitial pneumonitis) *(36,37)* or to the combination of gemcitabine and radiation. Radiation recall dermatitis is one of those toxicities reported to have occurred in relation to the combination of the two agents *(38,39)*. In one of the reported cases *(38)* a patient who had initial treatment with a lumpectomy, axillary node dissection, ipsilateral breast radiation, and adjuvant cyclophosphamide, methotrexate and 5-fluorouracil (CMF) chemotherapy for breast cancer presented 3 yr later with metastatic disease in the spine for which she received localized radiotherapy to the lumbosacral spine prior to starting systemic therapies. In the course of her illness she developed a confluent erythematous maculopapular rash on her back exactly corresponding to the area of the previous spine radiation within 2 wk of starting gemcitabine. This rash gradually receded with cessation of gemcitabine chemotherapy.

6. ONGOING CLINICAL EXPERIENCE

Although the systemic activity of gemcitabine has been examined in many tumor sites, the role of this drug in combined modality therapy remains undefined for a number of human tumors. The following is an overview of the current results of investigations involving gemcitabine in locally advanced tumors in combination with ionizing radiation.

Table 2
EORTC Gemcitabine Dose-Escalation Scheme

Dose level[a]	*Dose gemcitabine administered*	*Schedule of drug administration*	*Number of patients*
1	300 mg/m^2	d 1	3
2	300 mg/m^2	d 1, 15	3
3	300 mg/m^2	d 1, 15, 29	3
4	300 mg/m^2	d 1, 8, 15, 29	3
5	300 mg/m^2	d 1, 8, 15, 22, 29	3
6	300 mg/m^2	d 1, 8, 15, 22, 29, 36	3
7	450 mg/m^2	d 1, 8, 15, 22, 29, 36	3–6
8	600 mg/m^2	d 1, 8, 15, 22, 29, 36	3–6

[a]If unacceptable toxicity occurs with 300 mg/m^2, then the dose will be decreased to 200 mg/m^2 with the same intensification schedule.

6.1. Lung

The results of the initial reported clinical trial in the setting of the treatment of locally advanced NSCLC have had sobering effects on the oncologic community. Scalliet et al. *(40)* reported on their phase II experience conducted between October 1994 and August 1995. They enrolled eight patients in a protocol that planned to give gemcitabine in "full" doses of 1000 mg/m^2 weekly for 6 wk concurrently with thoracic radiation to a total dose of 60 Gy delivered in 2 Gy fractions daily for 6 wk. Of the eight treated patients, seven had a greater than 50% reduction in their primary tumors with four of five patients also responding in the nodes. These investigators also saw a parallel increase in toxicity. Three of the eight patients died of radiation-related toxicities and the other six patients suffered from either serious acute or chronic radiation side effects. There was no formal phase I data concerning drug and radiation dose or schedule prior to the start of this trial; however, this treatment approach proved to be unacceptable. A retrospective analysis *(41)* of the treatment fields revealed that they tended to be rather generous with the coverage of quite large primary tumors and prophylactic treatment of lymph node groups. It is generally felt that the large portals used in this trial may account for some of the excessive toxicity seen.

After this disappointing experience, investigators from the European Organization for Research and Treatment of Cancer (EORTC) have designed a phase I trial with an original escalation scheme *(42)* in order to more definitively examine the role of concurrent gemcitabine radiation for NSCLC. Given the impressive preclinical data shown earlier in this chapter that gemcitabine is a potent radiation sensitizer, it was felt that further trials were warranted prior to abandoning the use of the drug in a concurrent fashion. In this new trial (see schema in Table 2) several cohorts have been planned where the gemcitabine dosing (300 mg/m^2) is increased by adding to the number of weekly doses administered concurrently with radiation prior to escalating the dose of the chemotherapy. Additional constraints added to the trial in order to minimize toxicity include limiting the planning target volume to less than or equal to 2000 cm^3. The trial remains ongoing, and as of the last report the first six cohorts had been enrolled and in the first four cohorts there have been at least five partial or complete responses in 12 patients with only one case of significant acute pulmonary toxicity (RTOG Grade 3).

Table 3
Phase I and II Trials of Concurrent Gemcitabine and Radiation in Locally Advanced NSCLC

Study	*Chemotherapy details*	*Radiotherapy details*	*Number of patients*	*Toxicity*	*Response*	*Survival (months)*
Groen *(44)* (Phase I)	As outlined in Table 1	60 Gy delivered with concurrent chemo*	18 in cohorts 1–6	1 acute (Gr 3) sore throat, 4 late lung (Gr 2)	4 CR 7 PR 3 ?PR 3 SD 1 PD	N/A
Goss *(45)* (Phase I)	4 cycles IV Gem# + CDDP d 1, 8, 15 repeat d 28 Level 1-CDDP 20, Gem 150 mg/m^2, Level 2-CDDP 25, Gem 150 mg/m^2	60 Gy delivered concurrent with cycle 1 of chemo	9 total 3 level 1 6 level 2	Level 2 3/6 Gr 3-4 esophagitis, 2-Gr 3 skin reaction	N/A	8 of 9 alive at 80 wk of follow-up
Fossella *(46)* (Phase I)	IV Gem weekly × 7 wk starting at 125 mg/m^2 +4 cycles of Gem & CDDP	63 Gy delivered with concurrent 3D radiation	5 with 3D XRT 9 with 2D XRT	No grade 3 esophagitis 5 with Gr 3 esophagitis	2 PR, 2 SD 6 PR	Not reported

Blackstock *(47)* (Phase I/II)	Twice-weekly Gem during XRT q M and Th starting at 10 mg/dose	60 Gy conformal XRT delivered with concurrent chemo	14 total	2 Gr 3 esophagitis at 35 and 50 mg doses and 1 Gr 3 pneumonitis at 35 mg dosing	1 CR 10 PR 1 SD 1 PD	Not reported
Chrysofakis *(48)* (Phase I/II)	Weekly Gem and CDDP (15 mg/m^2) during XRT	60 Gy delivered with concurrent chemo	38 total esophagitis and neutropenia at 125 and 150 mg/m^2	Dose-limiting	24 PR	Not reported
Gonzales *(49)*	Weekly Gem during XRT (200–600 mg/m^2)	50 Gy with concurrent chemo	20 total		Not reported	Not reported
Vokes *(43)* (Phase II)	4 cycles: Cisplatin 80 mg/m^2 on d 1, 22, 43, 64 Gemcitabine 1250 mg/m^2 d 1, 8, 22, 29 600 mg/m^2 d 43, 50, 64, 71	66 Gy starts at d 43 with concurrent chemo	53 patients	49% Gr 3-4 esophagitis during concurrent phase	70% response rate	18.4 mo median survival

*The PTV is restricted to less than 2000 cm^3. $Gem^{\#}$ = gemcitabine, $^{@}$Cis = cisplatin.

This caution has been tempered by the results of a recent Cancer and Leukemia Group B (CALGB) study *(43)* that looked at concurrent chemoradiotherapy in a randomized phase II trial with three arms using the newer generation of chemotherapy agents with cisplatin. In this trial patients with inoperable stage III NSCLC with ECOG performance status 0 or 1 and no prior treatment entered the protocol and were randomized between the following arms: ARM 1—gemcitabine at a dose of 1250 mg/m^2 on d 1, 8, 22, and 29 and 600 mg/m^2 on d 43, 50, 64, and 71; ARM 2—paclitaxel at a dose of 225 mg/m^2 over 3 h on d 1 and 22 and 135 mg/m^2 on d 43 and 64; and ARM 3—vinorelbine at a dose of 25 mg/m^2 on d 1, 8, 15, 22, and 29 and 15 mg/m^2 on d 43, 50, 64, and 71. X-ray therapy (XRT) was initiated on d 43 at 200 cGy per fraction (total dose 66 Gy). Patients in all three arms received four cycles of cisplatin at 80 mg/m^2 on d 1, 22, 43, and 64. At the last report with 180 patients analyzed there were no statistical differences between the arms, although the patients treated on the cisplatin–gemcitabine arm appeared to have numerically superior outcomes in terms of median survival, 1-yr survival, and failure-free survival. The study investigators felt that this regimen was active in locally advanced NSCLC with acceptable toxicities (49% of patients experienced grade 3/4 esophagitis).

In a strategy that proposes to maximize radiation sensitization, Blackstock et al. at Wake Forest University have recently completed a phase I trial of twice-weekly gemcitabine and thoracic radiation *(47)*. The rationale for evaluating a twice-weekly dosing schedule was based on preclinical data suggesting gemcitabine possesses greater radiation-sensitizing activity if dosed more frequently. Lawrence et al., reporting data from the University of Michigan, have shown that the radiation-sensitizing effect of gemcitabine is lost 48–72 h after the drug is administered, leading the authors to suggest that a twice-weekly gemcitabine schedule may produce greater radiation sensitization than a less frequent dosing schedule *(20)*. Fields et al., evaluating gemcitabine and concurrent radiation in a squamous carcinoma xenograft, determined a twice-weekly dose of 100 mg/kg administered with radiation resulted in a greater antitumor effect than the same radiation given with a much higher once-weekly dose of 800 mg/kg *(32)*. A similar tumor growth delay with twice-weekly gemcitabine and radiation was observed in a colon adenocarcinoma xenograft in experiments performed by Blackstock et al. *(50)*. To date, the investigators at Wake Forest have enrolled 24 patients with stage IIIa/IIIb into a phase I/II study of twice-weekly gemcitabine and thoracic radiation. The gemcitabine was administered via a 30 min infusion twice-weekly for 6 wk concurrent with 60–66 Gy conformal thoracic radiation. Of the 24 patients entered, 17 were enrolled into the phase I portion of the study and were evaluable for toxicity. The dose-limiting toxicity at 50 mg/m^2 given twice-weekly (100 mg/m^2/wk) was grade III/IV esophagitis. The overall complete and partial response was an encouraging 88% and the median survival for the entire group was 18.0 mo. This study will soon enter phase II testing by the CALGB; patients will receive two cycles of induction gemcitabine and carboplatin followed by thoracic radiation to 70 Gy concurrent with twice-weekly gemcitabine at a dose of 35 mg/m^2 (70 mg/m^2/wk).

Several other small phase I or phase I/II studies looking at the concurrent administration of gemcitabine and radiation with or without other agents have been reported in abstract form (Table 3). In general these trials illustrate that gemcitabine can be safely administered with radiation in NSCLC patients. However, their small numbers and the fact that they are reported from only a few select institutions have not fully conquered the fears that many have about concurrent administration of this agent with radiation.

Table 4
Proposed RTOG Gemcitabine Dose-Escalation Schema

Level (Arm A)	*Gemcitabine dose ($mg/m^2/wk$)*	*Carboplatin dose (AUC)*	*Number of patients*
0	300	—	3–6
1A	300	2	3–6
2A	450	2	3–6
3A	600	2	3–6
4A	750	2	3–6
5A	900	2	3–6
Level (Arm B)	*Gemcitabine dose ($mg/m^2/wk$)*	*Paclitaxel dose ($mg/m^2/wk$)*	*Number of patients*
1B	300	30	3–6
2B	450	30	3–6
3B	450	40	3–6
4B	600	40	3–6
5B	600	50	3–6
6B	750	50	3–6
7B	900	50	3–6

Currently, the RTOG is planning what may serve to be the definitive dose finding trial in the area of concurrent gemcitabine and radiation *(1)*. This will be a two-arm phase I trial where one arm will be treated with carboplatin, gemcitabine, and concurrent radiation to a total dose of 63 Gy. While toxicity evaluations are occurring with patients in arm 1, new patients will be entered on the second arm where they will be treated with paclitaxel, gemcitabine, and radiation to 63 Gy. The proposed dose-escalation scheme is seen in Table 4. This trial will ultimately prove to be key to future efforts to incorporate gemcitabine into combined modality therapy with radiation in NSCLC.

6.2. Head and Neck

The limited experience to date in this tumor site combining external beam radiation with gemcitabine spans a variety of treatment strategies and dosing schemes. In phase I data from Jaremtchuk et al., patients with locally advanced (unresectable) head and neck cancer received increasing doses of weekly gemcitabine starting at a dose of 100 mg/m^2 *(51)*. Radiation was delivered using standard fractionation to a total dose of 70 Gy given over 7 wk. Owing to unacceptable grade IV mucositis observed in the first patient cohort, resulting in a subsequent dose deescalation, the MTD determined in this trial was 75 mg/m^2. The trial was again modified to allow for the administration of amifostine, a thiol-containing compound that protects against radiation-induced xerostomia and mucositis. The MTD for gemcitabine in the ongoing amended study has not been determined; patients have been successfully treated at the 100 mg/m^2 dose level and accrual continues at 125 mg/m^2. Although the data are preliminary, the investigators have observed complete and or partial response in 21 of the 23 patients enrolled thus far. Comparable results from a similar study evaluating single agent gemcitabine and radiation have been reported by Wildfang et al. *(54)*. Gemcitabine was delivered weekly at an initial dose of 200 mg/m^2 concurrent with either 70 Gy in patients with untreated disease or 26–40 Gy in patients previously treated. The authors report a response rate of 80% in previously untreated patients and conclude that weekly gemcitabine at a dose of 100 mg/m^2 and full dose radiation was tolerable. The results of a very important study evaluating concurrent gemcitabine and radiation were recently reported by Eisbruch et al. *(55)*. Twenty-nine patients with unresectable head and neck cancer received a course of radiation (70 Gy over 7 wk) concurrent with weekly infusions of gemcitabine; range 300 mg/m^2 to 10 mg/m^2. The authors report severe acute and late mucosal and pharyngeal-related toxicities that required deescalation of the initial 300 mg/m^2 gemcitabine dose in successive patient cohorts. No dose-limiting toxicities were observed in patients at the 10 mg/m^2 dose level. Consistent with the prior studies, the rate of complete tumor response was an encouraging 66% to 87% seen in the various patient cohorts. As a laboratory correlative to this clinical trial, the investigators sought to assess whether the intracellular tumor incorporation levels of the active drug metabolite, 2',2'-difluoro-2'-deoxycytidine triphosphate (dFdCTP), were compatible with levels that cause radiosensitization in vitro. In this effort, tumor biopsies were performed in patients after the first infusion of gemcitabine prior to all radiation and the intracellular concentrations of dFdCTP were determined. Although the authors report a trend toward higher amounts of dFdCTP at the 300-mg/m^2 compared with the 50- and 150-mg/m^2 dose levels, the difference in the average values among the three doses was not statistically significant. As suggested by the authors, these data indicate that gemcitabine is a potent radiosensitizer at concentrations well below cytotoxic levels.

Gemcitabine delivered concurrently with other chemotherapeutic agents and radiation has also been evaluated in limited studies. Benasso et al. have reported the preliminary results of a phase II study of concurrent gemcitabine, cisplatin, and radiation in a cohort of 14 patients with either stage IV or recurrent squamous cell carcinoma of the head and neck *(56)*. The treatment regimen consisted of cisplatin (20 mg/m^2) administered on d 1–5 during the first and fifth week with gemcitabine (800 mg/m^2) given on d 5, 12, 19, 33, 40, and 47 of therapy. Patients received standard radiation to doses in the range of 60–64 Gy during wk 2–4 and 6–8 of the concurrent chemotherapy. Although a complete response was seen in 85% of patients, significant gemcitabine dose modifications were required and toxicity was significant. Grade III/IV neutropenic fevers, anemia, and mucositis was seen in 57%, 29%, and 100% of patients, respectively. Two patients died of acute hemorrhages within 1 mo of completing therapy. Clearly this strategy attempting to incorporate full dose gemcitabine with weekly cisplatin and radiation in patients with head and neck cancer will require future dose/scheduling modifications to reduce toxicity. Investigators from the University of Chicago/Michael Reese Hospital have also recently reported the early results of their phase I/II trial evaluating concurrent radiation, gemcitabine, 5-fluorouracil, and paclitaxel *(57)*. As part of the phase I study, patients received increasing doses of gemcitabine, starting at 50 mg/m^2 then escalated in 50 mg/m^2 increments. Thus far, 18 patients with either recurrent or locally advanced cancers of the head and neck have been entered into the trial. Grade III/IV neutropenia was seen in five patients, while grade III and IV mucositis was seen in eight and four patients, respectively. In the 14 patients evaluable for response, a complete and/or partial response was observed in 10 patients. The investigators determined that toxicity was unacceptable at the 150 mg/m^2 dose level and have elected to reduce the number of cycles of gemcitabine given with radiation and continue to dose escalate.

In our review of the available data, concurrent gemcitabine and radiation possesses high activity in the treatment of advanced cancers of the head and neck. Unfortunately, the toxicity of this combination also appears to be significant. Strategies to reduce toxicity are needed in future clinical trials evaluating this combination.

6.3. Gastrointestinal

The treatment of pancreatic cancer continues to be challenging. Standard treatment with 5-FU-based regimens and radiation has resulted in 5-yr survival rates of 15–20%. In locally advanced and metastatic patients, the median survival is less than 10 mo. As such, investigators have tried to improve outcomes by incorporating novel agents like gemcitabine into therapy (Table 5).

During the 2000 American Society of Clinical Oncology meeting, the Wilkowski group presented their results on radiochemotherapy with gemcitabine and 5-FU for treatment of locally advanced pancreatic cancer. Patients received one cycle of GEM/cisplatin before and three cycles subsequent to radiation. (Gemcitabine 1000 mg/m^2 and cisplatin 50 mg/m^2 on d 1, and 15, q 29 days.) Thirteen patients were treated with concurrent radiotherapy including gemcitabine (300 mg/m^2, on radiation d 1, 15, and 29) and 5-FU (350 mg/m^2 continuous infusion). Radiation therapy fields included the pancreatic tumor and regional lymph nodes. The dose delivered was 45 Gy at 1.8 Gy per fraction. Among 12 evaluable patients, 42% showed clinical complete response (cCR), and 33% showed clinical partial response (cPR). While downstaging was shown in 70% (7/10) of patients, resectability as the primary goal of the trial was achieved in 5/13 (38%) patients (four R0-resection, one R1-resection) *(58)*.

The Kentucky group reported the results of their phase I/II dose escalation study. Gemcitabine was delivered at a dose of 50 mg/m^2 over 24 h with radiation. The dose was increased in 50 mg/m^2 increments. The radiation dose was 40 Gy plus a boost at 1.8 Gy fractions. The clinical tumor response was evaluable in 12 unresectable patients. Five patients had a cCR of (42%), four patients (33%) had cPR after being treated with gemcitabine and radiation concurrently *(59)*. Other ongoing phase I studies also found the concomitant delivery of GEM and radiation to be feasible *(60–63)*.

At Emory, a phase I/II study led by Landry et al. demonstrated that neoadjuvant treatment with gemcitabine/cisplatin/5-FU for two cycles followed by accelerated hyperfractionated radiation (1.5 Gy bid to 49.5 Gy) with continuous infusion 5-FU (225 mg/m^2) in advanced GI malignancies was feasible. The authors reported an encouraging 45% response rate (one cCR, one pCR) in 11 locally advanced pancreatic cancer patients. The maximum tolerated dose of gemcitabine with this combination regimen was 175 mg/m^2 on d 1 and 5 of a 5-d regimen for two cycles *(64)*. The combination regimen is now part of a randomized phase II trial being conducted by the Eastern Cooperative Oncology Group (ECOG).

Blackstock et al. reported a promising radiation–gemcitabine regimen in a phase I study. A dose of twice-weekly gemcitabine at 40 mg/m^2 for 5 wk concurrent with 50.4 Gy of radiation to the pancreas was tolerable in pancreatic cancer patients with a 20% response rate in 15 evaluable patients. Three out of eight patients with a minimum of 12 mo follow up were alive *(65)*. Based on these data, Cancer and Leukemia Group B (CALGB) conducted a phase II trial to examine the efficacy of concurrent twice-weekly Gemcitabine (40 mg/m^2) and radiation (50.4 Gy) treatment regimen in patients with locally advanced pancreatic cancer. The preliminary result showed 55% of the

Table 5
Gemcitabine-Based Chemoradiation for Pancreatic Cancer

Regimen	*Results*	*Ref.*
Phase I/II: Gemcitabine + RT (50.4 Gy)	Gemcitabine 40 mg/m^2 twice weekly with RT is well tolerated, median survival 7.9 mo	Blackstock, personal communication Blackstock, personal communication
Phase I/II: Gemcitabine + RT (40 Gy ± boost)	42% (5/12) cCR, 33% (4/12) cPR, no late toxicity	*(59)*
Phase I/II: Gemcitabine + Cisplatin + 5-FU + RT (49.5 Gy 1.5 Gy bid) → Surg	45% (5/11) response rate (1 cCR, 1 pCR)	*(64)*
Gemcitabine + Cisplatin RT + Gemcitabine + 5-FU → Gemcitabine + Cisplatin	12 patients, 42% cCR, 33% cPR 70% (7/10) downstaging 38% (5/13) become resectable (4 R0-resection, 1 R1-resection)	*(58)*
Pilot protocol: Post-op: RT (45–54 Gy) + 5-FU → Gemcitabine	Gemcitabine after Post-op ChemoRT is feasible	*(60)*
Phase I: Pre-op Gemcitabine + RT (50.4 Gy) + Post-op Gemcitabine	Surgical resection rate 68% Median survival 19 mo MTD 600 mg/m^2	
Phase I: Cisplatin + Gemcitabine + RT (45 Gy)	The MTD has not been reached	*(63)*
Phase I: Gemcitabine + RT (50.4 Gy)	The MTD has not been reached	*(62)*

patients completed the chemoradiation portion of the study without treatment delays. With a median follow-up of 10 mo, the median overall and failure-free survival was 7.9 mo and 5.7 mo, respectively. Of 38 evaluable patients, 25 had pretreatment CA 19-9 above 75 % and of these, 17 experienced a greater than 75% decrease during treatment. (Blackstock, personal communication.)

At Fox Chase, Hoffman et al. recently completed a phase I dose-escalation study of GEM given weekly with radiation therapy to 50 Gy preoperatively in marginally resectable pancreatic cancer. They treated 25 patients on the protocol, three patients at 300 mg/m^2, six at 400 mg/m^2, six at 500 mg/m^2, five at 600 mg/m^2, and five at 700 mg/m^2. Gemcitabine was given weekly over 30 min with the radiation (field size was 3 cm area around the gross tumor volume to 39.6 Gy, then reduced to 2 cm margin for the last 10.8 Gy for a total dose of 50.4 Gy). Seventeen patients underwent surgical resections (68%). Toxicities were primarily mild hematologic, but there was one localized perforation of a gastric ulcer in a patient who was very malnourished at 400 mg/m^2 and one patient at 700 mg/m^2 developed a two unit bleed from gastritis. These (the perforated and the bleeding ulcers) were in the treatment fields and happened 2–3 wk after radiation completion. The second toxicity at 700 mg/m^2, which defined the MTD, was thrombocytopenia (51,000) on two occasions during radiation, necessitating drug withholding twice. There was one in hospital postoperative death from a myocardial infarction 3 mo after resection. The median survival of those resected was 19 mo. The recommended phase II dose of gemcitabine is 600 mg/m^2. This trial supports gemcitabine as a potent radiation sensitizer resulting in an increased median survival and surgical resection rate. (Personal communications, John Hoffman, ECOG meeting July 2000.)

Gemcitabine has displayed activity in other aerodigestive tract malignancies such as both small- and nonsmall-cell lung cancer and squamous cell carcinoma of the head and neck. Given this information, it was logical to study this agent in esophageal carcinoma. In a phase II study, Sandler et al. observed no response in 17 evaluable patients with chemonaive metastatic esophageal carcinoma at a dose of 1250 mg/m^2 given over 30–60 min on d 1, 8, and 15 followed by 1 wk of rest with a maximum of six cycles *(66)*.

The reports of phase II trials of gemcitabine in other GI tumors except for pancreatic cancer have likewise been less encouraging. Abbruzzese et al. reported no major responses in advanced colorectal cancer when treating with gemcitabine at a dosage of 800 mg/m^2 three times a week *(67)*. Other phase II studies also showed gemcitabine had little antitumor activity (3%–4%) in colorectal cancer *(68,69)*. In two phase II studies of gemcitabine (800 mg/m^2–1000 mg/m^2 weekly) in patients with gastric cancer, the response rates ranged from 0% to 4%. At this tested schedule, the drug has no relevant antitumor activity in gastric cancer *(70,71)*. Gemcitabine does however show activity against advanced hepatocellular carcinoma and cholangiocarcinoma. In phase II studies, the response rate seems to be particularly promising with up to a 25% response and low toxicity profile *(72–74)*. In a Taiwanese study of hepatocellular carcinoma (HCC) patients, 28 patients with unresectable and nonembolizable HCC received gemcitabine 1250 mg/m^2 weekly × 3 q 4 wk. A 17.8 % response rate was seen but the response duration was short-lived *(73)*. Fuloria et al. obtained a response rate of 25% by adding cisplatin to gemcitabine *(75)*. Weissmann et al. using intraarterial gemcitabine 1200 mg/m^2 for eight cholangiocarcinoma patients found a 25% response rate in their pilot phase II study. This study showed that intra-arterial administration is feasible and well tolerated *(74)*. Given the overall lack of impressive activity in advanced disease in these disease sites there has not been a great impetus to pursue combined modality therapy treatment that might incorporate gemcitabine in locally advanced disease.

Based on the promising phase I/II result from Landry et al., ECOG is planning a randomized phase II study to compare gemcitabine with radiation vs gemcitabine/cisplatin/5-FU followed by radiation and 5-FU in marginally resectable pancreatic carcinoma patients. The Radiation Therapy Oncology Group (RTOG) study 9704 is a phase III study of postoperative adjuvant treatment of resected pancreatic carcinoma evaluating postoperative chemoradiation (50.4 Gy + 5-FU at 250 mg/m^2/d), preceded and followed by systemic chemotherapy with randomization to either 5-FU or gemcitabine. This trial will evaluate whether there is a survival advantage to giving gemcitabine compared to 5-FU in patients with resectable pancreatic cancer. To determine the pharmacokinetics of gemcitabine concurrent with radiation treatment, the NCI has initiated a phase II study of neoadjuvant intraperitoneal gemcitabine and intravenous gemcitabine with radiation followed by surgery and adjuvant intraperitoneal gemcitabine, intravenous gemcitabine, and 5-FU in patients with advanced pancreatic cancer.

Gemcitabine has proven activity in the treatment of pancreatic cancer, in terms of clinical benefit, response rate, and survival, and is rapidly becoming the standard therapy for advanced pancreatic cancer worldwide. Optimizing the treatment schedule both in single-agent and combination therapy deserves high priority. Gemcitabine seems to be a potent radiosensitizer; there are ongoing trials in which it is combined with radiation. Preliminary phase I and II clinical results show that concurrent gemcitabine and radiation is feasible and promising. However, the optimal schedule for concomitant delivery of drug and radiation remains to be determined.

6.4. Other Sites

In general little has been published on the use of this drug in combined modality therapy in other disease sites. Of note is one phase II study from Thailand showing that the external beam portion of treatment with radiation and gemcitabine (iv weekly 300 mg/m^2) yielded very high response rates (17 of 19 CRs) with minimal morbidity in stage IIIB carcinoma of the cervix. These very early results are encouraging *(76)*. Ultimately, the role of this drug and its administration with radiotherapy in other potentially curable diseases is undefined at this moment.

7. CONCLUSIONS AND THE FUTURE

Ultimately the future of combined modality therapy looks bright for several of the major tumor sites. The role of gemcitabine in combination with radiation remains to be determined in many malignancies largely because trials have progressed slowly because of the initial clinical experience with this combination. Oncologists will hopefully have learned from the initial worrisome experience in lung cancer that proper phase I trials designed with an understanding of the interaction between radiation and the drug in question really need to be undertaken prior to starting novel therapies. The current series of ongoing trials will help determine the ultimate utility of the gemcitabine and radiation combination. It is hoped that the results of preclinical studies showing the potency of gemcitabine's radiosensitizing properties will be realized while normal tissue toxicities can be minimized.

REFERENCES

1. Choy H. Combination chemoradiotherapy with gemcitabine: potential applications. *Oncology (Huntingt)* 2000; 14(7 Suppl 4):20–25.
2. Plunkett W, Huang P, Xu YZ, Heinemann V, Grunewald R, Gandhi V. Gemcitabine: metabolism, mechanisms of action, and self-potentiation. *Semin Oncol* 1995; 22(4 Suppl 11):3–10.
3. Heinemann V, Hertel LW, Grindey GB, et al. Comparison of the cellular pharmacokinetics and toxicity of 2',2'-difluorodeoxycytidine and 1-beta-D-arabinofuranosylcytosine. *Cancer Res* 1988; 48(14):4024–4031.
4. Grunewald R, Abbruzzese JL, Tarassoff P, et al. Saturation of 2',2'-difluorodeoxycytidine 5'-triphosphate accumulation by mononuclear cells during a phase I trial of gemcitabine. *Cancer Chemother Pharmacol* 1991; 27(4):258–262.
5. Abbruzzese JL, Grunewald R, Weeks EA, et al. A Phase I clinical, plasma and cellular pharmacology study of gemcitabine. *J Clin Oncol* 1991; 9:491–498.
6. Grunewald R, Kantarjian H, Du M, et al. Gemcitabine in leukemia: a phase I clinical, plasma and cellular pharmacology study. *J Clin Oncol* 1992; 10:406–413.
7. Bouffard DY, Laliberte J, Momparler RL. Kinetic studies on 2',2'-difluorodeoxycytidine (Gemcitabine) with purified human deoxycytidine kinase and cytidine deaminase. *Biochem Pharmacol* 1993; 45(9):1857–1861.
8. Plunkett W, Ghandi V, Chubb S, et al. 2',2'-difluorodeoxycytidine metabolism and mechanism of action in human leukemia cells. *Nucleosides Nucleotides* 1989; 8:775–785.
9. Heinemann V, Xu YZ, Chubb S, et al. Inhibition of ribonucleotide reduction in CCRF-CEM cells by 2',2'-difluorodeoxycytidine. *Mol Pharmacol* 1990; 38(4):567–572.
10. Huang P, Chubb S, Hertel LW, et al. Action of 2',2'-difluorodeoxycytidine on DNA synthesis. *Cancer Res* 1991; 51(22):6110–6117.
11. Huang P, Plunkett W. Induction of Apoptosis by Gemcitabine. *Sem Oncol* 1995; 22(4, Suppl 11): 19–25.
12. Huang P, Plunkett W. Fludarabine and gemcitabine induced apoptosis: Incorporation of analogs into DNA is a critical event. *Cancer Chemother Pharmacol* 1995; 36:181–188.
13. Hui YF, Reitz J. Gemcitabine: A cytidine analogue active against solid tumors. *Am J Health-Sys Pharm* 1997; 54:162–170.
14. Rothenberg ML, Moore MJ, Cripps MC, et al. A phase II trial of gemcitabine in patients with 5-FU-refractory pancreas cancer. *Ann Oncol* 1996; 7(4):347–353.
15. Burris HA, Moore MJ, Andersen J, et al. Improvements in survival and clinical benefit with gemcitabine as first-line therapy for patients with advanced pancreas cancer: a randomized trial. *J Clin Oncol* 1997; 15(6):2403–2413.
16. Gregoire V, Hittleman WN, Rosier JF, et al. Chemo-radiotherapy: Radiosensitizing nucleoside analogues (Review). *Oncol Reports* 1999; 6:949–957.
17. Milas L, Fujii T, Hunter N, et al. Enhancement of tumor radioresponse in vivo by gemcitabine. *Cancer Res* 1999; 59(1):1-7–114.
18. Gregoire V, Beauduin M, Bruniaux M, et al. Radiosensitization of mouse sarcoma cells by fludarabine (F-ara-A) or gemcitabine (dFdC), two nucleoside analogues, is not mediated by an increased induction or a repair inhibition of DNA double-strand breaks as measured by pulsed-field gel electrophoresis. *Int J Radiat Biol* 1998; 73(5):511–520.
19. Lawrence TS, Chang EY, Hahn TM, et al. Radio sensitization of pancreatic cells by 2',2'-difluro-2'-deoxycytidine. *Int J Rad Onc Biol Phys* 1996; 34:867–872.
20. Lawrence TS, Chang EY, Hahn TM, Shewach DS. Delayed radiosensitization of human colon carcinoma cells after a brief exposure to 2',2'-difluoro-2'-deoxycytidine (Gemcitabine). *Clin Cancer Res* 1997; 3(5):777–782.
21. Latz D, Fleckenstein K, Eble M, Blatter J, Wannenmacher M, Weber KJ. Radiosensitizing potential of gemcitabine (2',2'-difluoro-2'-deoxycytidine) within the cell cycle in vitro. *Int J Radiat Oncol Biol Phys* 1998; 41(4):875–882.
22. Mose S, Karapetian M, Juling-Pohlit L, et al. Radiation enhancement of gemcitabine in two human squamous cell carcinoma cell lines. *Anticancer Res* 2000; 20(1A):401–405.
23. Rosier JF, Beauduin M, Bruniaux M, et al. The effect of 2'-2' difluorodeoxycytidine (dFdC, gemcitabine) on radiation-induced cell lethality in two human head and neck squamous carcinoma cell lines differing in intrinsic radiosensitivity. *Int J Radiat Biol* 1999; 75(2):245–251.

24. Zhang XL, Yang SJ, Ashamalla H, et al. Gemcitabine induced radio sensitization of human breast cancer cells. *Pro Am Soc Clin Oncol* 1998; 17:abstract 1732.
25. Ostruszka LJ, Shewach DS. Gemcitabine and radio sensitization in two glioblastoma cells lines. *Proc Amer Soc Cancer Res* 1998; 39:abstract 2599.
26. Rockwell S, Grindey GB. Effect of 2'-2' difluorodeoxycytidine on the viability and radiosensitivity of EMT6 cells in vitro. *Oncol Res* 1992; 4:151–155.
27. Shewach DS, Hahn TM, Chang E, et al. Metabolism of 2'-2' difluorodeoxycytidine and Radiation Sensitization of Human Colon carcinoma cells. *Cancer Res* 1994; 54:3218–3223.
28. Tannock IF, Hill RP. The Basic Science of Oncology 3rd Edition. McGraw-Hill. St. Louis. 1998, pp. 295–419.
29. Chen M, Hough AM, Lawrence TS. The role of p53 in gemcitabine-mediated cytotoxicity and radiosensitization. *Cancer Chemother Pharmacol* 2000; 45(5):369–374.
30. Milas l, Milas MM, Mason KA. Combination of Taxanes with radiation: preclinical studies. *Sem Rad Oncol* 1999; 9(2, Suppl 1):12–26.
31. Joschko MA, Webster LK, Groves J, et al. Enhancement of radiation-induced regrowth delay by gemcitabine in a human tumor xenograft model. *Radiat Oncol Investig* 1997; 5(2):62–71.
32. Fields MT, Eisbruch A, Normolle D, et al. Radiosensitization produced in vivo by once- vs. twice-weekly 2'2'-difluoro-2'-deoxycytidine (gemcitabine). *Int J Radiat Oncol Biol Phys* 2000; 47(3):785–791.
33. Milas L, Fujii T, Hunter N, et al. Enhancement of tumor radioresponse in vivo by gemcitabine. *Cancer Res* 1999; 59(1):107–114.
34. Mason KA, Milas L, Hunter NR, et al. Maximizing therapeutic gain with gemcitabine and fractionated radiation. *Int J Radiat Oncol Biol Phys* 1999; 44(5):1125–1135.
35. Gregoire V, Cvilic S, Beauduin M, De Coster B, Gueulette J, Octave-Prignot M, Scalliet P. Effect of gemcitabine on the tolerance of the lung to single-dose irradiation in C3H mice. *Radiat Res* 1999; 151(6):747–749.
36. Attar EC, Ervin T, Janicek M, et al. Side effects of chemotherapy. Case 3. Acute interstitial pneumonitis related to gemcitabine. *J Clin Oncol* 2000; 18(3):697–698.
37. Pavlakis N, Bell DR, Millward MJ, et al. Fatal pulmonary toxicity resulting from treatment with gemcitabine. *Cancer* 1997; 80(2):286–291.
38. Burstein HJ. Side effects of chemotherapy. Case 1. Radiation recall dermatitis from gemcitabine. *J Clin Oncol* 2000; 18(3):693–694.
39. Castellano D, Hitt R, Cortes-Funes H, Romero A, Rodriguez-Peralto JL. Side effects of chemotherapy. Case 2. Radiation recall reaction induced by gemcitabine. *J Clin Oncol* 2000; 18(3): 695–696.
40. Scalliet P, Goor C, Galdermans D, et al. Gemzar (Gemcitabine) with thoracic radiotherapy—A phase II pilot study in chemonaive patients with advanced nonsmall-cell lung cancer (NSCLC). *Pro Am Soc Clin Oncol* 1998; 17:abstract 1923.
41. Vokes EE, Gregor A, Turrisi AT. Gemcitabine and radiation therapy for non-small cell lung cancer. *Semin Oncol* 1998; 25(4 Suppl 9):66–69.
42. Gregor A. Gemcitabine plus radiotherapy for non-small cell lung cancer. *Semin Oncol* 1997; 24(3 Suppl 8):S8-39–S8-41.
43. Vokes EE, Leopold KA, Herndon JE, et al. CALGB Study 9431: A randomized phase study of cisplatin with gemcitabine or paclitaxel or vinorelbine as induction chemotherapy and concomitant chemoradiotherapy for unresectable stage III non-small cell lung cancer. *Lung Cancer* 2000; 29(S1):49(abstract 158).
44. Groen H, Gregor A, van Putten J, et al. Phase I study of gemcitabine(G) and high dose thoracic radiation (RT) in Stage III Non-Small Lung Cancer. *Pro Am Soc Clin Oncol* 2000; 19:abstract 2123.
45. Goss G, Lochrin C, Perry G, et al. A phase I study of gemcitabine and Cisplatin with concurrent curative irradiation in Stage III Non-small cell lung cancer (NSCLC). *Pro Am Soc Clin Oncol* 1999; 18:abstract 1986.
46. Fossella FV, Zinner RG, Komaki R, et al. Gemcitabine with concurrent chest radiation followed by consolidation chemotherapy with gemcitabine plus cisplatin: A phase I trial for patients with stage III non-small cell lung cancer. *Lung Cancer* 2000; 29(Suppl 1):111 (abstract 368).
47. Blackstock AW, Lesser G, Tucker G, et al. Twice-weekly gemcitabine and concurrent thoracic radiotherapy-a phase I/II study in patients with advanced nonsmall-cell lung cancer. *Pro Am Soc Clin Oncol* 2000; 19:47a (abstract 1846).

48. Varveris C, Lyraraki E, Kachris S, et al. Phase I/II study of gemcitabine combined to cisplatin weekly with concurrent thoracic MV-radiotherapy for patients with stage III A/B nonsmall-cell lung cancer. *Proc Am Soc Clin Oncol* 2000;19:537a (abstract 2116).
49. Gonzales E, Sanchez-Rovira P, Jaen A, Nobody A. Phase I study concomitant gemcitabine (G) with radiotherapy (RT) in stage III NSCLC. *Eur J Can* 1999; 35(Suppl 4):A1054.
50. Blackstock AW, Lightfoot H, Kwock L, Leadon SA, Hess S, Tepper JE. Gemcitabine: in vitro and in vivo evidence of its radiation sensitizing activity and studies using fluorine-19 magnetic resonance spectroscopy to determine the optimal dosing schedule-pre-clinical observations relevant to gemcitabine clinical trials. *Int J Radiat Oncol Bio Phys* 1997; 39:205.
51. Jaremtchuk V, Zarba JJ, Keropian M, Castagnino R, Gonzalez Jazey P. Low dose gemcitabine plus concurrent therapy with or without amifostine in locally advanced head and neck cancer. Proc of 11th NCI-EORTC-ACCR Symposium on New Drugs in Cancer Therapy, November 7-10, 2000 *Proc ASCO* 2000; 19:424a (abstract 1674).
52. McDonald S, Meyerowitz C, Smudzin T, Rubin P. Preliminary results of a pilot study using WR-2721 before fractionated irradiation of the head and neck to reduce salivary gland dysfunction. *Int J Radiat Oncol Biol Phys* 1994; 29:747–754.
53. Buntzel J, Kuttner K, Frohlich D, Glatzel M. Selective cytoprotection with amifostine in concurrent radiochemotherapy for head and neck cancer. *Ann Oncol* 1998; 9:505–509.
54. Wildfang I, Raub M, Guner SA, Rades D, Karstens JH. Low-dose gemcitabine with radiotherapy in advanced head and neck and thyroid cancer. *J Can Res Clin Oncol* 2000; 126:R:40.
55. Eisbruch A, Shewach DS, Bradford CR, et al. Radiation Concurrent With Gemcitabine for Locally Advanced Head and Neck Cancer: A Phase I Trial and Intracellular Drug Incorporation Study. *J Clin Oncol* 2001; 19:792–799.
56. Benasso M, Merlano M, Corvo R, Sanguineti G, Numico G, Di Costanzo G, Ricci I, Rosso R. Alternating/concomitant gemcitabine (GEM), cisplatin (CDDP) and radiotherapy (RT) in advanced squamous cell carcinoma of the head and neck (SCC-HN). *Proc ASCO* 1998; 17:403a (abstract 1552).
57. Humerickhouse R, Haraf D, Brockstein B, Gordon G, Dolan ME, Mansur D, Elahi R. Gemcitabine, 5-fluorouracil, and paclitaxel with concomitant radiotherapy in recurrent or advanced head and neck cancer. *Can Invest* 2000; 18:32–33.
58. Wilkowski R, Heinemann V, Rau H, et al. Radiochemotherapy including gemcitabine and 5-FU for treatment of locally advanced pancreatic cancer. *Proc Am Soc Clin Oncol* 2000; 19:276a.
59. Kudromoti M, Regine W, John W, et al. Concurrent infusional gemcitabine and radiation in the treatment of advanced unresectable GI malignancy: A phase I/II study. *Proc Am Soc Clin Oncol* 1999; 18:242a.
60. Friedman NS, Brenner MJ, Linder JA, et al. Adjuvant radiation and continuous 5-FU followed by gemcitabine as adjuvant treatment for resected pancreatic cancer. *Proc Am Soc Clin Oncol* 1999; 18:283a.
61. Hoffman JP, McGinn CJ, Szarka C, et al. A phase I study of preoperative gemcitabine with radiation therapy followed by postoperative gemcitabine for patients with localized resectable pancreatic adenocarcinoma. *Proc Am Soc Clin Oncol* 1998; 17:283a.
62. McGinn CJ, Smith DC, Szarka CE, et al. A phase I study of gemcitabine in combination with radiation therapy in patients with localized, unresectable pancreatic cancer. *Proc Am Soc Clin Oncol* 1998; 17:264a.
63. Safar AM, Altamiro PS, Recht A, et al. Phase I trial of gemcitabine, cisplatin and external beam radiation therapy for pancreatic cancer. *Proc Am Soc Clin Oncol* 1999; 18:227a.
64. Landry JC, Harris W Yang GY, et al. Neoadjuvant treatment with GEM, cisplatin, 5-FU and accelerated hyperfractionated radiation therapy in advanced GI malignancy. *Radiology* 2000; 217:147.
65. Blackstock AW, Bernard SA, Richards F, et al. Phase I trial of twice-weekly gemcitabine and concurrent radiation in patients with advanced pancreatic cancer. *JCO* 1999; 17:2208–2212.
66. Sandler AB, Kindler HL, Einhorn LH, et al. Phase II trial of gemcitabine in patients with previously untreated metastatic cancer of the esophagus or gastroesophageal junction. *Ann Oncol* 2000; 11: 1161–1164.
67. Abbruzzese JL, Pazdur R, Ajani J, et al. A phase II trial of gemcitabine in patients with advanced colorectal cancer. *Proc Am Soc Clin Oncol* 1991; 10:456.
68. Mani S, et al. Phase II trial of 150-minute weekly infusion of gemcitabine in advanced colorectal cancer: Minimal activity in colorectal cancer. *Invest New Drugs* 1998; 16:275.
69. Fink U, Molle B, Daschner H, et al. Phase II study of gemcitabine in metastatic colorectal cancer. *Proc Am Soc Clin Oncol* 1992; 11:173.
70. Christman K, Kelsen D, Saltz L, et al. Phase II trial of gemcitabine in patients with advanced gastric cancer. *Cancer* 1994; 73:5–7.

71. Sessa C, Aamdal S, Wolff I, et al. Gemcitabine in patients with advanced malignant melanoma or gastric cancer: phase II studies of the EORTC Early Clinical Trial group. *Ann Oncol* 1994; 5:471–472.
72. Dragovich T, Ramanathan, Remick S, et al. Phase II trial of a weekly 150-minute gemcitabine infusion in patients with biliary tree carcinomas. *Proc Am Soc Clin Oncol* 2000; 19:296a.
73. Yang TS, Lin YC, Chen JS, et al. Phase II study of gemcitabine in patients with advanced hepatocellular carcinoma. *Cancer* 2000; 89:750–756.
74. Weissmann A, Ludwig H. Intrarterial gemcitabine for treatment of inoperable pancreatic and cholangiocarcinoma. *Proc Am Soc Clin Oncol* 1999; 18:305a.
75. Fuloria JF, Parikh PM, Prabhakaran PS, et al. A multicenter, phase II trial of gemcitabine and cisplatin in unresectable hepatocellular carcinoma. *Proc Am Soc Clin Oncol* 2000; 19:29.
76. Pattaranutaporn P, Thirapakawong C, Chansilpa Y, et al. Study of concurrent gemcitabine and radiotherapy in locally advanced stage IIIB cervical carcinoma. *Pro Am Soc Clin Oncol* 2000; 19:390a (abstract 1545).

III Clinical Applications

7 Chemoradiation Strategies for Patients with Malignant Gliomas

Heather A. Curry, MD
and Walter J. Curran, Jr., MD

Contents

1. INTRODUCTION

Malignant glioma afflicts approx 10,000 patients per year in North America. Since the publication of the Brain Tumor Study Group (BTSG) 6901 study results in the late 1970s, the standard management of patients with malignant glioma has been maximal surgical resection without compromise of neurologic function, followed by postoperative cranial radiation therapy (RT) to 60 Gy with or without nitrosourea-based therapy *(1)*. The term malignant glioma includes a heterogeneous group of tumors including anaplastic astrocytoma (AA), glioblastoma multiforme (GBM), anaplastic oligodendroglioma (AO), anaplastic mixed tumors, and malignant glioma not otherwise specified. These histologies are associated with different responses to chemotherapy and radiation therapy (RT) as well as different natural histories and survival expectations. Typical median survival times (MSTs) with therapy for patients with GBM and AA with standard therapeutic approaches are 10–12 mo and 30–40 mo, respectively *(2)*. Genetic characteristics of primary brain tumors have been correlated with treatment response and clinical outcomes as shown by Cairncross et al., who demonstrated that allelic loss of chromosome 1p predicted increased response to chemotherapy and longer survival *(3)*. Despite

From: *Chemoradiation in Cancer Therapy*
Edited by: H. Choy

improvements in operative and perioperative management, radiotherapeutic techniques, and supportive measures, little progress has been made in prolonging survival for the majority of patients with malignant glioma. The purpose of this chapter is to review the literature on the combined modality treatment of patients with malignant glioma, focusing on the data from prospective randomized trials, and to briefly discuss future directions in research to improve outcome for patients affected by this disease.

2. RESULTS WITH SURGERY AND RADIATION THERAPY

In the late 1960s and early 1970s, several trials randomized patients to postoperative regimens containing cranial RT or to surgery alone. In both BTSG 6901 and the trial conducted by the Scandinavian Glioblastoma Study Group, there was a doubling or greater of MST favoring the RT-containing arms. These trials established the critical nature of using full-dose RT as a component of postoperative therapy. Additionally, BTSG 6901 and its successor trial BTSG 7201, demonstrated a small but statistically significant difference in survival favoring the arms containing RT and chemotherapy over RT alone. In these two trials, the MSTs for patients receiving combined therapy vs surgery alone were 35 and 16 wk and 44 and 21 wk, respectively. Unfortunately, no substantial improvements in survival have been observed since those trials.

The BTSG conducted a multicenter prospective randomized trial from 1969 to 1972 (Trial 6901) to evaluate the efficacy after surgery of BCNU as single-agent chemotherapy, radiotherapy, and the combination of BCNU and radiation compared to best supportive care *(1)*. A total of 303 patients were entered of whom 222 (73%) met protocol criteria and were considered the valid study group (VSG). Patients were divided into four random groups, and received BCNU (80 mg/m^2/d on three consecutive days every 6–8 wk), and/or whole brain radiation therapy using doses of 50–60 Gy, or best conventional care exclusive of adjuvant chemotherapy or radiotherapy. Analysis was performed on all eligible patients and also on the adequately treated group of patients (ATG), defined as those who had received radiotherapy consisting of 50 Gy or more, two or more courses of chemotherapy, and had a minimum survival of at least 8 wk (the time interval required to complete such treatment). Median survival of VSG patients was 14 wk with best supportive care, 18.5 wk with BCNU, 35.0 wk with radiotherapy, and 34.5 wk with radiotherapy and BCNU. In the ATG the comparable survivals by treatment group were 17.0 wk, 25.0 wk, 37.5 wk, and 40.5 wk, respectively. The improvement in MST seen in patients treated with BCNU only compared to those treated with supportive care was of marginal significance ($p = 0.119$). However, the addition of whole brain radiation, alone or in conjunction with BCNU, provided a statistically significant improvement in median survival time ($p = 0.001$). There was no apparent survival difference between patients receiving BCNU and radiotherapy vs radiotherapy alone; however, there was a significantly greater surviving fraction of patients at the end of 18 mo among those who received combination therapy (4% in the radiotherapy group vs 19% in the BCNU plus radiation group).

The Scandinavian Glioblastoma Study Group reported the results of a prospective randomized trial for patients with grades II–IV supratentorial astrocytoma to evaluate the results of radiation therapy and combined chemoradiation treatment in the postoperative setting *(4)*. One hundred eighteen patients were randomized to one of three groups:

1. Whole brain irradiation plus IV bleomycin.
2. Whole brain irradiation and IV placebo.
3. No postoperative chemotherapy or irradiation.

All eligible patients underwent maximal possible tumor resection, central pathologic review, and postoperative and posttherapy evaluation of functional status. Radiation therapy consisted of 45.0 Gy in 1.8 Gy fractions to the whole supratentorial brain. Bleomycin was administered in 15 mg doses iv 1 h before radiation on the first, third, and fifth day of the first, second, fourth, and fifth week of radiation for a cumulative dose of 180 mg. The median survival time was 10.8 mo in the two groups receiving postoperative therapy vs 5.2 mo in the patients treated with surgery only. The two groups of postoperatively treated patients showed almost identical results with respect to the number of patients surviving longer than 6 mo. A greater percentage of patients who received postoperative therapy achieved full or partial working capacity and the only patients to retain this level of function at 12 mo from the time of surgery were those who had received adjuvant therapy. This study confirmed that postoperative radiation therapy increases survival time and functional ability in patients with high-grade glioma, but failed to demonstrate an effect of bleomycin on survival.

3. TRIALS OF CHEMOTHERAPEUTIC AGENTS

With the importance of postoperative radiation therapy established, subsequent trials in the late 1970s and early 1980s focused on identifying chemotherapy agents with greater activity against malignant glioma. Phase III studies during this era produced the following results:

1. Postoperative BCNU offers an additional modest survival benefit to radiation therapy only (BTCG 7201 and 7501).
2. High-dose steroid use does not improve survival (BTCG 7501).
3. Procarbazine and streptozocin showed similar efficacy to BCNU (Trials 7501 and 7702).
4. Multiple-drug chemotherapy regimens consisting of various combinations of BCNU, hydroxyurea, procarbazine, and/or VM-26 (epipodophyllotoxin) showed no significant survival advantage over BCNU alone (BTCG 8001).

In a follow-up study to BTSG Trial 6901, the BTSG further evaluated the relative benefits of radiotherapy and nitrosureas and compared four treatment regimens: single-agent semustine chemotherapy, radiotherapy alone, carmustine plus radiotherapy, and the combination of semustine plus radiotherapy (BTSG 72-01) *(5)*. Radiotherapy consisted of 60 Gy in 30–35 fractions of 1.71–2.0 Gy over 6–7 wk. Semustine was given orally at a dose of 220 mg/m^2 every 6–8 wk. Carmustine was administered iv at a dose of 80 mg/m^2 on three successive days every 6–8 wk. For patients receiving combined modality treatment, the first cycle of chemotherapy was delivered during the first few fractions of radiation. Four hundred sixty seven patients were randomized of which 358 comprised the valid study group. Median survival time of VSG patients was 24 wk with semustine alone, 94 wk with radiation only, 92 wk with carmustine plus radiotherapy, and 91 wk with radiotherapy and semustine. The combination of semustine plus radiation did not show any advantage over carmustine plus radiation. Although statistical tests did not detect a significant improvement with combined modality therapy, the study results suggested a modest benefit for the combination of chemotherapy and radiotherapy over radiation alone as seen in the increased number of long-term survivors. At 18 mo 10% of the semustine only group was alive compared with 15.1%, 27.2%, and 23.3% of the radiation, RT plus carmustine, and RT plus semustine groups, respectively.

Trial BTSG 75-01 evaluated the role of high-dose corticosteroids on survival in patients with malignant glioma *(6)*. Six hundred nine patients with histologically documented supratentorial malignant glioma were treated with 60 Gy whole brain irradiation and randomized to one of four treatment arms:

1. Carmustine (BCNU) iv at a dose of 80 mg/m^2/d on three successive days every 8 wk.
2. High-dose methylprednisolone (400 mg/m^2/d orally in three divided doses).
3. Oral procarbazine (150 mg/m^2/d in three or four divided doses for 28 consecutive days every 8 wk).
4. BCNU plus high dose methylprednisolone.

Median survival was 50 wk in the BCNU arm, 41 wk in the methylprednisolone arm, 43 wk in the procarbazine arm, and 41 wk in the BCNU plus steroid arm. A significantly larger proportion of patients treated with procarbazine or BCNU were long-term survivors compared to those receiving high-dose steroids alone with 2-yr survival rates of 19.5%, 8%, 22%, and 18%, respectively.

Trial 8001 compared three chemotherapy regimens:

1. Single-agent BCNU (80 mg/m^2 iv for 3 d every 8 wk).
2. BCNU as in arm 1 alternating with procarbazine (150 mg/m^2 in three or four equally divided oral doses for 28 d) every 8 wk.
3. BCNU plus oral hydroxyurea (1000 mg/m^2 every other day for 21 d) alternating with procarbazine plus VM-26 (130 mg/m^2 iv weekly) *(7)*.

A secondary objective of the trial compared whole brain irradiation with a regimen involving some whole brain combined with a focal coned-down boost. Patients accrued in 1980 and 1981 received 60.2 Gy to the whole brain in 1.72 Gy fractions concurrent with the first course of chemotherapy. Patients accrued after that time were randomly assigned to either whole-brain irradiation as above or 43.0 Gy whole-brain irradiation plus a 17.2 Gy boost to the tumor volume as determined by the preradiation tumor volume on CT scan plus a 2 cm margin. The data were analyzed for the 571 randomized study population and separately for the 510 VSG patients who met all eligibility requirements. MSTs for the VSG group were 13.1 mo, 11.3 mo, and 13.8 mo in arms one through three, respectively; these differences were not statistically significant. Analysis of survival by assigned radiotherapy group showed no significant difference between the two arms, demonstrating that giving a portion of the radiotherapy by coned-down boost is as effective as full whole brain irradiation. As noted in previous trials, younger patient age, higher performance status, and anaplastic astrocytoma histology were all correlated with improved survival. Based upon this trial and the earlier studies conducted by the BTSG, the authors concluded the standard therapy for malignant glioma should be maximal tumor resection followed by combination whole brain and coned-down radiation plus chemotherapy with a nitrosurea.

Further support for the use of chemotherapy in patients with malignant glioma has been gleaned from meta-analyses. Using the results from 16 randomized clinical trials involving over 3000 patients, Fine et al. compared survival rates of patients who received radiation alone or radiation plus chemotherapy *(8)*. For patients treated on the evaluated trials with radiation only, median survival ranged from 7 to 34 mo, with a median of 9.4 mo. Patients receiving both radiation and chemotherapy had median survivals ranging from 7 to 46 mo with a median of 12 mo. Median survival time was longer in the radiation-only treatment arm by 1 mo or more in only one study, but was longer in the RT plus chemotherapy arm in 12 studies. The use of adjuvant chemotherapy resulted in a significant increase in the proportion of patients surviving at 12, 18, and 24 mo after resection. While the absolute survival benefit attributable to chemotherapy was small, 10.1% and 8.6% at 12 and 24 mo, respectively, the relative survival advantage was high at 23.4% and 52.4%, respectively, due primarily to the low overall survival of patients with malignant glioma. Patients with either AA or GBM histology derived a survival benefit from the use of adjuvant chemotherapy; however, the time until maximal benefit from chemotherapy was seen at 12–18 mo for patients with AA vs 18–24 mo for patients with GBM. The authors postulated that long-term survivors with GBM represent a more favorable group of patients who tend to be younger, have better performance status, and have a lower tumor burden and thus would be more likely to benefit from therapy. When the group of trials was analyzed by median age of patients and fitted into a model for survival advantage, an approx 5% survival benefit was seen for younger patients, defined as less than 50 yr of age. A more recent meta-analysis reported by Stewart et al. analyzed individual patient data for over 2300 patients treated on 10 randomized clinical trials comparing radiotherapy alone to radiotherapy plus chemotherapy, mostly nitrosureas *(9)*. The use of adjuvant chemotherapy translated into a 16% relative reduction in the risk of death at two years, which was equivalent to an absolute improvement of 5% (from 15 to 20%, $p = 0.001$). Also noted was a 6% improvement in freedom from relapse (from 10 to 16%). This benefit appeared to be independent of age, histology, Karnofsky performance status (KPS), or extent of resection.

4. RECURSIVE PARTITIONING ANALYSIS

Many factors have been identified as significant prognosticators in patients with malignant glioma, including patient age, tumor histology, tumor grade, seizure symptoms, duration of symptoms, tumor vascularity, patient performance status, type of surgery performed, radiation therapy, corticosteroid administration, and chemotherapy. The BTSG series and other studies included patients with a variety of histologies, ages, and other prognostic factors thus confounding the actual patient outcome attributable to specific therapeutic interventions. In a novel statistical approach the RTOG analyzed data available on 1578 patients entered into three malignant glioma trials from 1974 to 1989 *(2)*. The technique was used to identify subgroups with survival rates sufficiently different to create improvements in the design and stratification of patients within future trials. A series of decision trees was constructed by performing individual Wilcoxon tests analyzing patient-, tumor-, and treatment-related variables such as age, gender, race, symptom duration, neurologic class, KPS, tumor size, histology, tumor location, extent of surgery, RT dose, RT fraction size, and chemotherapy use. The entire patient set was treated as the primary node and was split if the modified Wilcoxon statistic was significant for any variable beyond the 0.05 probability level. Each split produced two similar subgroups with respect to survival outcome. Terminal node groups were defined as those with fewer than 25 patients or when no additional significant partitions could be made. Twelve terminal nodes were created and then amalgamated into six classes, each having a distinct survival profile.

The results of the recursive partitioning analysis displaying the 12 terminal nodes and their amalgamation into six classes are shown in Fig. 1. The first major nodal split was identified as patient age. For the 541 patients under age 50 the most significant split was

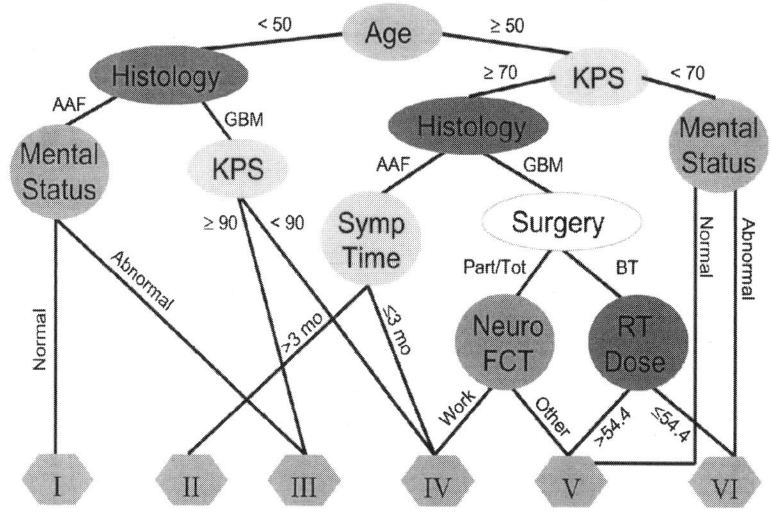

Fig. 1. Results of the recursive partitioning analysis showing the major nodal splits by prognostic factor and the amalgamation of terminal nodes into six distinct classes.

by histology, with anaplastic astrocytoma patients having a MST of 49.4 mo compared to 13.7 mo in the GBM patient population ($p < 0.000001$). Among the AA patients under 50 the only additional nodal split was seen when comparing normal vs abnormal mental status. GBM patients under 50 were further subdivided only by KPS. For the 1037 patients over 50 the primary split was defined by KPS, with a MST of 10.3 mo seen in those with a KPS 70 or more vs 5.3 mo in patients with KPS below 70. Patients with KPS below 70 were further split by normal vs abnormal mental status. Definition of the terminal nodes for patients with KPS above 70 was slightly more complex. The first split segregated patients by histology with MSTs of 21.7 mo for the AA patients and 9.7 mo for the GBM patients. AA patients were further divided only by duration of symptoms, whereas GBM patients were additionally divided by extent of surgery, neurologic function, and RT dose. The MSTs by patient classes ranged from 58.6 mo for the most favorable Class I patients (age < 50, AA histology, normal mental status) to 4.6 mo in the highly unfavorable group of Class VI patients (age >50, KPS <70, abnormal mental status). The validity of this statistical approach was further confirmed by updating the database, and this analysis technique has been utilized in other sites including nonsmall-cell lung cancer (NSCLC). This study has allowed identification of specific subgroups of patients with malignant glioma with similar prognoses so that clinical trials can be designed with comparable groups of patients and also serves as a benchmark of expected outcomes against which new therapeutic regimens can be measured.

5. SPECIFIC THERAPY CONSIDERATIONS IN NON-GBM MALIGNANT GLIOMAS

5.1. Anaplastic Astrocytoma

Nearly 25% of malignant glial neoplasms are of the AA histology with approx 2500 patients in the US diagnosed yearly *(10)*. The relative rareness of this disease makes accrual to clinical trials challenging. Histologic confirmation of the diagnosis and central pathologic review are essential in the design and interpretation of clinical studies. Many trials have included patients with all types of malignant glioma, the majority of which had GBM histology, thus complicating analysis of the impact of therapy in the subset of patients with AA histology.

Anaplastic astrocytomas are infiltrative in nature and lack clear borders on standard neuroimaging studies, thus making the extent of tumor difficult to define. Tumors are often associated with significant cerebral edema, indicating underlying tumor infiltration. Neurosurgical intervention for patients with presumed malignant glioma on the basis of radiographic appearance is appropriate to establish the histologic diagnosis and to relieve symptomatic mass effect; however, the clinical benefit of aggressive resection remains a subject of debate. Results from retrospective series are conflicting and there remains a lack of prospective studies to address this issue. Several retrospective studies have shown a benefit for resection vs biopsy among patients with malignant glioma, mostly showing an increase in progression-free survival but no improvement in overall survival *(2,11–16)*. Most of these studies included patients with malignant gliomas, the majority of whom had GBM histology. Winger et al. *(14)* found the extent of resection was of prognostic benefit in 285 patients with malignant glioma, 76 of whom had AA. Patients with AO had a median survival of 278 wk compared with 63 wk for AA and 32 wk for GBM. Of note they also observed the survival of patients with mixed OA to be similar to that of pure AA (MS = 7 wk). Curran et al. performed an independent analysis of AA patients treated with X-ray therapy (XRT) and BCNU on several RTOG protocols *(15)*. Among 103 AA patients, smaller tumor size and frontal location were found to favorably influence survival, even when stratified for age.

The role of adjuvant chemotherapy in the management of AA remains a topic of much debate. As discussed above, the first prospective randomized study to evaluate the use of BCNU (carmustine) in patients with malignant glioma was reported by the BTSG in 1978. Over 90% of the patients in that study had GBM histology. No significant advantage to the addition of carmustine to radiotherapy was seen *(1)*. The standard chemotherapy for AA is nitrosurea-based, but the issue of whether single-agent carmustine vs a multiagent regimen of procarbazine, CCNU (lomustine), and vincristine (PCV) is superior remains controversial. PCV had been considered the *de facto* standard after a report from the Northern California Oncology Group (NCOG) *(17)*, which demonstrated a survival advantage for patients with AA histology treated with PCV over BCNU. NCOG Protocol 6G61 compared the effects of following 60 Gy whole brain radiation and oral hydroxyurea treatment with either BCNU or the combination of procarbazine, CCNU, and PCV. This study included only a small number of selected patients with KPS between 70 and 100 and only those who completed at least one course of chemotherapy. Median survival was 157 wk in 36 AA patients treated with PCV vs 82 wk in 37 patients treated with BCNU ($p = 0.021$). A doubling of the median time to progression was also seen in the AA patients receiving PCV (125 wk vs 63 wk in the BCNU arm). GBM patients showed a slightly longer median survival and median time to progression with PCV treatment, however, this was not statistically significant. Recently, the Medical Research Council completed a study that randomized 674 patients with high-grade glioma to radiation or radiation and PCV *(18)*. No survival difference was observed. The difference in median survival of the AA cohort was 18 mo compared to previous study by NCOG of 36 mo has raised some concern over selection factors that might account for this discrepancy. A retrospective review using a matched-pair analysis of 422 AA patients treated on various RTOG protocols suggested that there was no advantage of PCV over BCNU, thus altering practice standards *(19)*. RTOG trial 9813 opened in June, 2000 and is a phase I/III randomized study designed to determine the appropriate dose and tolerance of combination BCNU and temozolomide and to compare the survival of patients with anaplastic astrocytoma treated with RT + BCNU to that achieved with RT + temozolomide. The superior treatment arm will then be compared to therapy with RT + BCNU + temozolomide.

5.2. Anaplastic Oligodendroglioma

The classic oligodendroglioma is characterized by a moderately cellular group of cells with round nuclei and perinuclear halos ("fried-egg" appearance) with branching or "chicken-wire" vasculature. These tumors were initially thought to be rare, comprising less than 5% of CNS tumors; however, it is becoming recognized that oligodendroglial tumors may represent a larger percentage of glial tumors than originally thought. Retrospective reviews of RTOG trials in malignant glioma have identified a significant number of patients with oligodendroglial tumors treated with surgery and radiation. The median survival time of these patients appears superior to that observed for patients with pure astrocytic tumors. In a review of RTOG 83-02 Donahue *(20)* noted patients with anaplastic pure or mixed oligodendrogliomas to have median survival of 7.3 yr vs 3.4 yr for pure anaplastic astrocytomas. On multivariate analysis, age, extent of surgery, and presence of an oligodendroglial component were all found to be independent prognostic factors for survival.

Molecular characterizations of oligodendroglial tumors have been reported. Smith *(21)* noted a significant correlation between 1p loss of heterozygosity, 19q loss of heterozygosity, and combined loss of 1p and 19q with an oligodendroglial phenotype in an analysis of 162 patients with diffuse glioma. Patients in the oligodendroglioma population who displayed combined loss of 1p and 19q had a prolonged overall survival even after correction for patient age and tumor grade. Similarly, Cairncross *(3)* observed an association between radiologic response to chemotherapy and improved survival for patients with AO demonstrating the specific loss of 19q heterozygosity. Loss of both 1p and 19q heterozygosity was associated with higher response rates to chemotherapy and improved survival compared to patients with preservation. CDKN2A gene deletion was associated with shorter survival times. Allelic loss of chromosomes 10q and TP53 gene mutation were not associated with survival or response rates in that series. Molecular markers such as 1p and 19q loss may improve our ability to appropriately classify oligodendroglial tumors as well as identify populations of patients expected to benefit from specific therapies. To this end, one aim of the current RTOG trial, discussed below, is the establishment of a tissue bank and blood sample repository of registered patients for subsequent genetic analysis.

A unique feature of anaplastic oligodendrogliomas and mixed oligoastrocytomas is their sensitivity to chemotherapy, particularly PCV. A prospective trial conducted by the National Cancer Institute of Canada (NCIC) evaluated 33 patients with pure anaplastic oligodendroglioma *(22)*. Of the 24 eligible patients, 18 (75%) showed a radiologic response to PCV with 38% achieving a complete response. Response rates were high even among patients who had received previous radiation therapy. The authors concluded that the high response rate even in recurrent tumors warranted further investigation of the use of PCV as an adjunct to surgery and XRT in patients with newly diagnosed lesions.

Additional studies using neoadjuvant PCV for patients with pure or mixed oligodendroglial tumors have shown similar high response rates, although the absolute number of patients in such studies has been small. Two-year survival rates for AO or anaplastic mixed tumors were 75% and 65%, respectively, in the series of 20 patients treated with surgery, radiation, and chemotherapy reported by Kyritsis *(23)*. In the series of malignant glioma patients treated with XRT and neoadjuvant PCV reported by Kirby et al., three of seven patients with AO or oligoastrocytoma had a response to chemotherapy and the 2-yr survival in this subset was 58% *(24)*. Kim et al. described results of 32 patients treated with surgery, PCV, and radiation *(25)*. The median survival times were 50 mo, 16 mo, and longer than 76 mo for patients with WHO grade III oligoastrocytoma, WHO grade IV oligoastrocytoma, and anaplastic oligodendroglioma, respectively. The difference in survival outcome was correlated with the percentage of oligodendroglial component within the tumor with those patients whose tumors had greater than 99% oligodendroglial elements surviving significantly longer than those patients with tumors comprised of predominantly astrocytic cells. Boiardi et al. reported on 71 patients with anaplastic glioma treated with neoadjuvant CCNU and cisplatin *(26)*. A median survival time of 6 yr was seen in the 30 patients with AO or oligoastrocytoma, which was significantly longer than the 3.2-yr median survival of the patients with AA. Patients with anaplastic oligodendrogliomas and oligoastrocytomas had similar survival. Jeremic et al. reported results of 23 patients with WHO grade III anaplastic mixed gliomas treated with PCV chemotherapy, surgery, and radiation. Response rate to therapy was 83% with a five-yr survival of 53% *(27)*.

A current intergroup trial (RTOG 9402; INT 0149) is underway to evaluate the role of PCV chemotherapy in patients with anaplastic oligodendroglioma. Patients are randomized to radiation alone vs induction PCV plus radiation. Inclusion criteria include at least 25% oligodendroglial component and two or more anaplastic features. Cases are further stratified as moderately or highly anaplastic depending upon the number of features of malignancy present including high cellularity, vascular proliferation, or necrosis. The primary study endpoint is overall survival with secondary endpoints of time to progression, incidence of severe complications, quality of life, and neurologic function. A current EORTC trial is investigating postoperative RT alone or followed by six cycles of PCV.

6. RADIATION THERAPY STRATEGIES

Since the publication of the initial BTSG and Scandinavian Glioblastoma trials, radiation therapy has been accepted as a necessary component in the overall management of patients with malignant glioma. As discussed above, trials to identify more efficacious systemic therapy have not significantly improved upon the survival rates noted in those initial studies. Alternate strategies to improve clinical outcomes for patients with malignant glioma have focused on intensifying radiotherapy through a variety of techniques such as dose escalation, accelerated hyperfractionation, and use of radiosensitizers to enhance the therapeutic ratio.

Walker et al. reported on the combined data from a series of BTSG trials and demonstrated a stepwise prolongation of survival with increasing dose. Median survival times for patients in the 50-, 55-, and 60-Gy subgroups was 28, 36, and 42 wk, respectively. The difference in survival observed between the 50 and 60 Gy groups was significant

($p = 0.004$) *(28)*. However, in a randomized study conducted by RTOG and ECOG (RTOG 7401/ECOG 1374) no survival benefit was demonstrated in patients receiving 70 Gy compared to those patients receiving 60 Gy *(29)*. Little data exist regarding specific radiation dose or volume effects for anaplastic astrocytoma, anaplastic oligodendroglioma, or mixed oligoastrocytomas. Treatment for patients with non-GBM malignant gliomas is typically planned with doses and volumes similar to those used in the management of GBM.

The optimal volume to be irradiated remains an issue of continued debate. Malignant gliomas are thought to be capable of infiltrating large distances into the normal brain. For patients with malignant gliomas, the gross tumor volume (GTV) is usually defined by the preoperative contrast-enhancing volume on CT/MRI, and the clinical target volume (CTV) is delineated by the area of edema on CT/MRI with a 2 cm margin. Malignant gliomas are typically treated with conformal, partial brain fields encompassing the contrast-enhancing volume with a 2–3 cm margin or treating the region of increased signal on T2-weighted MRI with a 1–2 cm margin to 45–50 Gy, followed by a field reduction to the enhancing volume with a 2–3 cm margin. Tighter margins may be utilized if the tumor is in close proximity to dose-limiting structures, e.g., the optic chiasm, or in an unlikely direction of tumor spread, such as across the tentorium or falx. A total dose of 59.4–60.0 Gy is given in 1.8–2.0 Gy daily fractions.

Halperin and colleagues compared tumor extent on CT and MRI and noted that the tumor area identified on T2-weighted images was larger that the abnormal zone seen on CT; autopsy studies revealed a significant portion of patients had tumor extending more than 2 cm beyond the CT contrast-enhancing region *(30)*. Serial biopsies through areas of edema surrounding the region of contrast enhancement on CT or MRI have demonstrated a gradient of tumor cells infiltrating normal brain *(31)*. The need to encompass regions at clinical risk for disease must be balanced against the potential toxicity of irradiating large volumes of central nervous system (CNS) tissue and the still predominant local failure pattern exhibited by malignant gliomas. Analysis of failure patterns in patients with malignant glioma have revealed the epicenter of recurrence to be most frequently within 1–2 cm of the original contrast-enhancing tumor *(32)*. The high preponderance for local failure has prompted interest in improving the therapeutic ratio of external beam radiation utilizing techniques such as altered fractionation schemes, 3D conformal therapy, stereotactic radiosurgery, interstitial brachytherapy, particle therapy, and radiosensitizers.

As discussed above, attempts at RT dose escalation with conventional external beam radiotherapy have been made. The lack of an observed dose response above 60 Gy may be attributable to the increased toxicity associated with therapy delivered using conventional fractionation and planning techniques. For most normal tissues, late morbidity from radiation treatment is dependent upon cumulative radiation dose, fraction size, and treatment volume. A clear dose–volume relationship for CNS injury and conventionally fractionated radiation therapy has not been established. However, Marks et al. have reported an 18% incidence of brain necrosis with doses greater than 64.8 Gy compared to 0% with radiation doses under 57 Gy *(33)*. Currently the RTOG is conducting a phase I/II study (RTOG 9803) to evaluate the feasibility and toxicity of escalating doses of conformal radiation therapy using 3D treatment planning techniques, to determine dose/volume and dose/anatomic factors that influence radiation-induced CNS toxicity, and to evaluate key endpoints such as local control, survival and failure patterns in patients treated with high-dose conformal radiation. Accrual continues to the third dose level of 78.0 Gy in the fall of 2001.

Focal radiation techniques such as radiosurgery and interstitial brachytherapy have been investigated as methods to increase radiation dose to selective volumes. These therapies offer the potential to selectively increase dose to a target volume while minimizing dose to adjacent normal tissues. However, given the infiltrative nature of most gliomas and the ability to use these techniques predominantly in noneloquent areas of the brain, such therapies are applicable to only a limited portion of patients with malignant glioma. In a prospective NCOG study (6G-82-2) the use of interstitial brachytherapy in the initial treatment of patients with malignant gliomas was shown to produce less of an increase survival in patients with AA compared to those with GBM histology *(34)*. Retrospective review of AA patients treated on a variety of NCOG studies and the UCSF database reported by Prados et al. found age and KPS had a significant influence on survival and time to tumor progression, whereas extent of surgery and the use of interstitial brachytherapy did not *(16)*. Prospective data from the UCSF experience showed a median survival of 36 mo from time of diagnosis utilizing a brachytherapy boost *(35)*. Since this was no better than the results with conventional EBRT alone, brachytherapy boost for AA patients was no longer offered at UCSF after 1989. The RTOG has recently completed the first phase III study to evaluate the role of a stereotactic boost in addition to conventional RT and BCNU in patients with supratentorial malignant glioma. All patients received conventional radiotherapy consisting of 60 Gy in 30 fractions and six cycles of BCNU 80 mg/m^2 iv for 3 d every 8 wk commencing with the initiation of radiation. Patients were randomized to receive either a single fraction stereotactic boost to be delivered within one week prior to initiation of conventional RT or no radiosurgery boost. Radiosurgery dose was dependent on tumor size. Study endpoints included overall survival, toxicity comparisons between the two arms, and evaluation of mental status and quality of life. The trial reached its accrual goal in June 2000 and the data will be available in 2002.

Altered fractionation schedules have the potential to allow for dose escalation by exploiting the differences in the capacity of radiation damage repair between tumor cells and normal brain tissue. Accelerated fractionation (AHF) and hyperfractionation (HF) were studied in several randomized trials all of which were negative *(15,36–39)*. Werner-Wasik et al. reported the final results of RTOG 83-02 a phase I/II study of HF and AHF radiation therapy and BCNU of 747 patients with malignant gliomas, 19% of whom had AA histology *(39)*. HF treatment consisted of 1.2 Gy twice daily to doses of 64.8, 72, 76.8, and 81.6 Gy. The AHF schedule consisted of 1.6 Gy twice daily to 48 or 54.4 Gy. This was not associated with any survival advantage when compared with historic controls and the subgroup of AA patients who received lower HF doses had a better median survival (50 mo) compared with those receiving higher HF doses (35 mo; $p = 0.35$). One suggested explanation for this finding was increased toxicity at the higher dose levels, a particularly important finding within the AA subgroup of patients who would be expected to have a more favorable natural history.

7. NOVEL CHEMOTHERAPEUTIC AGENTS

Several reasons have been cited for the limitations of the use of chemotherapy in the treatment of malignant glioma. Inherent and acquired drug resistance and the lack of good drug penetration through the blood-brain barrier have both been cited as obstacles. Several strategies have been employed to overcome these limitations including intraarterial (IA) drug administration and placement of chemotherapy directly within the resection cavity. More recent trials have focused on the use of novel chemotherapy agents including hypoxic cell sensitizers, inhibitors of angiogenesis, immune modulators as well as chemotherapeutic drugs shown to have efficacy against other solid tumor types.

In an effort to overcome the lack of solubility, poor penetration across the blood-brain barrier and decreased delivery of conventional systemic agents by a compromised intratumoral blood supply, several studies have evaluated various combinations of BCNU alone or with other agents delivered intraarterally. Unfortunately, response rates and median survival times observed in patients treated with intraarterial chemotherapy have not been significantly different than those seen in patients treated with standard intravenous nitrosurea-containing regimens, while increased rates of toxicity such as leukoencephalopathy, retinal injury, edema, myelosuppression, sepsis, and thrombotic complications have been noted *(40–46)*.

Bromodeoxyuridine (BUdR) is a halogenated pyrimidine analog that is incorporated as a substitute for thymidine into actively dividing cells during DNA synthesis; this substitution results in a two- to threefold increase in cell sensitivity to radiation in vitro. Encouraged by results of a NCOG phase II trial utilizing BUdR during radiation therapy followed by adjuvant PCV chemotherapy in patients with newly diagnosed GBM and AA, the RTOG conducted a randomized trial to evaluate the effect of BUdR as a radiosensitizer *(47)*. The study began as a NCOG trial in 1991, and became an Intergroup RTOG, SWOG, and NCCTG study in July 1994. Two hundred eighty-one patients with AA, gemistocytic astrocytoma, Grade 3 astrocytoma, and malignant glioma other than GBM were accrued to the study of which 189 were eligible/analyzable. In July 1996 accrual was suspended after preliminary analysis suggested that the addition of BUdR was unlikely to be associated with increased survival. The study was closed in February 1997 at which time the 1-yr survival estimates were 82% for the RT plus PCV group vs 68% for the RT/BudR plus PCV group ($p = 0.96$). The survival difference between the two arms was attributed to a larger number of early deaths in the BUdR arm, not related to treatment toxicity.

Preclinical laboratory data supported the theory that tirapazimine (WIN 59075), a benzotriazine compound exhibiting substantial differential toxicity for hypoxic cells, increased the efficacy of RT against hypoxic tumor cells possibly resulting in greater than additive hypoxic cell toxicity. These data coupled with clinical support for hypoxia as a contributor to the treatment-resistant nature of malignant gliomas prompted the RTOG to launch a Phase II trial (RTOG 9417) of tirapazimine with cranial RT in patients with radiosurgery-ineligible GBM. Survival in the patients treated with radiation and tirapazimine was equivalent to the control population *(48)*. Patients in RPA class II treated with radiation and tirapazamine at the 159 mg/m^2 dose level had a longer survival when compared to historical controls; however, this did not reach statistical significance.

RTOG 9602 evaluated weekly paclitaxel and conventional radiotherapy for patients with GBM. Previous studies had shown taxanes to be potent radiosensitizers. Thirty-five evaluable patients were reported *(49)*. With a median follow-up of 20 mo the overall median survival was 9.7 mo with median survival times for RPA classes II, IV, V, and VI being 16.3, 10.2, 9.5, and 2.5 mo, respectively. Median survival by RPA class with brief taxane therapy was comparable to RTOG historical controls treated with standard EBRT and BCNU (1-yr BCNU). Clinicopathologic evaluation did not disclose any correlation between tumor *p53* status or EGFr expression and patient survival, in contrast to previous observations suggesting improved outcomes in *p53*(+) GBM patients receiving concurrent radiation and weekly paclitaxel.

Owing to the lack of any single sufficiently promising phase II experience for radiosurgery-ineligible GBM patients, recent RTOG studies have focused on testing new systemic agents with cranial radiation. A phase I study of topotecan plus cranial radiation for GBM patients was completed, in an effort to enhance antitumor response by exploiting the strand break mechanisms of both topotecan and ionizing radiation. Preliminary toxicity data were acceptable and a dose level of 1.5 mg/m^2 was chosen *(50)*. Preliminary data from the phase II study 95-13 has been reviewed, and initial analysis has thus far not demonstrated a survival benefit. Malignant gliomas are generally highly vascular and angiogenic tumors and thus may be appropriate targets for angiogenesis inhibitors. Recent experimental evidence has shown that inhibition of angiogenesis leads to radiosensitization. A phase II trial (RTOG 98-06) has recently been completed using thalidomide, a basic fibroblast growth factor (bFGF) antagonist, in patients with newly diagnosed GBM receiving concomitant cranial radiation. RTOG 9710 was a phase II study of conventional radiation therapy followed by recombinant beta interferon for GBM to evaluate radiosensitizing effect. Median survival time was comparable to RTOG controls treated with standard EBRT and BCNU.

Temozolomide, a novel oral, second-generation alkylating agent, has shown significant promise as a cytotoxic agent in the treatment of a variety of solid tumors including melanoma, glioma, mycosis fungoides. Temozolomide is a prodrug of the active alkylating agent 5-(3-methyltriazen-1-yl)imidazole-4-carboximide (MTIC) that is spontaneously converted to the active form under physiologic conditions. The drug demonstrates 100% oral bioavailability and excellent tissue distribution including penetration of the blood-brain barrier and into cerebrospinal fluid *(51)*. Phase I/II studies have shown significant antineoplastic effect in patients with recurrent malignant glioma *(52,53)*. A randomized phase II trial comparing PCV to temozolomide in patients with supratentorial GBM at first relapse demonstrated improved progression free survival, overall survival, tumor response, and quality of life among the patients treated with temozolomide compared to those treated with PCV *(54)*. In a study of 33 patients with newly diagnosed GBM or AA, treatment with oral temodar, 200 mg/m^2 on a 5-d schedule every 28 d, resulted in a complete response in 3 patients, partial response in 15 patients, and disease stabilization in an additional 6 patients *(55)*. Preliminary data indicates that concomitant daily oral temozolomide (75 mg/m^2/d) and cranial radiotherapy is well tolerated *(56)*. Ongoing clinical trials are evaluating the role of temozolomide in conjunction with nitrosoureas, topoisomerase inhibitors and BCNU-impregnated interstitial wafers (Gliadel).

8. FUTURE DIRECTIONS

It is unlikely that any one systemic agent or multiagent regimen will substantially alter the natural history of malignant glioma. A significant improvement in survival will be realized only when improvements in loco-regional control are combined with progress in the systemic management of the disease. Specific opportunities to improve surgical and radiotherapy approaches to this disease need to be explored concurrent with development of novel agents targeted to modify the biologic response of these tumors to chemotherapy and radiation. Ongoing topics for future research include:

1. Elucidation of specific molecular pathways involved in the pathogenesis of gliomas and their response to chemotherapy and ionizing radiation.
2. The role of image-guided treatment planning and outcome evaluation.
3. Novel strategies of delivering chemotherapeutic agents.
4. Clarification of the role of radiation dose escalation particularly using innovative techniques such as intensity modulated radiation therapy (IMRT) and either single dose or fractionated stereotactic radiation.

REFERENCES

1. Walker MD, Alexander E, Hunt WE, et al. Evaluation of BCNU and/or radiotherapy in the treatment of anaplastic gliomas. *J Neurosurg* 1978; 49:333–343.
2. Curran WJ, Scott CB, Horton J, et al. Recursive partitioning analysis of prognostic factors in three Radiation Therapy Oncology Group malignant glioma trials. *J Natl Cancer Inst* 1993; 85:704–710.
3. Cairncross JG, Ueki K, Zlatescu MC, et al. Specific genetic predictors of chemotherapeutic response and survival in patients with anaplastic oligodendrogliomas. *J Natl Cancer Inst* 1998; 90:1473–1479.
4. Kristiansen K, Hagen S, Kollevold T, et al. Combined modality therapy of operated astrocytomas grade III and IV. Confirmation of the value of postoperative irradiation and lack of potentiation of bleomycin on survival time: a prospective multicenter trial of the Scandinavian Glioblastoma Study Group. *Cancer* 1981; 47:649–652.
5. Walker MD, Green SB, Byar DP, et al. Randomized comparisons of radiotherapy and nitrosureas for the treatment of malignant glioma after surgery. *N Engl J Med* 1980; 303:1323–1329.
6. Green SB, Byar DP, Walker MD, et al. Comparisons of carmustine, procarbazine, and high-dose methylprednisolone as additions to surgery and radiotherapy for the treatment of malignant glioma. *Cancer Treat Rep* 1983; 67:121–132.
7. Shapiro WR, Green SB, Burger PC, et al. Randomized trial of three chemotherapy regimens and two radiotherapy regimens in postoperative treatment of malignant glioma. *J Neurosurg* 1989; 71:1–9.
8. Fine HA, Dear KBG, Loeffler JS, Black PM, Canellos GP. Evaluation of BCNU and/or radiotherapy in the treatment of anaplastic gliomas. Cancer 1993; 71:2585–2597.
9. Stewart LA, Burdett S, Souhami RL. Chemotherapy in high-grade glioma: a meta-analysis using individual patient data from randomized clinical trials (RCTS). *Pro Am Soc Clin Oncol* 2000; 19:168.
10. Lands SH, Murray T, Bolden S. Cancer Statistics. *J Am Canc Soc* 1998; 48:6–29.
11. Prados MD, Scott C, Curran WJ, et al. Procarbazine, lomustine and vincristine (PCV) chemotherapy for anaplastic astrocytoma: a retrospective review of Radiation Therapy Oncology Group Protocols comparing survival with carmustine or PCV adjuvant chemotherapy. *J Clin Oncol* 1999; 17:3389–3395.
12. Kowalczuk A, Macdonald RL, Amidei C, et al. Quantitative imaging study of extent of surgical resection and prognosis of malignant astrocytomas. *Neurosurgery* 1997; 41:1028–1036.
13. Ciric I, Ammirati M, Vick N, Mikhael M. Supratentorial gliomas: surgical considerations and immediate postoperative results. Gross total resection versus partial resection. *Neurosurg* 1987; 21:21–26.
14. Winger MJ, Macdonald DR, Cairncross JG. Supratentorial anaplastic gliomas in adults: The prognostic importance of extent of resection and prior low-grade glioma. *J Neurosurg* 1989; 71:487–493.
15. Curran WJ Jr, Scott CB, Horton J, et al. Does extent of surgery influence outcome for astrocytoma with atypical or anaplastic foci (AAF)? A report of 3 Radiation Therapy Oncology Group trials. *J Neurooncol* 1992; 12:219–227.
16. Prados MD, Gutin PH, Phillips TL, et al. Highly anaplastic astrocytoma: a review of 357 patients treated between 1977 and 1989. *Int J Oncol Biol Phys* 1992; 23:3–8.
17. Levin VA, Silver P, Hannigan J, et al. Superiority of post-radiotherapy adjuvant chemotherapy with CCNU, procarbazine, and vincristine, (PCV) over BCNU for anaplastic gliomas: NCOG 6G61 final report. *Int J Oncol Biol Phys* 1990; 18:321–324.
18. Brada M, Thomas DGT, Bleehan NM. Medical Research Council (MRC) randomized trial of adjuvant chemotherapy in high grade glioma (HGG). *Proc Am Soc Clin Oncol* 1998; 17:400.
19. Prados MD,Scott CS, Curran WJ, et al. Procarbazine, lomustine and vincristine (PCV) chemotherapy for anaplastic astrocytoma: a retrospective review of Radiation Therapy Oncology Group protocols comparing survival with carmustine or PCV adjuvant chemotherapy. *J Clin Oncol* 1999; 17:3389–3395.

20. Donahue B, Scott CB, Nelson JS, et al. Influence of an oligodendroglial component on the survival of patients with anaplastic astrocytomas: A report of Radiation Therapy Oncology Group 83-02. *Int J Radiat Oncol Biol Phys* 1997; 38:911–914.
21. Smith JS, Perry A, Borell TJ, et al. Alterations of chromosome arms 1p and 19q as predictors of survival in oligodendrogliomas, astrocytomas, and mixed oligoastrocytomas. *J Clin Oncol* 2000; 18:636–645.
22. Cairncross G, Macdonald D, Ludwin S, et al. Chemotherapy for anaplastic oligodendroglioma. *J Clin Oncol* 1994; 12:2013–2017.
23. Kyritsis AP, Yung WK, Bruner J, Gleason MJ, Levin VA. The treatment of anaplastic oligodendrogliomas and mixed gliomas. *Neurosurgery* 1993; 32:365–371.
24. Kirby S, Macdonald D, Fisher B, Gaspar L, Cairncross G. Pre-radiation chemotherapy for malignant gliomas in adults. *Can J Neurol Sci* 1996; 23:123–127.
25. Kim L, Hochberg FH, Thornton AF, et al. Procarbazine, lomustine and vincristine (PCV) chemotherapy for grade II and grade IV oligoastrocytoma. *J Neurosurg* 1996; 85:602–607.
26. Boiardi A, Silvani A, Pozzi A, et al. Advantage of treating anaplastic gliomas with aggressive protocol combining chemotherapy and radiotherapy. *J Neurooncol* 1997; 34:179–185.
27. Jeremic B, Shibamoto Y, Gruijicic D, et al. Combined treatment modality for anaplastic oligodendroglioma: a phase II study. *J Neurooncol* 1999; 43:179–185.
28. Walker MD, Strike TA, Sheline GE. An analysis of dose-effect relationship in the radiotherapy of malignant gliomas. *Int J Radiat Oncol Biol Phys* 1979; 5:1725–1731.
29. Chang CH, Horton J, Schoenfeld D, et al. Comparison of post operative radiotherapy in combined post operative radiotherapy and chemotherapy in the multidisciplinary management of malignant gliomas. The Joint Radiation Therapy Oncology Group & The Eastern Cooperative Oncology Group study. *Cancer* 1983; 32:997–1007.
30. Halperin EC, Burger PC, Bullard DE. The fallacy of the localized supratentorial malignant glioma. *Int J Oncol Biol Phys* 1988; 15:505–508.
31. Kelly P, Daumas-Duport C, Kispert D, Imaging-based stereotactic biopsies in untreated intracranial glioneoplasm. *J Neurosurgery* 1987; 66:865–875.
32. Wallner KE, Galicich JH, Krol G, Arbit E, Malkin MG. Patterns of failure following treatment for glioblastoma multiforme and anaplastic astrocytoma. *Int J Oncol Biol Phys* 1989; 16:1405.
33. Marks JE, Wong J. The risk of cerebral radionecrosis in relation to dose, time and fractionation. *Prog Exp Tumor Res* 1985; 29:210–218.
34. Gutin PH, Prados MD, Phillips TL, et al. External irradiation followed by an interstitial high activity iodine-125 implant "boost" in the initial treatment of malignant gliomas: NCOG study 6G-82-2. *Int J Oncol Biol Phys* 1991; 21:601–606.
35. Sneed PK, McDermott MW, Gutin PH. Interstitial brachytherapy procedures for brain tumors. *Semin Surg Oncol* 1997; 13:157–166.
36. Payne DG, Simpson WJ, Keen C, Platts ME. Malignant astrocytoma: hyperfractionated and standard radiotherapy with chemotherapy in a randomized prospective clinical trial. *Cancer* 1982; 50:2301–2306.
37. Shin KH, Muller PH, Geggie PHS. Superfractionation radiation therapy in the treatment of malignant astrocytoma. *Cancer* 1983; 52:2040–2043.
38. Fulton DS, Urtasun RC, Shin KH, et al. Misonidazole combined with hyperfractionation in the management of malignant glioma. *Int J Radiat Oncol Biol Phys* 1984; 10:1709–1712.
39. Werner-Wasik M, Scott CB, Nelson DF, et al. Final report of a Phase I/II trial of hyperfractionated radiation therapy with carmustine for adults with supratentorial malignant gliomas: Radiation Therapy Oncology Group study 83-02. *Cancer* 1996; 77:1535–1543.
40. Stewart DJ, Grahovac Z, Hugenholtz H, et al. Feasibility study of intraarterial vs intravenous cisplatin, BCNU, and teniposide combined with systemic cisplatin, teniposide, cytosine arabinoside, glycerol and mannitol in the treatment of primary and metastatic brain tumors. *J Neurooncol* 1993; 17(1):71–79.
41. Kleinschmidt-DeMasters BK, Geier JM. Pathology of high-dose intraarterial BCNU. *Surg Neurol* 1989; 31(6):435–443.
42. Stewart DJ, Grahovac Z, Hugenholtz H, Russell N, Richard M, Benoit B. Combined intraarterial and systemic chemotherapy for intracerebral tumors. *Neurosurgery* 1987; 2:207–214.
43. Stewart DJ, Grahovac Z, Benoit B, et al. Intracarotid chemotherapy with a combination of 1,3-bis(2-chloroethyl)-1-nitrosourea (BCNU), cis-diaminedichloroplatinum (cisplatin), and 4'-O-demethyl-1-O-(4,6-O-2-thenylidene-beta-D-glucopyranosyl) epipodophyllotoxin (VM-26) in the treatment of primary and metastatic brain tumors. *Neurosurgery* 1984; 15(6):828–833.

44. Feun LG, Wallace S, Yung WK, et al. Phase-I trial of intracarotid BCNU and cisplatin in patients with malignant intracerebral tumors. *Cancer Drug Deliv* 1984; 1(3):239–245.
45. West CR, Avellanosa AM, Barua NR, Patel A, Hong CI. Intraarterial 1,3-bis(2-chloroethyl)-1-nitrosourea (BCNU) and systemic chemotherapy for malignant gliomas: a follow-up study. *Neurosurgery* 1983; 13(4):420–426.
46. Lehane DE, Bryan RN, Horowitz B, et al. Intraarterial cis-platinum chemotherapy for patients with primary and metastatic brain tumors. *Cancer Drug Deliv* 1983; 1(1):69–77.
47. Prados MD, Scott C, Sandler H, et al. A phase 3 randomized study of radiotherapy plus procarbazine, CCNU, and vincristine (PCV) with or without BUdR for the treatment of anaplastic astrocytoma: a preliminary report of RTOG 9404. *Int J Radiat Oncol Biol Phys* 1999; 45:1109–1115.
48. Del Rowe J, Scott C, Werner-Wasik M, et al. A single-arm open label phase II study of intravenously administered tirapazamine plus radiation therapy for glioblastoma multiforme. *J Clin Oncol* 2000; 18(6):1254–1259.
49. Langer CJ, Ruffer J, Rhodes H, et al. Phase II Radiation Therapy Oncology Group trial of weekly paclitaxel and conventional external beam radiation therapy for supratentorial glioblastoma multiforme. *Int J Radiat Oncol Biol Phys* 2001; 51:113–119.
50. MacDonald D. A Phase I study of Topotecan plus cranial radiation for glioblastoma multiforme: a report of Radiation Therapy Oncology Group (RTOG) study 95-07. Proc Am Soc Thera Rad Oncol. *Int J Radiat Oncol Biol Phys* 1997; 39:271.
51. Patel M, McCully C, Godwin K. Plasma and cerebrospinal fluid pharmacokinetics of temozolomide. *Proc Am Soc Clin Oncol* 1995; 14:461 (abstr 1485).
52. Newlands ES, O'Reilly SM, Glaser MG, et al. The Charing Cross Hospital experience with temozolomide in patients with gliomas. *Eur J Cancer* 1996; 32A:2236–2241.
53. Bower M, Newlands ES, Bleehen NM, et al. Multicentre CRC phase II trial of temozolomide in recurrent or progressive high grade glioma. *Cancer Chemother Pharmacol* 1997; 40:484–488.
54. Yung WKA. Temozolomide in malignant gliomas. *Semin Oncol* 2000; 27(Suppl 6):27–34.
55. Friedman HS, McLendon RE, Kerby T, et al. DNA mismatch repair and O6-alkylguanine-DNA alkyltransferase analysis and response to Temodal in newly diagnosed malignant glioma. *J Clin Oncol* 1998; 16:3851–3857.
56. Stupp R, Maillard I, Pica A. Daily temozolomide (TMZ) and concomitant radiotherapy followed by adjuvant TMZ for newly diagnosed glioblastoma multiforme (GBM). A well tolerated and promising regimen. *Proc Am Soc Clin Oncol* 1999; 18:154A (abstr 592).

8 Combined Modality Strategies in the Treatment of Head and Neck Cancer

Cathy Eng, MD *and Everett E. Vokes,* MD

Contents

1. INTRODUCTION

Head and neck cancer (HNC) comprises 5–6% of all malignancies *(1)*. Approximately 650,000 cases will be diagnosed worldwide in 2000 *(2)*. The American Cancer Society estimates that in the United States alone approx 40,300 new cases of HNC will be diagnosed annually with approx 11,700 deaths associated from this disease *(1)*. If cured, HNC patients are at increased risk of developing a second malignancy, estimated to occur at an annual incidence of 3–7% *(3)*. Field carcinogenesis, as initially proposed by Slaughter et al. in 1953, describes the concept of repetitive carcinogen exposure affecting the entire aerodigestive tract, resulting in cumulative toxicity to a large mucosal surface *(4)*. Squamous cell carcinomas constitute >90% of the histology of head and neck carcinomas. Therefore, this chapter will focus solely on this histology type unless specified otherwise.

One-third of patients present with early stage disease (AJCC stage I or II) with the remainder of patients presenting with locally advanced disease (AJCC stage III or IV).

From: *Chemoradiation in Cancer Therapy*
Edited by: H. Choy © Humana Press Inc., Totowa, NJ

Only a small fraction of patients present with distant metastases *(5)*. Single-modality therapy with surgery or radiation therapy with curative intent is the general method of treatment for early stage (stage I or II) patients. Approximately 80% of patients with stage I disease will be cured and 60% of patients with stage II disease will be cured. Previously, patients with locally advanced disease were offered surgery followed by radiation therapy; patients believed to have unresectable disease were treated with radiation therapy only. Despite treatment with curative intent, in the absence of frank metastatic disease, 3- and 5-yr survival rates for patients with unresectable disease were less than 30%. The majority of patients develop local recurrence within the first 2 yr indicating that surgery and/or radiation therapy cannot eliminate all tumor cells. The prognosis has recently improved through the use of concurrent chemoradiotherapy.

Recent advances changing the field of radiation oncology include hyperfractionated and intensity modulated radiation therapy (IMRT). In addition, incorporating chemotherapy agents as radiation sensitizers (the drug increases the effect of radiation therapy without having a direct cytotoxic effect) or enhancers (the drug has independent antitumor activity in addition to acting as a sensitizer) rather than primary administration of cytotoxic agents has advanced the treatment of locally advanced (as well as recurrent head and neck cancers). Novel cytostatic agents may also have a role in augmenting the effects of radiation therapy. Various preclinical models have shown that chemotherapy may enhance the cytotoxicity of radiation therapy by decreasing radioresistance, sensitize hypoxic cells, and synchronize cells in specific phases of the cell cycle.

Prior clinical trials have attempted to discern the best manner in which to administer chemotherapy when combined with radiation. It may be given concurrently with standard radiotherapy, an alternating or split-course radiotherapy schedule, or in a sequential fashion as induction (prior to definitive treatment) or adjuvant (following definitive treatment) chemotherapy. Concomitant chemoradiotherapy is the use of both modalities simultaneously. Alternating chemoradiotherapy is the use of systemic chemotherapy for a definitive duration, followed by radiotherapy for a specified period followed by repeated alternations of the two modalities. Split-course chemoradio-therapy usually involves concomitant systemic doses of chemotherapy combined with radiation therapy for a specified duration followed by a rest period, and then the regimen is repeated. This approach allows planned treatment breaks for toxicity recovery.

The purpose of this chapter will be to discuss the rationale for concomitant chemoradiation therapy, using standard and novel agents as well as promising molecular targets, and the encouraging strategies that may improve the overall survival, disease-free survival, and possibly the quality of life of a potentially debilitating and disfiguring disease.

2. SYNERGISTIC CYTOTOXIC ACTIVITY OF CHEMOTHERAPY WITH RADIATION THERAPY

Preclinical models have established various methods to increase the cytotoxic activity of radiation therapy. This methodology includes promoting activity against cells in the most radiation-sensitive phase of the cell cycle, the G_2/M phase, and eradicating hypoxic tumor cells to decrease radioresistance. The method of radiation therapy (conventional, accelerated, intensity-modulated, and/or hyperfractionated radiation therapy) may also have an impact on the rate of tumor cell growth and toxicity. It has been postulated that decreasing the time interval between cytotoxic treatment will decrease the ability of tumor cells to regenerate and in turn decrease locoregional recurrence. It should be noted that by promoting the tumoricidal activity of radiation therapy, the patient may develop acute (early) and chronic (late) side effects because the synergistic activity of concomitant chemoradiation therapy is not tumor specific. Acute toxicities include mucositis, radiation dermatitis, and myelosuppression. Chronic toxicities may be debilitating as a result of radiation fibrosis, xerostomia, trismus (tonic contraction or fibrosis of the muscles of mastication), dysfunction of the muscles of mastication, disfigurement, and psychosocial difficulties with these sequelae. Investigative approaches must pursue equilibrium between tumor cytotoxicity and associated acute and chronic sequelae that may ensue.

Radiation therapists have also attempted to increase the cytotoxicity of radiotherapy as a single-treatment modality by developing intensified schedules of radiation therapy. Accelerated fractionation irradiation decreases the total time of treatment, may decrease the rate of tumor cell regrowth, and in turn, may increase locoregional control *(6)*. The principle of hyperfractionated radiation therapy is to provide multiple small fractions of radiation therapy, increase the total dose, but decrease the long-term toxicities associated with radiation therapy. The European Organization for the Research and Treatment of Cancer (EORTC) performed a prospective, randomized trial in oropharyngeal carcinoma patients noting a 20% increase in locoregional control at 5 yr and a trend in prolonged overall survival ($p = 0.08$) with the use of hyperfractionated radiation therapy vs conventional daily therapy *(7)* No difference in chronic toxicities were noted.

The Radiation Therapy Oncology Group (RTOG) has recently reported a randomized phase III trial (RTOG 9003), comparing four arms of radiotherapy for patients with locally advanced HNC *(8)*. The four arms were as follows:

1. Standard radiotherapy.
2. Hyperfractionated twice daily radiotherapy.
3. Accelerated fractionated twice daily therapy.
4. Accelerated fractionated therapy with concomitant boost (Table 1).

The median follow-up was 23 mo for the 1073 evaluable patients. Patients that received hyperfractionated or accelerated radiation therapy with boost had increased locoregional control ($p = 0.045$ and $p = 0.05$, respectively) and a trend toward improved disease-free survival (DFS) ($p = 0.067$ and $p = 0.054$, respectively) in comparison to conventional radiation therapy. However, there was no improvement in overall survival(s). Patients given accelerated split-course fractionation had similar outcomes to those who had received conventional radiotherapy. Hyperfractionated radiation therapy is the method of choice for combined chemoradiotherapy in current investigative approaches for head and neck cancer.

A technological advance in the field of radiation therapy has been IMRT. IMRT uses the veloses of three-dimensional imagery by computed tomography (CT) allowing accommodation of radiation to the target tumor site, but decreases the beam intensity to the surrounding normal tissue, thereby potentially decreasing the risk of chronic sequelae.

Table 1
RTOG 9003

Arms	*Standard*	*Hyperfractionated*	*Accelerated with split*	*Accelerated with boost*
Dose/fraction	2 Gy	1.2 Gy, twice-daily	1.6 Gy, twice-daily	1.8 Gy, boost (1.5 Gy) for last 12 d of treatment
Days/week	5	5	5	5
Total dose (no. of fractions)	70 Gy (35 fractions)	81.6 Gy (68 fractions)	67.2 Gy (42 fractions): 2-wk rest following 38.4 Gy	72 Gy (42 fractions)
Compared to standard radiation therapy				
Locoregional control	—	$p = 0.045$	$p = 0.55$	$p = 0.05$
Overall survival	—	$p = 0.13$	$p = 0.86$	$p = 0.40$
Disease-free survival	—	$p = 0.067$	$p = 0.26$	$p = 0.054$

3. CONCOMITANT CHEMORADIOTHERAPY

3.1. Single Agents

Concomitant chemoradiation therapy has been investigated over the past 40 yr. Active single agents in HNC have included cisplatin, methotrexate, 5-fluorouracil (5-FU), bleomycin, mitomycin C, the taxanes, and ifosfamide. Early trials were composed of daily radiation therapy combined with single agent chemotherapy. Recent trials have included newer agents such as the taxanes, topoisomerase I inhibitors, and potential targets of signal transduction including tyrosine kinase inhibitors that will be discussed later in this chapter.

3.2. Hydroxyurea

Hydroxyurea is an oral agent that inhibits ribonucleotide diphosphate reductase and interferes with the synthesis of DNA, specifically the S phase of the cell cycle. Sinclair et al. have demonstrated in preclinical animal models that hydroxyurea may inhibit cells from leaving the G_1 radiosensitive phase and entering the radioresistant S phase *(9)*. Early studies have demonstrated little or no efficacy associated with the use of single-agent hydroxyurea *(10)*. It has received FDA approval in the use of head and neck cancer when administered concomitantly with radiotherapy based upon promising results from earlier studies *(11)*.

The foundation for further study of combination regimens with hydroxyurea and 5-FU is based on in vitro pharmacokinetics denoting modulation of 5-FU by depleting deoxyuridine monophosphate (dUMP), a metabolic product of 5-FU. In turn, this will allow increased binding of 5-FU to thymidylate synthase and augment the properties of 5-FU.

3.3. 5-Fluorouracil (5-FU)

Lo and colleagues completed a randomized study in 136 patients comparing radiation therapy with bolus 5-FU *(12)*. The 5-yr overall survival ($p = 0.08$) was 32% vs 14% in the concomitant arm vs the radiation only arm, respectively. In a subset analysis, patients with primary tumors of the oral cavity were found to have statistically significant local control and survival rates. Overall, the 2-yr DFS was significant ($p = 0.05$) in the concomitant chemoradiation arm at 49% in comparison to 18% in the radiation therapy only arm.

A large randomized Spanish study by Sanchiz and colleagues evaluated 859 patients over a 10-yr period with untreated stage III or IVA HNC *(13)*. The study was divided into three arms with arms A and B consisting of conventional and hyperfractionated therapy, respectively; arm C was conventional single daily radiation therapy with bolus 5-FU. Complete response (CR) rates were promising with 90% in arm B and 96% reported in arm C.

Browman and colleagues randomized 175 stage III or IV HNC patients to standard daily radiotherapy (total 66 Gy) with or without 72-h infusion of 5-FU (1.2 G/m^2) during weeks 1 and 3 *(14)*. Statistically worse toxicities were seen in the concomitant arm including stomatitis ($p = 0.001$), radiation dermatitis ($p = 0.03$), and weight loss of >15% of baseline over 10 consecutive weeks ($p < 10^{-6}$). However, the complete response rate was significantly improved on the combined chemoradiation arm in comparison to the single modality arm (68% vs 56%, $p = 0.04$). The concomitant chemoradiation arm demonstrated a trend toward improved survival when evaluating overall median survival (33 vs 25 mo, $p = 0.08$) and progression-free survival (PFS, $p = 0.06$). Browman has recently provided updated information regarding this trial *(15)*. After a median follow-up of 9.4 yr, the concomitant chemoradiotherapy arm continues to demonstrate an improved median survival of 27 mo vs 16 mo. However, the survival benefit for concomitant chemoradiotherapy was primarily gained in the first 2.5 yr, and was not found to be significant in comparison to the radiotherapy only arm at 5.5 yr ($p = 0.66$). Additionally, the initial trend toward progression-free survival continues to have no statistical significance.

These initial studies were the foundation for further exploration of 5-FU in combination with biomodulators, platinum agents, and other novel agents to increase locoregional control and possibly overall survival.

3.4. Mitomycin C

Preclinical animal studies have demonstrated the bioreductive alkylating agent mitomycin C to have selective cytotoxicity to hypoxic cells *(16)*. Haffty and colleagues at Yale University have addressed the radioresistance of hypoxic tumor cells by enrolling 203 patients onto two consecutive randomized trials of radiation therapy with mitomycin C (15 mg/m^2, on the fifth day of radiation therapy) between 1980 and 1992 *(17)*. Each trial utilized standard daily radiation therapy with the second trial adding dicumarol (500 mg) in an attempt to enhance the cytotoxic activity of mitomycin C. With a median follow-up of 138 mo, both trials clearly showed benefit on the concomitant arms vs radiation therapy alone in regards to local recurrence-free survival (85% vs 66%, $p = 0.002$) and locoregional recurrence-free survival (76% vs 54%, $p = 0.003$), but neither trial could demonstrate an improvement in the overall survival (48% vs 42%). As of 1999, at a median follow-up of more than 10 yr, locoregional control was found to be superior in the concomitant chemoradiation therapy in comparison to radiation alone (70% vs 51%, $p < 0.005$) *(18)*. Although not determined to be statistically significant, there continues to be a trend in overall survival in the mitomycin arm of 34% vs 26%.

The International Atomic Energy Agency is completing a large, randomized trial of the role of mitomycin in head and neck malignancies. Yale University continues to evaluated the possible superiority of porfiromycin (methyl mitomycin) in comparison to mitomycin in a randomized trial of greater than 120 HNC patients. Final results have yet to be published.

3.5. Nitroimidazole Compounds

Danish investigators have looked at the role of pure hypoxic cell radiosensitizers such as misonidazole and nimorazole in improving overall survival. Misonidazole was initially evaluated in a randomized study of split-course radiotherapy in the DAHANCA 2 study (Danish Head and Neck Cancer Study). Overall, the study failed to demonstrate an improvement with misonidazole in comparison to placebo with 26% of patients developing profound peripheral neuropathy resulting in its discontinuation for further investigation *(19)*. Overgaard and colleagues proceeded to evaluate nimorazole, a less toxic hypoxic cell radiosensitizer, in comparison to placebo in a phase III randomized study of conventional radiotherapy in supraglottic and pharyngeal head and neck tumors *(20)*. The nimorazole group had improved locoregional control vs placebo (49% vs 33%, $p = 0.002$) with a trend toward improved survival at 10 yr (26% vs 16%, $p = 0.32$) warranting further study.

3.6. Bleomycin

Based on preliminary studies, Shanta and Krishnamurthi chose to evaluate the effects of Bleomycin with three fractions of radiation therapy per week in a randomized trial of 157 patients with stage III and IV HNC *(21)*. The 5-yr recurrence-free (72% vs 17%) and disease-free survival rates (66% vs 24%) in the chemoradiation arm were found to be superior.

The Northern California Oncology Group randomized 104 patients with unresectable disease to standard daily radiation therapy with or without concomitant bleomycin (5-FU iv twice weekly) followed by 16 wks of adjuvant chemotherapy (methotrexate 25 mg/m^2 weekly) after the completion of radiation therapy *(22)*. A locoregional CR of 67% was seen in the concomitant arm vs 45% in the control arm ($p = 0.056$). The 2-yr locoregional control rate was 64% vs 26% ($p = 0.001$); and the development of metastases was 38% vs 24% ($p > 0.25$), respectively.

Despite the promising results of these two studies, the European Organization for the Research and Treatment of Cancer (EORTC) reported no difference in primary tumor response 6 wk after completing treatment in a randomized study of conventional radiotherapy with or without single agent bleomycin. No difference in tumor response was seen in either arm (67% for radiation therapy only vs 68% for the concomitant arm). At 6 yrs, a differencein OS could not be appreciated when bleomycin was added to standard radiation therapy vs a control group (24% vs 22%, respectively *(23)*. However, only 64% of patients on the bleomycin arm receiving the full recommended dose, which may have contributed to the failure of an improved response rate and survival time in the chemoradiation arm.

3.7. Cisplatin/Carboplatin

Early interest concerning the role of cisplatin as a radiosensitizer led to several randomized clinical trials. A National Cancer Institute (NCI) sponsored intergroup trial of 371 unresectable patients comparing conventional radiation therapy to the use of weekly low dose cisplatin (20 mg/m^2) as an adjunct to the same regimen of conventional radiotherapy found no statistical difference in complete response (34% for the concurrent modality vs 30% in the radiation therapy alone arm) or overall survival *(24)*. The final results of this study were never published.

A preliminary report on a randomized trial on 83 stage III or IV locally advanced squamous cell head and neck cancer (SCHNC) patients demonstrated improved 2-yr disease-free survival (65% vs 41%, $p = 0.01$) and increased rate of local control (85% vs 59%, $p < 0.05$) in the concomitant chemoradiation group (cisplatin 50 mg/m^2 weekly) in comparison to radiation therapy alone *(25)*. It should be noted that the DFS was improved overall in the concomitant arm despite 18% patients receiving only two-thirds of their scheduled dose of cisplatin as a result of nausea and vomiting. Mature results from this study have not been published to date.

A Radiation Therapy Oncology Group (RTOG) trial headed by Al-Sarraf, reported the results of concomitant single agent cisplatin (100 mg/m^2) and standard radiotherapy in 124 stage III or IV unresectable patients *(26)*. An impressive CR of 70% was seen in all patients with a subset analysis of nasopharyngeal patients (28 patients, 27 of which had stage IV disease) with CR of 89%. Compared to historical matched controls, the disease-free survival, overall survival, and the decreased development of distal metastatic disease was greater in the concomitant arm *(27)*.

Al Saraf and colleagues have changed the standard treatment of nasopharyngeal carcinoma based upon a large randomized, prospective, phase III intergroup trial of 185 patients randomized to radiation therapy alone or concomitant chemoradiation therapy *(28)*. The study population was stratified by T and N stage, pathology, and performance status. Patients received 35–39 fractions of daily radiotherapy and were randomized to concomitant cisplatin (100 mg/m^2 on d 1, 22, and 43) followed by three cycles of adjuvant cisplatin (80 mg/m^2, d 1) and continuous infusion 5-FU (1000 mg/m^2, d 1–4) every 28 d. Overall, superiority of treatment was seen in the concomitant chemoradiation therapy arm in comparison to radiotherapy alone with the 3-yr progression-free survival (PFS) of 69% vs 24% ($p < 0.001$) and 3-yr OS of 78% vs 47% ($p = 0.005$). Hence, the recommended standard of care in treating patients with nasopharygneal carcinoma is concomitant chemoradiotherapy.

Carboplatin, an analog of cisplatin, has been shown to have single-agent activity in recurrent head and neck cancers *(29)*. Carboplatin is an attractive alternative due to its more attractive profile of myelosuppression and peripheral neuropathy in comparison to the numerous toxicities often seen with cisplatin including nephrotoxicity, peripheral neuropathy, electrolyte imbalance, emetogenicity, and ototoxicity. Jacobs and colleagues evaluated 26 chemoradiotherapy naive patients with stage IV SCCA in a phase I/II trial of escalating doses of weekly carboplatin (60–400 mg/m^2) and conventional radiation therapy *(30)*. The maximal tolerated dose (MTD) was 100 mg/m^2 with favorable response rates (52% CR, 24% PR).

Kamioner and colleagues reported a small French study of 41 patients with advanced HNC that were randomized to receive concomitant conventional radiotherapy (70 Gy/39 fractions/8 wk) in group A with carboplatin 100 mg/m^2 per wk for 6 wk *(31)*. Group B received the same regimen of radiotherapy with cisplatin 20 mg/m^2 per wk for 6 wk. Twenty-nine patients were evaluable with CR of 55% in the cisplatin arm and 69% in the carboplatin arm. The mention of this small study cannot establish the superiority of carboplatin over that of cisplatin but advocates further study of carboplatin in head and neck malignancies.

3.8. Taxanes

The taxanes, paclitaxel and docetaxel, act by promoting the assembly of microtubules. The taxanes induce cell cycle arrest in the most radiosensitive phase, G_2/M thereby promoting radiosensitivity. In vitro studies have also demonstrated apoptosis in cell culture lines with paclitaxel *(32)*. Paclitaxel dose-dependent synergy is also seen in squamous carcinoma cell lines *(33)*. Much literature has been published regarding the use of taxanes when combined with radiotherapy.

Single-agent activity of paclitaxel was initially evaluated by the Eastern Cooperative Oncology Group (ECOG) in a select cohort of 34 patients with unresectable, recurrent, or metastatic disease *(34)*. The overall response rate was 40% (4 CR, 8 PR). Myelosuppression was the primary toxicity. The median survival was 9.2 mo with a 1-yr survival of 33%.

Hoffman and colleagues evaluated the effects of a 1 h weekly infusion of paclitaxel (20 mg/m^2, escalating by 10 mg/m^2 increments) with conventional radiotherapy *(35)*. The MTD was 30 mg/m^2/wk with the dose-limiting toxicity being mucositis.

In vitro studies suggested maximum radiosensitization could be achieved by prolonged infusion of paclitaxel *(36)*. A phase I NCI sponsored trial examined the MTD of a 7-wk continuous infusion of paclitaxel with standard radiotherapy in advanced HNC patients *(37)*. Moist desquamation was the primary dose-limiting toxicity encountered at 17 mg/m^2/d. The recommended phase II dose is 10.5 mg/m^2/d.

A phase II pilot study examined the effects of 120-h continuous infusion paclitaxel at two dose levels (105 mg/m^2 and 120 mg/m^2) when combined with conventional radiotherapy in 33 previously untreated patients with stage III/IV HNC *(38)*. At the conclusion of treatment, 70% of patients had achieved a CR. The dose level of paclitaxel did not have an effect on the CR ($p = 1$). After 36 mo, locoregional control was achieved in 55.7%, OS of 57.8%, and DFS of 51.1%; the median duration of survival was greater than 50 mo.

As a single agent in the setting of locoregional, recurrent, and metastatic disease, docetaxel is also tolerated fairly well with leukopenia as the primary dose-limiting toxicity *(39)*. Response rates have been favorable at approx 42% when administered docetaxel (100 mg/m^2) every 21 d. Hesse et al. reported on significant toxicities encountered in a phase I study of concomitant taxotere (initial dose = 15 mg/m^2)/conventional radiation therapy (70 Gy) grade 3/4 radiation dermatitis, neuropathy, and thrombocytopenia at dose level 1 *(40)*. Of five evaluable patients three patients achieved a CR and one patient achieved a PR. Based on the severity of these toxicities, this treatment schedule was not pursued further.

3.9. Gemcitabine

Gemcitabine is a deoxycytidine analog associated with minimal toxicity and has demonstrated in vitro radiosensitization properties in HNC at noncytotoxic concentrations *(41)*. Recent in vitro analysis suggests that the etiology may be a result of lowering the threshold for radiation-induced apoptosis *(42)*. The antitumor activity of gemcitabine occurs by intracellular activation by phosphorylation to gemcitabine triphosphate (dFdCTP), a direct inhibitor of DNA polymerization. The intracellular cytotoxic activity of gemcitabine triphosphate is maintained for 72 h allowing once a week administration.

The MTD of concurrent weekly gemcitabine to standard head and neck radiotherapy has been recently reported in a phase I trial from the University of Michigan *(43)*. Twenty-nine patients (28 with SCCA and 1 with medullary thyroid cancer) with unresectable HNC received 35 fractions of daily radiotherapy with escalating doses of weekly gemcitabine (10–300 mg/m^2/wk). Gemcitabine triphosphate levels in biopsy specimens were obtained after the first infusion of gemcitabine, prior to radiation therapy. This study failed to establish a feasible Phase II dose or dose-escalating correlation of intracellular concentrations of dFdCTP at 50–300 mg/m^2/wk. The intracellular concentration of dFdCTP at gemcitabine doses of 10 mg/m^2/wk was nondetectable or barely detectable. The most common dose-limiting toxicity (DLT) was grade 3/4 mucositis requiring dose deescalation. No DLT was seen at 10 mg/m^2/wk. The late toxicity of pharyngeal ulceration or obstruction was not uncommon resulting in gastric feeding tubes in eight patients. Endoscopies and biopsies were obtained 2–3 mo following the completion of treatment with no detectable disease in 66–87% of patients in the various cohorts. These promising results encourage the use of gemcitabine as a potent and effective radiosensitizer for further study as a single agent or in combination.

3.10. Irinotecan (Camptosar, CPT-11)

Irinotecan is a topoisomerase-I inhibitory agent that prevents the initiation and elongation of RNA transcription, DNA replication, and supercoiling of DNA *(44)*. Investigators at Vanderbilt University have demonstrated a schedule-dependent radiosensitization activity when camptothecin derivatives such as irinotecan are combined with radiotherapy *(45)*. Decreased radioresistance was observed when the tumor cell lines were exposed to irinotecan before and during radiotherapy, but not after radiation therapy.

Early studies of human lung xenografts demonstrated an increase of cells in the G_2/M-phase, after only 1 h of exposure to the lowest dose of SN-38 (the major metabolite of irinotecan) demonstrating promising radiosensitization properties for further study *(46)*. Clinical trials have been initiated *(47)*.

4. MULTIAGENT CONCOMITANT TREATMENT

With promising response rates seen with earlier concomitant single-agent chemoradiotherapy, a series of trials sought to determine if multiagent chemoradiotherapy would improve the locoregional control and decrease the development of systemic disease despite the increased risk of associated toxicities.

4.2. Combination Chemotherapy Regimens vs Radiation Alone

An early trial sponsored by the National Cancer Institute of Canada failed to establish a significant difference in locoregional control and overall survival when evaluating 212 patients with larnygeal or hypopharyngeal squamous cell carcinoma (SCCA) treated with 50 Gy in 20 fractions over 28 d or split-course radiotherapy of 25 Gy in 10 fractions over 14 d, followed by a 28-d rest and then 25 Gy in 10 fractions over 14 d beginning on d 43 with mitomycin C (10 mg/m^2 on d 1 and 43) in combination with continuous infusion 5-FU (1000 mg/m^2/d on d 1–4 and 43–46) *(48)*. Nevertheless, this study suggested that the addition of chemotherapy may overcome the decreased activity of split-course radiotherapy.

An Italian cohort comprised of 157 patients with unresectable stage III or IV carcinoma were randomized to a sequential regimen of four cycles of cisplatin (20 mg/m^2, d 1–5), continuous infusion 5-FU (200 mg/m^2/d, d 1–5), alternating with three cycles of radiotherapy (2 Gy/d, 5 d/wk × 2 wk) or conventional radiotherapy (2 Gy/d, 5 d/wk, total 70 Gy) *(49)*. Statistically significant responses were seen overall with CR (42% vs 22%, $p = 0.037$), median survival (16.5 mo vs 11.7 mo, $p < 0.05$), and 3-yr OS (41% vs 23%) in the chemoradiation arm vs the radiotherapy alone, respectively. Toxicities were similar in both tarms (19% vs 18%). A 5-yr estimate of overall survival has been reported noting improved OS in the concomitant chemoradiation group, 24% vs 10%, $p = 0.01$ *(50)*. Other statistically significant parameters in the chemoradiation arm were locoregional relapse-free survival (64% vs 32%, $p = 0.038$) and PFS (21% vs 9%, $p = 0.008$).

The combination of cisplatin and 5-FU was evaluated in a large prospective randomized multicenter trial comparing radiation therapy alone to that of radiation therapy with concomitant cisplatin (60 mg/m^2)/5-FU (350 mg/m^2, bolus)/leucovorin (LV) *(51)*. Three courses of accelerated fractionated twice-daily radiation therapy were in both arms with 13 fractions of 1.8 Gy. The second arm incorporated cisplatin/bolus 5-FU/LV (50 mg/m^2) on d 2, with continuous infusion 5-FU (350 mg/m^2)/LV (100 mg/m^2) on d 2–5. The cycle was repeated every 21 d for a total of three courses. Toxicities were augmented in the concomitant regimen with 38% of patients having grade 3/4 mucositis versus only 16% seen on the radiation only arm ($p < 0.001$). Grade 3/4 radiation dermatitis was also increased on the concomitant arm vs the radiation therapy only arm

(17% vs 7%, respectively, $p < 0.05$). Patients in the chemoradiation arm fared better in the 3-yr analysis of locoregional control and survival 35% vs 17%, ($p < 0.004$) and 49% vs 24% ($p < 0.0003$), respectively. However, appearance of distant disease was equivalent in both arms 10% and 9%.

Adelstein et al. have recently reported preliminary results of a randomized phase III trial in 295 patients with unresectable stage III or IV HNC comparing three treatment arms: arm A of standard fractionated therapy (2 Gy/d); arm B was the same regimen of radiotherapy with three cycles of concurrent cisplatin (100 mg/m^2 on d 1 of a 21-d cycle); and arm C was split-course radiotherapy given with three cycles of concomitant cisplatin (100 mg/m^2 on d 1) and continuous infusion 5-FU (1000 mg/m^2, d 1–4) to be repeated every 28 d *(52)*. Patients were offered surgical resection following cycle 2 and all were offered salvage surgery in all treatment arms. As expected, grade III or worse toxicities were frequently seen in the concomitant chemoradiation arms 52% vs 86% ($p < 0.0001$) vs 77% ($p < 0.001$) in arms A, B, and C, respectively. After a median follow-up of 25 mo, the concomitant chemoradiation arms fared better with projected 3-yr overall survival rates of 20% vs 37% ($p = 0.016$), vs 29% ($p = 0.013$) in arms A, B, and C, respectively; no difference in overall survival was seen between arms B and C; median survival was more favorable in the chemoradiation arms 19.1 mo in arm B, and 14 mo for arm C (12.6 mo in arm A). These data support the use of concomitant chemoradiotherapy with cisplatin as the minimum in standard therapy. Although encouraging, administration of concomitant chemoradiotherapy with standard agents of cisplatin and 5-FU provided only modest increases in overall survival indicating the need for improved techniques, methodology, and chemotherapy agents.

Adelstein and colleagues have also recently reported the 5-yr results of a small phase III of 100 patients with stage III or IV disease randomized to radiotherapy alone or to that of radiotherapy combined with 5-FU (1000 mg/m^2/d) and cisplatin (20 mg/m^2/d) given by continuous infusion on d 1–4 and repeated on d 22 *(53)*. Only patients with residual or recurrent disease were to be resected following therapy. Following the completion of treatment, 82% of patients were disease-free following radiotherapy alone, with 98% of patients remaining disease-free on the concomitant chemoradiotherapy arm ($p = 0.02$). After a median follow-up of 5 yr the OS was not statistically significant ($p = 0.55$) when comparing the two modalities of treatment. This study was also unable to demonstrate a decrease in distant disease involvement ($p = 0.09$). However, fewer patients required salvage surgery on the concomitant chemoradiotherapy arm, and the study suggested the importance of the role of chemoradiotherapy for primary-site preservation. Of statistical significance was the recurrence-free interval ($p = 0.04$), OS with primary-site preservation ($p = 0.004$), and locoregional control without surgical resection ($p < 0.001$) in the chemoradiotherapy arm. Incorporating similar regimens with the primary goal of site preservation is promising to decrease the disfigurement and complications that may ensue with initial surgery.

A randomized study comparing carboplatin/5-FU/radiotherapy vs radiotherapy in patients with locally advanced oropharyngeal carcinoma was recently reported by the French Group of Radiation Oncology for HNC (GORTEC) *(54)*. Two hundred twenty-six patients were randomized to conventional radiotherapy or identical radiotherapy combined with three cycles of the 4-d regimen of carboplatin (70 mg/m^2/d) and continuous infusion 5-FU (600 mg/m^2/d) on d 1, 22, and 43 of radiation. Increased mucositis was reported in the combined modality arm 67% vs 36%. No difference in skin toxicity was reported. The 3-yr OS (51% vs 31%, $p = 0.002$) and DFS (42% vs 19%, $p = 0.003$) were significantly improved in the concomitant chemoradiation arm.

5. VARIATIONS IN COMBINED MODALITY CHEMORADIATION SCHEDULES

5.1. Concomitant Split-Course Chemoradiotherapy Trials

Byfield demonstrated enhanced radiosensitization properties of 5-FU when exposed continuously for at least 48 h following radiation therapy *(55)*. Thus, the cytoxicity of 5-FU is dependent on the exposure time to 5-FU exceeding the doubling time of the tumor cell. Based on this premise, a small phase I/II pilot study by Byfield and colleagues evaluated 18 patients with advanced HNC to study the effects of dose-escalating continuous infusion 5-FU (20–30 mg/kg in 5 mg/kg increments) over a 5-d period with four sequential daily fractions (250 rads) on d 1–4 *(56)*. The cycle was then repeated after a 9-d rest period for a total of five treatment cycles. The completed response rate was reported at 75% for stage IV patients with the primary toxicity being mucositis.

Taylor and colleagues have published an 8-yr analysis of Rush Medical College's experience with stage III or IV patients that have received concomitant cisplatin (60 mg/m^2, d 1), continuous infusion 5-FU (800 mg/m^2, d 1–5), and single fraction radiation therapy (2 Gy) on d 1–5 *(57)*. The cycle was repeated every other week for a total of seven cycles. The sample size was small with 78 patients. Six weeks after initial therapy, 63% had no clinical evidence of disease, 37% had a partial response (PR). Overall, 31% of patients had recurred or progressed; 24% died from nontumor-related causes. The 5-yr PFS was 60% in this small cohort of patients with an overall survival reported to be 43%.

At the University of Chicago an analysis of a small cohort of 39 patients suggested activity in head and neck malignancies when hydroxyurea is combined with 5-FU and radiation therapy. Patients were given escalating doses of hydroxyurea (500–3000 mg/d in 500 mg/d increments) with fixed doses of continuous infusion 5-FU (800 mg/m^2/d for d 1–5) with accelerated fractionated radiotherapy *(58)*. Patients were then given a 9-d rest period; one cycle was equivalent to 14 d. The patients were divided into two subgroups with an initial subgroup of patients that had been previously treated with surgery and/or radiation therapy demonstrating clinical response rates (40% CR, 53% PR) with short time to (TTP) of 6 mo; 14 eventually progressed locally. A second subgroup of radiation therapy naïve patients demonstrated clinical response rates (71% CR, 29% PR) with a median time to progression of 14 mo; only three patients failed locally. Failure to recur locally in this small subgroup prompted continued investigation of hydroxyurea as an adjunct to other chemotherapy agents at the University of Chicago.

We proceeded with a multi-institutional phase II trial of a select cohort of 60 patients who had received limited or no surgery for stage II or III HNC between 1989 and 1996 *(59)*. High-risk patients with stage III base of tongue and piriform sinus cancer were excluded from this study. The most common primary lesion was of the larynx (33 patients). Patients received continuous infusion 5-FU (800 mg/m^2/d, d 1–5) and hydroxyurea (1000 mg BID × 11 doses, in the evening of d 0–5), radiotherapy was given as a single daily fraction on d 1–5 (FHX); d 6–14 were considered to be a rest week. The initial endpoint was to improve locoregional control and increase OS. The secondary endpoint in this study was to determine if chemotherapy before or during radiation would result in less surgery and allow organ preservation. Patients received a total of six to eight cycles of treatment. Thirty-nine patients had received no prior surgery excluding biopsy. Primary toxicities encountered were grade 3/4 mucositis and neutropenia. The OS, PFS, and locoregional control were 65%, 82%, and 86%, respectively after 5-yr follow-up. Two patients developed metastatic disease; eight patients developed a locoregional recurrence with three of these patients undergoing salvage surgery for a 5-yr locoregional control rate of 91%. We believe this is the only study of its kind using concomitant chemoradiotherapy for early stage HNSCC patients.

We then chose to expand on the FHX regimen with the addition of paclitaxel (TFHX) for poor-prognosis patients HNC patients in a phase I study *(60)*. Included in this study were patients that developed a relapse following radiotherapy or surgery with curative intent, unresectable disease, metastatic disease requiring localized radiotherapy, and a 2-yr survival of < 10% were eligible. Patients were allowed to receive daily or hyperfractionated radiotherapy on d 2–6 with concurrent paclitaxel (5–25 mg/m^2/d for 5 d, in escalating increments of 5 mg/m^2/d), hydroxyurea (1000 mg BID for 11 doses), and continuous infusion 5-FU (600–800 mg/m^2/d for 5 d). Granulocyte colony-stimulating factor (5 μg/kg) was administered on d 7–13. As expected, primary toxicities encountered included myelosuppression, dermatitis, mucositis, and diarrhea. Of the evaluable patients, 70% achieved a pathologically confirmed CR. At a median follow-up of 28 mo, the median PFS is 9.5 mo and the 2-yr survival rate is 32%. The median overall survival is 14.5 mo with the estimated 2-yr survival of 32%. No differences were seen when comparing previously treated to untreated patients. The recommended phase II schedule is paclitaxel (20 mg/m^2/d for 5 d), hydroxyurea (1000 mg BID for 11 doses), continuous infusion 5-FU (600 mg/m^2/d for 5 d), and twice-daily hyperfractionated radiotherapy.

Based on the impressive response rates obtained on the TFHX regimen, a multi-institutional phase II study was pursued in 64 untreated stage IV patients at the recommended phase II dose *(61)*. Chemoradiation was completed d 1–5, with resumption of the regimen on d 14 for a total of five cycles. Patients were also requested to complete evaluations pertaining to their quality of life. Eighty-four percent of the patients developed grade 3/4 mucositis. After a median follow-up of 34 mo, 3-yr estimates of locoregional control were 86% and systemic control was achieved in 79% of patients. At 1-yr, chronic sequelae included severe xerostomia in 61% of patients and swallowing dysfunction in 47% of patients. Fifteen percent of survivors required feeding tubes. Despite these side effects, global quality of life assessment scores changed little in comparison to pretreatment levels and had fully recovered by 12 mo. Emotional well being at 12 mo was improved in comparison to pretreatment ($p = 0.1$).

5.2. Alternating Chemoradiotherapy

Merlano and colleagues completed a phase III study comparing sequential vs alternating chemoradiotherapy *(62)*. One hundred sixteen patients were randomized to arm A of the sequential regimen of four cycles of Vinblastine (6 mg/m^2, h 0), bleomycin (30 mg, h 6), methotrexate (200 mg, h 24–26), and leucovorin (45 mg, h 48) followed within 3 wk by definitive radiotherapy or arm B composed of the same chemotherapy regimen alternating with three courses of daily fractionated therapy for 2 wk. The difference in response rates (52% for arm A vs 64.9% for arm B) was found to be statistically significant, $p < 0.03$, as well as the median PFS (26 vs 34 wk, $p = 0.046$) without differences seen in OS ($p = 0.64$).

5.3. Sequential vs Concomitant Chemoradiotherapy

Taylor and colleagues randomized unresectable patients to sequential chemoradiotherapy or concomitant chemoradiotherapy *(63)*. The sequential treatment schedule consisted of three cycles of cisplatin (100 mg/m^2 on d 1) with continuous infusion 5-FU (1000 mg/m^2, on d 1–5) repeated every 3 wks followed by standard daily radiotherapy. On the concomitant arm, patients were given seven cycles of cisplatin (60 mg/m^2 on d 1) and continuous infusion 5-FU (800 mg/m^2 on d 1–5) with daily radiotherapy on d 1–5; the cycle was repeated every other week. Following chemotherapy patients were given the option to be resected prior to receiving radiotherapy. Toxicities encountered in both arms were similar with increased instances of cisplatin-induced electrolyte imbalance in the concurrent arm. Complete response rates were similar in both arms (50% vs 52%) with an increased number of partial responses in the concomitant arm resulting in increased overall response rate ($p = 0.006$). More patients in the sequential arm eventually died from the disease ($p = 0.011$). Development of distal disease was similar in both arms (10% vs 7%) but increasing instances of locoregional recurrence developed in the sequential arm (55% vs 39%).

A German study randomized 98 patients with unresectable hypopharyngeal head and neck carcinoma to sequential or concomitant chemoradiotherapy *(64)*. Patients on the sequential arm received two courses of cisplatin (25 mg/m^2 for 5 d) and continuous infusion 5-FU (750 mg/m^2 for 5 d) followed by G-CSF for 6 d. The second cycle was repeated on d 14 and then followed by standard radiotherapy. Identical dosages of chemoradiotherapy were used in the concomitant arm but incorporated a 21-d interval between each chemotherapy cycle and G-CSF support. Sequential treatment resulted in a CR of 49% in comparison to the concomitant arm of 57%. At 2-yr, the median survival was improved in the concomitant arm (53% vs 33%). However, one-third of the initial patients enrolled were withdrawn from study due to medical or socioeconomic problems; whether this resulted in a significant disparity between the two different treatment arms was not noted. Mature data from this trial have not been published to date.

In a phase I dose escalation study in locally advanced HNC patients, a concomitant regimen of weekly docetaxel and irinotecan and conventional radiotherapy was combined *(47)*. Docetaxel was given over 20 min on d 1, irinotecan was administered as 30 min infusion on d 3. Three docetaxel/irinotecan dose levels were compared: 20/25 mg/m^2 (level 1), 20/40 mg/m^2 (dose level 2), and 25/55 mg/m^2 (dose level 3). Severe asthenia resulted in all patients at dose level 3. Myelosuppression was minimal. Complete responses were seen radiologically in 75% of patients and a partial response in 25% of patients.

6. INDUCTION CHEMOTHERAPY AND ORGAN PRESERVATION

The rationale of induction or neoadjuvant chemotherapy is to decrease the locoregional tumor burden, decrease the need for surgery, promote organ preservation, and fundamentally increase the quality of life. A potential secondary role of induction chemotherapy is to treat micrometastatic disease and in turn prevent the appearance of distant disease. The use of induction chemotherapy has an essential role in laryngeal and hypopharyngeal cancers where primary treatment modalities initially included total laryngectomy with neck dissection followed by radiation therapy. Hence, patients would possibly suffer from loss of voice, develop swallowing dysfunction, and numerous changes in their daily lifestyle. Other aspects include lack of social acceptance, changes in personal hygiene, personal appearance, and consequently depression.

Review of the literature demonstrates little justification for the use of induction (neoadjuvant) chemotherapy outside of a clinical trial, unless in the setting of laryngeal or hypopharyngeal carcinoma. Five well-controlled studies have evaluated induction chemotherapy with the traditional agents, cisplatin and 5-FU, with only one study demonstrating a survival advantage in the development of locoregional and distant disease control, and an improvement in overall survival *(65,66)*. Primarily, induction chemotherapy was not found to have an impact on the prevention of locoregional disease. However, in the scenario of laryngeal or hypopharyngeal cancer, induction chemotherapy has been shown to preserve laryngeal function *(65,66)*. Therefore, induction chemotherapy outside of a clinical trial cannot be justified unless in the setting of laryngeal or hypopharyngeal disease.

Two trials have established the role of induction chemotherapy in organ preservation. The Veterans Affairs Laryngeal Study randomized 332 patients with stage III or IV laryngeal carcinoma to receive three cycles of cisplatin/5-FU (PF) followed by conventional radiotherapy or laryngectomy and conventional radiotherapy *(65)*. Patients were evaluated following two cycles of chemotherapy. Patients with a PR received a third cycle of chemotherapy followed by radiotherapy. Those patients without initial response to induction chemotherapy received laryngectomy followed by radiation therapy. Patients with residual disease following the completion of radiotherapy underwent surgical resection. After two cycles of induction, the overall response rate (ORR) was 85% (31% CR, 54% PR). Histological specimens were obtained in 103 patients after completing chemotherapy validating a complete response in 88% of patients with a clinical CR; 45% of those presumed to have a clinical PR were confirmed histologically. Overall, 64% of patients had a histological complete response. At a median follow-up of 33 mo, the estimated 2-yr survival was 68% in both treatment groups failing to demonstrate a difference in overall survival ($p = 0.9846$). However, the majority of patients (64%) were able to preserve laryngeal function. Patterns of recurrence differed between the two groups with increased local-regional control ($p = 0.0005$) and decreased metastases ($p = 0.016$) in the induction chemotherapy group. Although there was no significant difference in overall survival this demonstrates that induction is feasible in the setting of laryngeal carcinoma allowing organ preservation without compromise of overall survival. It should be noted that of these 166 patients on the chemotherapy arm, 120 patients (72%) had N0 or N1 disease.

The European Organization for Research and Treatment of Cancer (EORTC) confirmed these findings by completing a prospective, randomized phase III assessing the efficacy of organ preservation in patients with hypopharyngeal cancer of the pyriform sinus or aryepiglottic folds *(66)*. One hundred ninety-four eligible patients were randomized to immediate surgery followed by radiotherapy (94 patients) or induction chemotherapy (100 patients) with cisplatin (100 mg/m^2, d 1) and continuous infusion 5-FU (1000 mg/m^2/d, d 1–5). Patients were assessed by an endoscopic exam after each cycle. Patients with a CR or PR following cycle 2 were offered a third cycle of chemotherapy. Patients achieving a complete response were treated with radiation therapy; patients with stable disease were offered surgery followed by radiotherapy. Induction chemotherapy resulted in CR of 54% at the primary site and 51% achieved a CR for locoregional disease. Overall, fewer failures were seen distantly ($p = 0.041$) and an increased median survival was seen in the induction arm (44 mo) vs the surgical arm (25 mo). Unfortunately, the two arms failed to show a difference in locoregional recurrence. Induction chemotherapy did manage to preserve the larynx in 42% and 35% of patients in 3- and 5-yr estimates of survival. Once again suggesting that induction chemotherapy is a feasible alternative if organ preservation is desired without compromising duration of survival. However, it should be noted that only 31% of patients had $N2/N_3$ disease of which only 6% were N_3. Furthermore, patients with N_3 disease were eventually excluded from this trial since the first six patients failed to achieve a CR following induction.

An interesting perspective to evaluate in each of these trials would have been to include a subset analysis of the quality of life in patients that were disease-free following initial therapy on the combined modality arms in comparison to those that received surgery upfront.

The Dana-Farber Cancer Institute has recently reported the maximal tolerated dose of cisplatin, when given in the combination of docetaxel, and 5-FU as induction chemotherapy in patients with locally advanced HNC *(67)*. Patients received docetaxel (75 mg/m^2, d 1), cisplatin at (75 mg/m^2 or 100 mg/m^2) and continuous infusion 5-FU (1000 mg/m^2 on d 1–4), to be repeated every 21 d taxoterel platinum and 5-FU (TPF). Patients were given antibiotics empirically on d 5–15. Of 43 patients, 13 received the docetaxel at 75 mg/m^2. Toxicities were similar at both dose levels consisting of cisplatin-associated electrolyte imbalance in 30% of the patients and grade 3/4 neutropenia in 95% of patients. Patients were considered evaluable for response if they completed two or more cycles. The overall clinical response rate was 94% (40% CR, 54% PR). Twenty-five patients (58%) agreed to have their response pathologically confirmed. Eleven of 12 patients (92%) with a primary site clinical CR had negative biopsies; 7 of 13 patients (54%) with a primary site PR had a negative biopsy. Based on these promising results in comparison to standard cisplatin/5-FU (PF) as induction, a randomized phase III trial comparing TPF to PF is currently underway followed by sequential chemoradiotherapy with carboplatin is currently underway.

At the University of Chicago we continue to minimize the degree of surgery that must be undertaken. Review of our previous combined chemoradiation trials concluded that locoregional control was increased at the expense of the development of distant disease. Based on this premise, we have incorporated intensive concomitant chemoradiotherapy as the primary treatment modality in locoregionally advanced stage III, IV HNC to address both locoregional control and distant disease. Recent emphasis on potential benefits of chemoprevention provided the impetus for a phase II trial of the combination regimen of cisplatin (100 mg/m^2) every 28 d (cycles 1, 3, and 5), and continuous infusion 5-FU (800 mg/m^2, d 1–5), hydroxyurea (1000 mg BID for 11 doses), twice-daily radiotherapy (1.5 Gy/d, d 1–5) every other week; one cycle was equivalent to 14 d *(68)*. Patients were then given granulocyte colony-stimulating factor (5 μg/kg) on d 7–13. Stage III patients were only eligible if the primary tumor involved the base of the tongue or hypopharynx. After the completion of treatment, patients with palpable lymphadenopathy underwent a neck dissection. Complete excision at the primary site was undertaken if residual disease was seen macroscopically. Primary toxicities encountered included grade 3/4 neutropenia (81%), thrombocytopenia (78%), and mucositis (57%). Three patients developed sepsis and expired. Supportive care including feeding tubes and both blood and platelet transfusions were required. Elective chemopreventive measures including α-interferon and *cis*-retinoic acid were offered with the majority of patients (34%) declining. Thirteen patients had surgery at the primary site and 39 patients had a neck dissection. After a median follow-up of 38 mo, the 3-yr progression-free survival (PFS) was 72%, locoregional control was achieved in 92%, and distal control (83%), with an overall survival of 55%. Hence, 17% of patients recurred distally despite administration of cytotoxic chemotherapy. Whether the addition of induction chemotherapy in this setting could further reduce the appearance of distant disease has continued to be addressed at our institution.

The encouraging results of the Veterans Affairs laryngeal preservation trial has provided the foundation for a phase III RTOG (91-11) three-arm study comparing the benefits of induction chemoradiotherapy with cisplatin/5-FU vs concomitant chemoradiotherapy with single agent cisplatin vs single modality radiation therapy alone. Arm 1 consists of standard administration of three cycles of cisplatin/5-FU (continuous infusion) every 3 wk followed by standard daily radiotherapy; arm 2 is comprised of three cycles of standard bolus infusion of cisplatin every 21 d with concomitant conventional radiotherapy; and arm 3 is conventional radiotherapy only. Forastiere and colleges *(68a)* have reported preliminary results. At 2 yr., the laryngectomy-free survival was improved in both Arms 1 and 2 (58% to 66%, respectively) vs 52% in Arm 3. There was no statistical significant difference in laryngectomy-free survival or OS when comparing Arm 2 and Arm 3 to Arm 1. This study concluded that indication chemotherapy did not differ from radiation therapy alone.

Investigative studies utilizing induction chemotherapy have provided ample evidence of decreased development of distant disease following initial treatment. Although failure to demonstrate an improvement in overall survival causes us to conclude that distant disease, variances in salvage therapy after recurrence, and other complications are factors that need to be addressed to increase overall survival.

7. META-ANALYSES

Over 70 randomized trials comparing radiation to chemoradiotherapy have been completed in the hopes of ascertaining the absolute benefits of chemotherapy when used as an adjunct to radiotherapy in local control, overall survival, and relapse-free survival. However, these studies often involved small cohorts. As such, meta-analyses were created to assess a larger patient population and to help determine the absolute benefits of the addition of chemotherapy *(69–71)*.

The largest meta-analysis is the Meta-Analysis of Chemotherapy in Head and Neck Cancer (MACH-NC) study evaluating 63 trials with a total of 10,741 patients (Table 2) *(69)*. MACH-NC assessed individual data rather than literature-based data with the inclusion of updated data and unpublished trials. For two-thirds of the trials, individual data were updated to a median follow-up of 6.8 yr. The meta-analysis was subcategorized into locoregional treatment with and without concomitant chemotherapy, induction/adjuvant chemotherapy, and laryngeal preservation with induction chemotherapy rather than definitive treatment for laryngeal and hypopharyngeal tumors.

The MACH-NC study included a subset analysis of six randomized trials of 861 patients evaluating neoadjuvant with or without adjuvant chemotherapy combined with radiotherapy vs concomitant/alternating chemotherapy. No significant benefit was associated with adjuvant or neoadjuvant chemotherapy. A trend in favor of concomitant or alternating chemoradiotherapy was found but was not determined to be statistically significant (p = 0.23). This analysis demonstrated an absolute benefit of 7% and 8% for concomitant therapy at 2 and 5 yr ($p = 0.16$), respectively, an overall benefit of 4%. In short, if 10,000 patients were diagnosed with locally advanced HNC, concurrent therapy may benefit 800 patients over 5 yr.

Table 2
Meta-Analyses Overview

	Meta-Analyses			
	Stell	*Munro*	*El-Sayed*	*MACH-NC*
Number of trials evaluated	28	54	42	63
Absolute benefits of chemotherapy				
Induction	–2% (NS)	3.7% ($p = 0.011$)	Not known (NS)	2% ($p = 0.10$)
Adjuvant	–2%	N/A	Not known	1% ($p = 0.74$)
Concomitant	7% ($p = 0.02$)	12.1% ($p < 0.001$)	8% ($p < 0.005$)	8% ($p < 0.0001$)
Overall	2.8% (NS)	6.5% ($p < 0.001$)	4% ($p < 0.001$)	4% ($p < 0.0001$)

N/A = not applicable, NS = not statistically significant.

Bourhis et al. have completed a recent review focusing on four previously written meta-analyses comparing chemotherapy (induction, adjuvant, and concomitant) plus locoregional treatment vs locoregional treatment alone with the end-point of each analysis being overall survival. Overall, a small but significant advantage with the addition of single-agent chemotherapy to radiotherapy was demonstrated *(70)*. It should be mentioned that this review included the MACH-NC trial written by Bourhis and colleagues.

Stell and colleagues assessed 28 randomized trials published only in the English literature *(72)*. Induction and adjuvant chemotherapy was found to have no additional benefit (–2% in each); the addition of concomitant chemotherapy provided a 7% increase in absolute benefit. Therefore, the overall benefit when assessing induction, adjuvant, and concomitant chemotherapy was 2.8%.

Munro and colleagues evaluated 54 trials including those prior to 1965 *(71)*. Two trials included were specifically for maxillary sinus carcinoma and nasopharyngeal carcinoma. Additionally, the Veteran's Laryngeal Cancer study with the end-point being organ preservation was also included. In this study, the overall benefit of adding chemotherapy was 6.5% (3.7% for induction, 12.1% for concomitant, adjuvant chemotherapy was not assessed).

El Sayed and Nelson reviewed 42 trials between 1963 and 1993 including six trials prior to 1965 and one trial using razoxane, a nonstandard chemotherapy agent *(73)*. A drawback to the El Sayed analysis is the inclusion of a single trial that had been accounted for twice because of its publication in two different journals. The addition of chemotherapy to locoregional treatment added an absolute benefit of 4.0%; absolute benefits of concomitant chemotherapy were 8% (neoadjuvant and adjuvant chemotherapy were not assessed).

8. TREATING RECURRENT DISEASE

Combination regimens utilizing standard chemotherapy as a single modality have been attempted with increased toxicities reported but impressive overall and complete response rates as high as 27% for patients with recurrent and metastatic disease *(74)*. Schrijvers and colleagues concluded that the addition of interferon α-2b (IFN-α) as a biomodulator of 5-FU and cisplatin in the recurrent or metastatic setting offered no benefit *(75)*. One hundred twenty-two patients were randomized to cisplatin (100 mg/m^2, d 1) and continuous infusion 5-FU (1000 mg/m^2, d 1–4) with or without the addition of IFN-α. The overall response rates (47.1% vs 38.4%, $p > 0.50$) and median survival (6.3 vs 6 mo, $p = 0.49$) with and without the addition of INF-α, respectively were similar in both arms and were not statistically significant.

A randomized phase II trial comparing weekly methotrexate (MTX, 40–60 mg/m^2) vs triweekly paclitaxel (175–225 mg/m^2 by 3-h or 24-h infusion) in the recurrent or metastatic setting was prematurely closed as a result of toxicity and minimal response *(76)*.

The Eastern Cooperative Oncology Group has studied the combination of high-dose paclitaxel and cisplatin with G-CSF support in comparison to low-dose paclitaxel and cisplatin in a recent phase III trial *(77)*. Patients with locally advanced, recurrent, or metastatic disease were randomly placed on arm A of paclitaxel (200 mg/m^2 over a 24-h infusion), cisplatin (75 mg/m^2), and G-CSF (starting d 3 until the ANC was >10,000/μL) or arm B of paclitaxel (135 mg/m^2 over a 24-h infusion) and cisplatin (75 mg/m^2). The treatment was repeated every 21 d until progression of disease or a total of 12 cycles.

Despite G-CSF support, neutropenia was frequently encountered (70% in arm A, 78% arm B). Thirty-one percent of patients failed to complete their recommended treatment due to toxicity or patient refusal. Overall response rates in both arms were comparable (35% high-dose combination vs 36% low-dose combination) and were determined to be suboptimal not warranting further investigation.

Murphy and colleagues have reported on a randomized phase III study in recurrent or metastatic HNC comparing the standard chemotherapy regimen of cisplatin (100 mg/m^2, d 1) and continuous infusion 5-FU (1000 mg/m^2, d 1–4) every 21 d vs cisplatin (75 mg/m^2) and paclitaxel (175 mg/m^2) every 21 d *(78)*. No difference in survival ($p = 0.22$) or quality of life was noted.

The relatively high rates of locoregional recurrence following definitive treatment require the reconsideration of further radiation in a previously irradiated field. A synopsis of previously completed and current trials is presented in Table 3. A phase I trial of intensive reirradiation in patients with unresectable recurrent HNC requiring local irradiation has recently finished accrual at our institution. Patients were administered five cycles of paclitaxel (100 mg/m^2, d 1), 5-FU (600 mg/m^2/d on d 1–5), hydroxyurea with hyperfractionated twice-daily radiotherapy wk 1 and 2 with the addition of escalating doses of gemcitabine (50–300 mg/m^2, d 1 only) wk 3–5. Dose-limiting toxicities frequently encountered included grade 3/4 radiation dermatitis and mucositis resulting in a protocol amendment advocating the use of gemcitabine for wk 4 and 5 only. The MTD of gemcitabine is 150 mg/m^2 in this combination regimen. A preliminary analysis reveals a CR of 61% of 44 valuable patients *(78a)*.

We are also currently conducting a phase I/II trial in patients with unresectable, advanced, or locally recurrent HNC with potential benefits from reirradiation (Table 4). We chose to evaluate the promising radiosensitization effects of irinotecan by combining it with our FHX regimen *(79)*. Patients were given five cycles of irinotecan (5–15 mg/m^2, d 1–5), continuous infusion 5-FU (600 mg/m^2, d 1–5), hydroxyurea (500 mg BID for 11 doses), and hyperfractionated twice-daily radiotherapy. Preliminary analysis of patients in the phase I setting established a MTD of irinotecan at 10 mg/m^2.

Conceptually, can patients benefit from further radiotherapy in the setting of chronic sequelae that they often must endure? A French study addressed this concept by administering split-course chemoradiotherapy based on a modified University of Chicago FHX regimen to patients with unresectable, locally recurrent HNC *(80)*. Of 33 evaluable patients, ORR clinically of 54% (40% CR, 15% PR) with stable disease (SD) in 15%. These results were not confirmed pathologically. Grade III mucositis developed in 27% of patients and as a result, four patients required a dose reduction. The mean duration of maintaining a CR was 16 mo. The sample size was small but demonstrated the feasibility of considering reirradiation in locally recurrent disease.

Based on encouraging results from an early pilot study completed by Rush-Presbyterian-St. Luke's Medical Center, ECOG evaluated previously irradiated patients who presented with locally recurrent and/or metastatic disease *(81)*. Patients received seven cycles of cisplatin (60 mg/m^2, d 1), continuous infusion 5-FU (800 mg/m^2, d 1–5), and standard daily radiotherapy (d 1–5) to be repeated every other week. All patients developed grade 2/3 mucositis. Clinically, the ORR was 74% (48% CR, 24% PR). Median TTP was 5 mo. Of interest were three patients that remained disease-free at 44 mo (T2N0), 86 mo (T0N2), and 88 mo (T2N0).

Table 3
Reirradiation for Recurrent Disease

Collaborators	N	*Regimen*	*Results*
Gandia	33	CIFU (800 mg/m^2, d 1–5)/Hydrea (1000–1500 mg daily)/ daily hyperfractionated XRT (2 Gy/fraction) (FHX), repeated every 14 d	CR = 40%, PR = 15%
Hartsell	21	Cisplatin (60 mg/m^2, d 1)/CIFU (800 mg/m^2, d 1–5), and daily XRT (20–70 Gy), every 14 d	CR = 48%, PR = 24%
Haraf	45	Cisplatin (100 mg/m^2, d 1)/CIFU (800 mg/m^2, d 1–5)/ Hydrea (1000 mg q12 × 11 doses)/ hyperfractionated twice-daily XRT (1.5 Gy/fraction) every 14 d	At 5 yr: OS = 14.6%, LRC = 20%
Haraf	48	Paclitaxel/CIFU/Hydrea/XRT (escalated from 2 Gy daily to 1.5 Gy BID)	At 2 yr: OS = 31%, PFS = 44%, LRC = 59%
RTOG 96-10	86	5-FU (300 mg/m^2 iv bolus, d 1–5)/Hydrea (1500 mg, d 1–5)/ hyperfractionated twice daily XRT (1.5 Gy/fraction, d 1–5), wk 1,3, 5, and 7	Median OS = 8.8 m, 1-yr OS = 43 ± 11%
University of Chicago	73	Paclitaxel/5-FU/Hydrea/Gemcitabine/ hyperfractionated twice-daily XRT	CR = 61%, PR = 16%
Humerickhouse		CPT-11/5-FU/Hydrea/hyperfractionated twice-daily XRT	Pending
RTOG 99-11	In progress	Paclitaxel (20 mg/m^2 over 1 h, d 1–5)/Cisplatin (15 mg/m^2, d 1–5)/ hyperfractionated twice-daily XRT (60 Gy total dose in 40 fractions: 1.5 Gy/fraction, d 1–5), wk 1, 3, 5, and 7	Pending

N = number of patients, CIFU = continuous infusion 5-FU, Hydrea = hydroxyurea, XRT = radiation therapy, LRC = locoregional control.

Table 4
Schema for Ongoing Trial at the University of Chicago for Patients Requiring Reirradiation

Within 4 wk of initiation therapy		*Within 1 wk of initiating treatment*			*D 0*
Initial H & P		Baseline physical exam			Hydrea
Performance status	→	Baseline laboratory work		→	Continuous infusion 5-FU
Chest X-ray					
Panendoscopy/biopsy					↓
Bone scan					*D 1–5*
CT or MRI					Hydrea
Swallowing evaluation					Continuous infusion 5-FU
					CPT-11
					Hyperfractionated twice-daily XRT
			Repeat every		
			14 d		↓
					Maximum of five cycles

A retrospective analysis of a subset of previously radiated patients with locoregional recurrence or progression who were treated with the split-course combination regimen of cisplatin-FHX (CFHX) has been reported *(82)*. After a median observation of 46 mo, the median survival was 8.5 mo. Patients that received ≥ 58 Gy, had improved 5-yr survival (22%), PFS (26%), and locoregional control (40%).

The RTOG has recently reported on RTOG 96-10, a phase I/II study of a split-course chemoradiation schedule of concomitant hydroxyurea (2000 mg prior to second daily radiation dose, d 1–5), 5-FU (300 mg/m^2 iv bolus prior to second daily radiation dose, d 1–5), and twice-daily hyperfractionated radiation therapy (1.5 Gy/fraction, d 1–5) to be administered wk 1, 3, 5, 7 *(83)*. Seventy-nine percent of the patients received all four cycles. Treatment delays of at least one week were required in 32% of patients. Six patients died from treatment-related toxicity. Of 81 evaluable patients, common grade 3/4 toxicities that developed included mucositis (19%), oropharyngeal toxicity (17%), and neutropenia (19%). Grade 5 neutropenia developed in 7%. After a median follow-up of 16.5 mo for living patientsthe median overall survival was 8.2 mo. When comparing a subset analysis of patients that were previously irradiated > 3 yr prior, the 1-yr survival was improved (48% vs 35%, $p = 0.17$).

These studies have demonstrated the improved response rates and feasibility of combined chemotherapy and reirradiation in comparison to standard chemotherapy in this setting of otherwise poor prognosis patients. Other chemotherapy agents currently undergoing investigation trials are those being evaluated in the primary setting including the taxanes, topoisomerase I inhibitors, and gemcitabine.

The RTOG has an ongoing phase II study analyzing the use of paclitaxel and cisplatin in combination with split-course concomitant radiotherapy in patients with recurrent squamous cell carcinoma requiring reirradiation. Cisplatin and paclitaxel are administered d 1–5 with concomitant hyperfractionated twice daily radiation therapy on wk 1, 3, 5, and 7.

9. NEW AGENTS

A variety of new chemotherapy agents are promising in the treatment of advanced HNC. Different combinations with new and old agents to promote decreased radioresistance, decreased toxicities, and diverse methodology including incorporation of induction continue to be investigated.

9.1. Tirapazamine

Novel mechanisms of interest include sensitizing hypoxic tumor cell lines to enhance radiotoxicity. Tirapazamine is a hypoxia-selective compound 1–2-fold greater in magnitude in comparison to mitomycin C or porfiromycin *(84)*. Its mechanism of action results in a one-electron reduction inducing DNA double-strand breaks and cell death under hypoxic conditions. The free radical is oxidized back to the parent compound under aerobic conditions. When combined with the platinum compounds, the cytotoxic effects may be equivalent to that seen with five times the dose of cisplatin without the toxicities that would be encountered if actually administered *(85)*.

Rishin and colleagues have recently reported results of a phase I trial of conventional fractionated radiotherapy with concurrent tirapazamine (290 mg/m^2), cisplatin (75 mg/m^2) wk 1, 4, and 7, and tirapazemine alone (160 mg/m^2, three times per wk) wk 2, 3, 5, and 6 for untreated stage IV HNC patients *(86)*. The cohort was small at 20 patients. Dose limiting toxicity of febrile neutropenia developed in 3 of 6 patients requiring a revision of the initial treatment schedule by omitting wk 5 and 6 of tirapazamine. Though, survival was a secondary endpoint in this phase I study, after a median follow-up of 2.7 yr the 3-yr OS rate was 69% with a 3-yr PFS rate of 88%.

Based on this initial study by Rischin et al., the University of Chicago is currently accruing for a phase I trial of previously irradiated patients. Patients will receive standard daily radiotherapy and tirapazamine (wk 1–3) combined with cisplatin (wk 3 and 5), converting to hyperfractionated radiotherapy for wk 4–6.

9.2. Novel Targets

The growth factor receptors have been recognized as promising potential cytostatic targets in tumor cell growth and survival. Overexpression of the epidermal growth factor receptor (EGFR) is recognized in 80–100% of squamous cell head and neck carcinomas. Ligand binding of the extracellular domain results in homo- or heterodimerization and activation of tyrosine kinase resulting in cell proliferation and activation. Inhibition of EGFR has been shown in cell lines to promote apoptosis *(87)*. It has been reported that an inverse correlation may exist between EGFR expression and radioresistance *(88)*. Administration of the chimeric monoclonal antibody against the EGFR, IMC-C225, has been shown to increase radiosensitization in HNC cell lines decreasing tumor cell line growth and increasing apoptosis *(89)*. Conceptually, inhibiting the extracellular domain and the intracellular domain of tyrosine kinase receptor in combination with radiotherapy may further promote tumoricidal activity.

Baselga and colleagues have provided results from their phase I study of C225 alone (5, 20, 50, and 100 mg/m^2) and in combination (C225 of 5–400 mg/m^2) with cisplatin (60 mg/m^2 every 28 d) in patients with solid tumors overexpressing EGFR *(90)*. The use of the combination regimen was limited to head and neck or nonsmall-cell lung carcinoma patients. The most frequent adverse events reported with C225 were flu-like symptoms and acneiform rash. Although response was not a primary endpoint, 11 of 19 patients (58%) had stable disease; two patients had a PR. Nine of 13 patients (69%) that had received ≥ 50 mg/m^2 of C225 achieved disease stabilization and received all 12 wk of therapy.

Promising results of the oral tyrosine kinase inhibitor ZD1839 (Iressa) were reported earlier this year *(90a)*. Final results are to be published shortly.

9.3. Vascular Endothelial Growth Factor (VEGF)

Other potential tumor targets for monoclonal antibodies include the vascular endothelial growth factor (VEGF), which may have a role in angiogenesis. Inhibition of VEGF has resulted in tumor shrinkage in earlier clinical trials. Conceptually, promoting angiogenesis and administration of cytotoxic chemoradiotherapy should promote tumor cell kill. Bevacizumab is a recombinant humanized anti-VEGF monoclonal antibody. At the University of Chicago we have begun accruing patients in a phase I study to assess the MTD of bevacizumab when combined with our standard regimen of FHX for patients with poor prognosis HNC including patients with locoregional recurrent disease or those with bulky locoregional disease.

9.4. Gene Therapy: Adenovirus

The mutation of the *p53* tumor suppressor gene has been well recognized to be associated in most head and neck malignancies. ONYX-015 is an adenovirus vector composed of the wild-type *p53* gene with preferential replication in *p53* deficient cells causing cell lysis. In the setting of recurrent disease, the intratumoral injection of ONYX-015 when combined with cisplatin/5-FU resulting in an improved overall response rate of 63% vs the standard regimen of cisplatin/5-FU at 37% *(91)*. Improved results when combined with chemotherapy suggest synergistic activity causing augmentation of chemotoxicity. In theory, incorporating ONYX-015 with radiosensitizing chemotherapeutic agents may result in increased cytotoxicity. Ongoing studies continue to evaluate ONYX-015 as a single-agent and in combination with cisplatin/5-FU by intratumoral injection and in the intravenous setting but have not been conducted in in vivo radiation combination studies.

10. THE ESSENTIAL ROLE OF SUPPORTIVE CARE

With more aggressive interventions in controlling locoregional and recurrent disease, patients require close surveillance. The importance of a teamwork approach to treating HNC patients cannot be underestimated. The expertise of a radiation oncologist, speech therapist, pathologist, otolaryngologist, nurse, and oncologist is fundamental in the care of these patients. Evaluating the quality of life in these patients is also essential when determining the nature of such aggressive chemoradiotherapy that may alter the daily lifestyle of these patients physically, including physical appearance and loss of their voice, and psychologically; patients may have to sacrifice simple capabilities such as their swallowing ability and appreciation of the texture of food. Additionally, the lifestyle of these patients has placed these patients at increased risk of developing a second malignancy of the aerodigestive tract. Consequently, we encourage monthly clinical exams on our patients following the completion of treatment for the first year unless otherwise indicated and quarterly CT scans for the first 2–3 yr. Owing to the treatment field that radiotherapy involves, quarterly thyroid function studies are suggested because of the increased incidence of hypothyroidism.

During treatment, other supportive measures may include chemoprotectants against xerostomia as amifostine for patients receiving radiotherapy. A phase III study completed by Brizel and colleagues demonstrated decreased xerostomia in patients receiving amifostine prior to standard daily single modality radiation therapy ($p = 0.002$) *(92)*.

Recent studies have advocated the importance of pretreatment hemoglobin in the local control and survival of advanced head and neck malignancies. In vitro data supports that under anoxic conditions increased doses of radiotherapy are needed to obtain the same biologic effect *(93)*. Fein and colleagues published results of 109 untreated patients with T1–T2/N0 laryngeal carcinoma treated with single daily radiotherapy (two patients with N2 were treated with twice-daily radiotherapy) *(94)*. The local control rate was significantly better in those patients with a hemoglobin of ≥13 g/dL (95%) in comparison to patients with hemoglobin ≤13 g/dL (66%, $p = 0.0018$). The 2-yr survival was also increased in those patients that maintained their hemoglobin ≥13 g/dL (88% vs 46%, $p < 0.0018$).

A retrospective analysis of anemia as a prognostic indicator and its impact on the efficacy of radiotherapy has been recently published. Patients who received concomitant cisplatin (150 mg/m^2/wk for 4 wk) and radiotherapy (RADPLAT protocol) for stage III or IV HNC were found to have less treatment interruptions, decreased locoregional failure, and improved overall survival if not anemic *(95)*.

New trials are needed to incorporate and support investigation of the impact of anemia as a primary endpoint since this may have a bearing on prognosis and overall survival. Surveying the degree of anemia through blood draws especially in a population of patients that is being observed closely for myelosuppression can be completed with relative ease. Additionally, if further studies continue to support these aforementioned trials, the amount of radiation may possibly be decreased due to increased radiosensitivity at an adequate hemoglobin level. In turn, this may result in less radiation fibrosis and decrease the chronic sequelae often associated with radiotherapy especially in the setting of reirradiation. A phase III trial by the RTOG (99-03) is currently underway where patients receiving radiation therapy alone are randomized to receive epoetin alfa (EPOGEN) 40,000 U 7–10 d prior to initiation of therapy. Patients will be categorized by stage, sex, and hemoglobin level (9–10.5 g/dL and 11.5–13.5 g/dL). Results are pending at this time.

11. FUTURE DIRECTIONS

Novel approaches when combining standard cytotoxic chemotherapy agents with new cytotoxic and cytostatic agents, and improved radiotherapy techniques are promising in promoting decreased radioresistance, toxicities, and possibly increased overall survival. Outside of an academic setting, cisplatin and 5-FU still remain the standard of treatment. Though more aggressive, the aforementioned studies, have overall demonstrated improved response rates in locally advanced and recurrent disease. Hence, patients should be encouraged to participate in academic clinical trials. Newer agents will continue to be discovered and provide a basis for further consideration in the treatment of HNC.

REFERENCES

1. Greenlee RT, Murray T, Bolden S, et al. Cancer statistics, 2000. *CA Cancer J Clin* 2000; 50:7–33.
2. Parkin DM, Pisani P, Ferlay J. Global cancer statistics. *CA Cancer J Clin* 1999; 49:33–64.
3. Khuri FRL, Lee JJ, Winn RJ. Interim Analysis of Randomized Chemoprevention Trial of HNSCC. *Proc Annu Meet Am Soc Clin Oncol* 1999; 18:A:1503.
4. Slaughter DP, Southwick HW, Smejkal W. "Field cancerization" in oral stratified squamous epithelium: clinical implications of multicentric origin. *Cancer* 1953; 6:963.
5. Vokes EE, Weichselbaum RR, Lippman SM, et al. Head and neck cancer. *N Engl J Med* 1993; 328:184–194.
6. Brizel DM, Albers ME, Fisher SR, et al. Hyperfractionated irradiation with or without concurrent chemotherapy for locally advanced head and neck cancer. *N Engl J Med* 1998; 338:1798–1804.
7. Horiot JC, Le Fur R, N'Guyen T, et al. Hyperfractionation versus conventional fractionation in oropharyngeal carcinoma: final analysis of a randomized trial of the EORTC cooperative group of radiotherapy. *Radiother Oncol* 1992; 25:231–241.
8. Fu KK, Pajak TF, Trotti A, et al. A Radiation Therapy Oncology Group (RTOG) phase III randomized study to compare hyperfractionation and two variants of accelerated fractionation to standard fractionation radiotherapy for head and neck squamous cell carcinomas: first report of RTOG 9003. *Int J Radiat Oncol Biol Phys* 2000; 48:7–16.
9. Sinclair WK. Hydroxyurea: effects on Chinese hamster cells grown in culture. *Cancer Res* 1967; 27:297–308.
10. Hussey DH, Abrams JP. Combined therapy in advanced head and neck cancer: hydroxyurea and radiotherapy. *Prog Clin Cancer* 1975; 6:79–86.
11. Richards GJ Jr, Chambers RG. Hydroxyurea in the treatment of neoplasms of the head and neck. A resurvey. *Am J Surg* 1973; 126:513–518.
12. Lo TC, Wiley AL, Ansfield FJ, et al. Combined radiation therapy and 5-fluorouracil for advanced squamous cell carcinoma of the oral cavity and oropharynx: a randomized study. *Am J Roentgenol* 1976; 126:229–235.
13. Sanchiz F, Milla A, Torner J, et al. Single fraction per day versus two fractions per day versus radiochemotherapy in the treatment of head and neck cancer. *Int J Radiat Oncol Biol Phys* 1990; 19: 1347–1350.

14. Browman GP, Cripps C, Hodson DI, et al. Placebo-controlled randomized trial of infusional fluorouracil during standard radiotherapy in locally advanced head and neck cancer. *J Clin Oncol* 1994; 12:2648–2653.
15. Browman GP, Cripps C, Hodson DI. Placebo-controlled randomized trial of infusional fluorouracil during standard radiotherapy in locally advanced head and neck cancer, Author Update. *Classic Papers and Current Comments* 1999; 4:625–630.
16. Rockwell S. Use of hypoxia-directed drugs in the therapy of solid tumors. *Semin Oncol* 1992; 19:29–40.
17. Haffty BG, Son YH, Papac R, et al. Chemotherapy as an adjunct to radiation in the treatment of squamous cell carcinoma of the head and neck: results of the Yale Mitomycin Randomized Trials. *J Clin Oncol* 1997; 15:268–276.
18. Haffty BG. Concurrent chemoradiation in the treatment of head and neck cancer. *Hematol Oncol Clin North Am* 1999; 13:719–742.
19. Overgaard J, Hansen HS, Andersen AP, et al. Misonidazole combined with split-course radiotherapy in the treatment of invasive carcinoma of larynx and pharynx: report from the DAHANCA 2 study. *Int J Radiat Oncol Biol Phys* 1989; 16:1065–1068.
20. Overgaard J, Hansen HS, Overgaard M, et al. A randomized double-blind phase III study of nimorazole as a hypoxic radiosensitizer of primary radiotherapy in supraglottic larynx and pharynx carcinoma. Results of the Danish Head and Neck Cancer Study (DAHANCA) Protocol 5-85. *Radiother Oncol* 1998; 46:135–146.
21. Shanta V, Krishnamurthi S. Combined bleomycin and radiotherapy in oral cancer. *Clin Radiol* 1980; 31:617–620.
22. Fu KK, Phillips TL, Silverberg IJ, et al. Combined radiotherapy and chemotherapy with bleomycin and methotrexate for advanced inoperable head and neck cancer: update of a Northern California Oncology Group randomized trial. *J Clin Oncol* 1987; 5:1410–1418.
23. Eschwege F, Sancho-Garnier H, Gerard JP, et al. Ten-year results of randomized trial comparing radiotherapy and concomitant bleomycin to radiotherapy alone in epidermoid carcinomas of the oropharynx: experience of the European Organization for Research and Treatment of Cancer. *NCI Monogr* 1988; 6:275–278.
24. Haselow RE, Warshaw MC, Oken MM, et al. Radiation alone versus radiation with weekly low dose cisplatinum in unresectable cancer of the head and neck. In: (Fee WE Jr. GH, Johns ME, eds). Head and Neck Cancer. Vol. 2. Philadelphia: BC Decker, 1990:279–281.
25. Bachaud JM, David JM, Boussin G, et al. Combined postoperative radiotherapy and weekly cisplatin infusion for locally advanced squamous cell carcinoma of the head and neck: preliminary report of a randomized trial. *Int J Radiat Oncol Biol Phys* 1991; 20:243–246.
26. Al-Sarraf M, Pajak TF, Marcial VA, et al. Concurrent radiotherapy and chemotherapy with cisplatin in inoperable squamous cell carcinoma of the head and neck. An RTOG Study. *Cancer* 1987; 59:259–265.
27. Al-Sarraf M, Pajak TF, Cooper JS, et al. Chemo-radiotherapy in patients with locally advanced nasopharyngeal carcinoma: a radiation therapy oncology group study. *J Clin Oncol* 1990; 8:1342–1351.
28. Al-Sarraf M, LeBlanc M, Giri PG, et al. Chemoradiotherapy versus radiotherapy in patients with advanced nasopharyngeal cancer: phase III randomized Intergroup study 0099. *J Clin Oncol* 1998; 16:1310–1317.
29. Al-Sarraf M, Metch B, Kish J, et al. Platinum analogs in recurrent and advanced head and neck cancer: a Southwest Oncology Group and Wayne State University Study. *Cancer Treat Rep* 1987; 71:723–726.
30. Jacobs MC, Eisenberger M, Oh MC, et al. Carboplatin (CBDCA) and radiotherapy for stage IV carcinoma of the head and neck: a phase I-II study. *Int J Radiat Oncol Biol Phys* 1989; 17:361–363.
31. Kamioner DH, E. Vallantin, X. Fourth International Congress on Anti-Cancer Chemotherapy, Paris, France, Feb 2–5, 1993.
32. Bhalla K, Ibrado AM, Tourkina E, et al. Taxol induces internucleosomal DNA fragmentation associated with programmed cell death in human myeloid leukemia cells. *Leukemia* 1993; 7:563–568.
33. Leonard CE, Chan DC, Chou TC, et al. Paclitaxel enhances in vitro radiosensitivity of squamous carcinoma cell lines of the head and neck. *Cancer Res* 1996; 56:5198–5204.
34. Forastiere AA, Shank D, Neuberg D, et al. Final report of a phase II evaluation of paclitaxel in patients with advanced squamous cell carcinoma of the head and neck: an Eastern Cooperative Oncology Group trial (PA390). *Cancer* 1998; 82:2270–2274.
35. Hoffmann W, Belka C, Schmidberger H, et al. Radiotherapy and concomitant weekly 1-hour infusion of paclitaxel in the treatment of head and neck cancer—results from a Phase I trial. *Int J Radiat Oncol Biol Phys* 1997; 38:691–696.

36. Liebmann J, Cook JA, Fisher J, et al. In vitro studies of Taxol as a radiation sensitizer in human tumor cells. *J Natl Cancer Inst* 1994; 86:441–446.
37. Rosenthal DI, Lee JH, Sinard R. Phase I study of paclitaxel given by seven-week continuous infusion concurrent with radiation therapy for locally advanced squamous cell carcinoma of the head and neck. *J Clin Oncol* 2001; 19:1363–1373.
38. Sunwoo JB, Herscher LL, Kroog GS. Concurrent paclitaxel and radiation in the treatment of locally advanced head and neck cancer. *J Clin Oncol* 2001; 19:800–811.
39. Dreyfuss AI, Clark JR, Norris CM, et al. Docetaxel: an active drug for squamous cell carcinoma of the head and neck. *J Clin Oncol* 1996; 14:1672–1678.
40. Hesse K, Heinrich B, Zimmermann F, et al. Combined radiochemotherapy with docetaxel in patients with unresectable locally advanced head and neck tumors. *Strahlenther Onkol* 2000; 176:67–72.
41. Shewach DS, Hahn TM, Chang E, et al. Metabolism of 2',2'-difluoro-2'-deoxycytidine and radiation sensitization of human colon carcinoma cells. *Cancer Res* 1994; 54:3218–3223.
42. Lawrence TS, Eisbruch A, McGinn CJ, et al. Radiosensitization by gemcitabine. *Oncology (Huntingt)* 1999; 13:55–60.
43. Eisbruch A, Shewach DS, Bradford CR. Radiation concurrent with gemcitabine for locally advanced head and neck cancer. *J Clin Oncol* 2001; 19:792–799.
44. Chen AY, Choy H, Rothenberg ML. DNA topoisomerase I-targeting drugs as radiation sensitizers. *Oncology (Huntingt)* 1999; 13:39–46.
45. Chen AY, Okunieff P, Pommier Y, et al. Mammalian DNA topoisomerase I mediates the enhancement of radiation cytotoxicity by camptothecin derivatives. *Cancer Res* 1997; 57:1529–1536.
46. Tamura K, Takada M, Kawase I, et al. Enhancement of tumor radio-response by irinotecan in human lung tumor xenografts. *Jpn J Cancer Res* 1997; 88:218–223.
47. Koukourakis MI, Bizakis JG, Skoulakis CE, et al. Combined irinotecan, docetaxel and conventionally fractionated radiotherapy in locally advanced head and neck cancer. A phase I dose escalation study. *Anticancer Res* 1999; 19:2305–2309.
48. Keane TJ, Cummings BJ, O'Sullivan B, et al. A randomized trial of radiation therapy compared to split course radiation therapy combined with mitomycin C and 5 fluorouracil as initial treatment for advanced laryngeal and hypopharyngeal squamous carcinoma. *Int J Radiat Oncol Biol Phys* 1993; 25:613–618.
49. Merlano M, Vitale V, Rosso R, et al. Treatment of advanced squamous-cell carcinoma of the head and neck with alternating chemotherapy and radiotherapy. *N Engl J Med* 1992; 327:1115–1121.
50. Merlano M, Benasso M, Corvo R, et al. Five-year update of a randomized trial of alternating radiotherapy and chemotherapy compared with radiotherapy alone in treatment of unresectable squamous cell carcinoma of the head and neck. *J Natl Cancer Inst* 1996; 88:583–589.
51. Wendt TG, Grabenbauer GG, Rodel CM, et al. Simultaneous radiochemotherapy versus radiotherapy alone in advanced head and neck cancer: a randomized multicenter study. *J Clin Oncol* 1998; 16:1318–1324.
52. Adelstein DJ, Adams GL, Li Y. A phase III comparison of standard radiation therapy (RT) versus RT plus concurrent cisplatin (DDP) versus split-course RT plus concurrent DDP and 5-fluorouracil (5FU) in patients with unresectable squamous cell head and neck cancer (SCHNC), *Proc Annu Meet Am Soc Clin Oncol* 2000; 19:A:1624.
53. Adelstein DJ, Lavertu P, Saxton JP, et al. Mature results of a phase III randomized trial comparing concurrent chemoradiotherapy with radiation therapy alone in patients with stage III and IV squamous cell carcinoma of the head and neck. *Cancer* 2000; 88:876–883.
54. Calais G, Alfonsi M, Bardet E, et al. Randomized trial of radiation therapy versus concomitant chemotherapy and radiation therapy for advanced-stage oropharynx carcinoma. *J Natl Cancer Inst* 1999; 91:2081–2086.
55. Byfield JE, Calabro-Jones P, Klisak I, et al. Pharmacologic requirements for obtaining sensitization of human tumor cells in vitro to combined 5-Fluorouracil or Florafur and X rays. *Int J Radiat Oncol Biol Phys* 1982; 8:1923–1933.
56. Byfield JE, Sharp TR, Frankel SS, et al. Phase I and II trial of five-day infused 5-fluorouracil and radiation in advanced cancer of the head and neck. *J Clin Oncol* 1984; 2:406–413.
57. Taylor SG, Murthy AK, Griem KL, et al. Concomitant cisplatin/5-FU infusion and radiotherapy in advanced head and neck cancer: 8-year analysis of results. *Head Neck* 1997; 19:684–691.
58. Vokes EE, Haraf DJ, Panje WR, et al. Hydroxyurea with concomitant radiotherapy for locally advanced head and neck cancer. *Semin Oncol* 1992; 19:53–58.

59. Haraf DJ, Kies M, Rademaker AW, et al. Radiation therapy with concomitant hydroxyurea and fluorouracil in stage II and III head and neck cancer. *J Clin Oncol* 1999; 17:638–644.
60. Brockstein B, Haraf DJ, Stenson K, et al. Phase I study of concomitant chemoradiotherapy with paclitaxel, fluorouracil, and hydroxyurea with granulocyte colony-stimulating factor support for patients with poor-prognosis cancer of the head and neck. *J Clin Oncol* 1998; 16:735–744.
61. Kies MS, Haraf DJ, Rosen F, et al. Concomitant infusional paclitaxel and fluorouracil, oral hydroxyurea, and hyperfractionated radiation for locally advanced squamous head and neck cancer. *J Clin Oncol* 2001; 19:1961–1969.
62. Merlano M, Rosso R, Sertoli MR, et al. Sequential versus alternating chemotherapy and radiotherapy in stage III-IV squamous cell carcinoma of the head and neck: a phase III study. *J Clin Oncol* 1988; 6:627–632.
63. Taylor SG, Murthy AK, Vannetzel JM, et al. Randomized comparison of neoadjuvant cisplatin and fluorouracil infusion followed by radiation versus concomitant treatment in advanced head and neck cancer. *J Clin Oncol* 1994; 12:385–395.
64. Sendler A, Schuchardt U, Waldfahrer F. A randomized study comparing intensified sequential to concomitant chemoradiotherapy for advanced hypopharyngeal cancer. *Proc Annu Meet Am Soc Clin Oncol* 1997; 16:A1396.
65. Induction chemotherapy plus radiation compared with surgery plus radiation in patients with advanced laryngeal cancer. The Department of Veterans Affairs Laryngeal Cancer Study Group. *N Engl J Med* 1991; 324:1685–1690.
66. Lefebvre JL, Chevalier D, Luboinski B, et al. Larynx preservation in pyriform sinus cancer: preliminary results of a European Organization for Research and Treatment of Cancer phase III trial. EORTC Head and Neck Cancer Cooperative Group. *J Natl Cancer Inst* 1996; 88:890–899.
67. Posner MR, Glisson B, Frenette G, et al. Multicenter phase I-II trial of docetaxel, cisplatin, and fluorouracil induction chemotherapy for patients with locally advanced squamous cell cancer of the head and neck. *J Clin Oncol* 2001; 19:1096–1104.
68. Vokes EE, Kies MS, Haraf DJ, et al. Concomitant chemoradiotherapy as primary therapy for locoregionally advanced head and neck cancer. *J Clin Oncol* 2000; 18:1652–1661.
68a. Forastiere A, Berkey B, Mai M, et al. Phase III trial to preserve the larynx induction chemotherapy versus concomitant chemotherapy versus radiotherapy alone inner group trial R911-M. *Proc Annu Meet Soc Am Clin Oncol* 2001; 20:A4.
69. Pignon JP, Bourhis J, Domenge C, et al. Chemotherapy added to locoregional treatment for head and neck squamous-cell carcinoma: three meta-analyses of updated individual data. MACH-NC Collaborative Group. Meta-Analysis of Chemotherapy on Head and Neck Cancer. *Lancet* 2000; 355:949–955.
70. Bourhis J, Pignon JP. Meta-analyses in head and neck squamous cell carcinoma. What is the role of chemotherapy? *Hematol Oncol Clin North Am* 1999; 13:769–775, vii.
71. Munro AJ. An overview of randomised controlled trials of adjuvant chemotherapy in head and neck cancer. *Br J Cancer* 1995; 71:83–91.
72. Stell PM. Meta-analysis confounded. *Lancet* 1992; 339:623.
73. El-Sayed S, Nelson N. Adjuvant and adjunctive chemotherapy in the management of squamous cell carcinoma of the head and neck region. A meta-analysis of prospective and randomized trials. *J Clin Oncol* 1996; 14:838–847.
74. Kish JA, Weaver A, Jacobs J, et al. Cisplatin and 5-fluorouracil infusion in patients with recurrent and disseminated epidermoid cancer of the head and neck. *Cancer* 1984; 53:1819–1824.
75. Schrijvers D, Johnson J, Jiminez U, et al. Phase III trial of modulation of cisplatin/fluorouracil chemotherapy by interferon alfa-2b in patients with recurrent or metastatic head and neck cancer. Head and Neck Interferon Cooperative Study Group. *J Clin Oncol* 1998; 16:1054–1059.
76. Vermorken J, Catimel G, Mulder PD, et al. Randomized phase II trial of weekly methotrexate (MTX) versus two schedules of triweekly paclitaxel (taxol) in patients with metastatic or recurrent squamous cell carcinoma of the head and neck (SCCHN). *Proc Annu Meet Am Soc Clin Oncol* 1999; 18:A 1527.
77. Forastiere A, Leong T, Rowisky E. Phase III comparison of high-dose paclitaxel + cisplatin + granulocyte colony-stimulating factor versus low-dose paclitaxel + cisplatin in advanced head and neck cancer: eastern cooperative oncology group study E1393. *J Clin Oncol* 2001; 19:1088–1095.
78. Murphy B, Li Y, Cella D, et al. Phase III study comparing cisplatin (C) and 5-Fluorouracil (F) versus cisplatin and paclitaxel (T) in metastatic/recurrent head and neck cancer (MHNC). *Proc Annu Meet Am Soc Clin Oncol* 2001; 20:A894.

78a. Eng C, Haraf D, Stenson K, et al. Phase I study of concomitant chemoradiotherapy with Gemcitabine (G) paditaxel (T) and 5-fluorouracil (5-FU) with poor prognosis head and neck cancer patients. *Lung Cancer* 2001; (Suppl 34):SS50
79. Humerickhouse RA, Haraf D, Stenson K, et al. Phase I study of irinotecan (CPT-11), 5-FU, and hydroxyurea with radiation in recurrent or advanced head and neck cancer. *Proc Annu Meet Am Soc Clin Oncol* 2000; 19:A1650.
80. Gandia D, Wibault P, Guillot T, et al. Simultaneous chemoradiotherapy as salvage treatment in locoregional recurrences of squamous head and neck cancer. *Head Neck* 1993; 15:8–15.
81. Hartsell WF, Thomas CR, Murthy AK, et al. Pilot study for the evaluation of simultaneous cisplatin/5-fluorouracil infusion and limited radiation therapy in regionally recurrent head and neck cancer (EST P-C385). *Am J Clin Oncol* 1994; 17:338–343.
82. Haraf DJ, Weichselbaum RR, Vokes EE. Re-irradiation with concomitant chemotherapy of unresectable recurrent head and neck cancer: a potentially curable disease. *Ann Oncol* 1996; 7:913–918.
83. Spencer SA, Harris J, Wheeler RH, et al. RTOG 9610: Reirradiation with concurrent hydroxyurea and 5-fluorouracil in patients with squamous cell cancer of the head and neck. *Int J Radiat Oncol Biol Phys* 2000; 51:1299–1304.
84. Rowinsky EK. Novel radiation sensitizers targeting tissue hypoxia. *Oncology (Huntingt)* 1999; 13:61–70.
85. Dorie MJ, Brown JM. Tumor-specific, schedule-dependent interaction between tirapazamine (SR 4233) and cisplatin. *Cancer Res* 1993; 53:4633–4636.
86. Rishchin D, Peters L, Hicks R, et al. Phase I trial of concurrent tirapazamine, cisplatin, and radiotherapy in patients with advanced head and neck cancer. *J Clin Oncol* 2001; 19:535–542.
87. Rodeck U, Jost M, Kari C, et al. EGF-R dependent regulation of keratinocyte survival. *J Cell Sci* 1997; 110:113–121.
88. Maurizi M, Almadori G, Ferrandina G, et al. Prognostic significance of epidermal growth factor receptor in laryngeal squamous cell carcinoma. *Br J Cancer* 1996; 74:1253–1257.
89. Huang SM, Bock JM, Harari PM. Epidermal growth factor receptor blockade with C225 modulates proliferation, apoptosis, and radiosensitivity in squamous cell carcinomas of the head and neck. *Cancer Res* 1999; 59:1935–1940.
90. Baselga J, Pfister D, Cooper MR, et al. Phase I studies of anti-epidermal growth factor receptor chimeric antibody C225 alone and in combination with cisplatin. *J Clin Oncol* 2000; 18:904–914.
90a. Cohen EEW, Rosen F, Dekker A, et al. Phase II study of 2D1839 (Iressa) in recurrent or metastic squamous cell carcinoma of the head and neck (SCCHN). *Proc Annu Meet Soc Am Clin Oncol* 21:A88.
91. Khuri FR, Nemunaitis J, Ganly I, et al. A controlled trial of intratumoral ONYX-015, a selectively-replicating adenovirus, in combination with cisplatin and 5-fluorouracil in patients with recurrent head and neck cancer. *Nat Med* 2000; 6:879–885.
92. Brizel DM, Wasserman TH, Henke M, et al. Phase III randomized trial of amifostine as a radioprotector in head and neck cancer. *J Clin Oncol*, 2000; 18:3339–3345.
93. Hollaender A, Stapleton GE, Martin FL, et al. X-ray sensitivity of E. coli as modified by oxygen tension. *Nature* 1951; 167:103–104.
94. Fein DA, Lee WR, Hanlon AL, et al. Pretreatment hemoglobin level influences local control and survival of T1-T2 squamous cell carcinomas of the glottic larynx. *J Clin Oncol* 1995; 13:2077–2083.
95. Kumar P. Importance of anemia as a prognostic factor in patients with head and neck cancer. *Anemia Oncol* 2000; 3:2–4.

9 The Role of Combined Modality Therapy for Stage III Nonsmall-Cell Lung Cancer

Roger W. Byhardt, MD, FACR

Contents

1. INTRODUCTION

Despite recent advances in treatment, lung cancer is still the number one cause of cancer mortality in the United States *(1)*. About 95% of the estimated 131,000 new cases of nonsmall-cell lung cancer (NSCLC) diagnosed in 2000 will die from their disease *(2)*. The focus of this chapter is on the patients who present with locally advanced or stage III NSCLC (about 46,000 patients yearly). Although it is tempting to think of stage III NSCLC as a uniform stage category, it really contains patient subgroups with disparate tumor burdens and prognosis. Included in stage III are patients with involvement ranging from potentially resectable T3N1 (small T3 and microscopically involved N1 lymph node) to unresectable, locally advanced T4N3 disease (large primary invading mediastinal structures and contralateral mediastinal adenopathy) *(3)*.

Obviously, this broad range of tumor extent requires an equally broad array of treatment approaches, ranging from surgery, with or without adjuvant radiation therapy (RT) or chemotherapy (ChT), to definitive chemoradiation combinations, to palliative

From: *Chemoradiation in Cancer Therapy*
Edited by: H. Choy © Humana Press Inc., Totowa, NJ

management with ChT and/or radiation. Although this chapter summarizes the range of treatment strategies, the majority of stage III patients are treated nonoperatively using chemoradiation *(4)*. Although the topic of this chapter is combined modality therapy, it is useful to review the impact of RT alone and surgery alone, both of which are essentially local therapies.

2. RADIATION THERAPY ALONE

Prior to the 1980s, RT was considered the standard treatment for most stage III NSCLC. In this pre-computed tomography era there was often little distinction made between the disease subsets that now distinguish IIIA and IIIB, since both were often considered inoperable. It was frequently difficult to make an accurate clinical assessment of mediastinal node status. Early studies of RT established that disease-related symptoms were often improved, but that overall disease control was little affected *(5)*. A dose-response relationship was established by a Radiation Therapy Oncology Group (RTOG) study, showing better local control and short-term, but not long-term, survival with 60 Gy in 6 wk than with lower doses *(6)*. Failure rates were still high both locally and at distant sites even after 60 Gy. Reported 5-yr survival rates were rarely above 5%. More effective local and systemic treatments were clearly needed. Analysis of these older data is difficult because actual initial nodal status was often not known. Subsequent efforts to improve local control with radiation alone by using hyperfractionation to higher total doses than 60 Gy were met with limited success *(7)*.

With the advent of more effective staging, some patients with N2 disease were selected out for surgical approaches. However, N2 patients not suitable for surgery because of poor performance status, weight loss, refusal, or other factors still usually underwent irradiation *(8)*. Radiation results are poor in patients with overt N2 disease, but these patients generally have bulkier disease than patients who undergo resection. A subset of N2 patients was identified in completed RTOG studies of radiation alone that theoretically would have been suitable for surgery (similar T stage, good performance status, and so on). There was no significant increase in 5-yr survival above 5% seen in this subset with standard radiation doses, but hyperfractionated radiation to 69.6 Gy had a 3-yr survival of 20% *(7,9)*. The outcome of radiation alone and surgery alone has never been directly compared in a randomized trial, nor is it likely to be. However, hyperfractionated RT alone (MST 12.3 mo) was not better than standard RT (MST 11.4 mo) in a subsequent RTOG phase III trial of patients with inoperable NSCLC, about half of which had IIIA (N2) disease *(10)*. Benchmark survival data for radiation alone to standard or hyperfractionated radiation alone are 1-yr survival of 45–50%, 3-yr survival of 20–24%, and 5-yr survival of 5–6% *(11)*. Local control rates remained disappointingly low, around 25% or less *(12)*.

Accelerated hyperfractionation has also been explored in an effort to increase the biologically effective tumor dose. A phase III trial conducted by the Medical Research Council of the United Kingdom of an aggressive three-times-daily regimen of continuous hyperfractionated accelerated radiation therapy (CHART) delivering 54 Gy in 12 continuous days had significantly better 2-yr survival (29%) than standard radiation to 60 Gy (20%) *(13)*. Although in this comparison CHART was better than standard RT, the 2-yr survival rates for both study arms seem to be somewhat lower than the benchmark data noted above.

No distinct advantage has been noted when other forms of external beam irradiation, other than photons, or brachytherapy have been used. Neutron irradiation has not proven to be better than photons for stage III inoperable NSCLC *(14,15)*. The use of brachytherapy has been limited to endobronchial treatment for palliation or as a boost after external beam. There have been institutional reports of interstitial brachytherapy, also usually done as a boost. Neither of these two approaches has been shown to be superior to external beam *(16,17)*.

By the mid-1980s it was evident that unless higher effective doses of radiation could be given to the primary disease, local control would be limited with conventional radiation alone. Also, effective treatment of occult systemic disease was needed to improve overall control. This observation led not only to investigations of high dose delivery using techniques such as 3D conformal radiation, currently under investigation, but to various combinations of radiation with surgery and/or chemotherapy. Subsequent paragraphs will summarize these investigations.

3. SURGERY ALONE

Accurate staging of stage III disease at diagnosis is a prerequisite for determining the appropriate treatment. The subdivision of stage III into subsets A and B roughly corresponds to tumors that are potentially resectable and those that are not. Also, because of the high risk of occult metastatic disease, stage III patients need thorough screening with computed tomography (CT) of the chest and abdomen, contrast CT or magnetic resonance imaging (MRI) of the brain, and bone scan. Positron emission tomography (PET) permits even more precise functional imaging of small tumor deposits not detectable on CT or MRI. It can also discern whether equivocal findings on CT or MRI are likely attributable to tumor involvement. Although PET imaging is not yet widely available, there is increasing evidence validating its utility in optimizing the preoperative evaluation of NSCLC patients for surgery with a consequent impact on outcome *(18)*.

In the absence of extrathoracic disease or evidence of overt N2 or N3 mediastinal node involvement on CT, and if surgery is being considered, the mediastinal nodes should be further evaluated for occult involvement, since neither CT nor MRI have better than a 65% overall accuracy *(19)*. Mediastinoscopy is preferred because it has an overall accuracy rate of 95%, a sensitivity of 87%, and a specificity of 100% *(20)*. CT and MRI can only suggest lymph node involvement when a threshold size is exceeded and cannot identify microscopic disease in a normal sized lymph node *(21)*. In addition, subcarinal and aortopulmonary nodes are not well imaged radiographically. Since resectability hinges on distinguishing between N2 and N3 involvement, mediastinoscopy is a critical step in the staging process and has only a 2.3% complication rate *(22)*. As noted above, PET scanning has the potential to detect occult nodal disease; however, the definitive studies to demonstrate that it can supplant mediastinoscopy have not yet been conducted *(23)*.

Several large surgical series suggest that surgery alone is of limited value for patients with N2 disease. Only about one-fifth of patients with N2 disease prove to have disease confined to the chest and are potentially eligible for resection. Of these, if the mediastinal node involvement is evident clinically, the results of surgery are poor with 10–20% survival at 3–5 yr *(21,24,25)*. Patients with multilevel or bulky nodal involvement have an even worse prognosis. Patients with radiographically negative mediastinal nodes, but with evidence of microscopic involvement found at mediastinoscopy or on pathologic analysis of the resected specimen, fare somewhat better with long-term survival up to 30%, if complete resection is done *(25)*.

Based on these results and the fact that only a small percentage of N2 patients have even the potential to benefit from a solely local treatment, surgery alone is rarely an appropriate treatment. The same applies to RT alone, which, in the past, was often the treatment of choice for this patient group. RT alone, using standard fractionation and doses, yielded only 5–7% 5-yr survival rates and median survivals of < 1 yr. Altered fractionation RT to higher doses provided only a slight improvement *(7,10,26)*. Distant metastases are the most common mode of failure (80%) in N2 patients treated solely with surgery or RT, with failure appearing early in the disease course (50% within 1 yr), consistent with the presence of pretreatment micrometastases. Nevertheless, both ChT and RT have been explored in the postoperative and preoperative settings. Postoperative ChT has been generally unrewarding, adding only toxicity during the vulnerable postoperative recovery period *(27)*. Postoperative RT has similarly been noted to add toxicity and, despite reducing local-regional failure rates, has not been shown to improve survival over surgery alone, although the topic remains somewhat controversial *(28)*. Preoperative, or neoadjuvant, ChT and RT, alone or in combination, has also been actively investigated and may hold greater promise. The following sections will discuss each of these areas in greater depth.

4. POSTOPERATIVE RADIATION THERAPY

For the purpose of this discussion, only patients with pN2 disease will be considered. The data from randomized trials are rather limited, since only several of the trials of postoperative RT have considered N2 patients apart from pN0 or pN1 disease.

In the Lung Cancer Study Group (LCSG) 773 study, subgroup analysis showed no survival benefit for the N2 patients and local recurrence analysis was not done for the N2 subgroup *(29)*. The larger Medical Research Council (MRC) study (190 N2 cases) showed a trend ($p = 0.07$) toward a lower local recurrence rate and a trend ($p = 0.18$) toward an improved survival rate (36% vs 21%) in the irradiated group compared to surgery alone *(30)*. However, the freedom-from-distant-metastases rate was significantly lower ($p = 0.03$) in the RT group. A recent MRC meta-analysis suggested neither a decrease nor an improvement in survival rate with postoperative RT for N2 patients *(31)*.

Each of these studies can be criticized for design flaws and for use of RT doses or techniques that many would consider nonideal *(28)*. The MRC study used midline spinal cord blocking and a suboptimal dose (the equivalent of 42 Gy at 2 Gy/fx) for microscopic disease *(30)*. Most consider the minimum RT dose for this purpose to be 50 Gy at 2 Gy/fx. The sample size for each individual study was too small to detect small survival differences. The MRC meta-analysis pooled data which included studies that used significantly older equipment with submegavoltage beam energy, inadequate treatment volumes, and substandard techniques. In some of the trials analyzed, the doses were too low for control of micrometastases (approx 40 Gy) and in others the doses were higher than needed (approx 60 Gy) putting the patients at greater risk for toxicity. Thus, the studies making up the meta-analysis were flawed. It is not possible that the meta-analysis corrected those flaws. Thus, it is not surprising that the meta-analysis did not find a survival benefit for postoperative RT or that the topic still remains controversial.

Ironically, some of the strongest support for postoperative RT is found in retrospective institutional reports *(32,33)*. For example, regression analysis of 224 patients receiving postoperative RT found that the administration of postoperative RT was the dominant independent prognostic factor in predicting both a lower rate of local-regional recurrence and a higher rate of survival ($p = 0.001$ for both) *(34)*. Four-year survival in the irradiated group was also twice that for surgery alone (40% vs 22%). Further analysis of the trial showed that the survival benefit applied with greater likelihood to patients with the highest risk of local-regional recurrence and mortality, namely, those with multiple N2 nodes involved. Although such evidence is suggestive, it does not carry the imprimatur of a randomized, controlled trial. The definitive randomized trial of postoperative RT alone has not yet been performed. Despite the absence of definitive evidence of a survival benefit, RT may be justified for the N2 subset of patients, especially those with multiple nodes involved, on the basis of a large body of strong but nondefinitive evidence.

5. POSTOPERATIVE CHEMOTHERAPY OR CHEMORADIATION

Three prior Lung Cancer Study Group (LCSG) studies have suggested postoperative cisplatin-based chemotherapy may have an impact on survival of NSCLC patients with *pathologically* documented stage II/III disease. Although a treatment effect has been detected for nonsquamous cancer, and is suggested for squamous cancer, the treatment effect has been of marginal significance *(35)*. Other studies have shown a modest improvement in disease-free survival with the use of chemotherapy after surgery, but little impact on overall survival *(36,37)*. A frequent problem with postoperative chemotherapy has been the inability to deliver all the planned amount of drug in patients recovering from lung resection. Drug delivery rates of around 50% are often the rule.

To investigate further the role of postoperative therapy, an intergroup trial (0115) was designed to determine if the combination of cisplatin/etoposide and RT was superior to RT alone in increasing local control and in prolonging survival in patients with completely resected Stage II and IIIA NSCLC *(38)*. The estimated baseline median survival for resected IIIA (N2) patients receiving postoperative RT was 20 mo and it was hoped that the adjuvant therapy might increase that by 40%. The study accrued 351 eligible patients for analysis with a median follow-up of 37 mo. Grade 3 and 4 toxicities were significantly higher in the combined treatment arm (leukopenia, 25% vs 9% and esophagitis, 65% vs 1.3%). Consequently, fewer patients received all of the prescribed protocol treatment on the ChT/RT arm than did patients on the SRT arm. Treatment-associated mortality was about 2.5% in both arms. Median survival in the RT arm was 41.1 mo and 38.6 mo in the ChT/RT arm ($p = 0.99$). Subgroup analysis showed no benefit to survival for either treatment arm. The conclusion was that ChT adjuvant to postoperative RT does not improve survival over postoperative RT alone for resected Stage II and IIIA NSCLC.

Unfortunately, the intergroup trial did not answer the question of whether postoperative radiation alone has an impact. It proved only that the addition of ChT to radiation did not improve the outcome over postoperative radiation alone and it added unnecessary toxicity. The issue is also being tested in an ongoing CALGB phase III trial in which all patients receive postoperative ChT and are randomized to receive postoperative RT or not following completion of the ChT. Future investigations of postoperative therapy will explore the addition of less toxic therapy to postoperative irradiation, such as low-dose long-term maintenance ChT, immunotherapy, angiogenesis inhibitors, or signal transduction inhibitors.

Table 1
Major Subsets in Stage III NSCLC

Group	*Subsets*
Minimal, nonbulky disease	• T3N0 or N1 • Nonenlarged N2 nodes on CT scan • Microscopic N2 only (negative CT scan)
Nonminimal, bulky disease	• Bulky N2 on CT scan or chest X-ray • T4 (no effusion) • N3

6. NEOADJUVANT THERAPY, IN GENERAL

Clearly, for this strategy, the patients must be considered operable at the time of preoperative staging. Thus, the majority of cases treated in this fashion will have IIIA disease. Mediastinoscopic documentation of N2 status is usually done.

Before effective ChT, preoperative RT was attempted based on the concept that it would decrease the primary tumor burden and might reduce the risk of distant dissemination at the time of surgery. Beginning with early studies by the Veterans Administration, the results of preoperative RT did not improve overall survival, although one-fourth of the patients had no viable tumor in the resected specimen *(39)*. On the basis of the above findings, the adjuvant role of systemic ChT has been actively investigated in stage III NSCLC over the past two decades. These investigations have demonstrated that neoadjuvant cisplatin-based regimens are well tolerated and offer the potential to reduce local tumor burden, as well as to eradicate regional and distant micrometastases. Preoperative ChT is better tolerated than ChT given during the postoperative recovery period.

Two basic strategies of neoadjuvant treatment have been employed, namely, induction ChT followed by surgery and induction chemoradiation followed by surgery. There were a number of Phase II feasibility studies of neoadjuvant therapy in the 1980s; however, their interpretation is hampered by variability of the regimens, differing patient eligibility, and the use of pre-1986 American Joint Committee on Cancer (AJCC) staging, which did not divide stage III into A and B, making it difficult to separate out N2 patients. The trials also differed in method of documentation of N2 status (radiographic vs histologic), by which patients underwent surgery (those with stable disease or those with responding tumors), and in the definition of a complete resection (removal of gross disease vs complete resection with negative margins). Definition of what is meant by "bulky" N2 disease has also varied, including, in some trials, the presence of a single N2 node with intranodal involvement, in other trials, involved nodal stations N5 or N6 only, and in others, positive N7 nodes (Table 1). Finally, in some of the surgical trials, resection rate and survival is stated only in terms of those undergoing thoracotomy, not including those that received preoperative treatment and were unable, for various reasons, to go to surgery.

Theoretically, preoperative ChT allows higher drug doses than when used with radiation, optimizing control of occult micrometastases. The disadvantage of excluding radiation is a reduced likelihood of control of bulky local/regional disease.

7. PREOPERATIVE RADIATION THERAPY

Several early investigations explored preoperative RT. In a comprehensive review, it was concluded that preoperative RT improves resectability and local control *(40,41)*. Preoperative RT regimens provide pathologic complete response in 15–45% of patients, but with increased operative complications (doses above 45 Gy). Randomized trials have failed to show a survival benefit when preoperative radiation was compared to surgery alone, but many of the trials are fairly old and modern staging techniques were not used. A more recent randomized phase II trial of the Lung Cancer Study Group (LCSG 881) gave preoperative RT of 44 Gy to patients with pathologically proven IIIA disease, yielding only a 12 mo median survival and pathologic complete response (CR) in only 1/33 patients *(42)*. Thus, despite more modern methods, results of preoperative RT and surgery do not appear to increase survival.

8. PREOPERATIVE CHEMOTHERAPY

Several institutional and cooperative group trials of preoperative cisplatin-based ChT established the feasibility of preoperative ChT patients with clinical N2 disease. Interpretation of the available data is difficult. A variety of induction regimens have been reported from trials using heterogeneous patient populations with variable performance status. Some of these trials have used rigorous mediastinal nodal staging and others have used only clinical staging. The bulk of mediastinal node involvement has varied and has sometimes included patients with N0 and N1 stage III disease because of the version of the AJCC staging system in use then. In some of the trials, postoperative radiation was given to patients with persistent mediastinal nodal disease at thoracotomy *(43,44)*. These early studies used first-generation ChT with low-dose cisplatin and the radiation was added variably after surgery. The major response rates were around 75%, with complete resection possible in about 35–65%, and complete clearance of tumor in the final pathology in up to 20% of patients. Treatment-related mortality ranged from 5 to 15% and overall survival rates were around 25% at 3 yr and 15% at 5 yr (Table 2).

No large phase III trials have yet been reported comparing surgery alone to neoadjuvant ChT and surgery for biopsy-proven N2 disease; however, several small randomized studies have suggested a survival benefit for preoperative ChT (Table 3) *(45–48)*. Rosell et al. used three cycles of mitomycin, ifosfamide, and cisplatin in 60 patients prior to surgery and reported a median survival of 26 mo for combined therapy compared to 8 mo for surgery alone *(45)*. Using three cycles of cyclophosphamide, etoposide, and cisplatin preoperatively and additional ChT postoperatively, Roth et al. reported significantly better median survival in 60 patients with combined therapy (64 mo) compared to surgery alone (11 mo) *(47)*. An even smaller phase III study of 28 patients suggested a trend toward improved survival with two cycles of induction cisplatin and etoposide followed by surgery. Conclusions from these trials are limited because of the lack of statistical power, lack of uniform staging, and the unusually poor survival of the surgery only patients in some of the trials. In 1994 the European Organization for Research and Treatment of Cancer (EORTC) launched a multicenter randomized trial (08941) to compare the efficacy of surgery vs radiotherapy after neoadjuvant ChT for stage III (N2) NSCLC. The trial is still ongoing, but, when complete, should provide an important insight regarding the role of both surgery and radiation *(49)*.

Table 2
Preoperative MVP or VP for Stage IIIA (N2) Nonsmall-Cell Lung Cancer

Study	*Number of patients*	*Radiation*	*Complete resection (%)*	*Operative mortality (%)*	*Median survival (mo)*
Memorial *(43,95)*	136	Variable (intraoperative, postoperative)	65	4.4	19
Toronto *(92)*	55	Postoperative	51	8.0	21
LCSG *(42)*	20	None	NA	17.0	13
CALGB *(44)*	74	Postoperative	62	3.1	15

CALGB, Cancer and Leukemia Group B; LCSG, Lung Cancer Study Group; MVP, mitomycin/vinblastine/cisplatin; VP, vinblastine/cisplatin; RT, radiation therapy.

9. PREOPERATIVE CHEMORADIATION

The objective of induction chemoradiation is that the ChT will both eradicate occult micrometastases and radiosensitize the local-regional disease to augment its response to radiation. The LCSG showed the feasibility of this approach in two phase II studies using cisplatin-based ChT with relatively low-dose RT (15–30 Gy) *(50,51)*. Operative mortality ranged from 0 to 7% with overall response rates of around 50% and complete response rates of about 34%. Median survival times were 11 and 13 mo. On the basis of these trials higher doses of RT were tested, again with cisplatin-based ChT, showing improved response rates and complete resection possible in 60–70% of patients *(52,53)*. Median survivals improved to 15 to 22 mo, although some patients with T3 disease were included.

The Southwest Oncology Group (SWOG) conducted the largest phase II trial (126 patients) of a somewhat intensified induction chemoradiation regimen, enrolling both IIIA and IIIB patients *(54)*. They used two cycles of cisplatin (50 mg/m^2, d 1 and 8) and etoposide with 45 Gy/25 fractions. All patients had mediastinoscopic documentation of nodal status and had thoracotomy unless there was disease progression. Both IIIA and IIIB patients had a high rate of resectability (85% and 80%) and two out of three patients had either no tumor or minimal residual tumor at final pathology. Surprisingly, both IIIA and IIIB patients had promising 3-yr survival rates (27% and 24%) and those with no tumor in the specimen had 3-yr survival of 44%. Patients with T4 disease had similar survival as those with N2 disease, but patients with N3 disease had poor survival. The preoperative treatment did not seem to significantly increase operative mortality (6%) and treatment-related mortality was 10%. Patterns of failure suggested that the local-regional component of treatment was quite effective, with the majority of failures at distant sites, especially brain.

Thus, the intensified SWOG induction regimen seemed to provide an improved outcome without a significant increase in morbidity/mortality compared to the earlier studies. Some attempts by other investigators to further intensify the induction regimen resulted in unacceptable toxicity *(55,56)*. However, two recent German phase II trials have safely used intensified regimens incorporating hyperfractionated accelerated RT *(57,58)*. The RT consisted of 45 Gy in 3 wk using 1.5 Gy bid concurrent with either cisplatin/etoposide or carboplatin/vindesine after the same drugs had been given alone at higher dosage. Acute toxicity was acceptable and treatment-related deaths were 9% or

Table 3
Randomized Trials of Surgery With or Without Preoperative Chemotherapy in Resectable Nonsmall-Cell Lung Cancer

					2- to 3-Yr Survival Rates		
Study	*Number of patients*	*Stage subset(s)*	*ChT*	*Radiation*	*ChT*	*No ChT*	p *Value*
NCI *(48)*	28	N2 by biopsy	EP × 2 preop.; × 4 postop.	Postop. only in non-ChT arm	46%	21%	.12
Japan *(46)*	83	Clinical IIIA & select IIIB	VdP preop.	50–60 Gy with ChT	37%	40%	NS
Roth *(47)*	60	Mixed III (N2 not required; some IIIB)	CyEP × 3 preop. and × 3 postop.	Only if residual disease at surgery	56%	15%	<.05
Rosell *(45)*	60	Mixed IIIA (N2 not required)	PIM × 3 preop.	Postop. for both arms	30%	0%	<.05

CyEP, cyclophosphamide/etoposide/cisplatin; EP, etoposide/cisplatin; NCI, National Cancer Institute; PIM, cisplatin/ifosfamide/mitomycin; VdP, vindesine/cisplatin; preop., preoperatively; postop., postoperatively; ChT, chemotherapy; NS, not significant.

Table 4
Concurrent Chemoradiation Followed by Surgery for Stage III Nonsmall-Cell Lung Cancer

Study	*Number of patients*	*T3N0-1/T4, N3 (%)*	*ChT*	*Complete resections (%)*	*Operative mortality (%)*	*Median survival (mo)*
SWOG *(54)*	126	0/40	EP	71	8	15
LCSG *(51)*	85	0/13	PF	52	7	13
Rush-Pres. *(52)*	85	21/6	PF/PEF	71	4	22
CALGB *(95)*	41	20/0	PVF	61	15	16
Eberhardt *(58)*	94	6/12	EP	53	6	19
Choi *(93)*	42	0/0	PVF	81	7	25
Granone *(94)*	82	0/11	Cbo/E	95	1	NS

CALGB, Cancer and Leukemia Group B; EP, etoposide/cisplatin; LCSG, Lung Cancer Study Group; PEF, cisplatin/etoposide/5-fluorouracil; PVF, cisplatin/vinblastine/5-fluorouracil; SWOG, Southwest Oncology Group; Cbo/E, carboplatin/etoposide; NS, not stated.

less. Overall 3-yr survivals were around 35% and were about 25% for IIIA patients and 17% for IIIB patients. Up to 50% of patients had a complete pathologic response, which predicted for improved long-term survival of around 75% at 3 yr (Table 4).

On the basis of the phase II experience with induction chemoradiation, in the early 1990s, two cooperative group phase III trials of chemoradiation for IIIA (N2) NSCLC were initiated. The trial started by the RTOG and the Eastern Cooperative Oncology Group (ECOG) compared chemotherapy + radiation therapy with chemotherapy + surgery (RTOG 89-01). The trial started by the SWOG compared chemoradiation alone to induction chemoradiation followed by surgery, using the SWOG 8805 regimen. In order to avoid poor accrual by having two phase III trials competing for the same patient population, in 1992, the two trials were merged into an RTOG-run intergroup phase III study (INT 0139) following the SWOG schema. INT 0139 included only IIIA (N2) patients and required rigorous mediastinal nodal staging. In both arms, two cycles of cisplatin (50 mg/m^2, d 1, 8, 29, 36) and etoposide (50 mg/m^2, d 1–5 and 29–33) were used concurrent with radiation therapy (45 Gy/5 wk). Patients were randomized to receive either surgery 2–4 wk later or to continue with two more cycles of ChT and an additional 16 Gy at 2.0 Gy/fraction. The study enrolled over 400 patients and it constitutes the largest study of the N2 subset.

The INT 0139 trial essentially asked whether the addition of surgery to chemoradiation is necessary. Until the trial is mature we cannot be certain of the role of surgery after chemoradiation. The International Association for the Study of Lung Cancer (IASLC) recently issued a consensus statement stating that it is premature to conclude that surgery is the standard of care after neoadjuvant therapy for patients with marginally resectable N2 disease, since it has not yet been proven to be superior to chemoradiation alone. The same could be considered true for the cohort of patients with minimal-bulk N2 disease, in view of the small numbers of patients studied and subset biases. Depending on the outcome of INT0139, future directions could include further study of the more intense regimens described in the German reports, expansion of the preoperative chemoradiation approach to include selected IIIB patients, 3D conformal radiation therapy, newer generation chemotherapy (paclitaxel, gemcitabine, and so on) and/or the addition of noncytotoxic adjuvants such as angiogenesis inhibitors or other biologics. The potential for toxicity of these induction regimens must not be overlooked as there remains the potential for an increased risk of postoperative complications (bronchial stump leak, ARDS, and so on) whenever more treatment is added to the mix.

10. CHEMORADIATION ALONE FOR INOPERABLE STAGE III NSCLC

10.1. Induction Chemotherapy and Radiation Therapy

It became evident in the 1980s that cisplatin-based chemotherapy improved the survival of patients with advanced NSCLC compared to supportive care *(59,60)*. The higher response rates for stage III compared to stage IV disease, suggested there could be a theoretic advantage to pretreat stage III patients with ChT before RT. Smaller tumors with better oxygenation would potentially be more radioresponsive. Using ChT before radiation would allow assessment of chemoresponsiveness and gage the likelihood of controlling occult micrometastases. Phase II studies of induction (neoadjuvant) ChT followed by standard RT (60–63 Gy/6–7 wk) reported up to 80% response rates, 16 mo median survivals, and 30% 2-yr survivals *(61)*. Based on these observations, a series of phase III trials followed comparing RT with and without induction ChT, usually targeting good performance patients (KPS ≥ 70 and weight loss < 5%).

The first of these trials (8433) was conducted by the Cancer and Leukemia Group B (CALGB) and randomized patients to an induction regimen of vinblastine (5mg/m^2 weekly × 5 wk) and cisplatin (100 mg/m^2 wk 1 and 5) plus standard radiation 60 Gy in 6 wk) or standard radiation alone. Although closed early when interim analysis showed superior median survival with chemoradiation (13.6 mo) compared to radiation alone (9.7 mo), long-term follow-up verified a persistent survival benefit for combined therapy at 5 yr of 19% vs 7% for radiation alone *(62)*. The RTOG essentially verified this finding by comparing the same two regimens in two arms of their three-arm phase III intergroup trial 88-08, showing that long-term survival was statistically superior with the combined regimen. Although the median survivals in RTOG 88-08 were nearly identical (11.4 and 13.2 mo) to CALGB 8433, the 5-yr survival rates were lower at 8% and 5%. Nevertheless, the trial verified the CALGB findings and helped set the stage for induction chemoradiation becoming the new benchmark treatment for inoperable stage III NSCLC.

Almost concurrently with the CALGB study, the French CEBI trial explored induction ChT followed by concurrent chemoradiation, using a four-drug cisplatin-based regimen before and during 65 Gy vs 65 Gy alone *(63)*. Despite inclusion of some patients with worse performance status (Zubrod 0-2) and no exclusion for weight loss, the results significantly favored the combined approach, although the survival rates were somewhat lower than in CALGB 8433.

Other trials attempted to improve the results of sequential chemoradiation by using newer ChT agents and/or intensifying the RT component by the use of accelerated fractionation, based on the success of the British CHART regimen. A phase II trial of paclitaxel and carboplatin followed by hyperfractionated accelerated radiation therapy (HART) to 57.6 Gy tid in 3 wk gave a 1-yr survival of 59% and a severe acute esophagitis rate of 63% *(64)*. At the time of the report, the median survival had not yet been reached. On the basis of this trial, ECOG phase III trial 2597 is comparing the HART regimen to standard radiation, both preceded by paclitaxel/carboplatin.

Failure pattern analysis of the CALGB and French trials showed that local persistence or failure still occurred in around 80% of patients despite the ChT; however, the incidence of distant metastases as a first site of failure was significantly lower in the combined modality group, confirming the theoretical potential that ChT could effect distant micrometastases. Subsequent meta-analyses confirmed the superiority of induction ChT, using a cisplatin-based regimen, and RT over radiation alone *(60,65)*. Thus, sufficient evidence was now in place to establish induction chemoradiation as a world-wide standard of care. To further improve outcome, steps would have to be taken to improve local disease control as well.

10.2. Concurrent Chemoradiation

The rationale for concurrent chemoradiation is that the ChT can augment local-regional control by both direct tumor cell killing and radiosensitization at the same time as it addresses systemic micrometastases. Unfortunately, this also has the potential to increase radiation-related mucosal acute toxicity, predominantly esophagitis and pneumonitis. Thus, some of the early trials of concurrent therapy used either attenuated dose ChT or split course RT to ameliorate potential cotoxicity. These trials showed that concurrent therapy is feasible and, as with the sequential approach, improves outcome.

In 1991, the EORTC reported significantly improved 3-yr survival with concurrent reduced-dose cisplatin (either 30 mg/m^2 weekly or 6 mg/m^2 5 d per week) and split course RT (30 Gy/2 wk + 25 Gy/2 wk) compared to the same RT alone (26% vs 13%) *(66)*. In contrast to the sequential chemoradiation strategy, failure analysis showed a reduced risk of in-field failure with the concurrent regimen (70% vs 81%). A smaller European phase III trial using twice daily RT with and without concurrent cisplatin and etoposide also reported more favorable outcome with the concurrent chemoradiation regimen and a similar reduction of local failure rates *(67)*.

In an effort to optimize the opportunity for systemic and local control, subsequent studies focused on testing higher-dose ChT, incorporating newer ChT agents, and using full-dose, nonsplit course RT.

To exploit intensified RT, the North Central Cancer Treatment Group (NCCTG) reported that full dose cisplatin/etoposide along with accelerated hyperfractionated thoracic radiation therapy (AHTRT) yielded a median survival of 18 mo, significantly better than observed with sequential chemoradiation *(68)*. Unfortunately, a phase III study comparing the regimen to standard RT was closed early since it was felt standard RT alone was no longer appropriate *(26)*.

After phase I trials had determined the safety of paclitaxel doses of 45–50 mg/m^2/wk and carboplatin of AUC 2/wk concurrent with standard RT of 66 Gy/7 wk, phase II trials yielded encouraging survival results *(69)*. Acute esophageal grade III or greater toxicity was high (30–50%); however, most patients fully recovered from these acute effects. Choy extended the experience with concurrent radiation and paclitaxel/carboplatin using hyperfractionated radiation to 69.6 Gy and observed a 1-yr survival of 63% *(70)*.

Despite the emerging data suggesting concurrent chemoradiation was superior to radiation alone, it was not until 1998 that phase III evidence became available that concurrent chemoradiation might provide superior survival outcome compared to the less toxic sequential chemoradiation approach. In a Japanese phase III trial, concurrent and sequential chemoradiation were compared using two cycles of full dose mitomycin, vindesine, and cisplatin (MVP) either before or during radiation therapy to 56 Gy/6 wk *(71)*. The radiation was continuous course in the sequential approach, but there was a 2 wk split between two courses of 28 Gy/3 wk for the concurrent regimen. The ChT doses were not reduced in the concurrent arm and the split course may have conferred some protection from ChT-enhanced acute radiation toxicity, since the rate of severe esophagitis was low in both study arms. There was better short-term survival (MST 16.5 mo vs 13.3 mo) and long-term survival (5-yr survival of 15.8% vs 8.8%) for the concurrent regimen compared to the sequential regimen. The similarity of the 13.3 mo median survival time for the sequential approach to the previously reported phase III experience with sequential chemoradiation seemed to validate the comparability of the Japanese data.

The RTOG recently completed a three-arm phase III trial (94-10) comparing sequential chemoradiation to two concurrent chemoradiation regimens, one using standard radiation, the other using hyperfractionated radiation. The ChT was cisplatin/etoposide in the arm with concurrent hyperfractionated radiation and vinblastine/cisplatin in the other two arms. From 7/94 to 7/98, 610 good performance (KPS >60; weight loss < 5%) patients were randomized on 94-10. At 2-yr follow-up of 592 patients, preliminary results showed significantly improved median survival (17.1 vs 14.6 mo) with concurrent ChT and standard radiation compared to sequential ChT and standard radiation ($p = 0.038$) *(72)*. Time to in-field progression was significantly longer for concurrent ChT and hyperfractionated radiation, but survival was not better than in the other two arms. There was significantly higher grade 3 or greater acute nonhematologic toxicity for concurrent ChT and hyperfractionated radiation (62%) compared to the other two arms (30% and 48%). Further follow-up is needed to assess long-term survival, but this large trial seems to confirm the Japanese trial and the phase II data favoring concurrent over sequential chemoradiation.

The last decade has led to the development of a number of new generation chemotherapeutic agents in addition to the taxanes, paclitaxel and docetaxel, already discussed above, many of which have novel mechanisms of action and significant single-agent activity against NSCLC. One advantage of the taxanes is that they are somewhat easier to administer than cisplatin-based regimens and may be associated with reduced toxicity. In some trials, carboplatin has supplanted cisplatin for similar reasons. Other new agents include the vinca alkaloid vinolrelbine, the topoisomerase I inhibitor irinotecan, and the nucleoside analog gemcitabine *(73)*. These new agents have all been combined in some form with cisplatin for treatment of metastatic NSCLC and have demonstrated improved response rates and survival *(74)*. Their other unique feature is a shared ability to have radiosensitizing properties and to have synergy with RT *(75–78)*. Based on this information a number of clinical trials are now planned or underway to combine these new agents with radiation for stage III NSCLC. These trials will help sort out issues regarding optimal dosing and scheduling of the new agents, and the best way to combine them with radiation. Another novel compound undergoing preliminary investigation is the benzotriazine tirapazamine (SR259075), which is a specific cytotoxic for hypoxic tumor cells. Hypoxia is felt to impart resistance to both radiation and ChT *(79)*. It is outside the scope of this chapter to discuss these new agents in detail and they are more thoroughly discussed elsewhere in this text.

There has been widespread acceptance of some of the new generation ChT agents like paclitaxel and carboplatin because of their more favorable toxicity profile and greater ease of administration. Although they appear to be as efficacious as cisplatin-based regimens when used in stage IV NSCLC, they have never been compared head-to-head in stage III patients. Nevertheless, this has not prevented their incorporation in new clinical trials. Efforts are underway to reduce the acute toxicity of the concurrent approach through the use of 3D conformal RT, radiation protectors (i.e., Amifostine), pulsed low dose ChT scheduling, and exploration of lower toxicity adjuvants (i.e., angiogenesis inhibitors, hypoxic cytotoxics, biologic modulators, and so on).

To date, the outcome benefit provided by concurrent chemoradiation has, in general, accrued only to patients with good functional status. Patients that are less fit and have had pretreatment weight loss > 5% do not tolerate aggressive therapy as well as their good performance counterparts. A secondary analysis done on an RTOG trial of chemoradiation completed in the early 1990s showed that good performance patients over 70 yr did not enjoy the same survival benefit, when adjusted for time spent with severe toxicity, from the addition of concurrent ChT as did patients under age 70 *(80,81)*. A similar analysis done on RTOG study 94-10 showed that fit elderly patients did benefit from chemoradiation although they had more pronounced, but acceptable, acute toxicity *(81a)*. It is likely that there are other factors, such as comorbidities, that influence outcome independent of performance status. This will be the focus of additional analysis. In addition, concurrent ChT does not seem to provide protection from CNS relapse, which remains a substantial risk for patients with nonsquamous NSCLC that otherwise enjoy good disease response to treatment and long-term survival *(82)*. This observation has lead to renewed interest in exploring prophylactic cranial irradiation in stage III NSCLC patients who have a good response to combined modality therapy and have prognostic factors predicting for a good chance of long-term survival.

In the meantime, there is continued interest in exploiting the use of induction ChT along with concurrent chemoradiation to maximize the opportunity to control occult micrometastases. There are potential downsides to this approach, as the induction ChT could reduce patient tolerance for the subsequent concurrent component. The induction ChT can also potentially stimulate accelerated tumor cell repopulation so that an additional burden of avidly dividing tumor is placed upon the subsequent concurrent chemoradiation.

10.3. Induction ChT Followed by Concurrent Chemoradiation

As noted above, the potential benefit of using both induction and concurrent ChT is to increase the overall exposure of micrometastases to cytotoxic therapy. It may also "pre-shrink" the primary disease and allow assessment of chemoresponsiveness, justifying continued use of the same drugs during radiation. Smaller radiation fields might be used following significant tumor regression, reducing the risk of toxicity during the concurrent portion. All the same benefits of concurrent chemoradiation noted previously should still apply. Possible disadvantages include reduced tolerance of the concurrent portion of treatment by "patient deconditioning" and accelerated tumor cell repopulation induced by the up-front ChT.

A number of phase II trials have investigated this approach, including RTOG studies 88-04 and 92-04, and suggested it was feasible *(83,84)*. CALGB trial 9310 used a cisplatin-based induction regimen followed by standard RT and weekly carboplatin *(85)*. There was no apparent survival advantage over sequential chemoradiation alone. A larger phase II randomized trial, CALGB 9431, evaluated induction ChT with three different doublets (gemcitabine/cisplatin, paclitaxel/cisplatin, and vinolrelbine/cisplatin) followed by standard radiation therapy (66 Gy/7 wk) *(86)*. The overall median survival of the three arms was 16.7 mo (range 14.1 to 17.7 mo), appearing better than that observed with sequential chemoradiation and similar to the Phase III concurrent chemoradiation results. Obviously, this conclusion can only be implied from a phase II result and requires verification in a phase III setting. At least two such phase III studies are ongoing.

An ongoing corporately sponsored multi-institutional phase II randomized trial uses paclitaxel, carboplatin, and standard RT and is comparing sequential chemoradiation, concurrent chemoradiation, and sequential followed by concurrent chemoradiation. Preliminary results are expected in the next year or two, but unless changed to a phase III design, will not have the statistical power to definitively discern between the three arms. CALGB is also conducting a phase III trial (39801) in good performance patients comparing chemoradiation with and without induction ChT *(87)*. The trial is expected to complete in mid-2001 and uses standard radiation to 66 Gy in 7 wk. The induction portion uses paclitaxel at 200 mg/m^2 every 3 wk and carboplatin at an AUC of 6. Drugs doses are reduced to 50 mg/m^2 and AUC of 2, both for seven weekly doses, during radiation. These two studies should help decide whether induction ChT truly augments immediate concurrent chemoradiation.

10.4. Concurrent Chemoradiation Followed by Consolidative ChT

Another approach to increasing patient exposure to ChT and potentially improving the control of micrometastases is to give ChT after concurrent chemoradiation. This so-called "posterior" or consolidative ChT can still be given in full dose and should not be confused with low-dose "maintenance" ChT.

A recent SWOG phase II trial demonstrated promising MST (22 mo) and 2-yr survival (50%) for consolidation docetaxel given after concurrent etoposide/cisplatin and RT *(88)*. These data have been compelling enough to generate a SWOG phase III trial that will add a bioactive adjuvant or not after concurrent etoposide/cisplatin/radiation and consolidation docetaxel. However, it must be noted that there is, as yet, no phase III data to validate that the strategy of consolidation ChT after concurrent chemoradiation is superior to concurrent chemoradiation alone. It is also intriguing to consider adding other noncytotoxic adjuvants after concurrent chemoradiation.

10.5. Cost Utility of Combined Chemoradiation

With the rising costs of health care, concerns have been voiced about the cost-effectiveness of combined modality treatment for stage III NSCLC. The available data, to date, show that cost-utility varies with the method of combining ChT and radiation. An analysis conducted in Canada concluded that neoadjuvant combined modality treatment for IIIA disease was cost effective and that cost should not be a barrier to its use *(89)*. An RTOG cost-utility analysis (US$/Quality adjusted life year) conducted on completed combined chemoradiation lung studies demonstrated that induction ChT and radiation was the most cost-effective treatment strategy for good performance stage III inoperable patients, a finding similar to the Canadian study *(90)*. However, although the concurrent strategy was cost-effective based on overall survival, when adjusted for time spent with severe toxicity, the additional cost of concurrent ChT/RT was not offset by the quality adjusted survival benefit.

11. CONCLUSIONS

When all the data are taken together, it is apparent that significant progress has been made in improving the outcome of treatment for stage III NSCLC, but that there is still a long way to go before victory can be declared. It is clear that radiation alone and surgery alone are inadequate for most stage III disease. Preoperative RT alone is of limited benefit. Postoperative radiation is controversial, but there may be a limited role in resected N2 patients. For selected stage III cases (N2), there may be a role for surgery after chemoradiation, but this conclusion awaits the outcome of a major phase III study. For inoperable stage III disease, concurrent ChT now appears to be the new standard of care. Large randomized trials of chemoradiation validate at least a twofold increase in short-term survival and perhaps a similar increase in long-term survival, although the data are less certain on this point. The available data suggest that the ChT be cisplatin-based; however, the widespread acceptance of less toxic and logistically more friendly newer agents, such as paclitaxel and carboplatin, have led to some "leap-frogging" to these new agents even though they have not been directly compared to cisplatin-based regimens in phase III trials. Concurrent chemoradiation seems to be superior to sequential chemoradiation, but combined sequential followed by concurrent chemoradiation remains under investigation as does consolidative ChT after concurrent chemoradiation. Current guidelines published by the American Society of Clinical Oncology state that chemoradiation is appropriate for selected patients with stage III NSCLC, but they do not specify a regimen or a sequence *(91)*. It is also important to remember that the benefit of combined modality treatment has only been demonstrated in stage III patients with good functional performance status. Another future challenge will be to determine how to design combined treatment strategies that can be safely and effectively given to poor performance patients, many of whom are elderly.

New approaches under investigation to improve results of combined modality treatment are aimed at reducing the toxicity of treatment and at exploring novel new agents, such as angiogenesis inhibitors and other bioactive agents, that are not cytotoxic in the traditional sense of ChT. There is considerable room to optimize the means by which the multiple available modalities can be combined. Even if the 5-yr survival rate could be improved by 100% over the best current combined modality approach, it would only go up to 25–30%. A pessimist might say that 32,000 patients will still die each year from stage III NSCLC. An optimist would point out that 6900 more patients will live. That's enough people to populate a small town.

REFERENCES

1. Greenlee RT, Murray T, Bolden S, et al. Cancer statistics 2000. *CA Cancer J Clin* 2000; 50:7–33.
2. Ginsberg RJ, Vokes EE, Raben A. Non-small cell lung cancer, in DeVita VT, Hellman S, Rosenberg SA (eds). Cancer, principles and Practices of Oncology, (ed 5). Philadelphia, PA, Lippincott-Raven, 1997, pp. 858–911.
3. Mountain CF. Revisions in the international system for staging lung cancer. *Chest* 1997; 111:1710–1717.
4. Vokes EE, Green MR. Current strategies for locoregionally advanced unresectable non-small cell lung cancer. *Semin Oncol* 1999; 26(Suppl 15):40–43.
5. Roswit B, Patno ME, Rapp R, et al. The survival of patients with inoperable lung cancer: A large scale randomized study of radiation therapy versus placebo. *Radiology* 1968; 90:688–697.
6. Perez CA, Stanley K, Grundy G, et al. Impact of radiation technique and tumor extent in tumor control and survival of patients with unresectable non-oat cell carcinoma of the lung: Report of the Radiation Therapy Oncology Group. *Cancer* 1982; 50:1091–1099.

7. Cox JD, Azarnia N, Byhardt RW, et al. A randomized phase I/II trial of hyperfractionated radiation therapy with total doses of 60.0 Gy to 79.2 Gy: Possible survival benefit with greater than or equal to 69.6 Gy in favorable patients with radiation oncology group stage III non small cell lung carcinoma: Report of Radiation Therapy Oncology Group 83-11. *J Clin Oncol* 1990; 8:1543–1555.
8. Lilenbaum RC, Green MR. Multimodality therapy for non-small-cell lung cancer. *Oncology* 1994; 8:25–36.
9. Cox JD, Azarnia N, Byhardt RW, et al. N2 (clinical) non-small cell carcinoma of the lung: Prospective trials of radiation therapy with total doses of 60 Gy by the Radiation Therapy Oncology Group. *Int J Radiat Oncol Biol Phys* 1991; 20:7–12.
10. Sause WT, Scott C, Taylor S, et al. Radiation Therapy Oncology Group (RTOG) 88-08 and Eastern Cooperative Oncology Group (ECOG) 4588: Preliminary results of a phase III trial in regionally advanced, unresectable non small cell lung cancer. *J. Nat. Cancer Inst* 1995; 87:198–205.
11. Sause W, Kolesar P, Taylor S, et al. Final results of phase III trial in regionally advanced unresectable non-small cell lung cancer. *Chest* 2000; 117:358–364.
12. Perez CA, Pajal TF, Rubion P, et al. Long term observations of the patterns of failure in patients with unresectable non-oat carcinoma of the lung treated with definitive radiotherapy. Report of the Radiation Therapy Oncology Group. *Cancer* 1982; 50:1874–1881.
13. Saunders MI, Dische S, Barrett A, et al. Continuous hyperfractionated accelerated radiotherapy (CHART) versus conventional radiotherapy in non-small cell lung cancer. A randomized multicentre trial. *Lancet* 1997; 350:161–165.
14. Koh W, Griffin TW, Laramore GE, et al. Neutron versus photon radiation therapy for inoperable non-small cell lung cancer: results of a multicenter randomized trial. *Int J Radiat Oncol Biol Phys* 1993; 27:499–505.
15. Duncan W. An evaluation of results of neutron therapy trials. *Acta Oncologica* 1994; 33:299–306.
16. Brach B, Buhler C, Hayman MH, et al. Percutaneous computed tomography-guided fine needle brachytherapy of pulmonary malignancies. *Chest* 1994; 106:268–274.
17. Aygun C, Weiner S, Scariato A, et al. Treatment of non-small cell lung cancer with external beam radiotherapy and high dose rate brachytherapy. *Int J Radiat Oncol Biol Phys* 1992; 23:127–132.
18. Gupta NC, Bishop HA, Rogers JS, et al. Treatment outcome of lung cancer patients as optimized by preoperative whole-body positron emission tomography fluorodeoxyglucose imaging. *Clinical Lung Cancer* 2000; 2:146–150.
19. Webb R, Gatsonis C, Zerhouni EA, et al. CT and MR imaging in staging non-small cell bronchogenic carcinoma. *Radiology* 1991; 178:705–713.
20. Patterson GA, Ginsberg RJ, Poon PY, et al. A prospective evaluation of magnetic resonance imaging , computed tomography, and mediastinoscopy in the preoperative assessment of mediastinal node status in bronchogenic carcinoma. *J Thorac Cardiovasc Surg* 1987; 94:679–684.
21. Watanabe Y, Shimizu J, Oda A, et al. Aggressive surgical intervention in N2 non-small cell cancer of the lung. *Ann Thorac Surg* 1991; 51:253–261.
22. Luke WP, Pearson FG, Todd TRJ, et al. Prospective evaluation of mediastinoscopy for assessment of carcinoma of the lung. *J Thorac Cardiovasc Surg* 1986; 91:53–56.
23. Valk PE, Pounds TR, Hopkins DM, et al. Staging non-small cell lung cancer by whole-body positron emission tomographic imaging. *AnnThor Surg* 1995; 60:1573–1582.
24. Martini N, Flehinger BJ, Zaman MB, et al. Results of resection in non-oat cell carcinoma of the lung with mediastinal lymph node metastases. *Ann Surg* 1983; 198:386–397.
25. Pearson FG, Delarue NC, Ilves R, et al. Significance of positive superior mediastinal nodes identified at mediastinoscopy in patients with resectable cancer of the lung. *J Thorac Cardiovasc Surg* 1982; 83:1–11.
26. Bonner JA, McGinnis WL, Stella PJ, et al. The possible advantage of hyperfractionated thoracic radiotherapy in the treatment of locally advanced non-small cell lung carcinoma: Results of the North Central Cancer Treatment Study Group Phase III trial. *Cancer* 1998; 82:1037–1048.
27. Socinski M. The current status of adjuvant chemotherapy for resected non-small cell lung cancer. *Semin Oncol* 1999; 26(Suppl 15):34–39.
28. Sawyer TE, Bonner JA. Postoperative irradiation in non-small cell lung cancer. *Sem Rad Oncol* 2000; 10:280–288.
29. Weisenburger TH, Gail M. The Lung Cancer Study Group: Effects of postoperative mediastinal radiation on completely resected stage II and stage III epidermoid cancer of the lung. *N Engl J Med* 1986; 315:1377–1381.

30. Stephens RJ, Girling DJ, Bleehen NM, et al. The role of post-operative radiotherapy in non-small-cell lung cancer: A multicentre randomized trial in patients with pathologically staged T1-2, N1-2, M0 disease. Medical Research Council Lung Cancer Working Party. *Br J Cancer* 1996; 74:632–639.
31. PORT Meta-analysis Trialists Group. Postoperative radiotherapy in non-small-cell lung cancer: Systematic review and meta-analysis of individual patient data from nine randomized controlled trials. *Lancet* 1998; 352:257–263.
32. Choi NC, Grillo HC, Gardiello M, et al. Basis for new strategies in postoperative radiotherapy of bronchogenic carcinoma. *Int J Radiat Oncol Biol Phys* 1980; 6:31–35.
33. Kirsh MM, Sloan H. Mediastinal metastases in bronchogenic carcinoma: Influence of postoperative irradiation, cell type, and location. *Ann Thorac Surg* 1982; 33:459–463.
34. Sawyer TE, Bonner JA, Gould PM, et al. The impact of surgical adjuvant thoracic radiation therapy for patients with nonsmall-cell lung carcinoma with ipsilateral mediastinal lymph node involvement. *Cancer* 1997; 80:1399–1408.
35. Lad TE. Post-surgical therapy in stage I, II, IIIA non-small cell lung cancer [Review]. *Hematology-Oncology Clinics of North America* 1990; 4:1111–1119.
36. Niiranen A, Niitamo-Korhonen S, Kouri M, et al. Adjuvant chemotherapy after radical surgery for non-small-cell lung cancer. A randomized study: *J Clin Oncol* 1992; 10:1927–1932.
37. Wada H, Hitomi S, Teramatsu T. Adjuvant chemotherapy after complete resection in non-small-cell lung cancer. *J Clin Oncol* 1996; 14:1048–1054.
38. Keller S, Adak S, Fossella F, et al. Randomized prospective comparison of adjuvant mediastinal radiation with or without concurrent chemotherapy with cisplatin and etoposide for patients with completely resected T1-3N1-2M0 NSCLC: US intergroup lung trial 0115. Proc Am Soc Thera Rad Oncol (ASTRO). IJROBP 45 ##, 1999 (abstr).
39. Shields TW, Higgins GA Jr, Lawton R, et al. Preoperative x-ray therapy as an adjuvant in the treatment of bronchogenic carcinoma. *J Thorac Cardiovasc Surg* 1970; 59:49–61.
40. Payne DG. Preoperative radiation therapy in non-small cell carcinoma of the lung. *Lung Cancer* 1991; 7:47–56.
41. Payne DG. Is preoperative or postoperative radiation therapy indicated in non-small cell cancer of the lung? *Lung Cancer* 1994; 10(Suppl 1):S205–S212.
42. Lad T, Wagner H, Piantadosi S. Randomized Phase II evaluation of preoperative chemotherapy alone and radiotherapy alone in stage IIIa non-small cell lung cancer. (Abstract) *Proc Amer Soc Clin Oncol* 1991; 10:258.
43. Martini N, Kris MG, Flehinger BJ, et al. Preoperative chemotherapy for stage IIIA (N2) lung cancer: The Sloan-Kettering experience with 136 patients. *Ann Thorac Surg* 1993; 55:1365–1374.
44. Sugarbaker DJ, Herndon J, Kohman LJ, and the Cancer and Leukemia Group B Thoracic Surgery Group. Results of Cancer and Leukemia Group B protocol 8935. A multiinstitutional phase II trimodality trial for stage IIIA (N2) non-small cell lung cancer. *J Thorac Cardiovasc Surg* 1995; 109:473–485.
45. Rosell R, Gomez-Codina J, Camps C, et al. A randomized trial comparing preoperative chemotherapy plus surgery with surgery alone in patients with non-small cell lung cancer. *N Eng J Med* 1994; 330:153–158.
46. Yoneda S, Hibino S, Gotoh I, et al. A comparative trial of induction chemoradiotherapy followed by surgery or immediate surgery for stage III NSCLC (abstract 1128). *Proc Am Soc Clin Oncol* 1995; 14:367.
47. Roth J, Fossella F, Komaki R, et al. A randomized trial comparing perioperative chemotherapy and surgery with surgery alone in resectable stage III non-small-cell lung cancer. *J Natl Cancer Inst* 1994; 86:673–680.
48. Pass H, Pogrebniak H, Steinberg SM, et al. Randomized trial of neoadjuvant therapy for lung cancer: Interim analysis. *Ann Thorac Surg* 1992; 53:992–1008.
49. Splinter TAW, va Schil PE, Kramer GWPM, et al. Randomized trial of surgery versus radiotherapy in patients with stage IIIA (N2) non-small cell lung cancer after a response to induction chemotherapy. EORTC 08941. *Clinical Lung Cancer* 2000; 2:69–72.
50. Eagan RT, Ruud C, Lee RE, et al. Pilot study of induction therapy with cyclophosphamide, doxirubicin, and cisplatin (CAP) and chest irradiation prior to thoracotomy in initially inoperable stage III non-small lung cancer. *Cancer Treat Rep* 1987, 71:895–900.
51. Weiden PL, Piantadosi S. Preoperative chemotherapy (cisplatin and fluorouracil) and radiation therapy in stage III non-small cell lung cancer: A phase II study of the Lung Cancer Study Group. *J Natl Cancer Inst* 1991; 83:266–272.

52. Faber LP, Kittle CF, Warren WH, et al. Properative chemotherapy and irradiation for stage III non-small cell lung cancer. *Ann Thor Surg* 1989; 47:669–675.
53. Strauss GM, Herndon JE, Sherman DD, et al. Neoadjuvant chemotherapy and radiotherapy followed by surgery in stage IIIA non-small cell carcinoma of the lung: Report of a Cancer and Leukemia Group B phase II study. *J Clin Oncol* 1992; 10:1237–1244.
54. Albain K, Rusch V, Crowley J, et al. Concurrent cisplatin/etoposide plus chest radiotherapy followed by surgery for stages IIIA (N2) and IIIB non-small-cell lung cancer: Mature results of Southwestern Oncology Group phase II study 8805. *J Clin Oncol* 1995; 13:1880–1892.
55. Yashar J, Weitberg AB, Glicksman AS, et al. Preoperative chemotherapy and radiation therapy for stage IIIa carcinoma of the lung. *Ann Thor Surg* 1992; 53:445–448.
56. Fowler WC, Langer CJ, Curran WJ, et al. Postoperative complications after combined neoadjuvant treatment of lung cancer. *Ann Thorac Surg* 1993; 55:986–989.
57. Thomas M, Rube C, Semik M, et al. Impact of preoperative bimodality induction including twice-daily radiation on tumor regression and survival in stage III non-small cell lung cancer. *J Clin Oncol* 1999; 17:1185–1193.
58. Eberhardt W, Wilke H, Stamatis G, et al. Preoperative chemotherapy followed by concurrent chemoradiation therapy based on hyperfractionated accelerated radiotherapy and definitive surgery in locally advanced non-small cell lung cancer. Mature results of a phase II trial. *J Clin Oncol* 1998; 16:622–634.
59. Rapp E, Pater JL, Willan A, et al. Chemotherapy can prolong survival in patients with advanced non-small cell lung cancer. Report of a Canadian multicenter randomized trial. *J Clin Oncol* 1988; 6:633–641.
60. Chemotherapy in non-small cell lung cancer: a meta-analysis using updated data on individual patients from 52 randomized clinical trials. Non-small Cell Lung Cancer Collaborative Group. *BMJ* 1995; 311:899–909.
61. Friess GG, Balkadi M, Harvey WH. Simultaneous cisplatin and etoposide with radiation therapy in loco-regional non-small cell lung cancer. Final results of a pilot trial. IN: Small Cell Lung Cancer and Non-small Cell Lung Cancer. Gralla RJ, Einhorn LH (eds). *Royal Society of Medicine Services Limited*, 1989, pp. 121–126.
62. Dillman RO, Herndon J, Seagren SL, et al. Improved survival in stage III non-small cell lung cancer: Seven-year follow-up of Cancer and Leukemia Group B (CALGB) 8433 trial. *J Natl Cancer Inst* 1996; 88:1210–1215.
63. Le Chevalier T, Arriagada R, Quoix E, et al. Radiotherapy alone versus combined chemotherapy and radiotherapy in resectable non-small cell lung cancer: First analysis of a randomized trial in 353 patients. *J Natl Cancer Inst* 1991; 83:417–423.
64. Wagner H, Antonia S, Shaw G, et al. Induction Chemotherapy with Carboplatin and Paclitaxel followed by Hyperfractionated Accelerated Radiation for Patients with Unresectable Stage IIA and IIB Non-Small-Cell Lung Cancer. *Proc Am Soc Clin Oncol* 1998; 17:469a (abstr).
65. Pritchard RS, Anthony SP. Chemotherapy plus radiotherapy compared with radiotherapy alone in the treatment of locally advanced, unresectable, non-small cell lung cancer: A meta-analysis. *Ann Intern Med* 1996; 125:723–729.
66. Schaake-Koning C, Van den Bogaert W, Dalesio O, et al. Effects of concomitant cisplatin and radiotherapy on inoperable non small cell lung cancer. *N Engl J Med* 1992; 326:524–530.
67. Jeremic B, Shibamoto Y, Acimovic L, et al. Hyperfractionated radiation therapy with or without concurrent low-dose daily carboplatin/etoposide for stage III non-small cell lung cancer: a randomized study. *J Clin Oncol* 1996; 14:1065–1107.
68. Shaw EG, McGinnis WL, Jett JR, et al. Pilot study of accelerated hyper-fractionated thoracic radiation therapy plus concomitant cisplatin chemotherapy in patients with unresectable stage III non small cell lung cancer. *J Natl Cancer Inst* 1993; 85:321–323.
69. Belani CP, Ramanathan RK. Combined modality treatment of locally advanced non-small cell lung cancer: Incorporation of novel chemotherapeutic agents. *Chest* 1998; 113(Suppl 1):53S–60S.
70. Choy H, DeVore RD, Hande KR, et al. Phase II study of paclitaxel, carboplatin, and hyperfractionated radiation therapy for locally advanced inoperable non-small cell lung cancer. A Vanderbilt Cancer Center Affiliate Network (VCCAN) Trial. *Proc Am Soc Clin Oncol* 1998; 17:467a (abstr).
71. Furuse K, Fukuoka M, Kawahara M, et al. Phase III study of concurrent versus sequential thoracic radiotherapy in combination with mitomycin, vindesine, and cisplatin in unresectable stage III non-small cell lung cancer. *J Clin Oncol* 1999; 17:2692–2699.

72. Komaki R, Seiferheld W, Curran W, et al. Sequential vs. concurrent chemotherapy and radiation therapy for inoperable non-small cell lung cancer (NSCLC): Analysis of failures in a Phase III study (RTOG 94-10) Proc Am Soc Thera Rad Oncol (ASTRO). *IJROBP* 2000; 48:5A (abstr).
73. Edelman MJ, Gandara DR. Promising new agents in the treatment of non-small cell lung cancer. *Cancer Chemother Pharmacol* 1996; 37:385–393.
74. Gandara DR, Edelman MJ, Lara PN, et al. Current status and novel therapeutic approaches in advanced non-small cell lung cancer. ASCO Educational Book, Spring: 362–369, 1999.
75. Tishler RB, Schiff PB, Geard CR, et al. Taxol: A novel radiation sensitizer. *Int J Radiat Oncol Biol Phys* 1992; 22:613–617.
76. Rockwell S, Grindley GB. Effect of 2',2'-difluorodeoxycytidine on the viability and radiosensitivity of EMT6 cell *in vitro*. *Oncol Res* 1992; 4:151–155.
77. Boothman DA, Wang M, Schea RA, et al. Post-treatment exposure to camptothecon enhances the lethal effects of x-rays on resistant human malignant melanoma cells. *Int J Radiat Biol Phys* 1992; 42:939–948.
78. Kim JH, Kim SH, Kolozsvary A, et al. Potentiation of radiation response in human carcinoma cells *in vitro* and murine fibrosarcoma cell *in vivo* by topotecan, an inhibitor of DNA topoisomerase I. *Int J Radiat Oncol Biol Phys* 1992; 22:515–518.
79. Von Pawel J, Von Roemeling T. Survival benefit from Tirazone (tirapazamine) and cisplatin in advanced non small cell lung cancer (NSCLC) patients: Final results from the phase III CATAPULT trial. *Proc Am Soc Clin Oncol* 1998; 17:454a (abstr 1749).
80. Langer C, Scott C, Byhardt R, et al. Effect of advanced age on outcome in Radiation Therapy Oncology Group studies of locally advanced NSCLC. *Lung Cancer* 2000; 29(Suppl 1)104:A-340.
81. Movsas B, Scott C, Sause W, et al. Age dramatically impacts on the quality-adjusted time without symptoms of toxicity (Q-Twist) in locally advanced non-small cell lung cancer - A Radiation Therapy Oncology Group (RTOG) analysis. Proc Am Soc Thera Rad Oncol (ASTRO). *IJROBP* 2000; 48:92A (abstr).
81a. Langer CJ, Hsu C, Curran W, Komaki R, Lee JS, Byhardt R, Sause W. Do elderly patients with locally advanced non-small cell lung cancer (NSCLC) benefit from combined modality therapy? A secondary analysis of RTOG 94-10. *IJROBP* 2001; 51:31A (abstr).
82. Komaki R, Scott CB, Byhardt RW, et al. Failure patterns by prognostic group determined by recursive partitioning analysis (RPA) of 1,547 patients on four Radiation Therapy Oncology Group studies in inoperable non-small cell lung cancer (NSCLC). *Int J Radiat Oncol Biol Phys* 1998; 42:263–267.
83. Sause WT, Scott C, Taylor S, et al. Phase II trial of combination chemotherapy and irradiation in non-small cell lung cancer, Radiation Therapy Oncology Group 88-04. *Am J Clin Oncol* 1992; 15:163–167.
84. Komaki R, Scott C, Ettinger D, et al. Randomized study of chemotherapy/radiation therapy combinations for favorable patients with locally advanced inoperable nonsmall-cell lung cancer: Radiation Therapy Oncology Group (RTOG) 92-04. *Int J Radiat Oncol Biol Phys* 1997; 38:149–155.
85. Clamon G. Herndon J. Cooper R, et al. Radiosensitization with carboplatin for patients with unresectable stage III non-small-cell lung cancer: A phase III trial of the Cancer and Leukemia Group B and the Eastern Cooperative Oncology Group *J Clin Oncol* 1999; 17:4–11.
86. Vokes EE, Leopold KA, Herndon JE II, et al. A randomized phase II trial of gemcitabine or paclitaxel or vinorelbine with cisplatin as induction chemotherapy and concomitant chemo-radiotherapy for unresectable stage III non-small cell lung cancer. *Proc Am Soc Clin Oncol* 1999; 18:459A (abstr).
87. Green MR, Rocha Lima CM, Sherman CA. Radiation and chemotherapy for patients with stage III non-small cell lung cancer. *Sem Rad Oncol* 2000; 10:289–295.
88. Gandara DR, Lovato LC, Albain KS, et al. Prolonged survival in pathologic stage IIIB non-small cell lung cancer with concurrent chemoradiotherapy followed by consolidation docetaxel: A phase II study (S9504) of the Southwest Oncology Group (SWOG). *Proc Am Soc Clin Oncol* 2000; 19:1916A (abstr).
89. Evans W, Will B, Berthelot J, et al. Cost of combined modality interventions for stage III non-small-cell lung cancer. *J Clin Oncol* 1997; 15:3038–3048.
90. Konski A, Scott C, Movsas B, et al. Cost-utility analysis of various treatments for non-small cell carcinoma of the lung (Abstract). *Eur J Cancer* 2000; 36:S19.
91. American Society of Clinical Oncology. Clinical practice guidelines for the treatment of unresectable non small cell lung cancer. *J Clin Oncol* 1997; 15:2996–3018.
92. Burkes R, Shepard F, Ginsberg R, et al. Induction chemotherapy with MVP in patients with stage IIIA (N2) unresectable non-small cell lung cancer. The Toronto experience (abstract 1078). *Proc Am Soc Clin Oncol* 1994; 13:327.

93. Choi N, Carey R, Daly W, et al. Potential impact on survival of improved tumor downstaging and resection rate by preoperative twice-daily radiation and concurrent chemotherapy in stage IIIA non-small-cell lung cancer. *J Clin Oncol* 1997; 15:712–722.
94. Granone P, Margaritora S, Cesario A, et al. Concurrent radio-chemotherapy in N2 non small cell lung cancer: interim analysis. *Eur J Cardio-thoracic Surgery* 1997; 12:366–371.
95. Strauss GM, Langer MP, Elias AD, et al. Multimodality treatment of stage IIIA non-small cell lung carcinoma: A critical review of the literature and strategies for future research. *J Clin Oncol* 1992; 10:829–838.

10 Combined Modality Treatment of Small-Cell Lung Cancer

Julie R. Brahmer, MD, *Larry Kleinberg,* MD, *and David S. Ettinger,* MD

Contents

1. INTRODUCTION

Small-cell lung cancer (SCLC) accounts for approx 18–25% of the estimated 169,500 cases of lung cancer in 2001 *(1,2)*. Most patients present with metastatic disease due to the aggressive nature of SCLC. SCLC is staged using a two-stage system identified by the Veterans Administration Lung Group (VALG). The VALG classified limited-stage disease (LD) as tumor limited to one hemithorax and its regional lymph nodes that can be encompassed by one radiation port. LD accounts for approx 40% of all SCLC cases. Extensive-stage disease (ED) is tumor spread beyond these boundaries *(2)*. The presence of pleural effusions and/or supraclavicular lymphadenopathy have been considered LD by some investigators and ED by others.

Radiation therapy's main role is in the treatment of LD. Because radiation only offers locoregional control, chemotherapy is necessary to destroy the micrometastatic disease that invariably is present. Multiple cooperative group trials have been performed to establish the role of radiation therapy in SCLC *(3–7)*.

However, many questions remain to be answered related to combined-modality therapies for LD-SCLC. These questions include: What is the best chemotherapy regimen? When should it be given?, In what dose, volume, and fractionation of radiation should be administered? What sequence (i.e., concurrent, sequential, or alternating) and time (i.e., cycle 1, 2, 3, or 4) should the radiation be given?

From: *Chemoradiation in Cancer Therapy*
Edited by: H. Choy © Humana Press Inc., Totowa, NJ

2. PATHOLOGY, BIOLOGY, DIAGNOSIS, AND STAGING

Rapid tumor growth and early dissemination characterize small-cell lung cancer. Common presenting symptoms such as cough, hemoptysis, chest pain, and dyspnea are caused by large tumor masses. Less common presenting symptoms include dysphagia caused by esophageal compression, hoarseness caused by laryngeal nerve paralysis, and facial swelling caused by superior vena cava compression *(2)*. Also, paraneoplastic syndromes such as Cushing's or Eaton–Lambert syndrome or inappropriate secretion of antidiuretic hormone can be present.

The diagnosis of SCLC is usually made using fiberoptic bronchoscopy. The value of fiberoptic bronchoscopy was established in the 1980s *(8,9)*. Ninety-three percent of SCLC cases are diagnosed by fiberoptic bronchoscopy while fine needle aspiration or mediastinoscopy diagnose the rest. The majority of time, the diagnosis of SCLC is made cytologically. Unfortunately, this limits the amount of tissue available for further studies, i.e., molecular markers and so on.

In the World Health Organization classification proposed in 1981, SCLC was subdivided into three pathologic subtypes.

1. Oat cell.
2. Intermediate (fusiform, polygonal).
3. Combined (small-cell lung cancer with squamous or adenocarcinoma features) *(10)*.

In 1988, because of the imprecision of this classification, the International Association for the Study of Lung Cancer (IASLC) revised the classification to include:

1. Pure small-cell lung cancer.
2. Mixed small-cell and large-cell carcinoma.
3. Combined (small-cell lung cancer with squamous or adenocarcinoma features) *(11)*.

Besides the pure small-cell lung cancer, the mixed small-cell and large-cell carcinoma comprises less than 6% of all small-cell lung cancer, and combined SCLC/nonsmall-cell lung cancer (NSCLC) comprises less than 3% of all SCLC *(11–14)*.

Because of early dissemination, staging of patients with small-cell lung cancer is more extensive than for patients with NSCLC. It is important to rule out distant metastasis because it will change the role of thoracic radiation in the treatment of these patients. Staging should include a complete history and physical examination, CAT scans of chest and upper abdomen to include the liver and adrenal glands, brain MRI scan, bone scan, complete blood count, and a possible bone marrow aspiration and biopsy.

A short cell cycle and a high cell proliferation fraction cause the rapid tumor growth and early metastasis. These factors account, in part, for the high sensitivity of SCLC to chemotherapy and radiation therapy. The mean doubling time of SCLC cell lines is 50 d (15–250 d) *(15–17)*. The response to chemotherapy alone is approx 80% but with a low complete response rate of 30–40% *(18)*. The complete response rate to combination chemotherapy and radiation therapy is up to 80% *(19)*.

3. DEVELOPMENT OF RADIATION TREATMENT FOR SCLC

Thoracic radiation was not established as a standard part of the treatment of limited-disease (LD) SCLC until the 1980s. In the early 1960s, surgery was the treatment of choice for patients with resectable SCLC. However, this practice was stopped when

Table 1

Studies of Chemotherapy vs Chemotherapy and Chest Radiation in Patients with LD-SCLC

Study	*Number of pt*	*Chemotherapy regimen*	*Radiation dose*	*Radiation schedule*
1. SECSG *(3)*	369	CAV	30 Gy/15 fractions/ wk 1, 2, 7	Alternating
2. CALGB *(4)*	399	CEV/CAV	50 Gy/25 fractions/ 5 wk Continuous	Concurrent starting on D 1 of cycle 1 thru D 4 of cycle 3 No RT
3. ECOG *(7)*	310	CCM/EA	50 Gy/25 fractions/ 5 wk Continuous	Sequential D 43
4. SWOG *(5)*	93	VMV/VAC	48 Gy/22 fractions/ 6.5 wk Split	Sequential wk 12
5. NCI *(23)*	96	CCM/VAP	40 Gy/15 fractions/ 3 wk bid Continuous	Concurrent D 1
6. NCIC *(6)*	308	CAV/PE Alternating	40 Gy/15 fractions per wk	Concurrent D 22 (cycle 2) D 106 (cycle 6)

CAV = cyclophosphamide/doxorubicin/vincristine; CEV = cyclophosphamide/epirubicin/vincristine; CCM = cyclophosphamide/lomustine/methotrexate; EA = etoposide/doxorubicin; VMV/VAC = vincristine, methotrexate, VP-16/vincristine, doxorubicin, cyclophosphamide; VAP = vincristine/doxorubicin/procarbazine; PE = cisplatin/etoposide.

Table 1A
Studies of Chemotherapy vs Chemotherapy and Chest Radiation in Patients with LD-SCLC

<table>
<tr><th></th><th colspan="2">Median survival time (mo)</th><th colspan="2">2-Yr Survival rate %</th></tr>
<tr><th>Study</th><th>CT</th><th>CRT</th><th>CT</th><th>CRT</th></tr>
<tr><td>1. SECSG (3)</td><td>10.6</td><td>11.9</td><td>21%</td><td>29%</td></tr>
<tr><td>2. CALGB (4)</td><td></td><td>11.2</td><td>8%</td><td>15%</td></tr>
<tr><td></td><td></td><td>11.8</td><td></td><td>25%</td></tr>
<tr><td></td><td>7.7</td><td></td><td>8%</td><td></td></tr>
<tr><td>3. ECOG (7)</td><td>12.4</td><td>14.4</td><td>13%</td><td>19%</td></tr>
<tr><td>4. SWOG (5)</td><td colspan="2">18.5</td><td>25%</td><td>35%</td></tr>
<tr><td>5. NCI (23)</td><td>11.6</td><td>15</td><td>12%</td><td>28%</td></tr>
<tr><td>6. NCIC (6)</td><td>15.4</td><td>21.2</td><td></td><td>40%</td></tr>
<tr><td></td><td></td><td></td><td></td><td>34%</td></tr>
</table>

results of a trial performed in the United Kingdom were available. This trial compared patients with limited disease treated with thoracic radiation alone versus surgery alone. The 10-yr survival for the surgery alone arm was zero, but the 10-yr survival for the radiation alone arm was 5% *(20)*. The mean survival was 199 d for the surgery alone arm, and the mean survival was 300 d for the radiation alone arm. In 1978, an extensive review on the outcome of surgery performed on patients with "resectable" SCLC was done in the United States. The review revealed no difference in survival if surgery was included in the treatment regimen *(21)*.

In the late 1960s, the systemic nature of SCLC was realized and treatment began to shift to the use of chemotherapy. In 1969, the Veteran's Association Lung Cancer Study Group demonstrated that cyclophosphamide increased the median survival in patients with extensive disease to 6 mo *(22)*. Thus, chemotherapy was the mainstay of treatment for SCLC in the 1960s and 1970s. However, a high rate of locoregional recurrence of disease and poor survival remained problems.

In the 1970s and 1980s, multiple cooperative group trials were performed to test the role of adding thoracic radiation therapy to chemotherapy (Table 1 and 1A). The SECSG *(3)*, CALGB *(4)*, SWOG *(5)*, NCIC *(6)*, ECOG *(7)*, and NCI *(23)* trials randomized patients with LD-SCLC to chemotherapy alone vs chemotherapy with radiation. The schedule of radiation and type of chemotherapy used varied between trials, but all the trials used prophylactic cranial irradiation (PCI). The combination of radiation therapy and chemotherapy decreased the locoregional recurrence rates compared to the use of chemotherapy alone in the treatment of LD-SCLC (Table 2). All of the trials except for the SWOG trial reported statistically significant improvements in survival. As a result of these studies, thoracic radiation therapy became a standard part of the therapy for patients with LD-SCLC.

Meta-analyses performed by Pignon et al. and Warde et al. evaluated the improvement of survival and local control with combined chemotherapy and radiation in LD-SCLC *(24,25)*. Local regional failure still remained a principal cause of failure in LD-SCLC occurring in 25–30% although combined local and/or distant recurrence was greater than 50%. Combined chemotherapy and radiation therapy improved survival by 5% and

Table 2
Local Recurrence Rates for Chemotherapy Alone vs Chemotherapy and Chest Irradiation in Patients with LD-SCLC

		Local recurrence rates %	
Study	*Radiation*	*CT*	*CRT*
1. SECSG *(3)*		79%	51%
2. CALGB *(4)*	Concurrent		74%
	No XRT	32%	60%
3. ECOG *(7)*		NR	
4. SWOG *(5)*		72%	50%
5. NCI *(23)*		33%	70%
6. NCIC *(16)*	D 22 (cycle 2)		59%
	D 106 (cycle 40)		61%

XRT = radiation; NR = Not reported.

decreased local recurrence by 50%. However, these meta-analyses demonstrated that local treatment is still suboptimal.

4. RADIATION THERAPY

4.1. General Considerations

A stepwise procedure is used when calculating a dose for an individual patient. First, the limits of the initial tumor and mediastinal lymphadenopathy involved are outlined on chest films taking into account radiologic, bronchoscopic, and clinical information. Second, the target volume is drawn on simulator films. Third, safety margins of the anterior and posterior and lateral or oblique fields are measured (the distance between the target volume and the border of the fields).

Once the volume is estimated, the dose, fraction size, and schedule are decided upon. All of these factors—volume, dose, fraction size, and the timing of chemotherapy—are considered and important in trying to reduce the local recurrence rate and improve overall survival in patients with LD-SCLC.

4.2. Dose

The optimal dose of radiation therapy for patients with limited stage disease is unknown. Full dose radiation therapy is critical to achieve the therapeutic gain of local tumor control. Effective chemotherapy may allow a decrease in the radiation dose needed for local control *(26)*. In the presence of chemotherapy, the radiation dose theoretically can be reduced 20% to control the tumor. Thus the dose for complete response, approx 70 Gy, can be decreased to 55 Gy *(26)*. Local recurrence is still around 40–50% *(27)*. Retrospective trials revealed that doses less than 40 Gy were not adequate for local control *(28)*.

In order to evaluate whether a higher dose is better, a dose-response relationship must be established between the total dose of radiation and locoregional control. The dose response relationship was established by Choi and Carey *(29)*. Doses of 30–35 Gy yielded a local control rate of 20–25%. Doses of 45–50 Gy resulted in a locoregional control rate of 60–70%. Beyond 50 Gy the level of local control is unclear. A Canadian group performed the only randomized trial in LD-SCLC patients comparing low-dose radiotherapy at 25 Gy given in 10 fractions over 2 wk (an equivalent dose of 28 Gy) or moderate dose radiation therapy of 37.5 Gy for 15 fractions over 3 wk (an equivalent conventional fraction dose of 42 Gy). The higher-dose radiation therapy delayed rather than decreased local recurrence *(30)*. Studies need to be performed to evaluate doses beyond 50 Gy.

Fractionation of radiation therapy effects dose. Conventional fractionation consists of five 2 Gy fractions per week, which allows up to 70 Gy to be delivered to a limited mediastinal volume. Pignon et al. performed a meta-analysis, and included 13 randomized trials *(24)*. The fractionation dose varied between 2 and 4 Gy. The analysis revealed that as the fraction got larger the toxicities increased *(24)*.

Hyperfractionated radiation decreases the fraction size but is repeated hours later. So, the overall days of treatment are decreased. The total dose is maintained similar to once-daily (conventional) radiation or a slightly higher dose is given. Theoretically, twice-daily radiation therapy decreases the repopulation of tumor cells. Choi established the maximum tolerated dose of hyperfractionated radiation therapy given twice-daily as 45 Gy in 30 fractions over three weeks and the maximum tolerated conventional dose was 70 Gy in 35 fractions over 7 wk *(31)*. Several phase II studies demonstrated the efficacy of hyperfractionated radiation therapy combined with chemotherapy *(31–34)*.

The only randomized phase III study evaluating hyperfractionated radiation therapy was an intergroup trial *(35)*. Patients were randomized to twice-daily radiation therapy (45 Gy over 3 wk) or conventional radiation therapy (45 Gy over 5 wk). Radiation therapy was started d 1, cycle 1 with four cycles of cisplatin and etoposide (CE). Local control trended better in the twice-daily arm. After a complete response, the recurrence rate was 75% in the daily radiation vs 42% in the twice-daily radiation. Local recurrence only rates were 52% vs 36%, respectively ($p = 0.058$). Median survival for the conventional radiation was 19 mo and for the hyperfractionated radiation was 23 mo. Five-year survival was 16% for conventional daily fractions and 26% for hyperfractionated radiation ($p = 0.04$). However, grade 3 or greater esophageal toxicity was higher for the twice-daily radiation (25.7% vs 10.9%, respectively). Thus, today, the standard radiation therapy regimen for patients with LD-SCLC should be twice-daily radiation therapy given in 1.8–2 Gy fractions for a total dose of 45–50 Gy when combined with cisplatin and etoposide chemotherapy. However, is it? The answer is probably not. Many patients with LD-SCLC and radiation oncologists do not favor the use of the hyperfractionated radiation therapy owing to the time spent (i.e., twice a day) receiving the therapy as well as the significant increase in the esophagitis.

4.3. Volume

In order to maximize the therapeutic ratio between efficacy and toxicity, a balance must exist between radiation dose and the volume of the radiation port. The volume of the radiation port affects the amount of radiation that can be given. In regards to toxicity of radiation, total radiation dose is inversely related to the volume of the radiation port *(36)*. Thus, to keep the toxicity at a minimum, the port size or the dose of radiation must be changed.

The standard for radiation port size without chemotherapy for limited-stage SCLC is a relatively large port, which includes the original tumor volume with a 1.5–2 cm free margin *(37,38)*. Included with the tumor are the involved lymph nodes as well as the neighboring uninvolved lymph nodes. A retrospective review of the SECSG trial revealed that, when the contralateral hilar lymph nodes where excluded from the radiation port, the failure rate increased from 33 to 69% ($p = 0.026$) *(3)*.

Several studies have tried to address the question of encompassing the pre- vs the postchemotherapy tumor volume *(3,5,39–41)*. Studies have been limited because of small patient numbers. In one such study, the radiation port only encompassed residual disease (the postchemotherapy tumor volume). Five of seven failures occurred outside of the port. This trial was the exception *(3)*. The Mayo Clinic performed a retrospective analysis comparing radiation ports encompassing the prechemotherapy or the postchemotherapy tumor volume. No marginal failures occurred. Locoregional failures occurred in 10 of 31 patients treated with a prechemotherapy port vs 9 of 28 patients treated with a postchemotherapy radiation port *(39)*. Locoregional recurrences occurred within the radiation port. SWOG performed a randomized study evaluating this same question *(5)*. Patients were randomized per their tumor response to induction chemotherapy. Those patients who achieved a complete response after chemotherapy were randomized to either a wide volume port followed by chemotherapy or chemotherapy alone. A wide volume port was defined as the prechemotherapy tumor volume plus mediastinal adenopathy and a surrounding margin. The radiation dose was 30 Gy given in 10 fractions over 2 wk. The patients were then given a 2-wk break and then given radiation therapy encompassing the postchemotherapy tumor volume plus a 2 cm margin. The radiation dose was 30 Gy given in 12 fractions over 2.5 wk. Local recurrence rate of the patients treated with the wide volume was 50% vs chemotherapy alone of 72% ($p = 0.01$). The median survival of the group of complete responders was 18.5 mo. Of the patients who achieved stable disease or a partial response to chemotherapy, they were randomized to either wide volume radiation therapy or a reduced field radiation, both of which were followed by more chemotherapy. The reduced field radiation port was defined as encompassing only the postchemotherapy tumor volume with 2 cm margins. The same radiation dose and fractionation scheme was used as above. Local recurrence rate of the group given wide field radiation therapy was 32% vs 28% for the reduced field radiation (not statistically different). The median survival of patients in this group who achieved a complete response after all therapy was completed was 18 mo. Patients who originally progressed on induction chemotherapy were taken off study. Another study reported that 86% of local regional recurrences occurred within the postchemotherapy volume *(40)*. A different study reported that radiation port margins around the tumor volume made no difference in locoregional recurrence *(41)*. This study compared a 1–1.5 cm margin vs a less than 1 cm margin. The locoregional recurrence was 33 vs 36%, respectively ($p = 0.86$). In conclusion, there is no difference in locoregional recurrence when the volume of the port size is varied between pre- vs postchemotherapy tumor volume or margin size. Thus, larger volumes do not necessarily mean better control. If combined chemotherapy and radiation therapy is used, only postchemotherapy tumor volumes need to be included within the radiation port. However, prophylactic radiation of regional lymph nodes is still a subject to be evaluated.

4.4. Combining Chemotherapy with Radiation Therapy

Several theoretical advantages exist for combining chemotherapy and radiation therapy for the treatment of limited stage SCLC:

1. Radiation can control the bulky disease earlier with chemotherapy eradicating the micrometastatic disease outside of the radiation field.

2. Radiation can improve survival because local progression itself can cause death, and improved local control may decrease further dissemination.
3. The combination can overcome the early emergence of chemoresistant cells since chemotherapy and radiation have independent mechanisms of action *(42)*.

The theory is that the earlier the combination is administered the better the chance for the resistance to be overcome. Unfortunately, cross-resistance can occur *(9,43,44)*. Several randomized studies have demonstrated that the combination of chemotherapy and radiation therapy improves overall survival compared to chemotherapy alone (Table 1 and 1A).

4.5. Timing and Sequence of Chemotherapy and Radiation

The optimal timing and sequence of combining chemotherapy and radiation therapy is unknown for the treatment of limited-stage small-cell lung cancer. Radiation can be combined with chemotherapy sequentially, alternating, or concurrently. When combined concurrently, radiation can be started early in the treatment or later during the treatment schedule.

Sequential combinations complete chemotherapy first and then follow it with radiation therapy. The advantages of this schedule are decreased toxicity and increased ability to deliver full doses of chemotherapy. The disadvantage is that there is an increased chance of developing therapy-resistant tumors *(36)*.

Three randomized phase III studies have been performed evaluating sequential chemotherapy followed by radiation therapy vs chemotherapy alone in patients with LD-SCLC (Table 3). The chemotherapy used in these studies was noncisplatin-based. One study performed by Carlson et al. randomized patients who responded to chemotherapy to chemotherapy only or radiation therapy *(45)*. The radiation therapy dose was 55 Gy given in 1.8–2.0 Gy fractions over 5–7 wk. No difference in overall survival was detected. Intrathoracic recurrence rates were 58% for the chemotherapy alone group and 29% for the patients who received chemotherapy followed by radiation ($p = 0.042$). A French group randomized 53 patients who achieved a complete response after chemotherapy to radiation of 46.5 Gy or no radiation therapy until disease relapse *(46)*. The local-regional recurrence rate was 33% for the sequential radiation therapy and 58% for chemotherapy but not statistically different ($p = 0.66$). The median survival was 10.5 mo for the radiation therapy group and 16.5 mo for the group who received radiation therapy at the time of relapse. The SWOG cooperative group randomized 93 patients who achieved complete responses postinduction chemotherapy to split course radiation therapy or chemotherapy alone *(5)*. The radiation dose was 48 Gy in 22 fractions. The radiation therapy did improve local control compared to chemotherapy alone (Local recurrence rate was 50% vs 72%, respectively). The Japanese Clinical Oncology group published a trial comparing concurrent and sequential chemotherapy and radiation, to be discussed subsequently *(47)*. The results favored the use of concurrent chemoradiation therapy compared to sequential therapy. This study was the only one in this group to use cisplatin-based chemotherapy.

Alternating schedule is defined as chemotherapy given conventionally with radiation given in between the chemotherapy cycles. An advantage of an alternating sequence is decreased toxicities, an increased ability to deliver full dose chemotherapy and radiation therapy, and a decreased probability of developing cross-therapy resistance. The disadvantages include splitting up the course of radiation therapy and loss of the possible advantages of concomitant chemoradiation sensitization of tumor cells *(36)*.

Table 3
Studies of Chemotherapy vs Sequential Chemotherapy Followed by Radiation Therapy in Patients with LD-SCLC

					Median survival time (mo)		*2-Yr Survival rate %*	
Study	*Number of pt.*	*Chemo*	*Radiation*	*Schedule*	*CT*	*CRT*	*CT*	*CRT*
Carlson *(44)*	48	CLVP/EAM	55 Gy/30 Fx/7 wk	Sequential after 6–9 mo	18.9	20.3	42%	42%
Le Beam *(45)*	53	CCAE	46.5 Gy/Equivalent	Sequential after 8 cycles	16.5	10.5	38%	26%
SWOG *(5)*	93	VMV/VAC	48 Gy/22 Fx/6.5 wk Split	Sequential wk 12	18.5		25%	35%

CLVP = cyclophosphamide/lomustine/vincristine/procarbazine; EAM = etoposide/doxorubicin/methotrexate; CCAE = cyclophosphamide/lomustine/doxorubicin/etoposide; VMV/VAC = VMV/VAC = vincristine, methotrexate, VP-16/vincristine, doxorubicin, cyclophosphamide; NR = not reported.

Two studies have evaluated this schema of treatment for LD-SCLC. Both trials used nonplatinum-based chemotherapy regimens. The SECSG trial randomized patients to chemotherapy alone or chemotherapy alternating with radiation therapy *(3)*. The chemotherapy regimen used was cyclophosphamide, doxorubicin, and vincristine. The addition of radiation therapy improved local control and 2-yr survival (64% vs 48% and 24% vs 16%, respectively) *(3)*. A French trial randomized patients between alternating and concurrent schedules *(48)*. In the concurrent arm, patients received 50 Gy of radiation in 20 fractions after the second cycle of chemotherapy (cyclophosphamide, doxorubicin, and etoposide-vindesine replaced doxorubicin during the second and third cycles). In the alternating schedule, patients received the same chemotherapy alternating with the radiation therapy given in three courses (d 36–47: 20 Gy in eight fractions; d 64–75: 20 Gy in eight fractions; d 92–101: 15 Gy in six fractions) *(48)*. The median survival for the concurrent arm was 13.5 mo and for the alternating arm was 14 mo. The 3-yr survival for the concurrent arm was 6% vs 11% for the alternating schedule arm. The differences were not statistically different *(48)*.

Concurrent schedule of chemotherapy and radiation therapy is defined as the delivery of radiation and chemotherapy simultaneously either early or late in the treatment schedule. The advantage of this schedule is that by giving the radiation and chemotherapy together early in the treatment course one can possibly prevent the development of resistant tumor cells. However, the disadvantages include increased toxicities and the decreased ability to deliver full dose chemotherapy *(36)*.

A Japanese trial compared sequential delivery of chemotherapy and radiation therapy to concurrent delivery of chemotherapy and radiation *(47)*. Patients were randomized to receive concurrent hyperfractionated radiation therapy (d 2 of cycle 1 of chemotherapy) or to sequential chemotherapy followed after the fourth cycle by hyperfractionated radiation therapy. The radiation dose was 45 Gy given in 1.5 Gy fractions twice daily for a total of 30 fractions in 3 wk. The chemotherapy given was cisplatin and etoposide. The median survival for the concurrent schedule was 29 mo and for the sequential schedule was 19 mo. The 2-yr survival was 50% for the concurrent therapy and 40% for the sequential therapy *(47)*. These results favored concurrent therapy and are the best results to date for patients with LD-SCLC.

Other studies evaluated the question of whether early delivery of radiation concurrently with chemotherapy was better than late delivery. A study performed by the CALGB randomized patients to early (d 1, cycle 1), late (d 64, cycle 4), or no radiation therapy. The radiation therapy dose was 50 Gy over 6 wk. Chemotherapy used in this trial was cyclophosphamide, etoposide, and vincristine. The local recurrence rate for the early, late, and no radiation therapy arms was 49%, 68%, and 82%, respectively. The 2-yr progression-free survival rate was 15% for the early schedule arm vs 25% for the late schedule ($p = 0.078$). The 5-yr survival rate for the early, late, and no radiation therapy arms was 6.6%, 12%, and 3%, respectively ($p = 0.007$). The poor 5-yr survival rate for the early schedule was felt to be due to the significant decrease in chemotherapy dose needed for the early schedule group *(4,49)*.

The NCIC randomized patients to radiation therapy started either early or late with concurrent chemotherapy (cyclophosphamide, doxorubicin, and vincristine alternating with cisplatin and etoposide) *(6)*. The radiation therapy dose was 40 Gy given in 15 fractions over three weeks with the cisplatin and etoposide portion of the chemotherapy. In the early arm the radiation was started on d 21 of cycle 2 (after the first cycle of cisplatin/etoposide). In the late arm, the radiation was started on d 106 (cycle 6) with the third cycle of cisplatin and etoposide. The local recurrence rate was 55% in both arms. The 5-yr survival in the early delivery arm and the late delivery arm was 20% and 11%, respectively ($p = 0.006$). The medial survival for the early delivery arm was 21.2 mo compared to 16 mo for the late delivery arm ($p = 0.008$). The early delivery arm also had a decreased incidence of brain metastasis (18% vs 28%-$p = 0.042$) which could explain the improved 5-yr survival *(6)*.

A Danish trial randomized 199 patients to either early radiation therapy or late radiation therapy given concurrently with chemotherapy *(50)*. The early arm delivered 20 or 22.5 Gy in eleven fractions followed by a cycle of cisplatin and etoposide followed by the same schedule of radiation and followed again by chemotherapy. The delayed radiation arm gave the chemotherapy first then started the radiation therapy in wk 18 and again in wk 23. The same chemotherapy and radiation doses were given. The 5-yr survival and local recurrence rate were not statistically different. The 5-yr survival for the early arm was 10.8% vs 12% for the delayed radiation therapy arm. The local recurrence rate for the early radiation arm was 76.6% vs 72.8% for the delayed arm *(50)*.

The EORTC randomized patients to either start radiation therapy during wk 6 (early) or after the chemotherapy during wk 14 (late). The chemotherapy regimen used was cyclophosphamide, doxorubicin, and etoposide. The dose of radiation given in the early arm was 50 Gy in 20 fractions in 89 d. The dose of radiation given in the late arm was 50 Gy in 20 fractions in 26 d. No significant differences were noted for local recurrence (50.5% early radiation vs 45.5% late radiation) or 3-yr survival (14% for both early and late radiation therapy) *(51)*.

Another CALGB study randomized patients to early vs late delivery of hyperfractionated radiation given with carboplatin and etoposide chemotherapy *(52)*. In the early radiation arm, patients received radiation with chemotherapy during wk 1–4. In the late radiation arm, patients received radiation with chemotherapy during wk 6–9. The radiation dose for both arms was 54 Gy given in 36 fractions over 4 wk. The radiation dose was also hyperfractionated with 1.5 Gy given twice daily for 5 d/wk. The locoregional recurrence rate for the early and late radiation was 42% and 65%, respectively. The median survival for the early radiation group was 34 mo compared to 26 mo in the late radiation group ($p = 0.052$). The 5-yr survival for the early radiation group was 30% vs 15% for the late radiation group ($p = 0.027$). The results favored the early delivery of radiation therapy concurrently with platinum-based chemotherapy *(52)*.

Current data support the use of concurrent over sequential or alternating chemotherapy and radiation therapy. The optimal delivery of concurrent chemoradiation is still under study. Early delivery of radiation therapy may decrease dissemination by killing the chemoresistant tumor cells prior to their distant seeding. Late delivery of radiation therapy possibly reduces toxicities and full chemotherapy doses can be delivered. However, even with increased toxicity, improved survival rates help establish as standard early delivery of concurrent radiation with platinum-based chemotherapy.

4.6. New Chemotherapeutic Agents

Further investigation of the benefits of three drugs over two drugs has been performed using newer agents. Using the standard regimen of etoposide and cisplatin (EP), investigators have added ifosfamide, paclitaxel, or other investigational drugs (Table 4). Glisson et al. added ifosfamide to EP while giving concurrent hyperfractionated radia-

Table 4
Studies Evaluating New Chemotherapeutic Agents for Treatment of Patients with LD-SCLC

Study	*Pts*	*Chemo*	*Radiation RR*	*Median survival*	*1-Yr Survival rate (mo)*	
Glisson RTOG *(52)*	54 evaluable	IEP	Concurrent hyperfractionated	63% (CR) 17% (PR)	21.4	—
Ettinger RTOG *(53)*	53 evaluable	PEP	Concurrent hyperfractionated 45 Gy with cycle 1 and 2	78%	24.4	83%
Sandler ECOG *(54)*	61 evaluable	PEP	Concurrent Daily Fx	64% (ORR) 18% (CR)	16.8	63%
Glisson *(55)*	18	TP with EP	1.5 Gy Fx × 30	100% (ORR) 41% (CR) 59% (PR)	17.0	—
Lyss *(56)*	75 (10 pt 60 Gy) (65 pt 70 Gy)	TP induction E Carbo concurrent	70 Gy	NR	9.4	—

IEP = ifosfamide, etoposide, cisplatin; PEP = cisplatin, etoposide, paclitaxel; EP = etoposide + cisplatin; TP = topotecan+ paclitaxel; E Carbo = etoposide + carboplatin.

tion therapy (45 Gy) in a RTOG phase II trial *(53)*. In the 54 evaluable patients, the complete response rate was 63% (34/54), and the partial response rate was 17% (19/54). The median survival was 21.4 mo and the median progression free survival was 11.6 mo. However, grade 4 esophagitis was 36%, grade 3–4 nausea and vomiting was 26%, and grade 4 neutropenia was 28%. In another RTOG phase II trial, Ettinger et al. added paclitaxel to EP while giving concurrent hyperfractionated radiation therapy (45 Gy) *(54)*. In the 53 evaluable patients, the complete response rate was 78%. The median survival was 24.4 mo. The 1-yr survival rate was 83%. However, grade 3–4 esophagitis was 32 and 4%, respectively, and grade 4 neutropenia was 43%. ECOG also added paclitaxel to EP, but gave the radiation therapy later with cycles 3 and 4 rather than immediately with cycles 1 and 2 *(55)*. In addition, in this trial, the radiation was given in daily fractions to 63 Gy. In the 61 evaluable patients, the overall response rate was 64% with a complete response rate of 18%. The median survival time was 16.8 mo and the time to progression was 8.6 mo. The 1-yr survival rate was 63%. Grade 4 neutropenia was 59% and the grade 3–4 esophagitis was 3%. Glisson et al. alternated topotecan and paclitaxel with etoposide and cisplatin and thoracic radiation *(56)*. The radiation was delivered at 1.5 Gy for 30 fractions. The dose of the etoposide was 120 $mg/m^2/d$ on d 1–3, and cisplatin was dosed at 60 mg/m^2 on d 1. The topotecan and paclitaxel doses were escalated. The topotecan dose was escalated to 1.4 $mg/m^2/d$ for 5 d and the paclitaxel dose was escalated to 175 mg/m^2 given as a 3-h infusion on d 1. The dose-limiting toxicities were pneumonia, febrile neutropenia, and prolonged thrombocytopenia. The maximally tolerated dose was determined to be topotecan 1.2 mg/m^2 and paclitaxel 160 mg/m^2. The response rate of the 18 patients enrolled to the topotecan and paclitaxel combination was 100% (6% CR, 94% PR). The response rate to the combination and alternation of the two chemotherapy regimens with radiation therapy was 100% (41% CR, 59% PR). More recently, CALGB added topotecan and paclitaxel for induction chemotherapy followed by concurrent carboplatin and etoposide with daily radiation therapy (70 Gy) *(57)*. The grade 3–4 neutropenia was noted in 48% of patients. Of the 44 patients who received 70 Gy of radiation therapy combined with chemotherapy, 82% had grade 3–5 toxicities. Grade 3–4 neutropenia was reported in 70% of those patients. Grade 3–4 thrombocytopenia was reported in 32% of the patients. Eleven percent had grade 3–4 dysphagia. One patient had grade 5 esophageal toxicity at 64 Gy secondary to hemorrhage and death after dilatation of an esophageal stricture. The median survival was 9.4 mo. Currently, SWOG is combining EP with concurrent radiation therapy (61 Gy) and following this with paclitaxel and carboplatin for three cycles. Other agents that are or should be investigated in combination with radiation therapy in the future include irinotecan, docetaxel, and vinorelbine. In addition, molecular targeting agents will be added to these regimens in the near future.

4.7. Prophylactic Cranial Irradiation

Prophylactic cranial irradiation (PCI) use for SCLC began in the 1970s. The CNS is a sanctuary from most chemotherapy agents, and for patients with SCLC, relapse in the CNS is common. At diagnosis, 10% of patients with SCLC have brain metastasis, and 20–25% of patients with SCLC are diagnosed later with brain metastasis *(2)*. PCI is thought to decrease disease relapse in the CNS. Several studies have randomized patients after receiving definitive therapy for their systemic disease and achieving a complete remission to PCI vs no PCI. Of three randomized trials, PCI improved overall relapse rate and brain only relapse rate (Table 5). A trend toward improved survival was also demon-

Table 5
Summary of Prophylactic Cranial Irradiation for SCLC Patients

		Occurrence of brain metastasis		
Trial	*PCI dose*	*PCI*	*No PCI*	
Arriagada *(58)*	24 Gy/8 Fx	41%	59%	$p < 0.0001$
Gregor *(61)*	36 Gy/18 Fx 30 Gy/10 Fx 24 Gy/12 Fx 8 Gy/1 Fx	29%	52%	$p = 0.0002$

strated *(58–60)*. A meta-analysis of PCI was performed including seven randomized trials *(61)*. A total of 847 patients with LD-SCLC and 140 patients with extensive disease SCLC were included in the meta-analysis. These patients were in complete remission and then randomized to PCI or observation. A 16% decrease in mortality was observed in those patients who received PCI. Also, a 5.4% increase in the three-year survival was demonstrated (15.3% controls vs 20.7% PCI). From these data, PCI should be considered for patients who achieve a complete remission or near complete remission after initial therapy. The optimal dose and fractionation for PCI is unknown. The most commonly used dose for PCI is 25 Gy given over 10 fractions.

5. CONCLUSION

The best results combining chemotherapy with radiation therapy were seen with concurrent radiation therapy and cisplatin-based chemotherapy *(6,47)*. At this time, standard treatment for patients with limited stage small-cell lung cancer is early concurrent twice daily radiation therapy of 1.8 Gy fractions for a total dose of 45 Gy and platinum-based chemotherapy. However, the most efficacious regimen is still in question. Several studies are still needed to evaluate the appropriate dose, volume, fractionation, and timing of radiation therapy. As newer chemotherapy regimens emerge for the treatment of small-cell lung cancer, these regimens must be evaluated combining them with radiation therapy.

REFERENCES

1. Cancer Facts and Figures, 2001. Atlanta: American Cancer Society, 14.
2. Murran J, Glatstein E, Pass HI. Small-cell Lung Cancer. In: (Devita VT Jr, Hellman S, Rosenberg SA eds). Cancer: Principles and Practice of Oncology, 6th ed. Philadelphia: JB Lippincott, 2001: 983–1018.
3. Birch R, Omura GA, Greco FA, et al. Patterns of failure in combined chemotherapy and radiotherapy for limited small-cell lung cancer: Southeastern Cancer Study Group experience. *NCI Monogr* 1988; 6:265–270.
4. Perry MC, Eaton WL, Propert KJ, et al. Chemotherapy with or without radiation therapy in limited small-cell carcinoma of the lung. *N Engl J Med* 1987; 316:912–918.
5. Kies MS, Mira JG, Crowley JJ, et al. Multimodal therapy for limited small-cell lung cancer: A randomized study of induction combination chemotherapy with or without thoracic radiation in complete responders, and with wide-field vs reduced-field radiation in partial responders: A Southwest Oncology Group Study. *J Clin Oncol* 1987; 5:592–600.
6. Murray N, Coy P, Pater JL, et al. Importance of timing for thoracic irradiation in the combined modality treatment of limited-stage small-cell lung cancer: The National Cancer Institute of Canada Clinical Trials Group. *J Clin Oncol* 1993; 11:336–344.

7. Creech R, Richter M, Finkelstein D, for the ECOG. Combination chemotherapy with or without consolidation radiation therapy (RT) for regional small-cell carcinoma of the lung (abstract 756). *Proc Am Soc Clin Oncol* 1988; 7:196.
8. Baldeyrou P, Marrash R, LeChevalier R, Arriagada R. L'endoscopie bronchique dans le bilan diagnostique et evolutif des concers broncho-pulmonaires a petites cellules. *Bull Cancer* 1987; 74:511–515.
9. Schwartz JL, Rotmensch J, Beckett MA, et al. X-ray and cis-diamminedichloroplatinum (II) cross-resistance in human tumor cell lines. *Cancer Res* 1988; 48:5133–5135.
10. World Health Organization: Histologic typing of lung tumors, 2nd ed. Geneva: World Health Organization, 1981.
11. Hirsch FR, Matthews MJ, Aisner S, et al. Histopathologic classification of small-cell lung cancer. Changing concepts and terminology. *Cancer* 1988; 62:973.
12. Aisner SC, Finkelstein DM, Ettinger DS, et al. The clinical significance of variant-morphology small-cell carcinoma of the lung. *J Clin Oncol* 1990; 8:402.
13. Fraire AE, Johnson EH, Yesner R, et al. Prognostic significance of histopathologic subtype and stage in small-cell lung cancer. *Hum Pathol* 1992; 23:520.
14. Mangum MD, Greco FA, Hainsworth JD, et al. Combined small-cell and non-small-cell lung cancer. *J Clin Oncol* 1989; 7:607.
15. Brigham BA, Bunn PA, Minna JD, Cohen MH, Ihde DC, Shachney SE. Growth rates of small-cell bronchogenic carcinomas. *Cancer* 1978; 42:2880–2886.
16. Charbit A, Malaise EP, Tubiana M. Relation between the pathological nature and the growth rate of human tumors. *Eur J Cancer* 1977; 7:307–315.
17. Straus MJ. Characteristics of lung cancer. In: Straus MJ, ed. Lung cancer; clinical diagnosis and treatment. New York: Grune & Stratton, 1977:19–32.
18. Hansen HH. Management of small-cell cancer of the lung. *Lancet* 1992; 339:846–849.
19. Arriagada R, LeChevalier TL. Regional disease. In: (Aisner J, Arriagada R, Green MR, Martini N, Perry MC eds). Comprehensive textbook of thoracic oncology. Baltimore: Williams & Wilkins, 1996: 456–495.
20. Fox W, Scadding JG. Medical Research Council comparative trial of surgery and radiotherapy for primary treatment of small-celled or oat-celled carcinoma of bronchus: Ten-year follow-up. *Lancet* 1973; 2:63–65.
21. Mountain CF. Clinical biology of small-cell carcinoma: Relationship to surgical therapy. *Semin Oncol* 1978; 5:272–279.
22. Green RA, Humphrey E, Close H, et al. Alkylating agents in bronchogenic carcinoma. *Am J Med* 1969; 46:516–525.
23. Bunn PA, Lichter AS, Makuch RW, et al. Chemotherapy alone or chemotherapy with chest radiation therapy in limited small-cell lung cancer. A prospective, randomized trial. *Ann Intern Med* 1987; 106:655–662.
24. Pignon JP, Arriagada R, Ihde D, et al. A meta-analysis of thoracic radiotherapy for small-cell lung cancer. *N Engl J Med* 1992; 327:1618–1624.
25. Warde P, Payne D. Does thoracic irradiation improve survival and local control in limited-stage small-cell lung cancer? A meta-analysis. *J Clin Oncol* 1992; 10:890–895.
26. Jenkin D, Chan H, Freedman J, et al. Hodgkin's disease in children: treatment results with MOPP and low-dose, extended-field irradiation. *Cancer Treat Rep* 1982; 66:949–959.
27. Bergsagel DE, Phil D, Jenkin RDT, et al. Lung cancer: clinical trial of radiotherapy alone versus radiotherapy plus cyclophosphamide. *Cancer* 1972; 30:621–627.
28. Turrisi A, Glover DJ. Thoracic radiotherapy variables: influence on local control in small-cell lung cancer limited disease. *Int J Radiat Oncol Biol Phys* 1990; 19:1473–1479.
29. Choi N, Carey R. Importance of radiation dose in achieving improved loco-regional tumor control in limited stage small-cell lung carcinoma: an update. *Int J Radiat Oncol Biol Phys* 1989; 17:307–310.
30. Coy P, Hodson BM, Payne D, et al. The effect of dose of thoracic irradiation on recurrence in patients with limited stage small-cell lung cancer. Initial results of a Canadian multicenter randomized trial. *Int J Radiat Oncol Biol Phys* 1987; 14:219–226.
31. Choi NC, Herndon JE II, Rosenman J, et al. Phase I study to determine the maximum-tolerated dose of radiation in standard daily and hyperfractionated-accelerated twice-daily radiation schedules with concurrent chemotherapy for limited-stage small-cell lung cancer. *J Clin Oncol* 1998; 16:3528–3536.
32. Turrisi A, Glover DJ, Mason B, et al. Long term results of platinum etoposide (PE) + twice daily thoracic radiotherapy (TRT) for limited small-cell lung cancer (abstract 975). *Proc Am Soc Clin Oncol* 1995; 14:363.

33. Armstrong JG, Rosenstein MM, Kris MG, et al. Twice daily thoracic irradiation for limited small-cell lung cancer. *Int J Radiat Oncol Biol Phys* 1991; 21:1269–1274.
34. Johnson BE, Salem C, Nesbit J, et al. Limited stage small-cell lung cancer (SCLC) treated with concurrent BID chest radiotherapy (RT) and etoposide, cisplatin (VP/PT) followed by chemotherapy (CT) selected by in vitro drug sensitivity testing (abstract 818). *Proc Am Soc Clin Oncol* 1991; 10:240.
35. Turrisi AT III, Kim K, Blum R, et al. Twice-daily compared with once-daily thoracic radiotherapy in limited small-cell lung cancer treated concurrently with cisplatin and etoposide. *N Engl J Med* 1999; 340:265–271.
36. Kumar P. The role of thoracic radiotherapy in the management of limited-stage small-cell lung cancer. *Chest* 1997; 112(Suppl):259S–266S.
37. Bleehen NM. Radiotherapy for small-cell lung cancer. *Chest* 1986; 89:268S–276S.
38. Choi NC. Reassessment of the role of radiation therapy relative to other treatments in small-cell carcinoma of the lung. In: (Choi NC, Grillo HC, eds). Thoracic oncology. New York: Raven Press, 1983: 233–256.
39. Liengswangwong V, Bonner J, Shaw E, et al. Limited-stage small-cell lung cancer: patterns of intrathoracic recurrence and the implications for thoracic radiotherapy. *J Clin Oncol* 1994; 12:496–502.
40. Brodin O, Rikner G, Steinholz L, et al. Local failure in patients treated with radiotherapy and multidrug chemotherapy for small-cell lung cancer. *Acta Oncol* 1990; 29:739–746.
41. Arriagada R, Pellac-Cosset B, Cueto Ladron de Guevara J, et al. Alternating radiotherapy and chemotherapy schedules in limited small-cell lung cancer: analyses of local chest recurrences. *Radiother Oncol* 1991; 20:91–98.
42. Auquier A, Rutqvist LE, Rotstein S, Arriogada R. Post-mastectomy megavoltage radiotherapy: the Oslo and Stockholm trials. *Eur J Cancer* 1992; 28:433–437.
43. Tubiana M, Arriagada R, Cosset JM. Optimizing combinations of drugs and radiation. The interdigitated alternating regimen. In: (Wither HR, Peters LJ, eds). Innovations in radiation oncology. Berlin: Springer-Verlag, 1988:265–276.
44. Ensley JF, Jacobs JR, Weaver A, et al. Correlation between response to cis-platinum combination and subsequent radiotherapy in previously untreated patients with advanced squamous cell cancers of the head and neck. *Cancer* 1984; 54:811–814.
45. Carlson RW, Sikic BI, Gandara DR, et al. Late consolidative radiation therapy in the treatment of limited-stage small-cell lung cancer. *Cancer* 1991; 68:948–958.
46. Lebeau B, Chastang C, Brechot JM, et al. A randomized trial of delayed thoracic radiotherapy in complete responder patients with small-cell lung cancer: Petites Cellules Group. *Chest* 1993; 104:726–733.
47. Takada M, Fukuoka M, Furuse K, et al. A Phase III study of concurrent versus sequential thoracic radiotherapy in combination with cisplatin and etoposide for limited-stage small-cell lung cancer: preliminary results of the Japan Clinical Oncology Group (abstract 1103). *Proc Am Soc Clin Oncol* 1996; 15:372.
48. Lebeau B, Urban T, Brechot JM, et al. A randomized clinical trial comparing concurrent and alternated thoracic irradiation for patients with limited small-cell lung carcinoma. *Cancer* 1999; 86:1480–1487.
49. Perry MC, Herndon JE, Eaton WL, et al. Thoracic radiation therapy added to chemotherapy for small-cell lung cancer: an update of Cancer and Leukemia Group B study 8083. *J Clin Oncol* 1998; 16:2466–2467.
50. Work E, Nielsen OK, Bentzen SM, et al. Randomized study of initial versus late chest irradiation combined with chemotherapy in limited-stage small-cell lung cancer. *J Clin Oncol* 1997; 15:3030–3037.
51. Gregor A, Drings P, Burghouts J, et al. Randomized trial of alternating versus sequential radiotherapy/chemotherapy in limited-disease patients with small-cell lung cancer: a European Organization for Research and Treatment of Cancer Lung Cancer Cooperative Group study. *J Clin Oncol* 1997; 15:2840–2849.
52. Jeremic B, Shibamoto Y, Acimovic L, et al. Initial versus delayed accelerated hyperfractionated radiation therapy and concurrent chemotherapy in limited small-cell lung cancer: a randomized study. *J Clin Oncol* 1997; 15:893–900.
53. Glisson B, Scott C, Komaki R, et al. Cisplatin, Ifosfamide, prolonged oral etoposide and concurrent accelerated hyperfractionated thoracic radiotherapy for patients with limited small-cell lung cancer: results of RTOG 93-12 (abstract 1733). *Proc Am Soc Clin Oncol* 1998, 17:450a.
54. Ettinger DS, Seiferheld WF, Abrams RA, et al. Cisplatin, etoposide, paclitaxel and concurrent hyperfractionated thoracic radiotherapy for patients with limited disease small-cell lung cancer: Preliminary results of RTOG 96-09 (abstract 1917). *Proc Am Soc Clin Oncol* 2000; 19:490a.

55. Sandler A, Declerck L, Wagner N, et al. A phase II study of cisplatin plus etoposide plus paclitaxel and concurrent radiation therapy for previously untreated limited stage small-cell lung cancer (E2596): An Eastern Cooperative Oncology Group trial (abstract 1920). 2000; 19:491a.
56. Glisson BS, Lee JS, Shin DM, et al. Topotecan/paclitaxel alternating with etoposide/cisplatin and thoracic radiation in patients with limited small-cell lung cancer (abstract 1929). 2000; 19:493a.
57. Lyss JE, Herndon JE, Bogart D, et al. Topotecan (Topo) + Paclitaxel (Tax) + G-CSF Induction followed by concurrent chemoradiotherapy for patients with limited stage small-cell lung cancer: preliminary analysis of CALGB 39808 (abstract 1270). *Proc Am Soc Clin Oncol* 2001; 20:318a.
58. Gregor A. Prophylactic cranial irradiation in small-cell lung cancer: Is it ever indicated? *Oncology* 1998; 12:19–24.
59. Arriagada R, Le Chevalier T, Borie F, et al. Prophylactic cranial irradiation for patients with small-cell lung cancer in complete remission. *J Nat Cancer Inst* 1995; 87:183–190.
60. Gregor A, Cull A, Stephens RJ, et al. Prophylactic cranial irradiation as indicated following complete response to induction therapy in small-cell lung cancer: Results of a multicentre randomized trial. *Eur J Cancer* 1997; 33(Suppl 1):1752–1758.
61. Auperin A, Arriagada R, Pignon JP, et al. Prophylactic cranial irradiation in patients with small-cell lung cancer in complete remission. *N Engl J Med* 1999; 341:476–484.

11 The Role of Chemoradiation in the Management of Esophageal Cancer

Arlene Forastiere, MD and Bapsi Chak, MD

CONTENTS

1. INTRODUCTION

It is estimated that there will be 13,200 new cases of esophageal cancer in the year 2001 and an estimated 500 deaths *(1)*. Over the past two decades, tumor registry data obtained from the Surveillance, Epidemiology, and End Results (SEER) program has shown a decrease in the age-adjusted incidence of squamous cell carcinoma, while there has been a steady increase in the incidence of adenocarcinoma. Since the mid-1970s the incidence of adenocarcinoma has risen >350%, surpassing that of squamous cell cancers around 1990. Although the rate among black males has increased, it remains at much lower levels *(2)*. While certain risk factors for the development of squamous cell carcinomas have been identified (smoking, alcohol, diet), these are less clear for adenocarcinoma of the esophagus. Smoking remains a risk factor, but there appears to be less of an association with alcohol *(3)*. Barrett's esophagus has been shown to be a predisposing factor for adenocarcinoma of the esophagus. In a population-based study from Sweden, the frequency, severity, and duration of reflux symptoms were found to be strongly correlated

From: *Chemoradiation in Cancer Therapy*
Edited by: H. Choy © Humana Press Inc., Totowa, NJ

with the risk of developing adenocarcinoma (odds ratio, 43.5) but not squamous cell carcinoma (odds ratio, 1.1) of the esophagus *(4)*. There is increasing clinical, as well as molecular, evidence suggesting that dysplasia in Barrett's esophagus is a precursor to esophageal adenocarcinoma. DNA replication errors and allelic losses of chromosomes 17p, 18q, and 5q were studied in 36 patients who underwent resection for adenocarcinoma of the esophagus. There was an accumulation of genetic alterations from dysplasia to adenocarcinoma. Allelic loss of both 17p and 18q was associated with the worst prognosis *(5)*. Obesity, which may predispose patients to reflux, is also emerging as a potential risk factor.

2. OVERVIEW OF TREATMENT OPTIONS

There are currently two approaches being utilized in the management of locally advanced esophageal cancer: surgery alone and primary chemoradiation. Although there are no randomized trials comparing these two treatment options, the overall 5-yr survival with either approach is approx 20%. Current trials have focused on adding neoadjuvant chemotherapy with or without radiation to surgical management to improve outcomes.

3. STAGING

The introduction of neoadjuvant therapy prior to surgical resection has made pretreatment clinical staging an important aspect of care. The goal of staging is to determine the TNM status of the patient using the current American Joint Commission Staging System (Table 1).

All patients with esophageal cancer should be staged with computed tomography (CT) scans of the chest and abdomen. These can be used to identify bulky disease invading mediastinal soft tissue (T4). CT scanning can also identify those patients with distant disease to lung, liver, or adrenal glands who would then not be considered candidates for aggressive therapies but rather should focus primarily on palliative measures of symptom relief. Unfortunately, CT scans are unable to differentiate between T1–3 diseases. Moreover, lymph node metastasis and length of tumor involvement are missed in almost half the cases. Endoscopic ultrasound can determine T status with almost 80–90% accuracy *(6–8)*. Although it is able to identify lymph nodes, it is difficult to distinguish benign from malignant nodes without tissue confirmation. With the addition of transesophageal lymph node biopsy to endoscopic ultrasound, regional lymph node status is correctly diagnosed in almost 90% of patients *(9)*. Laparoscopic staging for distal esophageal cancers and positron emission tomography (PET) are new staging modalities that are currently under clinical evaluation. In a recent prospective study of the utility of PET in staging for esophageal cancer, it was found to significantly improve the detection of Stage IV disease over conventional staging *(10)*. Diagnostic laparoscopy changed the treatment plan in 17% of patients in a prospective study of the role of laparoscopy in preoperative staging of esophageal cancer *(11)*.

4. SURGERY ALONE

Although the primary treatment for cancers of the esophagus for many years had been surgical resection, the optimal surgery remains controversial. One approach uses transhiatal esophagectomy with anastamosis of the stomach to the cervical esophagus,

Table 1
Staging of Esophageal Cancer

- Primary tumor (T)
  - Tis: Carcinoma *in situ*
  - T1: Tumor invades lamina propria or submucosa
  - T2: Tumor invades muscularis propria
  - T3: Tumor invades adventitia
  - T4: Tumor invades adjacent structures
- Regional lymph nodes (N)
  - NX: Regional lymph nodes cannot be assessed
  - N0: No regional lymph node metastasis
  - N1: Regional lymph node metastasis
- Distant metastasis (M)
  - MX: Distant metastasis cannot be assessed
  - M0: No distant metastasis
  - M1: Distant metastasis
    - Tumors of the lower thoracic esophagus
      - M1a: Metastasis in celiac lymph nodes
      - M1b: Other distant metastasis
    - Tumors of the midthoracic esophagus
      - M1a: Not applicable
      - M1b: Nonregional lymph nodes and/or other distant metastasis
    - Tumors of the upper thoracic esophagus
      - M1a: Metastasis in cervical nodes
      - M1b: Other distant metastasis
- Stage grouping
  - Stage 0—Tis N0M0
  - Stage I—T1N0M0
  - Stage II—T2N0M0, T3N0M0, T1N1M0, T2N1M0
  - Stage III—T3N1M0, T4 any NM0
  - Stage IVA—Any T, any N, M1a
    Any T, any N, M1b

and the other approach advocates abdominal mobilization of the stomach and transthoracic excision of the esophagus with anastomosis of the stomach to the upper esophagus. Prospective studies have not been able to document any difference in morbidity or mortality between these two procedures *(12,13)*. Survival closely correlates with stage. Patients with Stage I–II disease have 5-yr survivals of approx 70%, whereas, those with Stage III disease have 5-yr survivals closer to 20%. Most patients in the United States present with Stage III disease (tumor extending into the adventitia and/or invading adjacent structures with regional lymph node involvement). Therefore, despite aggressive surgical treatment, the overall 5-yr survival remains poor.

5. RADIATION ALONE: AS PRIMARY THERAPY

Although radiation alone has been utilized historically in the treatment of medically inoperable esophageal cancers and continues to be used today in the palliative setting, the standard of care for the nonsurgical management of localized esophageal cancer remains concurrent chemoradiation. For those patients who are unable to tolerate surgery or

Table 2
Randomized Trials of Preoperative Radiation Alone

Investigator	*Treatment*	*N*	*Resected*	*LF*	*Medn S*	*5 YS*
Launois *(18)*	Surgery	57	70	NR	8.2	12
	39–45 Gy → S	67	76	NR	4.5	10
Gignoux *(17)*	Surgery	114	73	33	12	20
	33 Gy → S	115	82	21	12	14
Arnott *(16)*	Surgery	86	72	NR	8	17
	20 Gy → S	90	74	NR	8	9
Wang *(20)*	Surgery	102	67	13	NR	30
	40 Gy → S	104	72	4	NR	35
Kelsen *(24)*	CT → S	48	58	8	10	20
	55 Gy → S	48	6	19	12	20
Nygaard *(19)*	Surgery	41	69	NR	NR	9
	35 → S	48	54	NR	NR	21
	CT → S	50	58	NR	NR	3
	CT → RT→ S	47	66	NR	NR	17

chemotherapy due to comorbid medical conditions, radical radiation may be used. In retrospective studies of patients treated with radiation alone, the 5-yr survival varies from as high as 21% *(14)* in recent studies, down to 10–15%, in older series *(15)*. This variation may be a reflection of improved staging in more recent years. Doses generally used for radical radiotherapy alone are 6000–6500 cGy, using multiple fields. In patients with known distant disease, treatment regimens vary from 30 Gy in 2 wk for the extremely poor performance patients, to 60 Gy in 6 wk for more durable palliation in those with excellent performance status but inability to receive concurrent chemotherapy.

6. SURGICAL APPROACHES

6.1. Preoperative Radiation Alone

The rationale for adding radiation (preoperative or postoperative) to surgery is based on the patterns of failure of esophageal cancer. Although the majority of patients will die of distant disease, over half will suffer local failure as a component of failure. These studies are summarized in Table 2. Although there have been several randomized trials that have compared surgical intervention alone to surgery preceded by preoperative radiation *(16–20)*, only one has shown a survival benefit *(19)*. This study was a four-arm trial in which patients were randomized to preoperative chemotherapy (cisplatin/bleomycin × two cycles), preoperative radiation therapy, preoperative combined chemoradiation, or surgery alone. Patients who received preoperative radiation (with or without chemotherapy) showed an improvement in 3-yr survival (18% vs 5%, $p = 0.009$). Although 20% of the 48 patients who received preoperative radiation alone (without chemotherapy) were alive at 3 yr, the difference when compared to those treated with surgery alone was not statistically different *(19)*.

There have been many valid criticisms of these preoperative radiation studies. These criticisms include the varied dose and fractionation schedules. No two trials have used the same radiation regimen. None of these trials have allowed an adequate interval between completion of radiation and surgery. In general, at least 4–6 wk are required for

Table 3
Randomized Trials of Postoperative Radiotherapy

Author	*Treatment*	*N*	*Resected*	*Medn Survival (mo)*	*5-yr Survival (%)*
Fok *(23)*	Surgery	65	30	15.2	
	S → 49–52.5 Gy	65	30	8.7[a]	
Teniere *(22)*	Surgery	119	All		44
	S → 45–55 Gy	102	All		42

[a]Significant.

maximal therapeutic effects of radiation. Many of these studies have gone on to surgery 1–2 wk after completing radiation. In a meta-analysis of 1147 patients from these randomized studies, there was an overall reduction in risk of death by 11% and an absolute survival benefit of 3% at 2 yr and 4% at 5 yr. These results were not statistically improved over surgery alone *(21)*. These data, therefore, do not support the use of preoperative radiation alone.

6.2. Postoperative Radiation Therapy Alone

There are two randomized studies of postoperative radiation (Table 3). In a study of 221 patients with squamous cell carcinoma who were randomized to postoperative radiation (4500–5500 cGy at 180 cGy/fraction) or surgery alone there was no change in survival. There was, however, a decrease in local failure (35% to 10%) in node negative patients receiving postoperative radiation *(22)*.

In a second randomized study of postoperative radiation (4900 cGy: curative resection and 5250 cGy: palliative resection, 350 cGy/fraction) vs surgery alone, the median survival was shorter for the radiated arm (8.7 mo vs 15.2 mo). The authors attributed the shorter survival of the postoperative radiation arm to irradiation-related deaths *(23)*. Local recurrence was significantly reduced in the patients who received radiation following palliative resection (20% vs 46%, $p = 0.04$), but no difference in local recurrence was noted in the patients resected for cure.

In conclusion, postoperative radiation may decrease local recurrence in node negative patients, but there is no impact on survival. These data indicate that postoperative radiation should be used only in a prospective study setting. It is recommended as a standard of care only in the setting of a curative resection with positive surgical margins.

6.3. Preoperative Chemotherapy Alone

The addition of neoadjuvant chemotherapy to surgical resection is another approach in attempting to ameliorate the sometimes disappointing results of surgery alone. Because the majority of patients present with locally advanced disease (T3 or T4 and/or lymph node involvement), surgery alone will be curative in only a minority of cases. Moreover, esophageal cancer is a disease where distant dissemination occurs early, and preoperative chemotherapy may help to eradicate micrometastatic disease, which is not visible on routine staging evaluation. In vivo testing of chemotherapeutic agents may help identify those patients who may benefit from additional postoperative chemotherapy. Studies comparing neoadjuvant chemotherapy to surgery alone are summarized in Table 4 *(24–28)*. These studies confirm that neoadjuvant chemotherapy is feasible and does not

Table 4
Randomized Trials of Preoperative Chemotherapy vs Surgery Alone

Series	*Preop chemo*	*Cell type*	*Number of pts.*	*Med Survival (mo)*	*2-yr Survival*
Roth *(28)*	C, B + V × 2 → S → C, V	Scc	39	9	25 (3 yr survival)
	S only			9	5 (3 yr survival)
Schlag *(27)*	CF × 3	Scc	75	10	
	S only			10	
Kelsen *(24)*	CF × 3	Scc & A	440	15	35
	S only			16	37
Kok *(26)*	CE × 2-4	Scc	161	18.5[a]	
	S only			11	
MRC *(29)*	CF × 2	Scc & A	802	17[a]	45[a]
	S only			13	35

[a]Significant difference.
C = Cisplatin, B = bleomycin, V = vindesine, F = 5-fluorouracil, S = surgery, Scc = squamous cell carcinoma, A = adenocarcinoma.

increase postoperative mortality or morbidity. In contrast to the negative results of the intergroup trial *(24)*, there are now two European studies that suggest that neoadjuvant chemotherapy alone may provide a survival advantage *(26,29)*. The Medical Research Council (MRC) randomized 802 patients to two cycles of cisplatin, 5-fluorouracil (5-FU) followed by surgical resection vs surgery alone. There was an improvement in median survival (17.4 vs 13.4 mo), and 2-yr survival (45% vs 35%) for patients on the neoadjuvant chemotherapy arm *(29)*.

There are a number of possible explanations for the largely negative US trials *(24,27,28)*. These could include the fact that some of these studies randomized only patients with squamous cell carcinomas *(27,28)*. The patterns of spread for squamous cell carcinomas of the upper and midesophagus may be different from the now more common adenocarcinoma of the distal esophagus. A second possibility is that despite 440 patients, the intergroup study was still not large enough to detect a small, yet clinically significant, difference in survival. Of note, the MRC had to randomize 802 patients to detect a 10% difference in 2-yr survival. Yet a third explanation is that in the intergroup study the effect of chemotherapy could not be fully evaluated since only 71% of the patients received all three cycles of planned neoadjuvant chemotherapy. Moreover, only 80% of the chemotherapy group had surgery. Therefore, the role of neoadjuvant chemotherapy alone remains controversial.

Studies have found that the patients who respond to neoadjuvant chemotherapy have prolonged survival over nonresponders (median 20 vs 6.2 mo) *(28)*. The pathologic complete response rates in studies of neoadjuvant chemotherapy alone have been a dismal 10%. More recent studies have involved the addition of neoadjuvant radiation to chemotherapy to improve on these results.

6.4 Postoperative Chemotherapy

There are very few studies evaluating the role of postoperative chemotherapy alone. In a randomized study of 205 patients with resected squamous cell cancer of the esopha-

Table 5
Randomized Studies of Preoperative Chemoradiation

Series	*Histology*	*Treatment*[a]	*Number*	*pCR (%)*	*Median (mo)*	*3-yr Survival (%)*
Urba *(31)*	Adeno	Surgery	50		17.6	16
	+ squamous	Pre-op chemo + 45 Gy	50	28	16.9	30
Walsh *(35)*	Adeno	Surgery	55		11	6
		Pre-op chemo + 40 Gy	58	25	16	32[b]
Bosset *(36)*	Squamous	Surgery	139		18.6	36
		Pre-op chemo + 37 Gy	142	26	18.6	36

[a]Cisplatin/5-FU based chemotherapy.
[b]Difference statistically significant.

gus, there was no significant benefit to 5-yr survival with adjuvant chemotherapy (cisplatin, 70 mg/m^2, and vindesine 3 mg/m^2) compared to surgery alone *(30)*. In a randomized study of neoadjuvant chemotherapy followed by surgery and then two additional cycles of postoperative chemotherapy, only 52% of patients were able to receive at least one cycle and only 38% were able to receive both cycles of postoperative chemotherapy *(24)*. The data do not support the use of postoperative chemotherapy outside of a study setting.

6.5. Preoperative Chemoradiation

There are a number of advantages to combining both radiation and chemotherapy in the preoperative setting:

1. Spatial cooperation: Radiation is more effective at controlling the primary bulky disease but is unable to affect distant micrometastases. Chemotherapy, on the other hand, can deal with micrometastases but is unable to affect the large primary tumor. The combination of both local (radiation) and systemic (chemotherapy) approaches then maximizes therapeutic impact.
2. Radiosensitization: Many of the chemotherapeutic agents that are utilized in the treatment of esophageal cancers are also potent radiosensitizers.
3. In the neoadjuvant setting, radiation, as well as chemotherapy, can be delivered to more well-oxygenated tissue and thereby enhance the ability to kill tumor cells.

Thus far, five randomized studies have been completed comparing chemoradiation followed by surgery to surgery alone. These are summarized in Table 5.

Investigators at the University of Michigan randomized patients to two treatment groups:

1. Preoperative cisplatin, 20 mg/m^2 d 1–5 and d 17–21, vinblastine 1 mg/m^2 d 1–4 and d 17–20, 5-FU 300 mg/m^2/24 h d 1–21 and concurrent radiation consisting of 150 cGy BID to 4500 cGy followed by definitive surgery.
2. Surgery alone.

With a median follow-up of 8.2 yr, neoadjuvant therapy did not improve survival over surgery alone. Median survival was 17.6 vs 16.9 mo. Three-year survival was 16% for surgery only vs 30% for preoperative chemoradiation ($p = 0.15$). Multivariate analysis showed a survival benefit to neoadjuvant therapy ($p = 0.09$). There was also a significant survival advantage for patients who achieved a complete pathologic response. Patients with complete pathologic response had a median survival of 49.7 mo vs 12 mo for patients with residual disease in the resected specimen. The 3-yr survival was also improved (64% vs 19%) *(31)*.

Although this study found that the 3-yr survival was 16% for surgery compared to 30% for preoperative chemoradiation, the trial had only a 50% power to determine that this was statistically significant. The statistical design of this study was based on the pilot study conducted at the University of Michigan which showed that median survival was doubled to 29 mo vs 12 mo for historical controls treated with surgery alone *(32,33)*. Therefore, the statistical design, which was powered to detect this large difference with at least 80% power, required only 100 patients. It is possible that if this study had been powered to detect a more modest difference, i.e., 10%, it may have been a positive trial requiring almost 450 patients *(34)*.

In a trial from Dublin, there was a significant survival benefit to the addition of neoadjuvant chemoradiation over surgical controls. In this study, 113 patients were randomized to:

1. Two cycles of neoadjuvant 5-FU 15 mg/kg/24 h d 1, 5, cisplatin 75 mg/m^2 d 7 and concurrent radiation 267 cGy/fraction to 4000 cGy followed by surgical resection.
2. Surgery alone.

The neoadjuvant therapy was well tolerated with only a 15% incidence of grade 3 toxicity. Operative mortality was comparable between the two groups (9% vs 4%). With a median follow up of 18 mo, there was a significant improvement in median survival (16 vs 11 mo, $p = 0.01$) and 3-yr survival (32 vs 6%, $p = 0.01$) *(35)*.

There are, however, a number of criticisms to this study. The surgical control arm had a 3-yr survival of only 6%, which was significantly worse than the surgery alone arm of INT0113 (3-yr survival, 23%) or MRC (2-yr survival 35%). Although there were few early-stage tumors in the surgical arm, the precise number of early-stage patients in the neoadjuvant chemoradiation arm is unknown since preoperative staging was based solely on clinical exam, chest radiography, abdominal ultrasound, and upper endoscopy. CT scans were performed only on patients with equivocal findings on CXR or ultrasound. This may have resulted in an imbalance of early-stage patients in the neoadjuvant chemoradiation arm. Finally, the radiation dose and techniques used in this study were significantly different from those commonly applied today. Conventional radiation doses of 1.8–2.0 Gy per fraction to total doses of 45–5040 cGy are commonly used in the United States. Using 267 cGy per fraction adds to normal tissue toxicity and decreases tumor effects. Initially all patients were treated with AP-PA fields which later was modified to a three-field technique. The use of multiple fields, computerized treatment planning, and customized blocks may have allowed higher doses to be delivered to the tumor while sparing surrounding normal tissue.

The third randomized study of neoadjuvant chemoradiation vs surgery alone was performed by the EORTC. Two hundred eighty-two patients were randomized to two groups:

1. Preoperative chemotherapy consisting of cisplatin 80 mg/m^2 given 0–2 d prior to radiation that consisted of 370 cGy × 5 followed by a 2-wk rest and another 370 cGy × 5.
2. Surgery alone.

With a median follow-up of 55 mo, the neoadjuvant chemoradiation resulted in a significantly higher 3-yr disease free survival (40% vs 28%). There was also improved local disease free survival (relative risk 0.6). However, there was no improvement in median survival or overall 3-yr survival (36% vs 36%) when compared to surgery alone. Although the 3-yr survival for the combined modality arm (36%) was better in this study over those of other large randomized studies (approx 25%), this was likely the result of including Stage I/II disease *(36)*.

This study, which included split-course radiation, as well as high dose per fraction, had several drawbacks. Radiobiological principles would predict increased normal tissue toxicity and less tumor control. Therefore, it is not surprising that there was no benefit in terms of survival and, in fact, it is not clear why there was an improvement in disease-free survival using such a regimen. The systemic therapy using such a small dose of cisplatin would also be considered inadequate for systemic control.

Despite suggestions of a survival advantage in at least two of the five randomized studies, the drawbacks in study design, small sample size, and short follow-up make the results far from clear. A well-designed Intergroup study (CALGB 9781), which had attempted to compare surgery alone to surgery preceded by more conventional doses of radiation and chemotherapy, was recently closed due to poor accrual. This is unfortunate as it is unlikely that a similar study of this magnitude will be mounted in the near future.

The data thus far suggest that triple modality therapy should still be considered investigational. In single-institution studies of concurrent chemoradiation, the pathologic complete remission (CR) rates are higher than preoperative chemotherapy alone. Several studies have suggested that patients who have pathologic complete responses have a better outcome over patients who do not *(33,37)*. Therefore, methods that improve pathologic complete response rates continue to be an area of active investigation.

6.6. Postoperative Chemoradiation: Gastroesophageal Adenocarcinoma

Although there are efforts at this time to stratify squamous vs adenocarcinoma, studies to date have not separated these two histologies and, therefore, treatment recommendations have been similar, regardless of histology. The only exception to this generalization is adenocarcinomas of the gastroesophageal junction.

Cancer of the cardia is now topographically classified into three types:

1. Type I tumor: Adenocarcinoma of the distal esophagus, which usually arises from an area with specialized intestinal metaplasia of the esophagus (i.e., Barrett's esophagus) and which may infiltrate the esophagogastric junction from above.
2. Type II tumor: True carcinoma of the cardia arising from the cardiac epithelium or short segments with intestinal metaplasia at the esophagogastric junction.
3. Type III tumor: Subcardial gastric carcinoma, which infiltrates the esophagogastric junction and distal esophagus from below.

The assignment of a lesion into one of these types is purely morphological and based on the anatomical location of the tumor or the best estimate of its epicenter for those with advanced disease. Classification can be performed easily based on a combination of contrast radiography, upper endoscopy, and CT *(38)*. In a retrospective analysis of 74 patients with gastric cancer, the preoperative classification had a high correlation (95%) to the final classification based on the resected specimen *(39)*.

Although only reported in abstract form, INT0116, a randomized study of postoperative modality therapy (5-FU, leucovorin, and RT) vs surgery alone in resected adenocarcinoma of the stomach and gastroesophageal junction, has found a statistically significant increase in 3-yr survival (52% vs 41%, $p = 0.03$) *(40)*. In esophageal cancer, there are no studies that show an advantage to postoperative therapy. This is the first study to show an advantage to adjuvant therapy in this setting. Although 20% of patients had tumors of gastric cardia or gastroesophageal junction adenocarcinoma, this is primarily a study of gastric adenocarcinoma. The pattern of failure of gastric cancer is different from proximal lesions of the cardia, gastroesophageal junction, and distal esophagus. The predominant site of first failure (80%) is local-regional for the former in contrast to distant metastases as the site of first failure for the latter. Therefore, although the results of INT0116 may be used to justify postoperative chemoradiation for node positive, completely resected cardia and gastroesophageal junction adenocarcinoma, benefit may be marginal for this subsite and toxicity may be significant. Postoperative therapy can be offered to those patients who have recovered well from surgery, have an excellent performance status and are at high risk for recurrence.

7. NONSURGICAL APPROACHES

7.1. Radiation Alone vs Chemoradiotherapy

Although, historically, esophageal cancer was treated with surgery, surgical mortality was high at approx 25% in series reported from the 1960s through the 1970s. Therefore, many patients were treated with nonsurgical modalities such as radiation alone for palliation of symptoms. The early studies of chemoradiation in esophageal cancer were based on the successful treatment of anal carcinoma with low doses of radiation and concurrent chemotherapy *(41)*. These early studies of patients with squamous cell carcinoma of the esophagus showed that a few patients did have complete responses. Therapy similar to that used for anal cancer consisted of mitomycin C (10 mg/m^2 d 1) and continuous infusion 5-FU (1000 mg/m^2/24 h 1–4, 29–32) and radiation 3000 cGy. These studies first suggested that concurrent chemoradiation may possibly take the place of surgical resection *(42)*.

In the 1980s numerous phase II pilot studies combining chemotherapy with radiation were conducted primarily using 5-FU and cisplatin chemotherapy. In general, the median survival (12–20 mo) and 2-yr survival (35–40%) were improved over historical controls. Despite these encouraging results, randomized studies were needed to determine whether chemoradiation was superior to radiation alone.

Table 6 shows the results of five randomized studies of chemoradiation vs radiation alone. It is important to note that these studies consisted primarily of squamous cell carcinoma of the midesophagus. No studies have adequately evaluated this approach in adenocarcinoma of the esophagus. Thus, nonsurgical treatment approaches for adenocarcinoma are extrapolated from data based on trials of squamous cell carcinoma.

A landmark trial was an intergroup study (RTOG 85–01) in which patients with locally advanced esophageal cancer were randomized to chemotherapy and radiation or radiation alone. Chemotherapy consisted of 5-FU (1000 mg/m^2/24 h × 4 d) and cisplatin (75 mg/m^2, d 1). Radiation therapy (5000 cGy/25 fractions) was initiated concurrently with d 1 of chemotherapy. Chemotherapy was given q 4 wk during radiation (cycles 1, 2) and q 3 wk following radiation (cycles 3, 4). The radiation alone arm consisted of 6400 cGy/32 fractions. Only 50% of patients were able to complete all four cycles of chemotherapy.

Table 6
Randomized Trials of Primary Chemoradiation vs Radiation Alone

Trial		*Number*	*Local failure (%)*	*Median survival (mo)*	*Survival (%)*
Herskovic *(45)*[a]	RT	62	68	9	0 (5 yr)
(RTOG)	RT + CDDP/5-FU	61	47	14[c]	27[c]
Smith *(46)*[a]	RT	69		9	7 (5 yr)
(ECOG)	RT + 5-FU/mitro	59		15[c]	9
Roussel *(72)*[b]	RT	111	66	8	10 (4 yr)
(EORTC)	RT + CDDP	110	59	10	8
Slabber (73)[b]	RT	36		5	
(Pretoria)	RT + CDDP/5-FU	34		6	

[a]Resectability not specified.
[b]Unresectable.
[c]Difference statistically significant.

Patients receiving concurrent chemoradiotherapy had a significant improvement in median survival (14 vs 9 mo) and 5-yr survival (26% vs 0%, $p < 0.0001$) *(43)*. Even with further follow-up, the 8-yr survival remained 22% *(44)*. The incidence of local failure (defined as persistent disease, as well as the first site of failure) was significantly decreased in the combined modality arm (45% vs 68%, $p = 0.0123$). Although randomization was discontinued early due to the positive results, an additional 69 patients treated with the same chemoradiation regimen had similar results (3-yr survival = 30%) *(43–45)*. A second randomized study of chemoradiotherapy to radiation alone found a significant improvement in median survival (14.8 vs 9.2 mo, $p = 0.04$), but no difference in 5-yr survival (9% vs 7%). The chemotherapy consisted of 5-FU, mitomycin-C, and radiation. This was not, however, purely a comparison of concurrent chemoradiation to radiation alone, as almost 50% of patients in each arm went on to surgery. The operative mortality was 17% *(46)*.

Although chemoradiation has significantly improved survival and local control compared to radiation alone, this came at a cost of an increase in acute grade 3 toxicity (44% vs 25%), acute grade 4 toxicity (20 vs 3%), and one grade 5 treatment-related death (2%). There were no differences in late toxicities (29% vs 23%) *(43,44)*.

Based on these studies, the standard of care for the nonsurgical management of esophageal cancer is concurrent chemoradiation. Radiation alone is reserved for those patients whose performance status or organ dysfunction precludes the use of chemotherapy. Despite a survival benefit, there was an unacceptably high local failure rate (45%) in RTOG 85-01. Therefore, new approaches continue to be developed. These include intensification of treatment by increasing the quality or quantity of chemotherapy and higher doses of radiation.

7.2. Intensified Neoadjuvant Chemotherapy Followed by Intensified Chemoradiotherapy

A phase II Intergroup study (INT0122, ECOG PE289, RTOG 9012) increased the intensity of both chemotherapy and radiation. The neoadjuvant chemotherapy consisted of three courses of cisplatin and 5-FU followed by concurrent chemoradiation consisting of two additional courses of cisplatin and 5-FU and radiation, 6480 cGy/36 fractions.

For the 38 eligible patients, there was a 47% complete response, 8% partial response, and 3% stable disease. The site of first failure was local/regional in 39% and distant in 24%. Median survival was 20 mo, 3-yr survival 30% and actuarial 5-yr survival 20%. There were six deaths of which four (9%) were treatment-related. The authors concluded that this intensive neoadjuvant chemotherapy followed by chemoradiotherapy was not significantly better over conventional chemoradiation *(47)*. The higher doses of radiation, however, were felt to be well tolerated, and therefore formed the basis of the Phase III intergroup study (INT 0123/RTOG 94-05) comparing concurrent chemoradiation using standard doses of radiation (5040 cGy) to intensified radiation (6480 cGy) and concurrent chemotherapy.

7.3. Intensified Radiation (External Beam) as a Component of Chemoradiation

The second approach: Intensifying radiation was tested in a phase III intergroup study (INT 0123/RTOG 94–05). This compared a modification of the best arm of RTOG 85-01 (standard therapy) to the same chemotherapy with a higher total dose of radiation.

Continuous infusion 5-FU was increased from 4 to 5 d; the radiation was changed from 5000 cGy/25 fractions to 5040 cGy/28 fractions, and the chemotherapy was given every 4 wk, during and after completion of radiation for a total of four cycles. The experimental arm used the same chemotherapy but a higher dose of radiation (6480 cGy/36 fractions). Preliminary results for the 216 eligible patients showed no significant difference between the high-dose and low-dose arms, in terms of median survival (12.9 vs 17.6 mo), 2-yr survival (29% vs 38%) and local/regional failure rates (59% vs 52%). The trial was closed early at first interim analysis because of the low probability of the higher-dose radiation arm demonstrating survival benefit if accrual continued. Moreover, the experimental arm was associated with increased toxicity. There were 11 treatment-related deaths in the high-dose arm, of which 8 occurred in patients who had received 5040 cGy *(48)*.

7.4. Intensified Radiation (Brachytherapy) as a Component of Chemoradiation

A second method of intensifying radiation is the use of brachytherapy. RTOG 9207 was a Phase II trial of 49 patients with localized esophageal cancer. Patients were given 15–20 Gy brachytherapy boost after 5-FU, cisplatin, and 50 Gy external beam. Local failure rates were 63% (37% local failure and 26% local persistence); median survival was estimated 11 mo and estimated 2-yr survival 31%. There was a 10% treatment-related death rate. The crude fistula rate was 12% with a cumulative rate of 17.5% a year *(49)*. There was no advantage to local control or survival when compared to the standard arm of RTOG 8501. The data thus far suggest that increasing the intensity of chemotherapy or radiation (via external or brachytherapy) adds toxicity without improving survival. Therefore, the standard of care is conventional doses of radiation 4500–5040 cGy and four courses of concurrent 5-FU and cisplatin for the primary nonsurgical treatment of esophageal cancer.

8. NEWER AGENTS IN COMBINED MODALITY THERAPY

8.1. The Taxanes

In an attempt to improve outcomes, newer agents, especially those that act synergistically with radiation, are being evaluated further. One such agent is paclitaxel, the first taxane to show antineoplastic activity in vitro. Paclitaxel was originally isolated from the bark of the western yew tree, *Taxus brevifolia (50)*. Phase I studies defined its toxicity profile, which included neutropenia, neuropathy, mucositis, arthralgias, hypersensitivity reactions, nausea, and alopecia *(51,52)*.

Phase II studies of paclitaxel, infused as a single agent over 24 h every 3 wk, showed promising results for patients with metastatic or locally unresectable esophageal cancer. The overall response rate was 32%, with a median survival of 13.2 mo *(53)*.

A Phase I study of docetaxel with concurrent radiation tested escalating doses of docetaxel given at different schedules to patients with advanced nonsmall-cell lung or esophageal cancer. Giving the drug once every 3 wk during standard radiotherapy, the maximum tolerated dose is 40 mg/m^2 per cycle. The dose-limiting toxicities are neutropenia and esophagitis. However, it is possible to escalate the total docetaxel dose to 60 mg/m^2 per cycle by weekly administration of 20 mg/m^2. The authors recommended phase II dose of docetaxel was 20 mg/m^2 administered weekly with concurrent chest radiotherapy for 6 wk *(54)*.

8.2. In Vitro Studies of Paclitaxel as a Radiation Sensitizer

In addition to trying to improve the results of standard chemoradiation by intensifying chemotherapy and/or radiation, a second approach has been to combine radiation therapy with some of the newer chemotherapeutic agents, which are also known to be potent radiation sensitizers. These agents have been used both in primary chemoradiation protocols, as well as in the preoperative setting.

Although the precise mechanism of action of paclitaxel in enhancing radiation effects is not clear, one of the proposed mechanisms is its effect on the cell cycle. Its effects on the microtubules result in an M-phase arrest *(55)*. Experiments done on synchronously dividing Chinese hamster cells have shown that cells in M and G2 are most sensitive to the effects of radiation *(56)*.

In vitro studies have shown that paclitaxel is a potent radiation sensitizer. Survival curves using grade 3 human astrocytoma cell lines showed a sensitizer enhancement ratio of 1.8 *(57)*. In a series of experiments using a human leukemic cell line (HL-60), a sensitizing enhancement ratio of 1.48 was noted *(58)*. Other studies have shown that G2/M block is not the only mechanism of paclitaxel-induced radiosensitization *(59)*.

8.3. Phase I/II Studies of Paclitaxel/RT: Esophageal Cancer

Table 7 summarizes selected phase I/II studies of paclitaxel/radiation in esophageal cancer. Although pathologic complete response rates have been encouraging, ranging from 11–41%, these regimens have not been tested in a randomized fashion against the more standard cisplatin, 5-FU based therapies.

Vanderbilt University Medical Center has recently completed accruing patients to a Phase II study of neoadjuvant chemoradiation, which consists of preoperative paclitaxel (175 mg/m^2, 3-h infusion) followed by cisplatin 75 mg/m^2 d 1 and 21. Concurrent radiation was given to a total dose of 3000 cGy, in 200 cGy/fraction. Patients who are resectable go on to surgery 4 wk after completion of chemoradiation, whereas those who are unresectable (i.e., cervical esophageal cancer) continue to a total dose of 60 Gy without treatment interruptions. One month following surgery, patients receive two cycles (q 21–28 d) of postoperative chemotherapy, which consists of paclitaxel 175 mg/m^2 over 3 h d 1, 5-FU 350 mg/m^2, d 1–3, and leucovorin 300 mg d 1–3. Preliminary analysis of this

Table 7
Taxane-Based Chemoradiation Regimens

Author	*Regimen*	*PCR (%)*	*3-Yr survival (%)*
Urba *(31)*	Paclitaxel + cisplatin/45 Gy	19	35
Adelstein *(65)*	Paclitaxel + cisplatin/45 Gy	23	30
Wright *(74)*	Paclitaxel + 5-FU/58.5 Gy	39	
Meluch *(75)*	Paclitaxel + carbo + 5-FU/45 Gy	41	
Weiner *(76)*	Paclitaxel + cisplatin + 5-FU/60 Gy	18	
Mauer *(54)*	Docetaxel + cisplatin × 3 Docetaxel/50 Gy	45	
Enzinger *(77)* (ASCO 99)	Paclitaxel + cisplatin × 2 Paclitaxel/50.4 Gy	11	

regimen had indicated that the predominant toxicities were myelosuppression (40%) and severe nausea/vomiting (25%) *(60,61)*.

Between 3/95 and 3/98, 47 patients were enrolled. At restaging, prior to surgery, eight (17%) were found to have progressed, while seven patients had metastases documented at surgery. Complete resection was achieved in 33 (70%) patients. At the time of surgery there were 5/33 patients with complete pathologic, pCRs (15%), and 9 (27%) had only microscopic residual foci. Only 25 patients were able to complete the two cycles of postoperative chemotherapy. Median survival was found to be 15 mo, and at 46 mo 16.5% of patients were alive *(62)*.

It is interesting to note that the results from our studies at Vanderbilt using lower doses of radiation have led to similar survival rates, local control, and less toxicity when compared to centers using higher doses of radiation. This dose of radiation was based on earlier studies that utilized two cycles of cisplatin, 5-FU, etoposide, and leucovorin with 3000 cGy of radiation followed by resection. The median survival of 24 mo and 2-yr survival of 51% was better than historical controls treated with surgery alone *(63,64)*.

There have been no randomized comparisons of these newer paclitaxel regimens to more standard chemotherapy regimens. Some investigators conducting nonrandomized comparisons of paclitaxel-based chemotherapy in a similarly staged cohort of cisplatin and 5-FU treated patients, report no advantage in overall survival *(65)*.

9. FUTURE DIRECTIONS

9.1. UFT

Fluorinated pyrimidines have played a role as radiation sensitizers in combined modality therapy in almost all gastrointestinal malignancies, including esophageal cancer. Although continuous infusion 5-FU has been shown to have a survival advantage only in the treatment of large bowel cancer *(66)*, theoretically, it has an advantage over bolus 5-FU, especially when it is being combined with radiation. In vitro and in vivo studies suggest that prolonged exposure of 5-FU is advantageous. A combination of uracil and tegafur (UFT) (in a molar ratio of 4:1) is an oral agent that can be safely combined with oral leucovorin. In early trials in gastrointestinal malignancies it has been found to be safe and effective. Vanderbilt University Medical Center is currently enrolling patients in a Phase I study of UFT, cisplatin, and concurrent radiation.

Data on UFT with RT is limited. However, 5-FU is a known radiosensitizer. Data from laboratory and clinical studies show that prolonged exposure seems to be more effective than bolus 5-FU *(67)*. Since UFT acts similarly to prolonged infusion of 5-FU when chronically administered, the combination of UFT with RT is logical. We are currently accruing patients on this study.

9.2. Irinotecan

Irinotecan is an active chemotherapeutic agent that has been used in esophageal cancer and is also a potent radiosensitizer. In vitro studies have shown activity in esophageal cancer cell lines. A Phase I study has demonstrated its safety and tolerability with cisplatin. Phase I/II studies are currently underway determining the maximum tolerated weekly dose of irinotecan combined with concurrent radiation for locally advanced esophageal cancer (MSKCC 99081).

9.3. Herceptin

The Brown University Oncology Group has reported results of a phase II study using neoadjuvant concurrent cisplatin, paclitaxel, and radiation therapy with encouraging response rates. Paclitaxel was given as a weekly 3-h infusion at 60 mg/m^2 with weekly cisplatin 25 mg/m^2 over 1 h. Radiation therapy consisted of 3960 cGy, 180 cGy/fraction, via parallel-opposed AP-PA fields with a 5 cm superior and inferior and a 2 cm circumferential margin. Toxicity was acceptable with 8/31 (26%) grade 3 neutropenia, 5/31 (16%) nausea/vomiting, 1/31 (3%) pneumonitis and 3/31 (9%) esophagitis. There was a single toxic death, and one patient required parenteral nutrition. There were 8 CR and 14 PR for an overall response rate of 71%. Pathologic CR rates were not reported *(68)*. A further modification of this study includes the addition of herceptin to paclitaxel and cisplatin and concurrent radiation in the neoadjuvant setting. In vitro studies have shown that treatment with rhuMAb HER-2, recombinant humanized monoclonal antibody to the HER-2 receptor, decreases cell proliferation in vitro and reduces tumor formation in nude mice. Therapy with rhuMAb HER-2 enhances tumor sensitivity to radiation at doses of 1–5 Gy. This benefit is specific to cells with HER-2 overexpression *(69)*.

9.4. Oxaliplatin

Oxaliplatin is a novel platinum compound that has shown promising activity in colorectal cancers. It has been associated with up to 60% response rates when used as front-line therapy, and 25–50% response rates in relapsed or refractory colorectal cancer. It is currently being evaluated in a Phase I study with 5-FU and radiation in patients with locally advanced esophageal cancer (NCI T99-0061).

10. RADIATION THERAPY TECHNIQUES

10.1. Volumes, Portals, and Beam Arrangement

Radiation therapy planning for patients with esophageal cancer is difficult for a number of reasons. These include:

1. The difficulty in clearly defining the target volume.
2. The proximity of several critical structures in the chest including spinal cord, heart, and lung.
3. The length of the field usually means that there is a rapidly sloping surface making it difficult to have a homogeneous dose distribution.

The volume to be treated and the configuration of the radiation portal depend not only on the size and location of the primary tumor but also the areas of known lymphatic drainage. The lymphatic drainage varies with the location of the primary tumor. Given that the target is deep within the chest, megavoltage equipment is required with minimum photon energies of 6 MV and preferably, higher (10 MV, 18 MV).

Patients are treated with multiple field techniques 5 d/wk at 180 cGy/d. The gross tumor volume is defined with the help of CT scans, endoscopy reports, and a barium swallow. Given the dual longitudinal interconnecting lymphatic system, esophageal metastases can have several centimeters of "skip areas" between gross tumor and draining nodes. Therefore, it is common practice to design treatment portals with a 2-cm radial margin but a 5-cm longitudinal margin.

Local regional nodes are included in the target volume. This varies with the location of the tumor. Regional nodes for tumors arising above the carina include scalene, internal jugular, upper cervical, periesophageal, supraclavicular, and cervical nodes. Therefore, involvement of nodes above the thoracic inlet would be considered regional (M1a) for cervical esophageal tumors but regarded as distant metastasis for tumor of the lower thoracic esophagus. Likewise, involvement of the celiac node would be considered regional metastases (M1a) for tumors of the lower esophagus, but distant disease if the primary was above the carina. For cervical primaries (those above the carina), bilateral supraclavicular nodes should be included. Depending on the tumor location and patient body habitus, occasionally a three-field technique (two anterior obliques, with a posterior field) will be able to include both primary tumor and draining lymphatics. More often, one needs to begin with AP-PA fields and switch to obliques at approx 3960 cGy to exclude the spinal cord. The supraclavicular field that has to be excluded can be supplemented with electrons to bring the final dose to tumor and regional nodes to 5040 cGy. Owing to the changing contour of the neck to the thoracic inlet, the location of the tumor in relation to the patient's shoulders, and the need to not exceed spinal cord dose, treating tumors of the cervical esophagus is particularly challenging. Another technique that has been devised at the University of Florida uses a four-field box technique. A wax bolus is used to build the lack of tissue above the shoulders *(70)*. Other methods include 140-degree arc rotations, anterior wedged pairs, and three-field approaches using two posterior obliques with a single anterior field. Although patients with resectable cancers who are in excellent medical condition can be treated with neoadjuvant chemoradiation with the intent of greater local control, patients who have early-stage disease should be considered for primary chemoradiation. Given the morbidity of surgery to this site, primary chemoradiation may be the preferred treatment for this site.

Midesophageal tumors (at or below the carina) are considerably easier to treat. The paraesophageal nodes need to be included but the supraclavicular and celiac nodes do not. These are often treated with AP-PA fields to 3960 cGy followed by obliques to 5040 cGy. Three-field techniques (posterior obliques, with single anterior fields) can also be utilized. Similar techniques are used in treating distal esophageal or gastroesophageal junction tumors. The fields, however, now must include the celiac nodes.

The sloping contour of the chest often requires the use of compensating filters or wedges to ensure dose homogeneity. If these are not available, consecutive cone downs should be utilized to maintain a homogenous dose and stay within normal tissue tolerances.

In summary, the superior and inferior margins are approx 5 cm above and below the primary tumor as defined by clinical and radiological studies. The fields are slightly larger for tumors above the carina so as to include the supraclavicular region and lower esophageal tumors so as to include the celiac node.

10.2. Normal Tissue Tolerances

Every effort needs to be made to keep within the normal tissue tolerances of several of the critical structures that may be within the treatment field. All normal tissue tolerances assume treatment at 180 cGy per fraction. The spinal cord should not exceed 4500 cGy. The entire heart should not receive more than 4500 cGy and ≥50% of the heart should not receive more than 5000 cGy. Normal lung, i.e., more than 2 cm outside the target volume, should not receive more than 4500 cGy. There is a strong correlation between the incidence of ≥grade 2 pneumonitis and the total volume of lung (both lungs) exceeding 20 Gy *(71)*. Therefore, the total volume of lung receiving more than 2000 cGy must be kept below 25%. The dose per fraction to the heart, lungs, spinal cord, and liver should be 2 Gy or less whenever possible. For lower esophageal tumors, the liver dose should be kept to a minimum. Half the liver should not exceed 3500 cGy. The whole liver should not exceed 3000 cGy.

10.3. Treatment Planning

Patients are generally treated in the supine position. If conventional simulation is used, a barium swallow should be done at the time of simulation to outline the target volume. Optimal immobilization such as an alpha cradle to improve daily set up reproducibility is used.

CT-based simulation is preferred whenever possible. Normal tissues (heart, lung, spinal cord) can then be contoured such that doses to these organs are kept to a minimum. If the tolerance dose is exceeded to any critical structure, alternate beam arrangements should be evaluated.

11. CONCLUSIONS

Despite improvements in surgery, radiation, and chemotherapy, the 5-yr survival for all patients with esophageal cancer is only 10%. Even for patients with locally advanced disease, the 5-yr survival is generally 20%. Currently, results from surgery alone or primary chemoradiation are equivalent, and both can be offered as options for patients with locally advanced esophageal cancer. The optimal treatment may be based on individual patient selection criteria such as the ability to undergo major surgery, histology, and the location of the tumor. The fact that local recurrence is high despite primary chemoradiation provides a rationale for trimodality therapy that includes surgery following preoperative chemoradiation.

The results of trials evaluating neoadjuvant chemotherapy followed by surgery are conflicting with two of five randomized studies suggesting a survival benefit. However, the results of the US studies have been negative and, therefore, neoadjuvant chemotherapy is recommended to be used only in the protocol setting. Pathologic complete response rates are improved with the combination of neoadjuvant radiation and chemotherapy, approx 25–30%, and local control is improved but results from randomized trials are conflicting. Triple modality therapy, therefore, remains investigational.

REFERENCES

1. Greenlee RT, Murray T, Bolden S, Wingo PA. Cancer statistics, 2000. *CA Cancer J Clin* 2000; 50(1):7–33.
2. Devesa SS, Blot WJ, Fraumeni JF Jr. Changing patterns in the incidence of esophageal and gastric carcinoma in the United States. *Cancer* 1998; 83(10):2049–2053.
3. Blot WJ, McLaughlin JK. The changing epidemiology of esophageal cancer. *Semin Oncol* 1999; 26(5 Suppl 15):2–8.
4. Lagergren J, Bergstrom R, Lindgren A, Nyren O. Symptomatic gastroesophageal reflux as a risk factor for esophageal adenocarcinoma. *N Engl J Med* 1999; 340(11):825–831.
5. Wu TT, Watanabe T, Heitmiller R, Zahurak M, Forastiere AA, Hamilton SR. Genetic alterations in Barrett esophagus and adenocarcinomas of the esophagus and esophagogastric junction region. *Am J Pathol* 1998; 153(1):287–294.
6. Heidemann J, Schilling MK, Schmassmann A, Maurer CA, Buchler MW. Accuracy of endoscopic ultrasonography in preoperative staging of esophageal carcinoma. *Dig Surg* 2000; 17(3):219–224.
7. Botet JF, Lightdale CJ, Zauber AG, Gerdes H, Urmacher C, Brennan MF. Preoperative staging of esophageal cancer: comparison of endoscopic US and dynamic CT. *Radiology* 1991; 181(2): 419–425.
8. Rice TW, Boyce GA, Sivak MV, Adelstein DJ, Kirby TJ. Esophageal carcinoma: esophageal ultrasound assessment of preoperative chemotherapy. *Ann Thorac Surg* 1992; 53(6):972–977.
9. Reed CE, Mishra G, Sahai AV, Hoffman BJ, Hawes RH. Esophageal cancer staging: improved accuracy by endoscopic ultrasound of celiac lymph nodes. *Ann Thorac Surg* 1999; 67(2):319–321.
10. Flamen P, Lerut A, Van Cutsem E, et al. Utility of positron emission tomography for the staging of patients with potentially operable esophageal carcinoma. *J Clin Oncol* 2000; 18(18):3202–3210.
11. Heath EI, Kaufman HS, Talamini MA, et al. The role of laparoscopy in preoperative staging of esophageal cancer. *Surg Endosc* 2000; 14(5):495–499.
12. Putnam JB Jr, Suell DM, McMurtrey MJ, et al. Comparison of three techniques of esophagectomy within a residency training program. *Ann Thorac Surg* 1994; 57(2):319–325.
13. Stark S, Romberg M, Pierce G, et al. Transhiatal versus Transthoracic Esophagectomy for Adenocarcinoma of the Distal Esophagus and Cardia. *Am J Surg* 1996; 172:478–482.
14. Sykes AJ, Burt PA, Slevin NJ, Stout R, Marrs JE. Radical radiotherapy for carcinoma of the oesophagus: an effective alternative to surgery. *Radiother Oncol* 1998; 48(1):15–21.
15. Slevin NJ, Stout R. Carcinoma of the oesophagus—a review of 108 cases treated by radical radiotherapy. *Clin Radiol* 1989; 40(2):200–203.
16. Arnott SJ, Duncan W, Kerr GR, et al. Low dose preoperative radiotherapy for carcinoma of the oesophagus: results of a randomized clinical trial. *Radiother Oncol* 1992; 24(2):108–113.
17. Gignoux M, Roussel A, Paillot B, et al. The value of preoperative radiotherapy in esophageal cancer: results of a study by the EORTC. *Recent Results Cancer Res* 1988; 110:1–13.
18. Launois B, Delarue D, Campion JP, Kerbaol M. Preoperative radiotherapy for carcinoma of the esophagus. *Surg Gynecol Obstet* 1981; 153(5):690–692.
19. Nygaard K, Hagen S, Hansen HS, et al. Pre-operative radiotherapy prolongs survival in operable esophageal carcinoma: a randomized, multicenter study of pre-operative radiotherapy and chemotherapy. The second Scandinavian trial in esophageal cancer. *World J Surg* 1992; 16(6):1104–1109.
20. Wang M, Gu XZ, Yin WB, Huang GJ, Wang LJ, Zhang DW. Randomized clinical trial on the combination of preoperative irradiation and surgery in the treatment of esophageal carcinoma: report on 206 patients. *Int J Radiat Oncol Biol Phys* 1989; 16(2):325–327.
21. Arnott SJ, Duncan W, Gignoux M, et al. Preoperative radiotherapy in esophageal carcinoma: a meta-analysis using individual patient data (Oesophageal Cancer Collaborative Group). *Int J Radiat Oncol Biol Phys* 1998; 41(3):579–583.
22. Teniere P, Hay JM, Fingerhut A, Fagniez PL. Postoperative radiation therapy does not increase survival after curative resection for squamous cell carcinoma of the middle and lower esophagus as shown by a multicenter controlled trial. French University Association for Surgical Research. *Surg Gynecol Obstet* 1991; 173(2):123–130.
23. Fok M, Sham JS, Choy D, Cheng SW, Wong J. Postoperative radiotherapy for carcinoma of the esophagus: a prospective, randomized controlled study. *Surgery* 1993; 113(2):138–147.
24. Kelsen DP, Ginsberg R, Pajak TF, et al. Chemotherapy followed by surgery compared with surgery alone for localized esophageal cancer. *N Engl J Med* 1998; 339(27):1979–1984.

25. Law S, Fok M, Chow S, Chu KM, Wong J. Preoperative chemotherapy versus surgical therapy alone for squamous cell carcinoma of the esophagus: a prospective randomized trial. *J Thorac Cardiovasc Surg* 1997; 114(2):210–217.
26. Kok T, Lanschot J, Siersema P, et al. Neoadjuvant Chemotherapy in Operable Esophageal Squamous Cell Cancer: Final Report of a Phase III Multicenter Randomized Controlled Trial. *Proc Am Soc Clin Oncol* 1997; 16:277a.
27. Schlag PM. Randomized trial of preoperative chemotherapy for squamous cell cancer of the esophagus. The Chirurgische Arbeitsgemeinschaft Fuer Onkologie der Deutschen Gesellschaft Fuer Chirurgie Study Group. *Arch Surg* 1992; 127(12):1446–1450.
28. Roth JA, Pass HI, Flanagan MM, Graeber GM, Rosenberg JC, Steinberg S. Randomized clinical trial of preoperative and postoperative adjuvant chemotherapy with cisplatin, vindesine, and bleomycin for carcinoma of the esophagus. *J Thorac Cardiovasc Surg* 1988; 96(2):242–248.
29. Clark PI, Medical Research Council. Randomized Trial of Surgery with or without Pre-Operative Chemotherapy in Resectable Cancer of the Esophagus. *Ann Oncol* 2000; 11:4.
30. Ando N, Iizuka T, Kakegawa T, et al. A randomized trial of surgery with and without chemotherapy for localized squamous carcinoma of the thoracic esophagus: the Japan Clinical Oncology Group Study. *J Thorac Cardiovasc Surg* 1997; 114(2):205–209.
31. Urba SG, Orringer MB, Turrisi A, Iannettoni M, Forastiere A, Strawderman M. Randomized trial of preoperative chemoradiation versus surgery alone in patients with locoregional esophageal carcinoma. *J Clin Oncol* 2001; 19(2):305–313.
32. Forastiere AA, Orringer MB, Perez-Tamayo C, et al. Concurrent chemotherapy and radiation therapy followed by transhiatal esophagectomy for local-regional cancer of the esophagus. *J Clin Oncol* 1990; 8(1):119–127.
33. Forastiere AA, Orringer MB, Perez-Tamayo C, Urba SG, Zahurak M. Preoperative chemoradiation followed by transhiatal esophagectomy for carcinoma of the esophagus: final report. *J Clin Oncol* 1993; 11(6):1118–1123.
34. Kelsen D. Preoperative chemoradiotherapy for esophageal cancer. *J Clin Oncol* 2001; 19(2):283–285.
35. Walsh TN, Noonan N, Hollywood D, Kelly A, Keeling N, Hennessy TP. A comparison of multimodal therapy and surgery for esophageal adenocarcinoma. *N Engl J Med* 1996; 335(7):462–467.
36. Bosset JF, Gignoux M, Triboulet JP, et al. Chemoradiotherapy followed by surgery compared with surgery alone in squamous-cell cancer of the esophagus. *N Engl J Med* 1997; 337(3):161–167.
37. Forastiere AA, Heitmiller RF, Lee DJ, et al. Intensive chemoradiation followed by esophagectomy for squamous cell and adenocarcinoma of the esophagus. *Cancer J Sci Am* 1997; 3(3):144–152.
38. Roder JD, Bottcher K, Busch R, Wittekind C, Hermanek P, Siewert JR. Classification of regional lymph node metastasis from gastric carcinoma. German Gastric Cancer Study Group. *Cancer* 1998; 82(4):621–631.
39. Fein M, Fuchs KH, Ritter MP, et al. Application of the new classification for cancer of the cardia. *Surgery* 1998; 124(4):707–713.
40. Macdonald JS, Smalley S, Benedetti J, et al. Postoperative Combined Radiation and Chemotherapy Improves Disease-free Survival (DFS) and overall Survival (OS) in Resected Adenocarcinoma of the Stomach and G.E. Junction. *Am Soc Clin Oncol* 2000; 19:1a.
41. Buroker TR, Nigro N, Bradley G, et al. Combined therapy for cancer of the anal canal: a follow-up report. *Dis Colon Rectum* 1977; 20(8):677–678.
42. Franklin R, Steiger Z, Vaishampayan G, et al. Combined modality therapy for esophageal squamous cell carcinoma. *Cancer* 1983; 51(6):1062–1071.
43. al Sarraf M, Martz K, Herskovic A, et al. Progress report of combined chemoradiotherapy versus radiotherapy alone in patients with esophageal cancer: an intergroup study. *J Clin Oncol* 1997; 15(1):277–284.
44. Cooper JS, Guo MD, Herskovic A, et al. Chemoradiotherapy of locally advanced esophageal cancer: long-term follow-up of a prospective randomized trial (RTOG 85-01). Radiation Therapy Oncology Group. *JAMA* 1999; 281(17):1623–1627.
45. Herskovic A, Martz K, al Sarraf M, et al. Combined chemotherapy and radiotherapy compared with radiotherapy alone in patients with cancer of the esophagus. *N Engl J Med* 1992; 326(24): 1593–1598.
46. Smith TJ, Ryan LM, Douglass HO Jr, et al. Combined chemoradiotherapy vs. radiotherapy alone for early stage squamous cell carcinoma of the esophagus: a study of the Eastern Cooperative Oncology Group. *Int J Radiat Oncol Biol Phys* 1998; 42(2):269–276.

47. Minsky BD, Neuberg D, Kelsen DP, et al. Final report of Intergroup Trial 0122 (ECOG PE-289, RTOG 90-12): Phase II trial of neoadjuvant chemotherapy plus concurrent chemotherapy and high-dose radiation for squamous cell carcinoma of the esophagus. *Int J Radiat Oncol Biol Phys* 1999; 43(3):517–523.
48. Minsky BD, Berkey B, Kelsen D, et al. Hamilton Reg Cancer Ctr, Sacramento Rad Onc Ctr. Preliminary Results of Intergroup INT 0123 Randomized Trial of Combined Modality Therapy (CMT) for Esophageal Cancer: Standard vs. High Dose Radiation Therapy. *Proc Am Soc Clin Oncol* 2000; 19:239a.
49. Gaspar LE, Winter K, Kocha WI, Coia LR, Herskovic A, Graham M. A phase I/II study of external beam radiation, brachytherapy, and concurrent chemotherapy for patients with localized carcinoma of the esophagus (Radiation Therapy Oncology Group Study 9207): final report. *Cancer* 2000; 88(5):988–995.
50. Wani MC, Taylor HL, Wall ME, Coggon P, McPhail AT. Plant antitumor agents. VI. The isolation and structure of taxol, a novel antileukemic and antitumor agent from Taxus brevifolia. *J Am Chem Soc* 1971; 93(9):2325–2327.
51. Rowinsky EK, Donehower RC. Paclitaxel (taxol). *N Engl J Med* 1995; 332(15):1004–1014.
52. Wiernik PH, Schwartz EL, Einzig A, Strauman JJ, Lipton RB, Dutcher JP. Phase I trial of taxol given as a 24-hour infusion every 21 days: responses observed in metastatic melanoma. *J Clin Oncol* 1987; 5(8):1232–1239.
53. Ajani JA, Ilson DH, Daugherty K, Pazdur R, Lynch PM, Kelsen DP. Activity of taxol in patients with squamous cell carcinoma and adenocarcinoma of the esophagus. *J Natl Cancer Inst* 1994; 86(14):1086–1091.
54. Mauer AM, Masters GA, Haraf DJ, et al. Phase I study of docetaxel with concomitant thoracic radiation therapy. *J Clin Oncol* 1998; 16(1):159–164.
55. Schiff PB, Horwitz SB. Taxol stabilizes microtubules in mouse fibroblast cells. *Proc Natl Acad Sci USA* 1980; 77(3):1561–1565.
56. Sinclair WK, Morton RA. X-ray sensitivity during the cell generation cycle of cultured Chinese hamster cells. *Radiat Res* 1966; 29(3):450–474.
57. Tishler RB, Schiff PB, Geard CR, Hall EJ. Taxol: a novel radiation sensitizer. *Int J Radiat Oncol Biol Phys* 1992; 22(3):613–617.
58. Choy H, Rodriguez FF, Koester S, Hilsenbeck S, Von Hoff DD. Investigation of taxol as a potential radiation sensitizer. *Cancer* 1993; 71(11):3774–3778.
59. Liebmann J, Cook JA, Fisher J, Teague D, Mitchell JB. In vitro studies of Taxol as a radiation sensitizer in human tumor cells. *J Natl Cancer Inst* 1994; 86(6):441–446.
60. Blanke CD, Chiappori A, Epstein B, et al. A Phase II Trial of Neoadjuvant Paclitaxel (T) and Cisplatin (P) with Radiotherapy, Followed by Surgery (S) and Postoperativve T with 5-Fluorouracil (F) and Leucovorin (L) in Patients (pts) with Locally Advanced Esophageal Cancer (LAEC). *Proc Annu Meet Am Soc Clin Oncol* 1997; 16:A1006.
61. Blanke CD, Choy H, Teng M, et al. Concurrent paclitaxel and thoracic irradiation for locally advanced esophageal cancer. *Semin Radiat Oncol* 1999; 9(2 Suppl 1):43–52.
62. Berlin J, Kubba S, Blanke CD, et al. Phase II Study of Neoadjuvant Cisplatin (P), and Taxol (T) with Concomitant Radiotherapy Followed by Surgery and then Taxol and 5FU, Leucovorin (L) in Patients with Locally Advanced Esophageal Cancer. ASCO 2000; Abstract #1246.
63. Hoff SJ, Stewart JR, Sawyers JL, et al. Preliminary results with neoadjuvant therapy and resection for esophageal carcinoma. *Ann Thorac Surg* 1993; 56(2):282–286.
64. Stewart JR, Hoff SJ, Johnson DH, et al. Improved survival with neoadjuvant therapy and resection for adenocarcinoma of the esophagus. *Ann Surg* 1993; 218(4):571–576.
65. Adelstein DJ, Rice TW, Rybicki LA, et al. Does paclitaxel improve the chemoradiotherapy of locoregionally advanced esophageal cancer? A nonrandomized comparison with fluorouracil-based therapy. *J Clin Oncol* 2000; 18(10):2032–2039.
66. O'Connell MJ, Martenson JA, Wieand HS, et al. Improving adjuvant therapy for rectal cancer by combining protracted- infusion fluorouracil with radiation therapy after curative surgery. *N Engl J Med* 1994; 331(8):502–507.
67. Meta-Analysis Group in Cancer. Efficacy of intravenous continuous infusion of fluorouracil compared with bolus administration in advanced colorectal cancer. *J Clin Oncol* 1998; 16(1):301–308.
68. Safran H, Gaissert H, Akerman P, et al. Neoadjuvant Paclitaxel, Cisplatin and Radiation for Esophageal Cancer. *Proc Am Soc Clin Oncol* 1998; 17:259a.

69. Pietras RJ, Poen JC, Gallardo D, Wongvipat PN, Lee HJ, Slamon DJ. Monoclonal antibody to HER-2/neureceptor modulates repair of radiation-induced DNA damage and enhances radiosensitivity of human breast cancer cells overexpressing this oncogene. *Cancer Res* 1999; 59(6):1347–1355.
70. Mendenhall WM, Sombeck MD, Parsons JT, Kasper ME, Stringer SP, Vogel SB. Management of Cervical Esophageal Carcinoma. *Semin Radiat Oncol* 1994; 4(3):179–191.
71. Graham MV, Purdy JA, Emami B, et al. Clinical dose-volume histogram analysis for pneumonitis after 3D treatment for non-small cell lung cancer (NSCLC). *Int J Radiat Oncol Biol Phys* 1999; 45(2):323–329.
72. Roussel A, Jacob JH, Haegele P, et al. Controlled clinical trial for the treatment of patients with inoperable esophageal carcinoma: a study of the EORTC Gastrointestinal Tract Cancer Cooperative Group. *Recent Results Cancer Res* 1988; 110:21–29.
73. Slabber CF, Nel JS, Schoeman L, Burger W, Falkson G, Falkson CI. A randomized study of radiotherapy alone versus radiotherapy plus 5-fluorouracil and platinum in patients with inoperable, locally advanced squamous cancer of the esophagus. *Am J Clin Oncol* 1998; 21(5):462–465.
74. Wright CD, Wain JC, Lynch TJ, et al. Induction therapy for esophageal cancer with paclitaxel and hyperfractionated radiotherapy: a phase I and II study. *J Thorac Cardiovasc Surg* 1997; 114(5): 811–815.
75. Meluch A, Greco F, Burris H III, et al. Preoperative Paclitaxel, Carbonplatin, 5-FU and Radiation Therapy for Localized Esophageal Cancer. *Proc Annu Meet Am Soc Clin Oncol* 2001; 20:A636.
76. Weiner LM, Colarusso P, Goldberg M, Dresler C, Coia LR. Combined-modality therapy for esophageal cancer: phase I trial of escalating doses of paclitaxel in combination with cisplatin, 5-fluorouracil, and high-dose radiation before esophagectomy. *Semin Oncol* 1997; 24(6 Suppl 19):S19.
77. Enzinger P, Ilson D, Minsky BD, et al. Neoadjuvant Concurrent 96 Hour Taxol, Cisplatin, and Radiation Therapy: Promising Toxicity Profile and Response in localized Esophageal Cancer. *Am Soc Clin Oncol* 1999; 18:271a.

12 Combined Modality Therapy in Locally Advanced Breast Cancer

Silvia C. Formenti, MD *and Matthew Volm,* MD

Contents

1. INTRODUCTION

The management of locally advanced breast cancer requires the integration of surgery, chemotherapy, and radiation therapy. This chapter summarizes the existing experience and addresses some of the remaining issues in combined modality therapy of locally advanced and inflammatory breast cancer.

2. COMBINED MODALITY OF LOCALLY ADVANCED BREAST CANCER

Historically, locally advanced breast cancer (LABC) was defined as disease deemed inoperable on the basis of physical tumor characteristics associated with surgical failure to consistently achieve resection with negative margins: edema, skin fixation, ulceration, and chest wall involvement. These characteristics, which comprise T4 disease in the current American Joint Cancer Commission (AJCC) classification system, were identified by Haagensen and Stout at a time when radical mastectomy was the recognized treatment for breast cancer. As clinical practice evolved in the 1970s and 1980s to include the option of lumpectomy or segmental excision plus radiotherapy, many physicians came to consider tumors greater than 5 cm (AJCC T3) to be "locally advanced" because

From: *Chemoradiation in Cancer Therapy*
Edited by: H. Choy © Humana Press Inc., Totowa, NJ

their size usually precludes breast-conserving surgery. Thus the term LABC now describes a more heterogeneous group of patients with AJCC Stages IIB, IIIA, and IIIB. While all of these patients may be said to have LABC, they have a spectrum of prognoses. This is important to recognize when reviewing the results of clinical trials that include varying proportions of patients with good or poor prognosis tumors. In addition, many reported series include patients with inflammatory breast cancer, which is characterized by a distinct, aggressive clinical course and is best considered a separate entity. In this chapter, we will use the term "LABC" to denote tumors considered to be locally advanced based on T3, T4, or N2 status, but excluding inflammatory breast cancer. Although patients with LABC comprise a heterogeneous group with respect to outcome, they share a high rate of both local and distant failure compared to patients with earlier stage disease. To achieve success, treatment strategies for LABC must accomplish local control and eradicate distant micrometastases.

3. LOCALLY ADVANCED BREAST CANCER: SEQUENTIAL THERAPIES

Three prospective randomized trials reported in the 1980s compared local therapy alone to local therapy followed by systemic therapy. Two of the studies included patients with T3b or T4 disease; local therapy was radiation therapy (RT) only. It is noteworthy that, although in one of these two studies the addition of systemic therapy improved disease-free survival compared to RT alone, in neither study did the addition of systemic therapy show a significant survival benefit compared to RT *(1,2)*. The failure of systemic therapy to improve overall survival in these studies may be related to the fact that the use of conventional dose RT without surgery was inadequate to ensure local control, a determinant of outcome in LABC. The third randomized study investigating adjuvant systemic therapy in LABC enrolled patients with somewhat earlier stage, operable disease: T3, N0–2. All patients underwent a modified radical mastectomy followed by one of three treatment arms: RT alone, chemotherapy alone (doxorubicin, vincristine, and cyclophosphamide), or RT followed by chemotherapy *(3)*. Combined therapy produced better relapse-free survival than RT or chemotherapy alone. In terms of overall survival, both combined therapy and chemotherapy were significantly superior to RT alone. Conversely, significantly better local control was maintained in both arms including radiation compared to the chemotherapy alone group.

3.1. Neoadjuvant Chemotherapy

The large experience with neoadjuvant chemotherapy (also called induction, primary, or preoperative chemotherapy) in patients with LABC allows us to derive the following conclusions:

- Objective response rates are significantly higher than those observed when the same chemotherapy is given to patients with overt metastatic disease.
- It appears to improve the overall survival of patients with LABC, but most patients remain at high risk for the development of distant metastases.
- Without additional radiation therapy only a minority of patients achieve pathological response in the breast and axillary nodes.
- The response to induction therapy provides prognostic information.

Neoadjuvant chemotherapy has become a standard of care for LABC based on multiple nonrandomized trials demonstrating excellent clinical response rates and improved survival compared to historic controls. Standard anthracycline-based chemotherapy induces responses in 60–90% of patients, as shown in Table 1. However, in spite of high response rates, induction chemotherapy only rarely eradicates the primary tumor in the breast and axilla with most patients found to have significant residual disease at surgery.

4. LOCALLY ADVANCED BREAST CANCER: CONCURRENT CHEMORADIATION

Encouraged by the promising results achieved in other tumor types *(4–6)*, in the early 1990s we hypothesized that locally advanced breast cancer could also be treated by primary concurrent chemoradiation (chemo-RT). Moreover, LABC could be a clinical setting to conduct interesting translational research. A series of observations justified this position:

1. Because of the accessibility of large breast cancers it is relatively easy to obtain tissue for molecular studies *(7)*.
2. Preoperative/neoadjuvant treatment is the conventional approach, allowing for a reliable pathological quantification of response to therapy.
3. LABC propensity to local recurrence makes local control a priority, in order to preserve the best quality of life in these patients.

Based on these presumptions, during the past decade we have tested in two prospective Phase I-II clinical trials the role of concurrent chemo-RT as the primary therapy in LABC. In both trials pretreatment biopsies of the tumor were included in the study design to explore correlations between original molecular markers and the extent of pathological response achieved at surgery, after chemo-RT.

4.1. Concurrent 5-Fluorouracil (5-FU) and Radiation

The first trial combined concurrent 5-FU and radiation, as a continuation of the experience acquired at our institution by combining the radiosensitizing properties of 5-FU *(8,9)* with radiation in gastrointestinal cancers *(10,11)*. We selected the continuous infusion (CI) schedule, both with the purpose of optimizing drug exposure during the course of radiation and because of its promising results in metastatic breast cancer *(12)*. Figure 1A displays the original study design of this trial *(13,14)*. Eligible for this study were patients with particularly large LABC, defined "inoperable" at presentation because in order to resect the primary tumor the wound could be closed only with the interposition of a skin graft or a myocutaneous flap *(14)*. Preoperative CI infusion 5-FU, 200 mg/m^2/d was delivered for 8 wk with radiotherapy, wk 3–8, 50 Gy at 2 Gy fractions.

For each patient pretreatment breast cancer biopsies were analyzed by immunohistochemistry for ER/PR hormonal receptors, HER2/neu and *p53* overexpression. This study pilot-tested a definition of pathological response to chemo-RT. At mastectomy pathological findings were classified based on persistence of invasive cancer: pathological complete response (pCR) = no residual invasive cells in the breast and axillary contents; pathological partial response (pPR) = presence of microscopic foci of invasive cells in either the breast or nodal specimens; no pathological response (pNR) = pathological persistence of tumor. Presence of ductal carcinoma *in situ* (DCIS) in the specimen did not modify this classification. All patients responded enough to become operable with primary wound closure. A high clinical and pathological response rate characterized this trial in large inoperable breast cancers, with 71% of patients achieving objective clinical response (CR + PR) and 34% achieving either complete or partial pathological response.

Table 1
Contemporary Phase I-Ii Trials of Primary Anthracycline-Based Chemotherapy, Followed by Surgery and Radiation

Author, year	*Number of pts.*	*Treatment regimen*	*Response rate*	*Survival*
Zambetti, 1999 *(20)*	88	Preoperative doxorubicin, post-op CMF, XRT	OR = 70% path CR = 2%	At 52 mo, RFS 52%, OS 62%
Thomas, 1999 *(45)* (MDAC)	377	Pre-op chemo (variety of regimens), XRT for all patients with > 1 cm residual tumor	OR = 85%	10 yr DFS 58% for IIIA, 29% for IIIB
Honkoop, 1999 *(46)*	42	Pre-op dose intense AC, post-op XRT	OR = 98%, path CR = 14%	3 yr DFS 57%, OS 79%
Dhingra, 1999 *(47)*	202	Pre-op standard FAC vs dose intense FAC, post-op vinblastine, methotrexate	FAC: OR = 76% path CR 9% dose intense FAC: OR = 90% path CR 14%	5 yr DFS 53% for standard FAC, 57% for dose intense FAC
Karlsson, 1998 *(19)*	128	Pre-op FEC, post-op FEC and XRT	Overall response rate 60%, pathologic CR 5%	5 yr DFS 36%, OS 49% (Inflammatory pts. fared poorly.)
Eltahir, 1998 *(48)*	77	Pre-op chemo, followed by XRT then surgery	OR = 90%	5 yr DFS 48%
DeMatteis, 1998 *(49)*	87	Pre-op epirubicin, surgery, post-op XRT	OR = 84%	5 yr OS 54%
Kuerer, 1999 *(15)*	372	Doxorubicin-based CT, surgery/XRT	Path CR = 16%	5 yr DFS pathologic CR 87%, others 58%
Morrell, 1998 *(17)*	49	Doxorubicin-based CT, surgery/XRT	OR = 89%, path CR = 20%	5 yr DFS 51%

A

Biopsy -Proven, LABC,Inoperable+,Informed Consent, Staging (CT Chest Abdomen And Pelvis)Placement Of Central Line. First Pre-Treatment Tumor Core Biopsies

Start c.i. 5-FU, 200 mg/ m^2/day for 2 weeks.

Day 14, Second core biopsy; Start RT50 Gy @2Gy/fraction

/ \

Operable patients
Surgery (MRM#)
/
ACX4

Inoperable patient
Core Biopsies for
Biological Studies

B

Biopsy-Proven LABC,TNM Stage IIB (T3 N0 Only) And III. Informed Consent, Staging (CT Chest Abdomen And Pelvis). Pre-Treatment Tumor Core Biopsies

Start Paclitaxel 30 mg/m^{2}Twice -Weekly (1 H Infusion)

A Week Later, Start Rt 45 Gy @1.8 Gy/Fraction

No Change Or Clinical Response
|
Twice A Week Paclitaxel X 2 Weeks
|
Surgery (MRM#)

Progression
|
AC X 4

CR/PR:
/
AT X 4

SD/NR:
\
AC X 4

Fig. 1. (A) Study design of concurrent CI 5-Fluorouracil and radiation in LABC. **(B)** Study design of concurrent paclitaxel and radiation in LABC.

The pathological response rate of chemo-RT compares favorably with that of any reported contemporary chemotherapy neo-adjuvant trial in this patient population *(15–20)*. In addition, this study proved the feasibility of using biological correlates from pretreatment tumor biopsies to explore associations with pathological response. In fact, 11/21 patients (52%) with no evidence of *p53* overexpression at immunohistochemistry achieved a pathological response to the regimen, compared to 1/14 patients (7%) with overexpressed *p53* ($p = 0.010$, Fisher exact text).

At multivariate analysis, lack of *p53* overexpression was the only independent predictive factor for pathological response. Nevertheless, because the majority of patients who overexpressed *p53* failed to achieve a pathological response, it became important to investigate agents less likely to be affected by tumor *p53* status. Taxanes became the next drugs to combine in a concurrent use with radiation.

4.2. Background for Combining Taxanes and Radiation

In vitro and preclinical models support the combination of taxanes with radiation. For instance, Whal et al. have shown that loss of normal *p53* function actually confers sensitivity to paclitaxel in some cell types because of an increased G2/M arrest leading to *p53* independent cell death *(21)* explaining the preferential activity of paclitaxel against cancer cells compared to normal cells *(22)* as well as its activity against tumors that are *p53* mutated *(23)*. Moreover, accumulation of cells at the G2/M checkpoint explains some of the in vivo radiosensitizing effects of the drug *(24)*. Interestingly, our group was able to document in human tumor tissue the kinetics of paclitaxel induced apoptosis and mitotic arrest *(25)*. The findings supported the use of twice/week regimen as the optimal radiosensitizing schedule in the clinic *(26)*.

Another reason for studying taxanes in a chemo-RT approach to LABC is the fact that several potential markers of sensitivity to taxanes have been identified. Since the microtubule (MT) is a well-described target of paclitaxel, biochemical mediators that could impact microtubule stability are expected to affect paclitaxel activity. For instance, the components of mammalian microtubules are α and β-tubulin: the latter is the main target of paclitaxel action *(27)* and elevated class III and class IV β-tubulin isoforms were found in paclitaxel-resistant ovarian tumor cells *(28)*. Metablastin (also termed p19 and stathmin) is also a regulator of MT dynamics *(29)* and thus could influence paclitaxel activity. Similarly, MAP4 protein overexpression, which is known to stabilize MT and thus would be expected to antagonize paclitaxel, was found to predict for paclitaxel-resistance in vitro *(30)*. Interestingly, MAP4 is one of the few genes known to be downregulated by wild-type *p53*, possibly explaining the observed inverse relationship of *p53* status and paclitaxel activity *(30)*. Other potential determinants for response to paclitaxel are genes associated with the apoptotic or cell cycle regulation pathways. Paclitaxel has been demonstrated to cause the phosphorylation of Bcl-2, which is supposed to abrogate the anti-apoptotic function of Bcl-2 by dissociating it from the pro-apoptotic molecule Bax *(31)*. Finally, HER2/neu overexpression was shown to both alter β-tubulin isoform expression and confer resistance to paclitaxel *(32)*. Interestingly, Pietras et al. reported resistance to radiation when HER2/neu overexpression was induced in vitro and in vivo in a breast xenografts tumor model. They also generated preliminary evidence that a monoclonal antibody directed against the HER-2/neu receptor affects repair of radiation-induced DNA damage and enhances radiosensitivity of human breast cancer cells overexpressing HER2 *(33)*.

4.3. Concurrent Paclitaxel and Radiation: A Phase I-II Study

Based on this background, the second concurrent chemo-RT study combined a taxane with RT *(23,26)*. The trial design is described in Fig. 2. For each patient studied, pretreatment breast cancer biopsies were prospectively analyzed by immunohistochemistry for *p53* overexpression. Estrogen receptor (ER), HER2/neu, metablastin, β-tubulin III and IV, MAP 4, Bcl-2, Bax gene expression were measured using real-time quantitative polymerase chain reaction (PCR). The regimen consisted of preoperative concurrent paclitaxel (30 mg/m^2 twice/week) for a total of 8 wk while radiation was delivered wk 2–7, 45 Gy at 1.8 Gy per fraction to the breast, and regional nodes. Forty-four patients accrued to the trial: The regimen was well tolerated with grade 3 toxicity limited to confluent wet desquamation in 10% and no grade 4 toxicities. Figure 2 exemplifies a case of a patient recovering from confluent wet desquamation a few days before mastectomy. This patient had residual cancer in the mastectomy specimen. Thirty-three percent achieved pathological response (pCR + pPR). Figures 3A and 3B document the microscopic findings from the tumor of a patient undergoing core biopsies before starting chemoradiation. In the same patient, Fig. 4A–C illustrate the microscopic findings after chemoradiation: This patient achieved a pathological CR. When associations of pathological response with molecular markers were explored, tumors with low HER2/neu gene expression and negative estrogen receptors were more likely to respond to the tested regimen ($p = 0.009$ and $p = 0.006$, respectively). Conversely, *p53* protein expression measured by immunohistochemistry (IHC) did not appear to be associated with pathological response ($p = 0.67$) *(34)*.

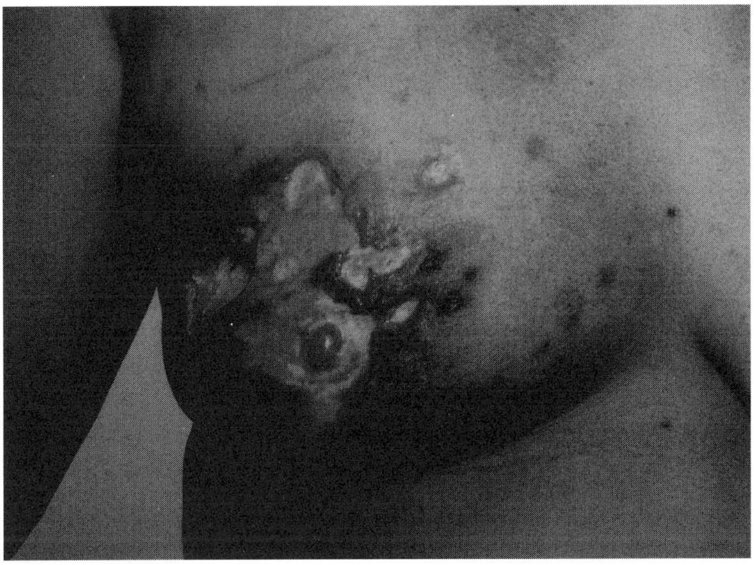

Fig. 2. Recovering wet desquamation after completion of concurrent paclitaxel and radiation in a patient who presented with stage IIIB breast cancer.

5. PATHOLOGICAL RESPONSE IN LABC: A SURROGATE ENDPOINT FOR SURVIVAL

Several lines of evidence exist to support the fact that in LABC the extent of pathological response after primary, neoadjuvant therapy is a surrogate for disease-free survival and possibly for overall survival. Bonadonna et al. first reported significantly different survival among patients achieving pathological response after doxorubicin-based primary treatment when compared to patients who had persistent disease *(35)*. Similarly, Kuerer et al. reported the clinical course of 372 patients treated with doxorubicin-based regimens at M.D. Anderson with a median follow-up of 58 mo both disease-free survival (DFS) and overall survival (OS) were statistically significantly better among patients who had achieved a pathological response compared to nonresponders ($p < 0.01$) *(15)*.

With regard to the 5-FU/RT trial, with a median follow-up of 5 yr, OS of the entire group of patients is 74% and DFS is 58%. With the limitations associated with the small number of patients in this study (35 patients), it is reassuring to note that postponing anthracycline-based treatment after mastectomy did not compromise DFS and OS among these women with large LABC, as shown in Table 2.

We asked the question of whether a pathological response to a regimen of chemo-RT could also be a surrogate endpoint for survival in LABC. With a median follow-up of 5 yr, we found that the patients who had achieved a pathological response (pCR + pPR) to 5-FU/RT had both a better DFS and OS than the nonresponders ($p = 0.023$, and $p = 0.06$, respectively), with only one failure among the women who achieved pathological response. In addition, no isolated chest wall/nodal recurrences have occurred so far *(36)*. It becomes compelling to explore strategies to optimize pathological response to chemo-RT.

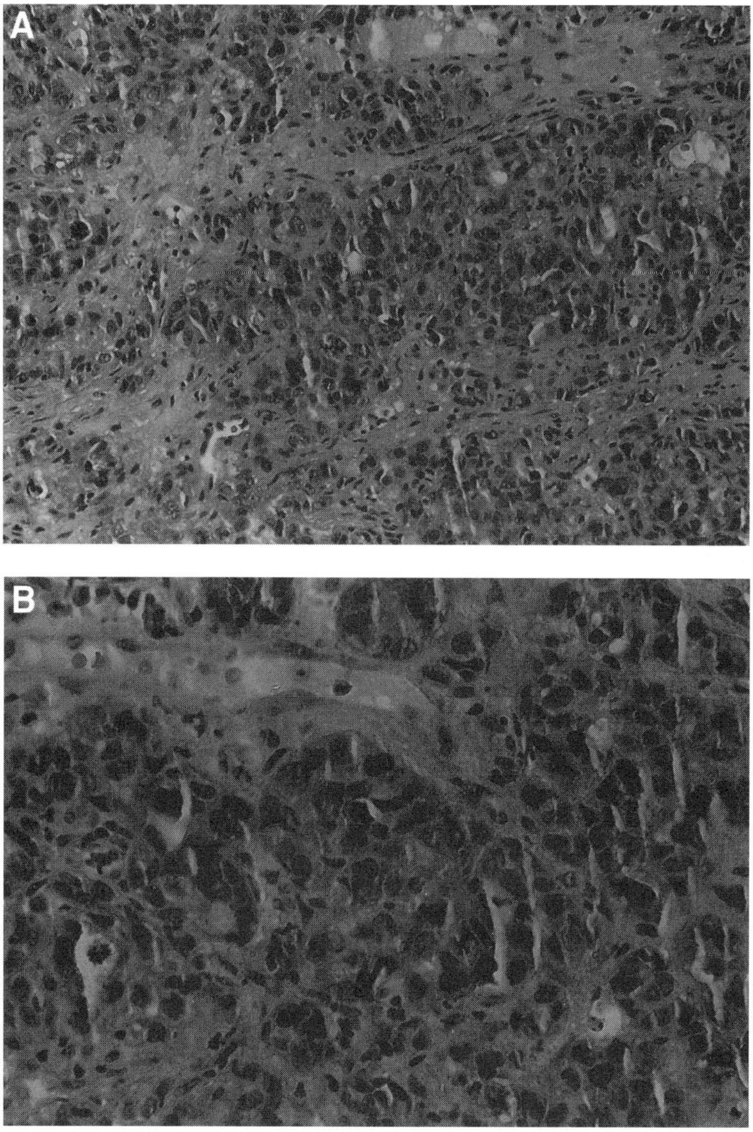

Fig. 3. (**A** and **B**) Breast carcinoma, in a core biopsy of a patient, pretreatment. Hematoxylin-eosin (H&E)-stained histological sections show a poorly differentiated ductal carcinoma with evident nuclear pleomorphism and numerous mitotic figures. (A) H&E, magnification ×200; (B) H&E, magnification ×400.

5.1. Future Studies

The two consecutive chemo-RT Phase I-II studies conducted showed that different molecular markers were associated with pathological response: The finding supports the hypothesis that different drugs combined with concurrent radiation are effective on different tumor types. If this hypothesis is correct, selecting up-front which patient should be treated with one type of chemo-RT vs the other, based on the molecular characteristics of the tumor, may optimize pathological response rates, thus potentially reflecting on

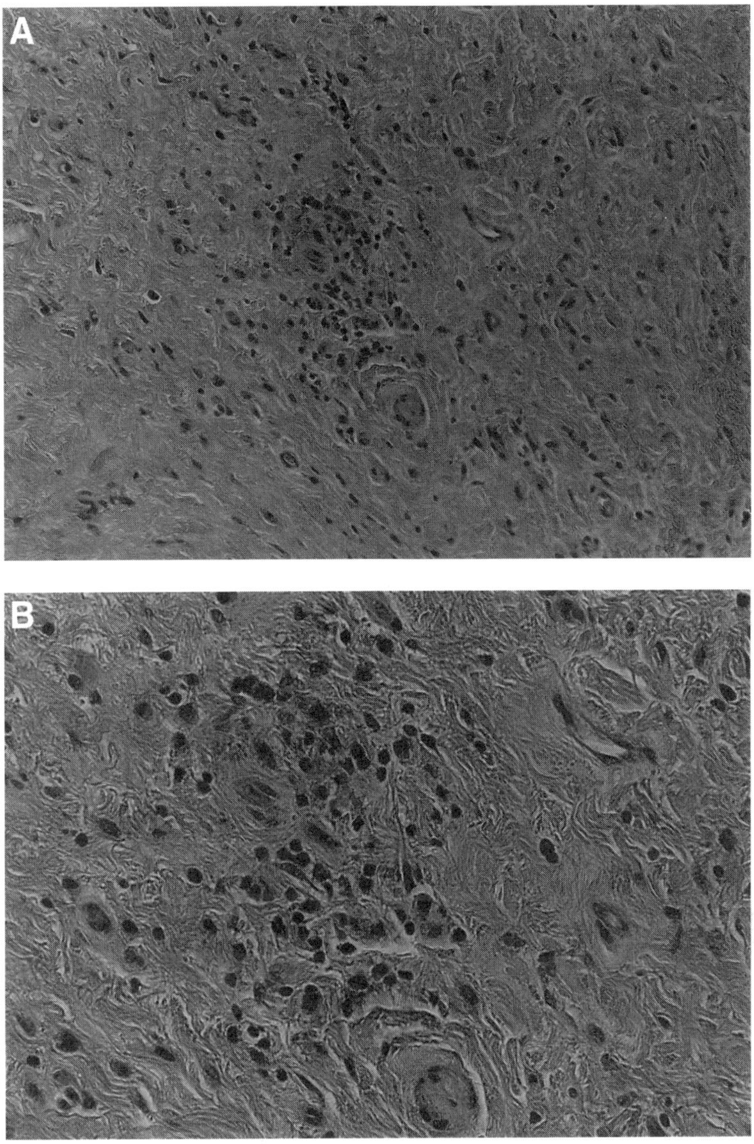

Fig. 4. (**A** and **B**) Breast tissue from the same patient, posttreatment. Section of the tumor bed posttreatment shows reactive changes consisting of cellular fibrous tissue with numerous vessels (granulation tissue) and infiltration by lymphocytes, plasma cells and numerous iron-loaded macrophages. No residual carcinoma cells are seen. (A) H&E, magnification ×200; (B) H&E, magnification ×400.

survival. Besides, the addition of a monoclonal antibody against HER2/neu in patients with tumors overexpressing this marker could overcome their observed resistance to paclitaxel and radiation, as suggested by experimental models *(33)*. To test these new hypotheses, we have started a clinical protocol that preselects LABC patients based on their tumor characteristics and assigns them to different chemoradiation regimens (taxane or fluoropyrimidine-based, combined with anti-HER2neu receptor monoclonal antibodies if HER2/neu positive). If this strategy is successful it could reflect in higher pathologi-

Table 2
Pathological Response and Outcome in Phase I-II Studies of LABC

Author, year	*Number of pts.*	*Treatment*	*% Path response*	*5 Y DFS*	*5 Y OS*
Powles, 1995 *(18)*	105	Chemo-endocrine therapy/surgery/RT	10%	NA	NA
Schwartz, 1994 *(50)*	158	Doxorubicin-Based CT/surgery/RT	10%	61%	69%
Merajver, 1997 *(16)*	89	Prolonged chemo-hormonal therapy/surgery or RT	NA	44%	54%
Formenti, 1997 *(14,36)*	35	Concurrent FU/RT/surgery/post-op AC	35%	58% pCR 90% Others 65%	74%
Karlsson, 1998 *(19)*	128	FEC/surgery/FEC/RT	NA	36% (actuarial)	49% (actuarial)
Morrell, 1998 *(17)*	49	Doxorubicin-based CT, surgery/RT	16%	51%	63%
Ayash, 1998 *(51)*	37	High dose CT with stem cell support/surgery/radiation	14%	64% at 30 mo	NA
Kuerer, 1999 *(52)*	372	Doxorubicin-based CT, surgery/RT	12%	p CR 87% Others 58%	pCR 89% Others 64%
Zambetti, 1999 *(20)*	88	Doxorubicin-based CT surgery/CMFX6/RT	2%	52%	62%
Formenti, 2001 *(34)*	44	Concurrent paclitaxel/RT/surgery/post-op Doxorubicin-based CT	35%	NA	NA

cal response rates that, based on the preliminary association with outcome found in the first chemo-RT study *(36)*, it is likely to reflect on DFS and OS.

6. COMBINED MODALITY TREATMENT IN INFLAMMATORY BREAST CANCER

Inflammatory carcinoma of the breast (IBC) is a unique syndrome characterized by extensive erythema of the breast, dermal lymphatic invasion, and an aggressive clinical course. There is a high likelihood of distant metastatic deposits, even though routine staging procedures are often negative at presentation. The multimodality therapy of inflammatory breast carcinoma thus emphasizes early aggressive systemic therapy. As is the case with noninflammatory LABC, the response to primary chemotherapy provides prognostic information. For example, investigators at M.D. Anderson reported a 10-yr DFS of 48%, 28%, and 10% for those with a CR, PR, and less than PR, respectively, in patients with inflammatory breast cancer treated with anthracyline-based therapy followed by surgery and/or radiation *(37)*. Maloisel et al. reported response to primary chemotherapy to be the most significant prognostic factor determining DFS *(38)*.

Selected series are shown in Table 3. It should be noted that much of the literature on IBC reports on retrospective data obtained by reviewing the records of patients treated with a variety of sequential combination regimens, often over a period of 10 yr or more, and that randomized trials are lacking. Radiation therapy is usually given after induction chemotherapy; there are no reported series of concurrent chemotherapy and RT in IBC. Five-year DFS remains under 50% in the large majority of series. This has led to investigational approaches that emphasize the eradication of microscopic metastatic disease, including high-dose chemotherapy with stem cell support. Early results from nonrandomized studies of high-dose therapy are encouraging, but further data are needed to support the use of high-dose therapy outside the setting of a clinical trial *(39,40)*.

The role of surgery in the management of IBC has been controversial. The high rate of systemic failure supports the relative importance of effective systemic therapy in IBC, and the difficulty in obtaining clear surgical margins when there is diffuse dermal lymphatic involvement has raised concern that surgery might not be useful and could even contribute to local recurrence if involved skin is transected. Although there are no randomized data evaluating the role of surgery in LABC, retrospective studies suggest that surgery is safe following successful induction chemotherapy and may improve local control and survival *(41)*.

7. CONCLUDING REMARKS

The management of locally advanced breast cancer and inflammatory breast cancer has evolved over the past twenty years. In general, surgery has maintained a role in the combined management of this disease but most studies have tested strategies to increase the extent of pathological response, especially in view of its prognostic implications.

Protocols based on individualization of therapy based on molecular characteristics of the original tumor and their likelihood to be associated with response to a specific regimen are under active investigation. It is likely that in the future, novel, high-throughput technologies for tumor molecular profiling may have a significant impact on the outcome of LABC and IBC patients.

Table 3
Phase I-II Clinical Trials of Inflammatory Breast Cancer

Author, year	*Number of pts.*	*Treatment regimen*	*Survival*	*Comment*
Fields, 1989 *(42)*	37	CAF X 2-3 cycles → XRT → mastectomy → maintenance chemo	5 yr DFS 37%, OS 48%	Patients had much better survival than historical controls that received RT. Mastectomy associated with improved local control and survival.
Thoms, 1989 *(43)*	61	Doxorubicin-based induction → mastectomy → adjuvant chemo → RT	5 yr DFS 27%	39% of patients failed to respond to induction chemotherapy. Mastectomy not associated with improved local control or survival.
Rouesse, 1986 *(44)*	170	Doxorubicin-based induction → RT → maintenance chemo	4 yr DFS, 32–54%	4 yr DFS for patients who received RT alone at the same institution 15%.
Maloisel, 1990 *(38)*	43	FAC → mastectomy for responders → FAC → RT	5 yr DFS 48%	
Chevallier, 1993 *(41)*	178	Anthracycline based induction → RT +/- surgery	Median DFS 17–22 mo	

C = cyclophosphamide, A = doxorubicin, F = 5FU.

REFERENCES

1. Schaake-Koning C, van der Linden EH, Hart G, Engelsman E. Adjuvant chemo- and hormonal therapy in locally advanced breast cancer: a randomized clinical study. *Int J Radiat Oncol Biol Phys* 1985; 11:1759–1763.
2. Rubens RD, Bartelink H, Engelsman E, et al. Locally advanced breast cancer: the contribution of cytotoxic and endocrine treatment to radiotherapy. An EORTC Breast Cancer Co-operative Group Trial (10792). *Eur J Cancer Clin Oncol* 1989; 25:667–678.
3. Grohn P, Heinonen E, Klefstrom P, Tarkkanen J. Adjuvant postoperative radiotherapy, chemotherapy, and immunotherapy in stage III breast cancer. *Cancer* 1984; 54:670–674.
4. Al-Sarraf M, LeBlanc M, Giri PG, et al. Chemoradiotherapy versus radiotherapy in patients with advanced nasopharyngeal cancer: phase III randomized Intergroup study 0099. *J Clin Oncol* 1998; 16:1310–1317.
5. Furuse K, Fukuoka M, Kawahara M, et al. Phase III study of concurrent versus sequential thoracic radiotherapy in combination with mitomycin, vindesine, and cisplatin in unresectable stage III non-small-cell lung cancer. *J Clin Oncol* 1999; 17:2692–2699.
6. Peters WA 3rd, Liu PY, Barrett RJ 2nd, et al. Concurrent chemotherapy and pelvic radiation therapy compared with pelvic radiation therapy alone as adjuvant therapy after radical surgery in high-risk early-stage cancer of the cervix. *J Clin Oncol* 2000; 18:1606–1613.
7. Johnston PG, Lenz HJ, Leichman CG, et al. Thymidylate synthase gene and protein expression correlate and are associated with response to 5-fluorouracil in human colorectal and gastric tumors. *Cancer Res* 1995; 55:1407–1412.
8. Byfield JE, Calabro-Jones P, Klisak I, Kulhanian F. Pharmacologic requirements for obtaining sensitization of human tumor cells in vitro to combined 5-Fluorouracil or ftorafur and X rays. *Int J Radiat Oncol, Biol, Phy* 1982; 8:1923–1933.
9. Lawrence TS, Davis MA, Maybaum J. Dependence of 5-fluorouracil-mediated radiosensitization on DNA- directed effects. Int J Radiat Oncol Biol Phys 1994; 29:519–523.
10. Janjan NA, Crane CN, Feig BW, et al. Prospective trial of preoperative concomitant boost radiotherapy with continuous infusion 5-fluorouracil for locally advanced rectal cancer. *Int J Radiat Oncol Biol Phys* 2000; 47:713–718.
11. Cafiero F, Gipponi M, Peressini A, Bertoglio S, Lionetto R. Preliminary analysis of a randomized clinical trial of adjuvant postoperative RT vs. postoperative RT plus 5-FU and levamisole in patients with TNM stage II-III resectable rectal cancer. *J Surg Oncol* 2000; 75:80–88.
12. Jabboury K, Holmes FA, Hortobagyi G. 5-Fluorouracil rechallenge by protracted infusion in refractory breast cancer. *Cancer* 1989; 64:793–797.
13. Formenti SC, Uziely B, Dunnington G, et al. Continuous infusion (ci) 5-fluorouracil (FU) with radiation in locally advanced breast cancer: clinicopathological and biological correlates (Meeting abstract). *Proc Annu Meet Am Soc Clin Oncol* 1995; 14:A358.
14. Formenti SC, Dunnington G, Uzieli B, et al. Original *p53* status predicts for pathological response in locally advanced breast cancer patients treated preoperatively with continuous infusion 5-fluorouracil and radiation therapy. *Int J Radiat Oncol, Biol, Physics* 1997; 39:1059–1068.
15. Kuerer HM, Newman LA, Smith TL, et al. Clinical course of breast cancer patients with complete pathologic primary tumor and axillary lymph node response to doxorubicin-based neoadjuvant chemotherapy. *J Clin Oncol* 1999; 17:460–469.
16. Merajver SD, Weber BL, Cody R, et al. Breast conservation and prolonged chemotherapy for locally advanced breast cancer: the University of Michigan experience. *J Clin Oncol* 1997; 15:2873–2881.
17. Morrell LE, Lee YJ, Hurley J, et al. A Phase II trial of neoadjuvant methotrexate, vinblastine, doxorubicin, and cisplatin in the treatment of patients with locally advanced breast carcinoma. *Cancer* 1998; 82:503–511.
18. Powles TJ, Hickish TF, Makris A, et al. Randomized trial of chemoendocrine therapy started before or after surgery for treatment of primary breast cancer. *J Clin Oncol* 1995; 13:547–552.
19. Karlsson YA, Malmstrom PO, Hatschek T, et al. Multimodality treatment of 128 patients with locally advanced breast carcinoma in the era of mammography screening using standard polychemotherapy with 5-fluorouracil, epirubicin, and cyclophosphamide: prognostic and therapeutic implications. *Cancer* 1998; 83:936–947.
20. Zambetti M, Oriana S, Quattrone P, et al. Combined sequential approach in locally advanced breast cancer. *Annals Oncol* 1999; 10:305–310.

21. Wahl AF, Donaldson KL, Fairchild C, et al. Loss of normal *p53* function confers sensitization to Taxol by increasing G2/M arrest and apoptosis. *Nature Med* 1996; 2:72–79.
22. Woods CM, Zhu J, McQueney PA, Bollag D, Lazarides E. Taxol-induced mitotic block triggers rapid onset of a *p53*-independent apoptotic pathway. *Mol Med* 1995; 1:506–526.
23. Kandioler-Eckersberger D, Ludwig C, Rudas M, et al. T*P53* mutation and *p53* overexpression for prediction of response to neoadjuvant treatment in breast cancer patients. *Clin Cancer Res* 2000; 6:50–56.
24. Milas L, Hunter NR, Kurdoglu B, et al. Kinetics of mitotic arrest and apoptosis in murine mammary and ovarian tumors treated with taxol. *Cancer Chemother Pharmacol* 1995; 35:297–303.
25. Symmans W, Volm M, Shapiro R, et al. Paclitaxel-induced apoptosis and mitotic arrest assessed by serial needle aspiration: implications for early prediction of breast cancer response to neoadjuvant treatment. *Clin Cancer Res* 2000; 6:4610–4617.
26. Formenti SC, Symmans WF, Volm M, et al. Concurrent paclitaxel and radiation therapy for breast cancer. *Semin Radiat Oncol* 1999; 9:34–42.
27. Horwitz S, Zambetti M, Oriana S, et al. Taxol: Mechanisms of action and resistance. *JNCI Monographs* 1993; 15:55–61.
28. Kavallaris M, Kuo DYS, Burkhart CA, et al. Taxol-resistant epithelial ovarian tumors are associated with altered expression of specific beta-tubulin isotypes. *J Clin Invest* 1997; 100:1282–1293.
29. Nguyen HL, Chari S, Gruber D, Lue CM, Chapin SJ, Bulinski JC. Overexpression of full- or partial-length MAP4 stabilizes microtubules and alters cell growth. *J Cell Sci* 1997; 110:281–294.
30. Zhang C. Genetic susceptibility to microtubule-active cancer chemotherapeutic drugs: *p53* action and the role of MAP4. *Proceedings of AACR* 1998; 1308.
31. Haldar S, Chintapalli J, Croce CM. Taxol induces Bcl-2 phosphorylation and death of prostate cancer cells. *Cancer Res* 1996; 56:1253–1255.
32. Montgomery RB, Guzman J, O'Rourke DM, Stahl WL. Expression of oncogenic epidermal growth factor receptor family kinases induces paclitaxel resistance and alters beta-tubulin isotype expression. *J Biol Chem* 2000; 275:17,358–17,363.
33. Pietras RJ, Poen JC, Gallardo D, Wongvipat PN, Lee HJ, Slamon DJ. Monoclonal antibody to HER-2/neu receptor modulates repair of radiation-induced DNA damage and enhances radiosensitivity of human breast cancer cells overexpressing this oncogene. *Cancer Res* 1999; 59:1347–1355.
34. Formenti S, et al. Low HER 2/NEU Gene Expression is Associated with Pathological Response to Primary Paclitaxel and Radiation in Locally Advanced Cancer (LABC). *Proceedings of ASTRO* 2000; 63.
35. Bonadonna G, Valagussa P, Brambilla C, et al. Primary chemotherapy in operable breast cancer: eight-year experience at the Milan Cancer Institute. *J Clin Oncol* 1998; 16:93–100.
36. Formenti SC, Cohen D, Tsao-Wei DD, et al. Clinical Course of Locally Advanced Breast Cancer (LABC) Patients with pathological response to primary concurrent 5-fluorouracil and radiation (FU/RT). *Int J Radiat Oncol Biol Phys* 2001; 51:195–196 (abstract 1039).
37. Buzdar AU, Singletary SE, Booser DJ, Frye DK, Wasaff B, Hortobagyi GN. Combined modality treatment of stage III and inflammatory breast cancer. M.D. Anderson Cancer Center experience. *Surg Oncol Clin N Am* 1995; 4:715–734.
38. Maloisel F, Dufour P, Bergerat JP, et al. Results of initial doxorubicin, 5-fluorouracil, and cyclophosphamide combination chemotherapy for inflammatory carcinoma of the breast. *Cancer* 1990; 65:851–855.
39. Viens P, Penault-Llorca F, Jacquemier J, et al. High-dose chemotherapy and haematopoietic stem cell transplantation for inflammatory breast cancer: pathologic response and outcome. *Bone Marrow Transplant* 1998; 21:249–254.
40. Cagnoni PJ, Nieto Y, Shpall EJ, et al. High-dose chemotherapy with autologous hematopoietic progenitor-cell support as part of combined modality therapy in patients with inflammatory breast cancer. *J Clin Oncol* 1998; 16:1661–1668.
41. Chevallier B, Bastit P, Graic Y, et al. The Centre H. Becquerel studies in inflammatory non metastatic breast cancer. Combined modality approach in 178 patients. *Br J Cancer* 1993; 67:594–601.
42. Fields JN, Perez CA, Kuske RR, Fineberg BB, Bartlett N. Inflammatory carcinoma of the breast: treatment results on 107 patients. *Int J Radiat Oncol Biol Phys* 1989; 17:249–255.
43. Thoms WW Jr, McNeese MD, Fletcher GH, Buzdar AU, Singletary SE, Oswald MJ. Multimodal treatment for inflammatory breast cancer. *Int J Radiat Oncol Biol Phys* 1989; 17:739–745.
44. Rouesse J, Friedman S, Sarrazin D, et al. Primary chemotherapy in the treatment of inflammatory breast carcinoma: a study of 230 cases from the Institut Gustave-Roussy. *J Clin Oncol* 1986; 4:1765–1771.

45. Thomas E, Buzdar A, Hortobagyi G, et al. Long-Term Follow Up of Stage III Breast Cancer-Combined Modality Treatment with Anthracycline Containing Chemotherapy (CT): The MD Anderson Experience (Meeting abstract). *Proc Annu Meet Am Soc Clin Oncol* 1999; 18:A284.
46. Honkoop AH, Luykx-de Bakker SA, Hoekman K, et al. Prolonged neoadjuvant chemotherapy with GM-CSF in locally advanced breast cancer. *Oncologist* 1999; 4:106–111.
47. Dhingra K, Esparza-Guerra L, Valero V, et al. A Phase III Randomized Trial of Dose-Intensive, Neoadjuvant 5FU, Doxorubicin, Cyclophosphamide (FAC) with G-CSF (filgrastim) in Locally Advanced Breast Cancer (LABC)-Efficacy and Safety Data (Meeting abstract). *Proc Annu Meet Am Soc Clin Oncol* 1999; 18:A278.
48. Eltahir A, Heys SD, Hutcheon AW, et al. Treatment of large and locally advanced breast cancers using neoadjuvant chemotherapy. *Am J Surg* 1998; 175:127–132.
49. De Matteis A, Montella M, Iannuzzo M, et al. Multimodal treatment strategy for locally advanced breast cancer. *J Chemother* 1998; 10:476–483.
50. Schwartz GF, Birchansky CA, Komarnicky LT, et al. Induction chemotherapy followed by breast conservation for locally advanced carcinoma of the breast. *Cancer* 1994; 73:362–369.
51. Ayash LJ, Elias A, Ibrahim J, et al. High-dose multimodality therapy with autologous stem-cell support for stage IIIB breast carcinoma. *J Clin Oncol* 1998; 16:1000–1007.
52. Kuerer HM, Newman LA, Buzdar AU, et al. Residual metastatic axillary lymph nodes following neoadjuvant chemotherapy predict disease-free survival in patients with locally advanced breast cancer. *Am J Surg* 1998; 176:502–509.

13 Combined Modality Therapy for Gastric, Pancreatic, and Biliary Tract Carcinomas

Alexandria Phan, MD *and Jaffer A. Ajani,* MD

Contents

1. COMBINED MODALITY THERAPY

Localized cancers are not often treated using a single modality. Rather, they are approached in a multidisciplinary manner. This approach has evolved over the past 15 yr to include medicine, surgery, radiation oncology, and gastroenterology.

2. GASTRIC CANCER

2.1. Background

2.1.1. Epidemiology

Gastric cancer is more common than esophageal cancer is in western countries. An estimated 22,000 new cases of gastric cancer were expected to be diagnosed and 13,000 deaths were expected to result from it in the United States in the year 2001. However, worldwide, gastric cancer is the second most common neoplasm, representing approx 10% of new cancer cases and accounting for more than 12% of all cancer deaths although the incidence and mortality rates of this disease have been declining in most countries. Men are more frequently afflicted by gastric cancer than women at a ratio of approx 2:1. Also, the incidence of gastric cancer increases with age with most cases occurring between the ages of 65 and 74 yr. Gastric cancer is most prevalent in Asian countries with almost 40% of newly diagnosed cases found in China. However, when adjusted for age, the highest occurrence rate of new gastric cancer cases is in Japan.

From: *Chemoradiation in Cancer Therapy*
Edited by: H. Choy

In addition, from 1992 to 1997, only 21% of patients having gastric cancer presented with localized disease, and in all patients as a whole the 5-yr survival rate is 20% or less *(1)*.

2.1.2. Etiology and Risk Factors

Diet and environment have been implicated in the development of gastric cancer. Specifically, a diet low in vegetables and fruits and high in salts and nitrates has been associated with an increased risk of gastric carcinoma *(2)*. Occupational exposure to carcinogens in coal mining and processing of nickel, rubber, and timber has also been reported to increase the risk of gastric cancer *(3–6)*. Studies have also reported an association between gastric adenocarcinoma and intestinal metaplasia *(7)*. In yet another study, intestinal metaplasia was found in 94% of resected gastric cancers, suggesting that it is a premalignant condition *(8)*. Furthermore, both prior gastric resection of benign disease and pernicious anemia have been anecdotally reported to be associated with an increased risk of gastric malignancies. *Helicobacter pylori* infection may be a contributing factor in gastric carcinogenesis. The genetic abnormalities associated with gastric cancer have not been successfully elucidated, although a number of abnormalities have been described, particularly those of the *p53* and *APC* genes.

2.1.3. Clinical Manifestations

Most gastric cancers are at an advanced stage when diagnosed. Presenting signs and symptoms are often nonspecific and typically include pain, early satiety, weight loss, vomiting, and anorexia; hematemesis is the presenting manifestation in 10–20% of patients. Peritoneal implants, abdominal mass, ascites, hepatomegaly, and nodal involvement are among the other possible physical findings.

2.1.4. Screening and Diagnosis

Routine screening of gastric cancer is generally not performed in western countries. However, routine mass screening for gastric cancers is performed in Japan. Methods of screening include endoscopy and barium X-ray. Once a diagnosis is obtained, the staging work-up may include computed tomography (CT) scans and endoscopic ultrasound. Laparoscopic staging is also used commonly.

2.1.5. Pathology

Adenocarcinoma is the predominant form of gastric cancer, accounting for approx 95% of all cases. Histologically, adenocarcinomas are classified as intestinal or diffuse; the mixed type occurs rarely. Intestinal-type cancer is characterized by cohesive cells that form gland-like structures and is often preceded by intestinal metaplasia. Diffuse-type cancer is composed of infiltrating cells that infrequently form masses or ulcers. Other histologic types, including squamous cell carcinomas, lymphomas, small cell carcinomas, carcinoid tumors, leiomyosarcomas, and gastrointestinal soft tissue sarcomas are infrequent.

2.1.6. Staging and Prognosis

Currently, the most frequently used staging system for gastric cancers is the TNM system (Table 1). The Japanese staging system relies on anatomic distribution but the American Joint Committee on Cancer (AJCC) system relies on the number of involved nodes. Traditional prognostic factors for gastric cancer include tumor size and number of involved nodes. It had been suggested that aneuploidy and diffuse-type adenocarci-

Table 1
TNM Staging System for Gastric Cancer

Primary tumor (T)				
Tx	Primary tumor cannot be assessed			
T0	No evidence of primary tumor			
Tis	Carcinoma *in situ*: intraepithelial tumor with invasion of the lamina propria			
T1	Tumor invades lamina propria or submucosa			
T2	Tumor invades mucularis propria or subserosa			
T3	Tumor penetrates the serosa (visceral involvement) without invasion of adjacent structures			
T4	Tumor invades adjacent structures			
Regional lymph nodes (N)				
Nx	Regional node(s) cannot be assessed			
N0	No regional lymph node metastasis			
N1	Metastasis in 1–6 regional lymph nodes			
N2	Metastasis in 7–15 regional lymph nodes			
N3	Metastasis in >15 regional lymph nodes			
Distant metastases (M)				
Mx	Distant metastasis cannot be assessed			
M0	No distant metastases			
M1	Distant metastases			
Stage grouping				5-Yr survival rate (%)
Stage 0 (*in situ*)	Tis	N0	M0	>90
Stage IA	T1	N0	M0	60–80
Stage IB	T1	N1	M0	50–60
	T2	N0	M0	
Stage II	T1	N2	M0	30–40
	T2	N1	M0	
	T3	N0	M0	
Stage IIIA	T2	N2	M0	20
	T3	N1	M0	
	T4	N0	M0	
Stage IIIB	T3	N2	M0	10
Stage IV	T4	N1-2	M0	<5
	Any T	N3	M0	
	Any T	Any N	M1	

noma have a poorer outcome. Finally, the prognostic significance of various oncogenes and tumor suppressor genes is currently under investigation.

2.1.7. Treatment

The only potentially curative treatment modality for localized gastric cancer is surgery; however, overall 5-yr survival rate often does not exceed 40%. Patients having unresectable localized gastric cancers but no evidence of metastatic disease can be expected to survive 5–6 mo. Palliative measures for advanced gastric cancer can include

Table 2
Standard Treatment According to Stage of Gastric Cancer

Stage	*Standard treatment option*
0	Surgery
IA	Surgery
IB	Surgery +/- chemoradiation
II	Surgery +/- chemoradiation
IIIA	Surgery +/- chemoradiation
IIIB	Palliative chemotherapy, radiotherapy +/- surgery, neoadjuvant chemoradiation
IV	Palliative chemotherapy, radiotherapy +/- surgery, neoadjuvant chemoradiation

surgery, radiotherapy, and chemoradiotherapy; palliative resection or bypass is often not recommended. Also, the treatment of gastric cancer depends on the disease stage at the time of diagnosis (Table 2).

2.1.8. Locoregional Disease—Surgery

The current treatment recommendation for patients having local-regional gastric cancer is surgical resection. The objectives of this treatment are to confirm resectability, completely remove the cancer, provide pathologic staging, and reestablish gastrointestinal continuity. Laparoscopy has emerged as an excellent tool for evaluating the extent of disease prior to surgery. However, subtotal gastrectomy is preferred over total gastrectomy, as it leads to comparable survival but lower morbidity. Additionally, the recommended margin of resection is 5 cm of normal gastric tissue. The extent of gastric resection depends on the location and size of the primary tumor.

The extent of lymph node dissection at the time of gastrectomy continues to be controversial. D1 lymphadenectomy involves only the removal of pericardial or perigastric lymph nodes, while D2 lymphadenectomy involves the removal of lymph nodes along the celiac, left gastric, splenic, and hepatic arteries. Retrospective data have shown that extended lymphadenectomy (D2 dissection or greater) is associated with more precise staging, improved locoregional control, and enhanced survival in comparison with historical controls. The more extensive lymph node resection is safe and does not increase morbidity *(9)*. However, it also has been shown that resection of the higher echelon of lymph nodes should be done only by experienced surgeons in large centers. In addition, prospective western studies comparing D1 and D2 lymphadenectomy have demonstrated higher postoperative morbidity and mortality without a significant improvement of long-term survival *(10–12)*.

Patients with T3–T4 tumors are at the highest risk for locoregional recurrence after potentially curative surgery regardless of their nodal and metastatic status. Even patients having node-negative disease (T3N0) have a gastric cancer-related mortality rate of about 50% within 5 yr. However, mortality is significantly worse in patients having positive nodes.

2.1.9. Locoregional Disease—Preoperative Therapy

Because surgical resection is the only curative treatment modality, several clinical trials have been carried out to improve the success of gastric cancer. Furthermore, prompted by the promising results and acceptable toxicity of preoperative chemoradiation in other parts of the gastrointestinal tract, such as the esophagus and rectum, there is growing enthusiasm for this modality in gastric cancer. Preoperative therapy used for this disease has included radiotherapy, chemotherapy, and chemoradiotherapy.

In addition, Safran et al. *(13)* presented preliminary data on preoperative chemoradiotherapy using paclitaxel (Taxol) in patients having T2-T4 N0-N3 adenocarcinoma. They found an overall response rate of 63% with acceptable toxicity.

2.1.10. Locoregional Disease—Adjuvant Therapy

The 5-yr survival rate after "curative resection" for gastric cancer is only 30–40%. Treatment failure in these cases stems from a combination of local or regional recurrence and distant metastasis. This has stimulated interest in adjuvant and postoperative therapy in the hope of improving treatment results.

The role of postoperative chemotherapy for gastric carcinoma is still not clearly defined. Numerous prospective, randomized trials have been conducted in the United States and Europe, producing conflicting results. For example, Hermans et al. *(14)*, in a meta-analysis of 123 trials, 11 of which could be analyzed for crude mortality odds, showed no improvement in survival after adjuvant chemotherapy. However, at the 1998 American Society of Clinical Oncology (ASCO) meeting, Earle et al. *(15)* presented a reanalysis of the literature. Twelve trials met the criteria for inclusion in this meta-analysis. They found a small survival benefit in the group that received adjuvant chemotherapy. Currently, postoperative adjuvant chemotherapy is not recommended.

The results of a large clinical trial designed to evaluate the role of chemoradiotherapy in patients having resected gastric cancer were presented at the 2000 ASCO meeting. The study, INT-0116, was designed to evaluate postoperative adjuvant chemoradiation in these patients. A total of 556 patients having adenocarcinoma of the gastroesophageal junction were randomized to either receive postoperative chemoradiation or undergo observation after curative resection. The chemoradiotherapy regimen consisted of one cycle of 5-fluorouracil (5-FU) (425 mg/m^2)/leucovorin (LV) (20 mg/m^2) given daily for five cycles followed by 4500 cGy of radiation (180 cGy/day) given with 5-FU/LV (400 mg/m^2 and 20 mg/m^2) on d 1–4 and the last 3 d of irradiation. One month after the completion of irradiation, two cycles of daily 5-FU/LV (425 and 20 mg/m^2, respectively) were given five times daily at monthly intervals. At a median follow-up of 3.3 yr, the 3-yr disease-free survival rate was 49% in the treatment group and 32% in the observation group, while the 3-yr overall survival rate was 52% in the treatment group and 41% in the observation group. These differences were statistically significant. The median survival duration was also improved from 27 to 42 mo in the two arms of patients. As a result of this large trial, postoperative chemoradiation is now considered a standard of care for R0 resected high-risk locally advanced adenocarcinoma of the stomach and gastroesophageal junction *(16)*.

2.1.11. Discussion

The major advance in the treatment of local-regional gastric carcinoma had been the new standard of adjuvant chemoradiotherapy following a curative resection. Laparoscopy is more or less established as a staging procedure prior to surgery. Staging with endoscopic ultrasonography has improved. New strategies will include the use of preoperative approaches and incorporation of new agents. Similar to the carcinoma of the esophagus, the use of molecular markers to predict response and survival is needed. Preoperative chemoradiotherapy needs to be further investigated in this disease.

3. PANCREATIC CANCER

3.1. Background

3.1.1. Epidemiology

Pancreatic cancer is a relatively rare malignancy, with approx 29,000 new cases diagnosed in the United States in 1998. Its incidence has decreased slightly over the past two decades, primarily due to a steady decline in the incidence among white male individuals. Furthermore, carcinoma of the pancreas is mainly a disease of the elderly, as more than 80% of cases occur between the ages of 60 and 80, and cases below the age of 40 are rare. In 1998, approx 28,900 deaths in the United States were attributed to pancreatic cancer, making it the fourth most common cause of cancer death in both men and women. The prognosis is dismal for patients having pancreatic cancer: The median survival duration is 6 mo from diagnosis, and less than 5% of patients survive 5 yr. Carcinoma of the pancreas is one of the most aggressive solid tumors, representing a major public health problem and significant clinical challenge *(17–19)*.

3.1.2. Etiology and Risk Factors

Many dietary and environmental factors have been implicated as possible etiologic factors in the development of pancreatic cancer, but no definite causal relationships have been established. The strongest evidence points to cigarette smoking as a risk factor associated with pancreatic cancer *(20–24)*. Occupational exposure to certain chemicals has also been linked to pancreatic carcinoma *(25)*. Others in the high-risk group include stone miners, cement workers, gardeners, textile workers, and leather tanners *(17,26)*.

Recent advances in the understanding of human genetics have brought about increasing appreciation of hereditary as a cause of pancreatic cancer. Abnormal changes in the oncogene *K-ras*, and tumor suppressor genes *p53*, *p16*, *DPC4*, and *BRCA2* have been linked with carcinoma of the pancreas *(27-28)*.

3.1.3. Pathology

The pancreas is both an endocrine and exocrine organ. However, most cancers (95%) occur in the exocrine portion. Histologically, ductal adenocarcinoma accounts for more than 80% of all pancreatic malignancies. Approximately 60% of all pancreatic cancers occur in the head of the pancreas, with 15% occurring in the body or tail and 20% diffusely involving the gland *(29)*.

Cancers in the head of the pancreas are usually less than 5 cm in diameter and are often associated with pancreatic and common bile duct obstruction, adjacent duodenum invasion, and portal vein or superior mesentery artery occlusion. Cancers in the tail of the pancreas are usually larger (5–10 cm) at the time of diagnosis and associated with splenic vein obstruction. Also, early subclinical metastases are characteristic of pancreatic cancer as less than 20% of patients have disease confined to the pancreas at the time of diagnosis. In addition, 40% of patients have locally advanced disease (regional lymph node and adjacent organ involvement), and more than 40% have distant metastases at diagnosis *(30)*. The most commonly involved distant organ is the liver, followed by the lungs, bone, and brain.

3.1.4. Clinical Manifestations

The early symptoms of pancreatic cancer tend to be nonspecific, thus delaying diagnosis in 80–90% of patients. Pain is the single most common presenting symptom;

specifically, the pain is constant and radiates to the middle and upper back, and it is due to invasion of the celiac and mesenteric plexuses *(31–33)*. Obstructive jaundice occurs in approx 50% of all patients and up to 90% of those having cancer in the head of the pancreas *(34)*. However, obstructive jaundice may represent less advanced cancer because patients seek medical attention early. Nausea, anorexia, weight loss, and fatigue also occur frequently.

Currently, contrast-enhancing helical CT is considered a mainstay in detecting a suspected pancreatic mass and determining its resectability *(35)*. Many studies have confirmed the accuracy of helical CT in predicting resectability, with a resectability rate approaching 80% *(36)*.

Other important diagnostic procedures are angiography, endoscopic retrograde cholangiopancreatography (ERCP), endoscopic ultrasound (EUS), and laparoscopy; angiography is not used frequently. ERCP is not helpful if a pancreatic mass is seen on a CT scan, but it is needed to place a stent to relieve obstructive jaundice. EUS is a relatively new diagnostic tool for staging pancreatic cancer that can detect small intrapancreatic masses missed by CT. It may also become useful for obtaining tissue biopsy samples and instituting celiac plexus neurolysis for pain control *(86)*. Also, some have advocated using laparoscopy with peritoneal cytology to further assess resectability *(38,39)*. Direct laparoscopic visualization of the peritoneum, omentum, and liver surface can spare patients unnecessary surgery. Once a pancreatic mass is considered to be unresectable or if metastasis occurs, then a histologic diagnosis should be established by using direct fine-needle aspiration.

Currently, there are a number of potential serum markers, including carcinoembryonic antigen (CEA), tumor-associated carbohydrate antigen (CA 19-9), CA 125 antigen, and monoclonal antibody products (DUPAN-2, SPAN-1). The level of CEA is elevated in approx 50% of pancreatic cancer patients, but it is also increased in patients having many benign and malignant disorders *(40)*. Also, the CA 19-9 level is elevated in approx 80% of pancreatic cancer patients. Although it has some limitations, CA 19-9 is a reasonable marker for the management of pancreatic cancer as a diagnostic adjunct, prognostic indicator, and monitoring tool *(41,42)*.

3.1.5. Staging and Prognosis

The AJCC staging system, also known as the TNM staging system, is based on the extent of the primary tumor, regional lymph node involvement, and metastasis (Table 3). Unfortunately, this system is not clinically useful as it is only applicable when surgery is performed. For prognosis prediction and therapy selection, most centers rely on a clinical or radiographic staging system. The TNM system classifies pancreatic cancer into three groups: stage I, localized to the pancreas and surgically resectable; stage II, locally advanced and not surgically resectable; and stages III-IV, metastatic spread. Less than 15% of patients have stage I pancreatic cancer, and less than 10% of patients are expected to survive to 1 yr.

3.1.6. Treatment

Surgery, radiotherapy, and chemotherapy are the treatment options for patients having pancreatic cancer. These treatment modalities have had a limited impact.

3.1.7. Resectable Disease—Surgery

For a resectable mass located in the head of the pancreas, pancreatoduodenectomy (Whipple procedure) is considered the standard of care *(43)*. This operation involves the

Table 3
TNM Staging System for Pancreatic Cancer

Primary tumor (T)			
Tx	Primary tumor cannot be assessed		
T0	No evidence of primary tumor		
Tis	Carcinoma *in situ*		
T1	Tumor limited to the pancreas ≤ 2 cm in greatest dimension		
T2	Tumor limited to the pancreas > 2 cm in greatest dimension		
T3	Tumor extends directly into any of the following: duodenum, bile duct, peripancreatic tissue		
T4	Tumor extends directly into any of the following: stomach, spleen, colon, adjacent large vessels		
Regional lymph nodes (N)			
Nx	Regional node(s) cannot be assessed		
N0	No regional lymph node metastasis		
N1	Regional lymph node metastasis		
pN1a	Metastasis in a single regional lymph node		
pN1b	Metastasis in multiple regional lymph nodes		
Distant metastases (M)			
Mx	Distant metastasis cannot be assessed		
M0	No distant metastases		
M1	Distant metastases		
Stage grouping			
Stage 0 (*in situ*)	Tis	N0	M0
Stage I	T1-2	N0	M0
Stage II	T3	N0	M0
Stage III	T1-3	N1	M0
Stage IVA	T4	Any N	M0
Stage IVB	Any T	Any N	M1

en bloc removal of the distal stomach and duodenum, the first portion of the jejunum, and the head and part of the body of the pancreas. However, despite successful surgery performed with curative intent, the prognosis remains unfavorable, even in this selected group of patients, with 5-yr survival rate of only 10–30% *(44)*. Long-term postoperative morbidity further reduces quality of life.

3.1.8. Resectable Disease—Postoperative Therapies

The incidence of local recurrence of pancreatic cancer after curative resection is 50–80%. Patients who undergo pancreatoduodenectomy alone have a median survival duration of 12 mo. However, a regimen combining external-beam radiotherapy (EBRT) with concomitant 5-FU chemotherapy has been shown to prolong survival in patients having locally advanced disease *(45)*. Based on these data, the Gastrointestinal Tumor Study Group (GITSG) conducted a prospective, randomized study of adjuvant chemoradiation (5-FU at 500 mg/m^2 for 6 d plus 40-Gy radiotherapy therapy) following pancreato-duodenectomy *(46)*. This study demonstrated that EBRT and concomitant 5-FU improved survival after curative resection. The GITSG study also observed a median survival duration of 18 mo. However, because of the prolonged recovery time after surgery, 24% of the patients in the adjuvant arm of this study could not begin receiving chemoradiation until more than 10 wk after undergoing pancreatoduodenectomy. Other studies reported similar improved survival durations and delays in the administration of therapy *(47–49)*.

3.1.9. Resectable Disease—Preoperative Therapies

Despite its benefits, the administration of postoperative multimodality therapy is not possible in 24% of pancreatic cancer patients due to prolonged recovery time after pancreatoduodenectomy *(50)*. However, several facts support the preoperative use of chemoradiation. First, positive gross and microscopic margins of resection along the right lateral border of the superior mesenteric artery are common following pancreatoduodenectomy, suggesting that surgery alone may be inadequate for local tumor control *(51)*. Second, peritoneal dissemination due to surgical manipulation may be prevented by preoperative therapies. Third, because chemoradiation is administered before surgery, an extended postoperative recovery time does not affect recovery from multimodality therapy. Fourth, patients having disseminated disease that is evident upon restaging after chemoradiation are not subjected to unnecessary surgery. Finally, recent data suggest that preoperative chemoradiation may decrease the incidence of pancreaticojejunal anastomotic fistula, the most common complication following pancreatoduodenectomy *(50)*.

In a nonrandomized trial, Spitz et al. *(50)* compared the preoperative chemoradiation approach with standard adjuvant chemoradiotherapy. Preoperative radiotherapy was delivered either in the standard regimen of 50.4 Gy over 5.5 wk or at 30 Gy as rapid fractionation over 2 wk; postoperative irradiation was given up to a total dose of 50.4 Gy in standard fractionation. Both preoperative and postoperative radiotherapy were delivered concurrently with a continuous infusion 5-FU at 300 mg/m^2/d for 5 d weekly. At a median follow-up of 19 mo, patients who underwent preoperative and postoperative chemoradiation had similar treatment toxicity, patterns of recurrence, and survival.

Recent preoperative chemoradiation studies of resectable pancreatic cancer have demonstrated improved survival. One of the first of these evaluated preoperative therapy using 50.4 Gy standard fractionation irradiation with a concurrent continuous infusion of low-dose 5-FU in patients having resectable pancreatic adenocarcinoma *(52)*. The recurrence rate and median survival duration were better than those historically reported for patients only undergoing pancreatoduodenectomy *(53)*. These findings prompted further studies evaluating the role of preoperative chemoradiation in patients having resectable pancreatic cancer. Data on 132 consecutive patients who received preoperative 5-FU and 30.0–50.4 Gy of irradiation demonstrated a median survival duration of 21 mo *(54)*. Using similar preoperative therapies, smaller studies demonstrated similar findings of improved survival *(50,55,56)*.

Despite the potential for better local-regional control using preoperative or adjuvant chemoradiotherapy, the prognosis of pancreatic cancer remains poor. Treatment failure is primarily due to distant metastases. Also, the progress in the treatment of pancreatic cancers is hindered by the absence of effective systemic agents. New approaches continue to be developed that hopefully will alter the natural history of this disease.

Gemcitabine, a new pyrimidine antimetabolite, is of substantial interest as a radiosensitizer in the treatment of pancreatic cancer. An ongoing multi-institutional Phase II study of preoperative EBRT and concomitant gemcitabine therapy for resectable adenocarcinoma will provide useful information *(57–60)*.

Several Phase II and III trials are currently accruing patients for evaluation of the role of different preoperative and postoperative chemoradiotherapy regimens for resected pancreatic cancers. Specifically, Radiation Therapy Oncology Group (RTOG) protocol 97-04 was designed for patients with complete resection of adenocarcinoma of the pancreas. Patients are being randomized to receive one cycle of either 5-FU or gemcitabine followed by continuous infusion 5-FU plus radiotherapy (50.4 Gy) followed by additional 5-FU or gemcitabine depending on the randomization. This study has accrued its initial target of 330 patients, but the total accrual target has now been extended to 500 or more patients to improve statistical power of the analysis. Another trial, RTOG 00-20, is being conducted to determine the efficacy of combined chemoradiation using gemcitabine and paclitaxel alone or with farnesyl transferase inhibitor R115777 for locally advanced pancreatic cancer. Results of these studies should elucidate the role of combined modality therapy in patients having resectable, locally advanced pancreatic cancer.

3.1.10. Discussion

Pancreatic carcinoma is one of the most rapidly fatal malignancies. The highest benefit will come from studies to detect early disease. Even in patients with localized pancreatic carcinoma, the curative resection rate is much less than desired and curatively resected tumors do not often result in prolonged survival of patients. A great deal of work is necessary. It would also be important to further understand molecular biology of this disease to facilitate early detection and potentially for developing more effective treatments.

4. GALLBLADDER AND BILIARY SYSTEM CANCERS

4.1. Background

4.1.1. Epidemiology

Malignancies of the biliary tract are uncommon in the United States, with approx 8000 cases reported annually; nearly two-thirds of these cases arise in the gallbladder, while the remainder (cholangiocarcinoma) originate from the bile ducts and periampullary region. However, gallbladder cancer occurs in epidemic proportions in many South American and Asian countries, particularly affecting women.

Gallbladder carcinoma is diagnosed approx 5000 times a year in the United States, making it the most common biliary tract cancer and fifth most common gastrointestinal tract cancer. Also, approx 4500 cases of bile duct cancer occur each year in the United States. Women are more commonly afflicted than men, with a female-to-male ratio of 2.7:1.0. The median age at presentation of gallbladder cancer is 73 yr. In addition, an incidence five to six times that in the general population is seen in southwestern Native Americans, Mexicans, Hispanics, and Alaskans.

Bile duct malignancy is diagnosed approx 3000 times a year in the United States and is found equally in men and women. Extrahepatic bile duct cancers occur primarily in older individuals, with a median age at diagnosis of 70 yr.

4.1.2. Etiology and Risk Factors

The risk of gallbladder cancer is higher in patients having cholelithiasis or a calcified gallbladder and typhoid carriers, while ulcerative colitis is a clear risk factor for bile duct cancer. Patients having ulcerative colitis have an incidence of bile duct cancer that is 9–21 times higher than that in the general population.

Primary sclerosing cholangitis, congenital anomalies of the pancreaticobiliary tree, and parasitic infections are also associated with bile duct cancer.

4.1.3. Pathology

About 85% of gallbladder malignancies are adenocarcinomas, whereas the remaining 15% are squamous cell or mixed cancers. The major route of extension of gallbladder cancer is locoregional rather than distant, with 25% of patients having lymphatic involvement and 70% having direct extension into the liver. Similarly, more than 90% of bile duct malignancies are adenocarcinomas. The subtypes of bile duct adenocarcinomas include papillary, nodular, and sclerosing. The papillary and nodular types occur more frequently in the distal bile duct, whereas the sclerosing type is found most often in the proximal bile duct. Papillary adenocarcinomas of the bile duct have the best prognosis.

4.1.4. Clinical Manifestations

Gallbladder cancers are often diagnosed incidentally or in late stages. The symptoms can include pain, vomiting, fatty food intolerance, anorexia, jaundice, and weight loss. Unlike gallbladder cancer, however, the most common symptom of bile duct cancer is painless jaundice, especially in patients having cancer involving the proximal bile duct. Nonspecific symptoms also can be manifested.

Additionally, ultrasound may show a thickened gallbladder wall or tumor extension into the liver. However, CT scans are more helpful in assessing adenopathy and the spread of disease into the liver, porta hepatis, or adjacent structures. ERCP or transhepatic cholangiography (THC) may be useful in the presence of obstruction to localize primary tumor.

Cholangiocarcinomas may present with biliary obstruction and can be mistaken for metastatic adenocarcinoma of unknown primary origin. Ultrasound should be used in the primary evaluation of jaundice. CT is complementary to ultrasound, but both tests are accurate in staging in only 50% of patients and in determining resectability in less than 45% of patients. However, cholangiography can define cholangiocarcinomas more clearly. In addition, percutaneous transhepatic cholangiography is used for proximal lesions, and ERCP is used for distal lesions. Magnetic resonance cholangiopancreatography (MRCP) may replace invasive studies in the near future. Histologic confirmation of cancer can be obtained in 45–85% of patients with the use of exfoliate or brush cytology during cholangiography.

4.1.5. Staging and Prognosis

Gallbladder cancer is staged primarily at the time of surgery. Specifically, the stage is determined by lymphatic involvement and extension to adjacent structures (Table 4). The 5-yr survival rate is 83% in patients having T1 lesion, and only 33% in patients having T3 lesions. In patients who have involvement of the lymph nodes or metastatic disease, the 5-yr survival rate ranges from 0–15%.

More than 70% of patients having bile duct cancer have local extension, lymph node involvement, or distal spread. The AJCC staging system for bile duct cancer is shown in Table 5. The median survival duration is approx 12 mo in patients having localized cancer but less than 8 mo in those having metastatic disease. Survival is also related to cancer location, with patients having distal lesions doing better than those having mid or proximal cancers. Also, curative resection and negative margins result in improved survival.

4.1.6. Treatment

The treatment options for localized gallbladder carcinoma and cholangiocarcinoma include surgery and chemoradiation.

Table 4
TNM Staging System for Gallbladder Cancer

Primary tumor (T)				
Tx	Primary tumor cannot be assessed			
T0	No evidence of primary tumor			
Tis	Carcinoma *in situ*			
T1	Tumor invades the lamina propria or muscle layer			
T1a	Tumor invades the lamina propria			
T1b	Tumor invades the muscle layer			
T2	Tumor invades the perimuscular connective tissue; no extension beyond the serosa or into the liver			
T3	Tumor perforates the serosa (visceral peritoneum), directly invades one adjacent organ, or both (extension ≤ 2 cm into the liver)			
T4	Tumor extends > 2 cm into the liver and/or into two or more adjacent organs (stomach, duodenum, colon, pancreas, omentum, extrahepatic bile ducts, any involvement of the liver)			
Regional lymph nodes (N)				
Nx	Regional node(s) cannot be assessed			
N0	No regional lymph node metastasis			
N1	Metastasis in the cystic ducts, pericholedochal lymph nodes, and/or hilar lymph nodes (i.e., in the hepatoduodenal ligament)			
N2	Metastasis in the peripancreatic (head only), periduodenal, periportal, celiac, and/or superior mesenteric lymph nodes			
Distant metastases (M)				
Mx	Distant metastasis cannot be assessed			
M0	No distant metastases			
M1	Distant metastases			
Stage grouping				5-Yr survival rate (%)
Stage 0 (*in situ*)	Tis	N0	M0	>95
Stage I	T1	N0	M0	85–100
Stage II	T2	N0	M0	50–80
Stage III	T1-3	N1	M0	40–60
	T3	N0	M0	
Stage IVA	T4	N0	M0	30–40
	T4	N1	M0	
Stage IVB	Any T	N2	M0	<10
	Any T	Any N	M1	

4.1.7. Treatment—Surgical Management

Surgical management of gallbladder carcinoma is based on local extension of the cancer. For example, T1 lesions require cholecystectomy alone, while many experts have advocated radical cholecystectomy for T2 lesions. There are several reasons for this recommendation. Specifically, Yamaguchi and Tsuneyoshi *(61)* reported 44% positive microscopic margins in patients having T2 lesions who underwent only simple cholecystectomy. Additionally, T2 lesions are associated with an increased incidence of nodal

Table 5
TNM Staging System for Bile Duct Cancer

Primary tumor (T)			
Tx	Primary tumor cannot be assessed		
T0	No evidence of primary tumor		
Tis	Carcinoma *in situ*		
T1	Tumor invades the subepithelial connective tissue or fibromuscular layer		
T1a	Tumor invades the subepithelial connective tissue		
T1b	Tumor invades the fibromuscular layer		
T2	Tumor invades the perifibromuscular connective tissue		
T3	Tumor invades adjacent structures: liver, pancreas, duodenum, gallbladder, colon, stomach		
Regional lymph nodes (N)			
Nx	Regional node(s) cannot be assessed		
N0	No regional lymph node metastasis		
N1	Metastasis in the cystic ducts, pericholedochal lymph nodes, and/or hilar lymph nodes (i.e., in the hepatoduodenal ligament)		
N2	Metastasis in the peripancreatic (head only), periduodenal, periportal, celiac, superior mesenteric, and/or posterior pancreaticoduodenal lymph nodes		
Distant metastases (M)			
Mx	Distant metastasis cannot be assessed		
M0	No distant metastases		
M1	Distant metastases		
Stage grouping			
Stage 0 (*in situ*)	Tis	N0	M0
Stage I	T1	N0	M0
Stage II	T2	N0	M0
Stage III	T1-2	N1	M0
	T1-2	N2	M0
Stage IVA	T3	Any N	M0
Stage IVB	Any T	Any N	M1

metastases and higher local-regional recurrence rate after curative resection *(62,63)*. Furthermore, radical cholecystectomy should include wedge resection of the gallbladder bed and porta hepatis lymphadenectomy. With more aggressive surgical resection, the overall survival duration is improved in patients having T2 gallbladder cancer *(64)*, and cancer with only gallbladder nodal metastases may be curable and should be resected. Cancer with nodal metastases beyond the pericholedochal nodes is often incurable.

The rate of resectability is only 15–20% for proximal bile duct carcinomas but up to 70% for distal lesions. In addition, there is little benefit to preoperative decompression of the biliary tree in patients having obstructive jaundice *(65,66)*. However, this procedure is frequently practiced. For proximal cancers, local excision is often possible. In particular, hepatic resection is indicated for upper bile duct cancers with quadrate lobe invasion or unilateral intrahepatic ductal or vascular involvement, and distal and midductal lesions may require pancreatoduodenectomy. Also, biliary–enteric continuity can be achieved using Roux-en-Y anastomosis. Finally, liver transplantation has significant morbidity and no demonstrated survival benefit; thus, it is not a routine option *(67–69)*.

4.1.8. Treatment—Chemoradiation

The role of preoperative therapy for resectable disease remains ill defined. Local recurrence after curative resection of gallbladder cancer can be as high as 86% *(70)*. Resected bile duct cancers have a rate of local recurrence of 25–40% *(71)*.

Clinical trials are being performed to evaluate the role of preoperative therapy in improving the overall survival duration in patients having localized gallbladder cancer and cholangiocarcinoma. For example, one prospective nonrandomized Phase II study involved a preoperative continuous infusion of 5-FU and concomitant radiotherapy in 18 potentially resectable gallbladder cancer patients. At a median follow-up of 2 yr, 39% of the patients were still alive, and only 9% had a local recurrence after curative resection *(72)*. A retrospective analysis of patients having extrahepatic cholangiocarcinoma in one institution suggested that preoperative chemoradiation for potentially resectable disease resulted in a complete pathologic response rate of 33% with a significantly improved rate of margin-negative resection *(73)*. There are still no prospective data to support adjuvant radiotherapy or chemotherapy for gallbladder cancers or cholangiocarcinomas, though. However, based on some preliminary data, preoperative chemoradiation is recommended frequently for patients having resected biliary tract cancer that is at T3 and/or is node positive.

4.1.9. Discussion

Gall bladder carcinoma is rampant in certain parts of the world. For example, it is the number one cause of death in women in Chile. Little has been known about these diseases. Since local relapse and low resectability remain major problems, more efforts are necessary to study preoperative chemoradiotherapy approaches and better staging techniques.

ACKNOWLEDGMENT

Supported in part by grants from Smith, Cantu, Dallas, and Ziffer Families and the Rivercreek Foundation.

REFERENCES

1. Anonymous, SEER Cancer Statistics Review, 1973–98. 1998.
2. Neugut AI, Hayek M, Howe G. Epidemiology of gastric cancer. *Semin Oncol* 1996; 23(3):281–291.
3. Gonzalez CA, et al. Occupation and gastric cancer in Spain. *Scand J Work Environ Health* 1991; 17(4):240–247.
4. Kneller RW, et al. Occupational risk factors for gastric cancer in Shanghai, China. *Am J Ind Med* 1990; 18(1):69–78.
5. Parent ME, Siemiatycki J, Fritschi L. Occupational exposures and gastric cancer. *Epidemiology* 1998; 9(1):48–55.
6. Tsuda T, et al. A case-control study of the relationships among silica exposure, gastric cancer, and esophageal cancer. *Am J Ind Med* 2001; 39(1):52–57.
7. Sugimura T, Matsukura N, Sato S. Intestinal metaplasia of the stomach as a precancerous stage. *IARC Sci Publ* 1982; 39:515–530.
8. Lei DN, Yu JY. Types of mucosal metaplasia in relation to the histogenesis of gastric carcinoma. *Arch Pathol Lab Med* 1984; 108(3):220–224.

9. Brennan MF, Karpeh MS Jr. Surgery for gastric cancer: the American view. *Semin Oncol* 1996; 23(3):352–359.
10. Bonenkamp JJ, et al. Extended lymph-node dissection for gastric cancer. Dutch Gastric Cancer Group. *N Engl J Med* 1999; 340(12):908–914.
11. Cuschieri A, et al. E.A.E.S. multicenter prospective randomized trial comparing two-stage vs single-stage management of patients with gallstone disease and ductal calculi. *Surg Endosc* 1999; 13(10):952–957.
12. Cuschieri A, et al. Patient survival after D1 and D2 resections for gastric cancer: long-term results of the MRC randomized surgical trial. Surgical Co-operative Group. *Br J Cancer* 1999; 79(9–10):1522–1530.
13. Safran H, et al. Paclitaxel and concurrent radiation therapy for locally advanced adenocarcinomas of the pancreas, stomach, and gastroesophageal junction. *Seminars in Radiation Oncology* 1999; 9(2 Suppl 1):53–57.
14. Hermans J, et al. Adjuvant therapy after curative resection for gastric cancer: meta- analysis of randomized trials. *J Clin Oncol* 1993; 11(8):1441–1447.
15. Earle CC, Maroun A. Adjuvant chemotherapy after curative resection for gastric cancer: Revisiting a meta-analysis of randomized trials (abstract). *Proc Am Soc Clin Oncol* 1998.
16. Macdonald JS, et al. Chemoradiotherapy after surgery compared with surgery alone for adenocarcinoma of the stomach or gastroesophageal junction. *N Engl J Med* 2001; 345(10):725–730.
17. Gold EB, Goldin SB. Epidemiology of and risk factors for pancreatic cancer. *Surg Oncol Clin N Am* 1998; 7(1):67–91.
18. Landis SH, et al. Cancer statistics, 1998. (erratum appears in CA Cancer J Clin 1998 May–Jun;48(3):192; CA Cancer J Clin 1998 Nov–Dec;48(6):329). Ca: a Cancer *Journal for Clinicians*, 1998; 48(1):6–29.
19. Wingo PA, et al. Annual report to the nation on the status of cancer, 1973–1996, with a special section on lung cancer and tobacco smoking. *J Natl Cancer Inst* 1999; 91(8):675–690.
20. La Vecchia C, et al. Smoking and cancer with emphasis on Europe. *Eur J Cancer* 1991; 27(1):94–104.
21. Mack TM, et al. Pancreas cancer and smoking, beverage consumption, and past medical history. *J Natl Cancer Inst* 1986; 76(1):49–60.
22. Olsen GW, et al. A case-control study of pancreatic cancer and cigarettes, alcohol, coffee and diet. *Am J Public Health* 1989; 79(8):1016–1019.
23. Silverman DT, et al. Cigarette smoking and pancreas cancer: a case-control study based on direct interviews. *J Natl Cancer Inst* 1994; 86(20):1510–1516.
24. Zheng W, et al. A cohort study of smoking, alcohol consumption, and dietary factors for pancreatic cancer (United States). *Cancer Causes Control* 1993; 4(5):477–482.
25. Mancuso TF, el-Attar AA. Cohort study of workers exposed to betanaphthylamine and benzidine. *J Occup Med* 1967; 9(6):277–285.
26. Pietri F, Clavel F. Occupational exposure and cancer of the pancreas: a review. *Br J Ind Med* 1991; 48(9):583–587.
27. Hruban RH, et al. Genetics of pancreatic cancer. From genes to families. *Surg Oncol Clin N Am* 1998; 7(1):1–23.
28. Nomoto S, et al. Clinical application of K-ras oncogene mutations in pancreatic carcinoma: detection of micrometastases. *Semin Surg Oncol* 1998; 15(1):40–46.
29. Wilentz RE, Hruban RH. Pathology of cancer of the pancreas. *Surg Oncol Clin N Am* 1998; 7(1):43–65.
30. Wingo PA, et al. Cancer incidence and mortality, 1973-1995: a report card for the U.S. Cancer, 1998; 82(6):1197–1207.
31. Kelsen DP, et al. Pain and depression in patients with newly diagnosed pancreas cancer. *J Clin Oncol* 1995; 13(3):748–755.
32. Krech RL, Walsh D. Symptoms of pancreatic cancer. *J Pain Symptom Manage* 1991; 6(6):360–367.
33. Passik SD, Breitbart WS. Depression in patients with pancreatic carcinoma. Diagnostic and treatment issues. *Cancer* 1996; 78(3 Suppl):615–626.
34. Lillemoe KD, Pitt HA. Palliation. Surgical and otherwise. *Cancer* 1996; 78(3 Suppl):605–614.
35. Bluemke DA, Fishman EK. CT and MR evaluation of pancreatic cancer. *Surg Oncol Clin N Am* 1998; 7(1):103–124.
36. Fuhrman GM, et al. Thin-section contrast-enhanced computed tomography accurately predicts the resectability of malignant pancreatic neoplasms. *Am J Surg* 1994; 167(1):104–111; discussion 111–113.

37. Stevens PD, Lightdale CJ. The role of endosonography in the diagnosis and management of pancreatic cancer. *Surg Oncol Clin N Am* 1998; 7(1):125–133.
38. Fernandez-del Castillo CL, Warshaw AL. Pancreatic cancer. Laparoscopic staging and peritoneal cytology. *Surg Oncol Clin N Am* 1998; 7(1):135–142.
39. Steinberg WM, et al. Workup of a patient with a mass in the head of the pancreas. *Pancreas* 1998; 17(1):24–30.
40. Posner MR, Mayer RJ. The use of serologic tumor markers in gastrointestinal malignancies. *Hematol Oncol Clin North Am* 1994; 8(3):533–553.
41. Nakao A, et al. Clinical usefulness of CA-19-9 in pancreatic carcinoma. *Semin Surg Oncol* 1998; 15(1):15–22.
42. Ritts RE, Pitt HA. CA 19-9 in pancreatic cancer. *Surg Oncol Clin N Am* 1998; 7(1):93–101.
43. Evans DB, Jessup JM, Colacchio T. Pancreatic cancer surgical practice guidelines. Pancreatic Cancer Practice Guideline Committee. *Oncology (Huntingt)* 1997; 11(7):1074–1079.
44. Nitecki SS, et al. Long-term survival after resection for ductal adenocarcinoma of the pancreas. Is it really improving? *Ann Surg* 1995; 221(1):59–66.
45. GITSG, A multi-institutional comparative trial of radiation therapy alone and in combination with 5-fluorouracil for locally unresectable pancreatic carcinoma. The Gastrointestinal Tumor Study Group. *Ann Surg* 1979; 189(2):205–208.
46. GITSG, Further evidence of effective adjuvant combined radiation and chemotherapy following curative resection of pancreatic cancer. Gastrointestinal Tumor Study Group. *Cancer* 1987; 59(12):2006–2010.
47. Sohn TA, et al. Resected adenocarcinoma of the pancreas-616 patients: results, outcomes, and prognostic indicators. *J Gastrointest Surg* 2000; 4(6):567–579.
48. Kalser MH, Ellenberg SS. Pancreatic cancer. Adjuvant combined radiation and chemotherapy following curative resection. *Arch Surg* 1985; 120(8):899–903.
49. Klinkenbijl JH, et al. Adjuvant radiotherapy and 5-fluorouracil after curative resection of cancer of the pancreas and periampullary region: phase III trial of the EORTC gastrointestinal tract cancer cooperative group. *Ann Surg* 1999; 230(6):776–782; discussion 782–784.
50. Spitz FR, et al. Preoperative and postoperative chemoradiation strategies in patients treated with pancreaticoduodenectomy for adenocarcinoma of the pancreas. *J Clin Oncol* 1997; 15(3): 928–937.
51. Willett CG, et al. Resection margins in carcinoma of the head of the pancreas. Implications for radiation therapy. *Ann Surg* 1993; 217(2):144–148.
52. Staley CA, et al. Preoperative chemoradiation, pancreaticoduodenectomy, and intraoperative radiation therapy for adenocarcinoma of the pancreatic head. *Am J Surg* 1996; 171(1):118–124; discussion 124–125.
53. Griffin JF, et al. Patterns of failure after curative resection of pancreatic carcinoma. *Cancer* 1990; 66(1):56–61.
54. Breslin TM, et al. Neoadjuvant chemoradiation for adenocarcinoma of the pancreas. *Frontiers Biosci* 1998; 3:E193–203.
55. Hoffman JP, et al. Phase II trial of preoperative radiation therapy and chemotherapy for patients with localized, resectable adenocarcinoma of the pancreas: an Eastern Cooperative Oncology Group Study. *J Clin Oncol* 1998; 16(1):317–323.
56. Pisters PW, et al. Preoperative chemoradiation for patients with pancreatic cancer: toxicity of endobiliary stents. *J Clin Oncol* 2000; 18(4):860–867.
57. Hidalgo M, et al. Phase I-II study of gemcitabine and fluorouracil as a continuous infusion in patients with pancreatic cancer. *J Clin Oncol* 1999; 17(2):585–592.
58. Lawrence TS, et al. Radiosensitization of pancreatic cancer cells by 2',2'-difluoro-2'-deoxycytidine. *Int J Radiat Oncol Biol Phys* 1996; 34(4):867–872.
59. Miller AR, et al. Neoadjuvant chemoradiation for adenocarcinoma of the pancreas. *Surg Oncol Clin N Am* 1998; 7(1):183–197.
60. Robertson JM, Shewach DS, Lawrence TS. Preclinical studies of chemotherapy and radiation therapy for pancreatic carcinoma. *Cancer* 1996; 78(3 Suppl):674–679.
61. Yamaguchi K, Tsuneyoshi M. Subclinical gallbladder carcinoma. *Am J Surg* 1992; 163(4):382–386.
62. Oertli DU, Herzog, Tondelli P. Primary carcinoma of the gallbladder: operative experience during a 16 year period. *Eur J Surg* 1993; 159(8):415–420.
63. Fong Y. Aggressive therapy is warranted for gallbladder cancer. *Cancer Invest* 1998; 16(1):64–65.

64. de Aretxabala XA, et al. Curative resection in potentially resectable tumours of the gallbladder. *Eur J Surg* 1997; 163(6):419–426.
65. Shepherd HA, et al. Endoscopic biliary endoprosthesis in the palliation of malignant obstruction of the distal common bile duct: a randomized trial. *Br J Surg* 1988; 75(12):1166–1168.
66. Andersen JR, et al. Randomised trial of endoscopic endoprosthesis versus operative bypass in malignant obstructive jaundice. *Gut* 1989; 30(8):1132–1135.
67. Meyer CG, Penn I, James L. Liver transplantation for cholangiocarcinoma: results in 207 patients. *Transplantation* 2000; 69(8):1633–1637.
68. Strong RW. Transplantation for liver and biliary cancer. *Semin Surg Oncol* 2000; 19(2):189–199.
69. Wall WJ, Liver transplantation for hepatic and biliary malignancy. *Semin Liver Dis* 2000; 20(4): 425–436.
70. Bartlett DL, et al. Long-term results after resection for gallbladder cancer. Implications for staging and management. *Ann Surg* 1996; 224(5):639–646.
71. Yamamoto M, et al. Recurrence after surgical resection of intrahepatic cholangiocarcinoma. *J Hepatobiliary Pancreat Surg* 2001; 8(2):154–157.
72. de Aretxabala X, et al. Preoperative chemoradiotherapy in the treatment of gallbladder cancer. *Am Surg* 1999; 65(3):241–246.
73. McMasters KM, et al. Neoadjuvant chemoradiation for extrahepatic cholangiocarcinoma. *Am J Surg* 1997; 174(6):605–608; discussion 608–609.

14 Chemoradiation in Therapy for Colon and Rectum Carcinoma

Jason H. Lee, MD
and Christopher G. Willett, MD

Contents

1. INTRODUCTION

Chemotherapy and radiation therapy play an important role in the management of colorectal carcinoma. Significant improvements in tumor control and overall survival have been demonstrated with the use of combined-modality therapy in several randomized clinical trials performed over the past 25 yr. This chapter reviews the role of adjuvant chemotherapy and radiation therapy for colon and rectal cancer. Issues surrounding chemoradiation for rectal cancer, including sphincter preservation, total mesorectal excision, local excision, and newer chemotherapy agents, are also discussed.

2. EPIDEMIOLOGY AND BIOLOGY OF COLORECTAL CANCER

Carcinomas of the colon and rectum are the second most common cause of death in the United States. Approximately 130,000 cases of colorectal carcinoma are diagnosed annually, and 56,000 patients will die of their disease *(1)*. A number of genetic mutations detected in familial adenomatous polyposis and hereditary nonpolyposis cancer syndromes predispose individuals to a high and early risk of developing colorectal cancer, but the majority of cases are sporadic. A diet high in fiber and low in fat as well as regular use of nonsteroidal antiinflammatory agents appears to have a protective effect. Despite public health efforts at routine screening for colorectal disease, a substantial proportion of patients are diagnosed with advanced stage disease.

From: *Chemoradiation in Cancer Therapy*
Edited by: H. Choy © Humana Press Inc., Totowa, NJ

Table 1
AJCC Stage Grouping and Equivalent Modified Astler-Coller Staging

AJCC TMN stage grouping					*Modified Astler-Coller staging*
Stage I	T1	N0	M0	A	Limited to mucosa (T1 lesions may invade submucosa)
	T2	N0	M0	B1	Invades muscularis propria
Stage II	T3	N0	M0	B2	Penetrates muscularis propria
	T4	N0	M0	B3	Tumor invades through serosa (colon) or adjuvant organs
Stage III	T1-2	N1-2	M0	C1	Positive nodes; within bowel wall
	T3	N1-2	M0	C2	Positive nodes; penetrates muscularis propria
	T4	N1-2	M0	C3	Positive nodes; invades through serosa (colon) or adjuvant organs
Stage IV	Any T	Any N	M1	D	Distant metastases

Surgical resection is the mainstay of therapy, and the most important prognostic factors following resection are the depth of penetration through the bowel wall and involvement of lymph nodes. The current American Joint Commission for Cancer (AJCC) and modified Astler-Coller staging systems are defined based on depth of penetration and number of lymph node metastases (Table 1). Other clinical and pathologic factors that determine the clinical course of disease include the preoperative serum level of carcinoembryonic antigen (CEA), lymphatic and blood vessel invasion, and histologic grade *(2)*. More recently, there has been intense activity in correlating clinical outcome and response to treatment with molecular markers and genetic alterations such as microsatellite instability *(3)*, cell proliferation indices, and loss of chromosome 18q *(4)*. In the future, identification of subgroups of patients at high risk for relapse by these techniques may guide treatment recommendations.

Although surgery is a vital component of patient management, resection alone is curative in approx 50% of patients with operable tumors. The presence of invasion through the muscularis propria (T3 or T4) or involvement of regional lymph nodes places patients at high risk for distant dissemination and local recurrence. The predominant site of distant failure in colorectal carcinoma is the liver, and less commonly, lungs, and peritoneum. Patients with transmural or node-positive rectal cancer, or locally advanced colon cancer, are also at significant risk for local recurrence *(5)*. Tumors arising at or below the peritoneal reflection are classified as rectal carcinomas. The location of the rectum within the bony confines of the pelvis and its proximity to adjacent organs make resection of tumors with wide radial margins difficult. Because of these factors, tumors originating in the rectum are associated with a higher risk of local failure compared with extrapelvic colon cancers on a stage by stage basis. With the exception of limited pelvic or hepatic relapse, salvage treatment is seldom feasible, and the majority of patients with recurrent disease ultimately die of cancer. Adjuvant therapy for colorectal carcinoma is delivered at the time of minimal disease burden for properly selected patients to eradicate microscopic residual or metastases, avoid recurrences, and improve cure rates over surgery alone. Oncologists have also recognized the role of adjuvant therapy before surgery to increase the chances of sphincter preservation and the resectability of locally advanced disease.

3. ADJUVANT THERAPY OF COLON CARCINOMA

3.1. Chemotherapy

The pattern of failure following resection of colon carcinoma is predominantly distant, and less commonly peritoneal or local. Whereas long-term survival for stage I and II colon cancer is greater than 80%, the presence of nodal metastases reduces survival by one-half. Patients with more than four lymph nodes involved (N2 disease) have a poor prognosis, with fewer than 30% surviving 5 yr following surgery alone. In response, a number of combinations of chemotherapy and immunotherapy strategies have been investigated. The National Surgical Adjuvant Breast and Bowel Project (NSABP) C-01 trial was the first to suggest an impact on overall survival (67% vs 58%, $p = 0.05$) with adjuvant semustine (methyl-CCNU), vincristine (Oncovin®), and 5-fluorouracil (MOF) compared with observation *(6)*. Landmark studies evaluating 5-fluorouracil (5-FU) with the immunomodulator levamisole showed a 40% reduction in disease recurrence and 33% reduction in mortality for node-positive patients *(7,8)*. Five-year survival in Intergroup study 0035 was improved from 54% without treatment to 65% with 5-FU and levamisole *(8)*. Early findings from more recent trials also support adjuvant 5-FU and leucovorin as a briefer and perhaps superior alternative option *(9–11)*.

Whereas the value of adjuvant chemotherapy has been well demonstrated in patients with stage C colon carcinoma, adjuvant chemotherapy for transmural but node-negative (stage B2) disease remains controversial. Randomized trials of adjuvant chemotherapy failed to reveal a survival advantage for patients with node-negative disease *(12)*. To overcome the low statistical power to detect a difference in outcome in stage B2 patients, investigators from two study groups have presented results from pooled data with conflicting conclusions *(13,14)*. Observation remains a reasonable management strategy for stage II patients; however, patients with tumors exhibiting adverse features such as lymphovascular invasion or bowel perforation may be considered for treatment. The current Intergroup trial randomizes high-risk stage II patients to monoclonal antibody 17-1A (edrecolomab) vs no treatment.

3.2. Radiation Therapy

Stage for stage, local recurrences occur less frequently for patients following resection of colon cancer vs rectal cancer. However, there are subsets of patients who appear to be at significant risk for local relapse, based on extent of bowel penetration and location of disease. A comprehensive retrospective review from the Massachusetts General Hospital compared patterns of failure in patients receiving postoperative radiation therapy to a historical cohort of 395 patients undergoing surgery alone *(15)*. After surgery alone, approximately one-third of patients with stage B3 or C2 disease, and one-half of patients with stage C3 disease, bowel perforation, or fistula formation experienced local-regional recurrence. Two hundred three patients received 50.4–55 Gy of radiation using shrinking-field technique to the tumor bed, and 63 patients also received some form of bolus

5-FU. Local control and 5-yr disease-free survival were significantly improved in patients with stage B3 or C3 disease, and those with perforation or fistulization. Acute and long-term grade 3+ bowel toxicity was 8% and 4.5%, respectively.

Based on promising retrospective data, an Intergroup trial comparing adjuvant chemotherapy alone versus chemotherapy and local irradiation was initiated for patients with stage B3, selected C2, and C3 disease, but was closed early because of slow accrual. Analysis of the 189 eligible patients showed no difference in the rates of recurrence or death with the addition of radiation therapy *(16)*. Because of the underpowered nature of this study, definitive conclusions regarding the efficacy of this treatment cannot be achieved. Other trials of regional or whole abdominal irradiation with systemic or intraperitoneal chemotherapy have been largely disappointing. A pilot study conducted by the Southwest Oncology Group subjected 41 patients with locally advanced colon cancer to whole abdominal irradiation (30 Gy), 16 Gy local tumor boost, and continuous-infusion 5-FU *(17)*. A post-hoc comparison to a separate adjuvant trial without radiation therapy suggested favorable disease-free and overall survival for those with more than four nodes involved. In the absence of more compelling evidence, the use of adjuvant radiation therapy in completely resected high-risk colon cancer patients remains investigational.

Patients with locally advanced colon cancer and suspected microscopic or gross residual disease after surgery pose a difficult management problem. Postoperative radiation therapy in addition to standard chemotherapy may have some utility in sterilizing residual disease. In retrospective studies, local radiation therapy with or without concurrent chemotherapy achieves local control in 46–70% of patients with microscopic residual *(15,18,19)*, and 20–45% of patients with gross residual disease *(18,19)*. Intraoperative electron radiotherapy has been advocated particularly in the setting of microscopic or gross residual disease.

4. ADJUVANT THERAPY OF RECTAL CARCINOMA

Standard treatment for patients with clinically operable carcinoma of the rectum involves surgical resection and selective administration of adjuvant therapy. Conventional operative procedures are a low anterior resection with or without coloanal anastamosis for tumors of the proximal two-thirds of the rectum and abdominoperineal resection (APR) for more distal tumors. As in colon carcinoma, adjuvant therapy for rectal cancer is designed to decrease the risk of local and distant recurrence, and ultimately improve survival. Because of the high risk of pelvic failure following surgery alone in patients with advanced primaries or node-positive disease, radiation therapy has proven an integral component of an adjuvant therapy program. Combined-modality therapy with pelvic irradiation and 5-FU-based chemotherapy maximizes disease-free and overall survival in high-risk patients. Adjuvant therapy is most commonly delivered postoperatively, thus allowing accurate pathologic evaluation of the surgical specimen. The desire to improve treatment efficacy while maintaining quality of life has led to the emergence of newer chemotherapy regimens and schedules, less radical surgery, and motivation for preoperative therapy.

Previous reviews of surgery alone for rectal cancer have demonstrated a stage-dependent risk of local failure. This risk is approx 15–30% for T3N0 disease, 35–50% for T3N1 disease, and even greater for T4 disease *(20,21)*. Retrospective studies of adjuvant pelvic radiation therapy demonstrate an absolute reduction of 15–30% in local recurrence compared with historical controls. At the Massachusetts General Hospital, postoperative radiation therapy using doses of 45–50.4 Gy was administered to 165 patients felt to be at high risk for local failure *(22)*. Compared with historical controls, adjuvant radiation reduced local failure from 31% in stage B2/B3 disease to 8%, and from 50% in stage C disease to 25%. In addition, overall survival without evidence of disease was improved in most patients, with the exception of those with stage C3 disease whose outlook remained poor. Only 8% of patients in this series received chemotherapy, which subsequent randomized trials would prove to be a valuable adjunctive therapy.

4.1. Postoperative Therapy

There have been multiple prospective trials evaluating the use of adjuvant radiation therapy with or without chemotherapy in both the preoperative and postoperative setting. The clinical trials in the United States have randomized patients following surgery to allow pathologic staging and risk assessment. Early trials conducted by the Gastrointestinal Tumor Study Group (GITSG) and NSABP compared surgery alone vs surgery followed by pelvic irradiation or 5-FU-based chemotherapy in patients with stage B2 or C disease *(23,24)*. In addition, the GITSG 7175 study included a fourth arm, which contained both radiation and chemotherapy. Local recurrence was approx 25% with only surgery, but not affected by chemotherapy alone. Local recurrence was reduced by radiation therapy (16–20% vs 25%), and overall survival was increased by 10–15% with the addition of chemotherapy. Interestingly, the benefit of chemotherapy in the NSABP R-01 trial appeared to be limited to males *(24)*. The use of combined modality adjuvant therapy, as in the GITSG trial, had the greatest impact on reducing local recurrence (11%) and improving overall survival (56% vs 42%) *(23)*. Although this trial had several limitations due to its relatively small patient numbers and poor compliance, these results have been confirmed in later studies. In 1990, the National Institutes of Health issued a clinical announcement recommending adjuvant 5-FU-based chemotherapy and radiation therapy for patients with stage B2, B3, and C rectal cancer *(25)*.

Subsequent trials have been designed to define the optimal chemotherapy regimen and to better assess the need for combined modality therapy. The North Central Cancer Treatment Group (NCCTG) conducted a trial comparing radiation therapy alone (50 Gy) vs radiation and 5-FU with semustine (methyl-CCNU) *(26)*. The addition of chemotherapy enhanced local control (87% vs 75%) and overall survival (53% vs 43%) compared with radiation alone. The chemotherapy regimens in the early adjuvant therapy trials incorporated several months of semustine with 5-FU. A follow-up GITSG study randomized patients to radiation therapy and 5-FU followed by additional chemotherapy with or without semustine, and found no advantage to the addition of semustine *(27)*. A second NCCTG study compared two schedules of 5-FU with or without semustine, and confirmed the lack of benefit of semustine *(28)*. Similarly, the three-drug regimen of semustine, vincristine, and 5-fluorouracil (MOF) was found to be no more effective than 5-FU in males enrolled on the NSABP R-02 trial *(29)*.

Based on the successful experience in colon carcinoma, the most recent Intergroup trial (INT-0114) explored the role of biomodulation of 5-FU in rectal cancer. This four-arm trial randomized patients to pelvic irradiation and 6 mo of bolus 5-FU vs bolus 5-FU and levamisole, leucovorin, or both *(30)*. There was no significant difference in disease-free survival and overall survival (78–80%) among the four treatment arms in a prelimi-

Table 2
Survival in Adjuvant Therapy Trials Using Chemotherapy

Study	*Chemotherapy*[b]	*Survival*[a] *Surgery ± RT (%)*	*Surgery + CT ± RT (%)*	*Follow up (yr)*
NSABP R-01 *(24)*	MOF	42	53	5
GITSG 7175 *(23)*	Bolus 5-FU	32–45	48–57	8
NCCTG 79-47-51 *(26)*	Bolus 5-FU + semustine	38	53	7
GITSG 7180 *(27)*	Bolus 5-FU ± semustine	—	66–75	3
NCCTG 86-47-51 *(28)*	Bolus 5-FU	—	60	4
	Infusional 5-FU	—	70	4
NSABP R-02 *(29)*	Bolus 5-FU or MOF	—	62–65	5
INT 0114 *(30)*	Bolus 5-FU ± LCV ± LVM	—	78–80	3

[a]RT = radiation therapy, CT = chemotherapy.
[b]MOF = semustine, vincristine, 5-fluorouracil; LCV = leucovorin; LVM = levamisole.

nary analysis, and toxicity was greatest with the three-drug regimen. Disease-free survival was 68% with 5-FU and leucovorin compared with 62–63% with other regimens, although this difference was not statistically significant. The potential benefit of leucovorin will require further follow-up.

Optimizing the combination of 5-FU and radiation therapy remains under active investigation. Typically, a radiation dose of 50.4 (range 45–54) Gy is delivered concurrently with 5-FU after surgery, or sandwiched between several cycles of systemic chemotherapy. Trials have continued systemic chemotherapy for 6–18 mo, although in current practice, this is generally limited to a total of 6 mo. During radiation therapy, 5-FU has traditionally been given as a bolus dose of 500 mg/m^2 for 3 d during the first and last weeks of treatment. The NCCTG initiated a multicenter trial comparing bolus 5-FU (+/– semustine) versus protracted venous infusion (PVI) 5-FU (225 mg/m^2/d) during the entire radiation therapy portion of treatment *(28)*. In this trial, there was a 10% increase in overall survival (70% vs 60%, $p = 0.04$) and decrease in distant metastases, suggesting a greater impact on systemic micrometastases. Table 2 summarizes survival outcomes from prospective trials incorporating chemotherapy in the adjuvant regimen.

Protracted venous infusion (PVI) of 5-FU modifies the toxicity profile, delivers a higher cumulative dose of drug, and maintains sensitization for each radiation fraction. Compared with bolus 5-FU, PVI 5-FU was associated with greater grade 3 diarrhea but less myelosuppression. Although not directly compared, the outcome with 5-FU and leucovorin from INT-0114 was felt to be similar to that achieved with PVI 5-FU. The preliminary results of a trial from the UK suggested superior relapse-free and overall survival with PVI 5-FU (300 mg/m^2/d) compared with 5-FU and leucovorin, as well as less toxicity among the 216 patients with rectal cancer *(31)*. However, only a minority of patients in this UK trial received radiation therapy. The current Intergroup (INT-0144) randomizes patients to a regimen using PVI 5-FU during the radiation therapy portion only, a regimen using PVI 5-FU during the entire 6 mo of adjuvant therapy, and a regimen using modulated bolus 5-FU with leucovorin and levamisole. All arms utilize pelvic irradiation beginning at wk 8. This trial will

Table 3
Local Recurrence Following Surgery Alone or Surgery and Adjuvant Therapy[a]

Study	*Surgery (± CT) (%)*	*Surgery + RT (%)*	*Surgery + RT + CT (%)*	*Follow up (yr)*
GITSG 7175 *(23)*	24–27	20	11	8
NSABP R-01 *(24)*	21–25	16	—	5
NCCTG 79-47-51 *(26)*	—	25	14	5
NCCTG 86-47-51 *(28)*	—	—	9–11	4
INT 0114 *(30)*	—	—	9–13	3
NSABP R-02 *(29)*	13	—	8	5

[a]CT = chemotherapy, RT = radiation therapy.

hopefully answer important questions regarding the utility of PVI 5-FU relative to modulated bolus 5-FU.

The improvement in local control with adjuvant radiation therapy demonstrated in randomized trials does not reach the magnitude seen in retrospective studies. In the postoperative setting, trials have shown a moderate but statistically significant reduction in local failure when comparing radiation to no-radiation arms, but no impact on overall survival (Table 3). In the absence of chemotherapy, pelvic irradiation reduced local failure from 25% to 16% in the first NSABP R-01 trial *(24)*. In the NSABP R-02 study, all patients received some form of 5-FU-based chemotherapy (MOF was available for males), and patients were randomized to pelvic radiation or no radiation. Approximately 75% of patients had transmural primary lesions, although an exact T-stage breakdown was not provided. Local failure was reduced from only 13% to 8% with radiation therapy *(29)*. Overall, severe or life-threatening toxicity was equivalent between the two treatment arms, but four (1.2%) on-treatment deaths occurred in the patients receiving radiation therapy. Retrospective studies suggest a detrimental effect of postoperative radiation therapy on sphincter function, particularly following coloanal anastamosis *(32)*; however, this important endpoint has not been assessed prospectively in a major trial. Clearly, the potential toxicity from radiation therapy needs to be weighed against the increased risk of locoregional recurrence without radiation and its associated morbidity.

Total mesorectal excision (TME) involves sharp resection around the integral hindgut, which envelopes the mid-rectum, as opposed to conventional blunt dissection. Proponents report low rates of local failures after TME and advocate widespread adoption of this procedure *(33)*. A series from Memorial Sloan-Kettering reported a 7.3% pelvic recurrence rate in 246 patients with Dukes' B and C disease *(34)*. In an updated analysis of the Basingstoke experience, the 5-yr local failure rate in 405 patients was 3%, with less than 10% of patients receiving radiation therapy *(35)*. Of note, these figures include 102 patients with Dukes' A disease and 167 with Dukes' B disease (T stage not stated), and excludes 108 patients with "non-curative" resections. Although impressive, these results should be interpreted with caution as many series are comprised of carefully selected patients and the risks of surgical complications, including anastomotic leaks, may be increased.

Whether the use of TME obviates the need for adjuvant radiation therapy is a topic of intense debate. It should be noted that a substantial proportion of patients undergoing TME may have received adjuvant radiation therapy and/or chemotherapy *(36)*. In a

Table 4
Accepted Adjuvant Therapy Regimens for High-Risk Rectal Cancer Patients

Systemic chemotherapy	*Chemotherapy with radiation*	*Ref.*
Bolus 5-FU 500 mg/m^2 × 5 d every 4 wk for 6 cycles	Bolus 5-FU 500 mg/m^2 × 3 d during wk 1 and 5	GITSG *(27)*
Bolus 5-FU 425 mg/m^2 and leucovorin 20 mg/m^2 × 5 d every 4 wk; 2 cycles administered before and after chemoradiation	Bolus 5-FU 400 mg/m^2 and leucovorin 20 mg/m^2 × 3 d during wk 1 and 5	INT-0114 *(30)*
Bolus 5-FU 500 mg/m^2 and leucovorin 500 mg/m^2 weekly × 6 followed by 2 rest weeks; total of 4 cycles	Bolus 5-FU 500 mg/m^2 × 3 d during wk 1 and 5	NSABP *(29)*
Additional bolus 5-FU as above	Infusional 5-FU 225 mg/m^2/d during entire course of irradiation	NCCTG *(28)*

prospective Dutch trial, patients are randomized to upfront TME or an intensive course of preoperative radiotherapy followed by TME *(37)*. Although all patients were felt to have clinically resectable disease (T4 tumors were excluded), approx 23% of patients had either microscopically-involved margins, tumor spillage, or gross residual disease following TME. Postoperative adjuvant therapy was permitted in these patients, suggesting a limit to local tumor control achieved by TME alone in patients who traditionally received adjuvant radiation therapy.

Although several issues remain unresolved, patients with T3 or T4 primary disease or nodal metastases should be considered for adjuvant 5-FU-based chemotherapy and radiation therapy following surgical resection of rectal carcinoma. 5-FU is effective in reducing the development of metastatic disease and augments the effect of radiotherapy on pelvic control. Outside of a clinical trial, acceptable chemotherapy regimens consist of several cycles of bolus 5-FU, usually with leuocovorin (Table 4). Most patients should be eligible to receive pelvic irradiation concurrently with bolus 5-FU, beginning either after surgery or after two cycles of systemic chemotherapy. Alternatively, 5-FU can be given as a continuous infusion during irradiation. While adjuvant radiation therapy maximizes pelvic control, there may be certain subgroups of patients for whom such treatment is unnecessary. It is possible that chemotherapy alone may be adequate for certain patients, such as those with microscopic transmural extension (stage B2m) or intramural disease with minimal nodal spread (stage C1) *(38,39)*. Further investigation will be essential to confirm the results from the NSABP R-02 study and to properly identify such patients.

4.2. Preoperative Therapy

Although most trials in the United States have evaluated adjuvant chemoradiation in the postoperative setting, there has been growing interest in the use of preoperative treatment. Preoperative chemotherapy and radiation therapy offers the advantages of downstaging of disease, increasing the possibility for sphincter preservation, and limiting the volume of small bowel exposed to radiation. Patients with locally advanced tumors that are marginally resectable or unresectable at presentation may be rendered operable

Table 5
Advantages and Disadvantages of Preoperative vs Postoperative Radiation Therapy

Preoperative therapy	*Postoperative therapy*
Advantages	
Downstage; increase resectability	Selection of patients based on pathology
Better oxygenation	Identify high-risk areas or residual disease
Increased chance for sphincter preservation	
Sterilization from surgical seeding	
In vivo assessment of response to treatment	
Disadvantages	
Overtreatment of early stage patients	Treatment of perineum following APR
Delay in definitive surgical resection	More small bowel in field
Wound healing complications	

by preoperative chemoradiation. Furthermore, preoperative radiation may allow a sphincter-sparing procedure in patients with low-lying rectal carcinomas who would have otherwise required APR.

Patients with clinically resectable disease may electively receive surgical adjuvant therapy preoperatively. Pelvic irradiation prior to surgery appears to reduce small bowel complications by avoiding abdominal adhesions and fixation of bowel within the field. The disadvantages of a preoperative adjuvant approach include the loss of information on pathologic staging, possibility of unnecessary treatment of early stage (T1-2N0) disease, and increase in surgical and wound healing complications. These concerns have been addressed with attention to radiation dose fractionation and the use of modern pretreatment imaging techniques that can predict pathological staging with reasonable accuracy. The accuracy of endoscopic ultrasound (EUS) to stage primary tumor ranges from 70% to 90% when compared to pathologic T stage. Cross-sectional imaging such as computed tomography and magnetic resonance with endorectal coil provide wide pelvic views and may be less operator-dependent than EUS. The advantages and disadvantages of either preoperative or postoperative treatment are summarized in Table 5.

Numerous early trials of preoperative treatment randomized patients to upfront surgery or radiation therapy alone followed by surgery. Many of these trials utilized low radiation doses or an accelerated course with large fraction sizes and suboptimal technique. These studies usually have demonstrated a reduction in local failure without improvement in survival. Recently, the Swedish Rectal Cancer Trial showed an improvement in overall 5-yr survival (58% vs 48%) with preoperative radiotherapy *(40)*. In this trial, pelvic irradiation (25 Gy in 5 fractions) was administered followed by a brief interval to surgery. The Dutch trial randomized patients to a similar intensive course of radiation followed by TME vs TME alone *(37)*. Although there was no difference in overall survival (82% at 2 yr), local failure was reduced from 8% to 2% with preoperative radiation. In stage III patients, the reduction in local failure was more substantial (4% vs 15%). A meta-analysis of preoperative radiation therapy trials concluded a significant reduction in mortality, with an odds ratio of 0.84 ($p = 0.03$) *(41)*. Despite these favorable results, preoperative regimens using unconventional radiation schedules without chemotherapy are usually not practiced in the United States.

Patients who are treated preoperatively typically receive a regimen of standard chemotherapy and radiation therapy similar to that administered in postoperative trials. Given the varying clinical inclusion criteria, the results of nonrandomized or retrospective preoperative therapy studies are difficult to compare to expected results from trials employing postoperative adjuvant therapy, which are based on pathologic staging. Other endpoints can be assessed to evaluate the efficacy of preoperative chemoradiation regimens. The extent of clinical, radiographic, or pathologic downstaging and conversion to resectability can be measured in patients with locally advanced or unresectable disease at presentation. For patients who have resectable but distal tumors and are at risk of requiring an APR, the ability to perform a sphincter-sparing procedure after preoperative chemoradiation is a desirable goal.

Locally advanced, unresectable (fixed), or recurrent rectal carcinoma can be significantly downstaged by combined modality therapy prior to attempted resection of disease. Trials of preoperative radiation therapy alone demonstrate a trend toward lesser stage disease *(40)* and a complete pathologic response rate usually less than 10%. With the addition of concurrent chemotherapy, response rates are higher and the majority of patients can be curatively resected. A variety of 5-FU-based regimens have been used, although most combinations include bolus 5-FU (325–500 mg/m^2) with or without leucovorin (20 mg/m^2) for 3–5 d during the first and last weeks of radiation *(42,43)*. Other investigators have incorporated continuous infusion 5-FU *(44,45)*, low-dose cisplatin *(46)*, or mitomycin *(47)*.

Janjan et al. reported the M.D. Anderson experience with continuous-infusion 5-FU (300 mg/m^2/d, M–F) during radiation therapy in predominantly clinically stage T3 disease *(48)* Perioperative complications (fistula, abscess, wound healing) following chemoradiation occurred in 14% of patients, and only one required reoperation. Clinical tumor downstaging was observed in 61% of patients, and 27% had documented complete response. The variation in complete response in other single-institution studies probably reflects the differences in patient selection and definition of "locally advanced" (Table 6). As expected, better pathologic response is associated with improved disease-free and overall survival. One of the major research goals over the next several years will be the identification of patients with rectal cancers that will exhibit complete response to preoperative chemoradiation strategies.

Preoperative combined modality therapy can induce sufficient shrinkage of distal rectal cancers to allow sphincter-sparing procedures in those who were originally felt to require APR. The determination to sacrifice the sphincter is often made definitively in the operating room; however, clinical estimation correlates reasonably well with intraoperative assessment and serves as a useful benchmark to evaluate preoperative therapy. Minsky has recently reviewed a number of trials that studied preoperative radiation therapy with and without chemotherapy following prospective clinical assessment of the need for APR *(49)*. A trial of preoperative bolus 5-FU (325 mg/m^2) and leucovorin (20 mg/m^2) for 5 d during wk 1 and 5 of pelvic radiation therapy (50.4 Gy) was recently updated with 72 patients enrolled. All patients had T3 lesions based on endoscopic ultrasound. Thirty-five patients were judged to require APR based on anatomic location and treated with the goal of sphincter-preservation (others were felt to require APR regardless of degree of downstaging). Sphincter-sparing surgery was performed in 31 (89%) patients, and 3-yr local failure for the entire cohort was only 2%. Other preoperative regimens have produced sphincter-preservation rates of 63–77% (Table 7).

Table 6

Resectability, Pathologic Response Rates, and Survival Following Preoperative Chemoradiation Therapy Regimens

Study	*Patients*	*Preoperative regimen*[a]	*Resectable*	*Complete response*	*Survival*
MDACC *(48)*	117 (96% T3)	Infusional 5-FU (300 $mg/m^2/d$) RT 45 Gy	100%	32 (27%)	83% (3-yr)
MSKCC *(42)*	36 (10 fixed)	Bolus 5-FU + LCV RT 50.4 Gy	97%	4 (11%)	76% (4-yr)
U. Kentucky *(45)*	77	5-FU (bolus or infusional) RT 50-63 Gy	100%	12 (16%)	76% (5-yr)
Duke *(46)*	43	Bolus 5-FU + cisplatin RT 45 Gy	41 (95%)	11 (27%)	91% (crude)
Calgary *(47)*	156	RT 40 Gy + 5-FU/MMC RT 50 Gy + 5-FU/MMC/LCV	91–100% 100%	4–15% 25%	52% (5-yr) 84% (5-yr)
EORTC *(43)*	66	Bolus 5-FU + LCV RT 45 Gy	58 (88%)	9 (16%)	60% (5-yr)

[a]5-FU = 5-fluorouracil, RT = radiation therapy, LCV = leucovorin, MMC = mitomycin C.

Table 7

Prospective Trials of Preoperative Radiation Therapy With and Without Chemotherapy and Rate of Sphincter-Sparing Procedures

	MSKCC (51)	*MSKCC* (42)	*NSABP R-03* (50)	*Rome* (52)
Patients enrolled	36	72	59	83
Pretreatment stage	5 T2, 31 T3	T3	Stage B or C	98% T3
Preoperative treatment[a]	RT 50.4 Gy	5-FU/LCV + RT 50.4 Gy	5-FU/LCV then RT + 5-FU/LCV	5-FU/MMC + RT 37.8 Gy
Patients felt to require APR	36	35	22 (69% of 32)	47
Patients undergoing complete resection	35	NR	32	81
Patients who actually underwent APR	8 (23%) of 35	4 (11%) of 35	16 (73%) of 22	16 (34%) of 47
Local failure (%)	17%	1%	NR	10%
Survival (%, 5-yr)	64%	88%	NR	72%

[a]RT = radiation therapy, 5-FU = 5-fluorouracil, LCV = leucovorin.

Preoperative therapy is well tolerated in the majority of patients. Grade 3 or higher toxicity during chemoradiation occurs in 13–28% of patients *(49,52)*. Nearly half of 49 patients experienced grade 3–4 toxicity during the course of therapy in the NSABP R-03 trial, although in this protocol patients received two cycles of 5-FU and leucovorin prior to commencing combined modality therapy *(50)*. Functional results following preoperative therapy and sphincter-sparing procedures appear acceptable in 80% or more of patients in studies assessing this endpoint.

Cooperative study groups have recognized the need for a randomized trial comparing preoperative chemoradiation with postoperative treatment. Two trials of similar design but slightly different chemoradiation schedules opened in the United States by the Intergroup (INT-0147) and the NSABP (R-03). Both trials required pretreatment clinical and radiographic staging and utilized concurrent chemotherapy and conventional radiation therapy. Because of formidable physician biases, both trials failed to enroll sufficient patients and were closely prematurely well short of accrual goals. A German trial randomizes patients after staging by endoscopic ultrasound to preoperative or postoperative radiation concurrent with 5-FU (1 gm/m^2/24 h × 120 h, wk 1 and 5) followed by maintenance 5-FU. An interim analysis of toxicity reported less grade 3+ diarrhea with preoperative chemoradiation, and no difference in postsurgical complications *(53)*. Hopefully, this study will provide important answers regarding tumor control, sphincter preservation, and survival between these two approaches.

In the absence of definitive data demonstrating a superiority of preoperative vs postoperative treatment for clinically resectable rectal carcinoma, preoperative adjuvant therapy is a reasonable alternative for patients judged to have transmural disease or nodal involvement by clinical or radiologic evaluation. For patients with distal rectal carcinomas, preoperative chemoradiation may be preferable in order to allow tumor downstaging and permit a sphincter-sparing operation. In this situation, a radiation dose of 45–50.4 Gy using conventional fractionation, concurrent 5-FU-based chemotherapy, and an interval to surgery of at least 4 wk appears to be most effective *(54)*. Following surgery, patients with persistent transmural or node-positive disease should receive additional cycles of systemic chemotherapy. Postoperative chemotherapy in those who have experienced significant downstaging to pT0-2N0 disease remains an open question, and is being addressed by ongoing European trials. Since standard adjuvant therapy consists of 6 mo of chemotherapy, most patients with high-risk features before surgery are offered chemotherapy postoperatively.

4.3. Local Excision and Adjuvant Therapy

Traditional surgical management of distal rectal carcinoma has been the abdominoperineal resection. This procedure results in loss of sphincter function with a permanent colostomy and is associated with a high incidence of genitourinary as well as sexual dysfunction. Alternative conservative surgical and nonsurgical approaches have been developed to obtain local tumor control without sacrificing anal sphincter function. Single-institution experiences with electrocoagulation *(55)*, endoluminal radiation therapy alone *(56)*, or local excision with or without adjuvant therapy *(57,58)* demonstrate certain patients with early-stage disease may be adequately managed with these techniques.

Wide local excision and selective postoperative therapy have been used in patients with early-stage distal carcinomas. Retrospective studies have identified patients with tumors less than 3 cm in size, limited to the superficial muscularis propria, and favorable

Table 8
Selected Prospective and Retrospective Studies of Wide Local Excision and Adjuvant Therapy

Study	*Patients*	*Adjuvant therapy*[a]	*Local failure*	*Survival*
CALGB *(59)*	59 T1	None	3 (5%)	87% (6-yr)
	51 T2	RT 54 Gy + 5-FU	7 (14%)	85% (6-yr)
Deaconess *(57)*	48 (21 T1, 21 T2, 6 T3)	RT 54 Gy + 5-FU	4 (8%)	94% (crude)
MDACC *(58)*	46 (15 T3)	RT 53 Gy, 5-FU in 7 pts.	4 (8%)	93% (3-yr)
MGH *(60)*	56 (34 T1, 22 T2)	RT 50.4–67.5 Gy ± 5-FU	17–20%	72%[b]
MGH/Emory *(61)*	52	None	28% (5-yr)	66%[b]
	47	RT 50–65 Gy; 5-FU in 26 pts.	10% (5-yr)	74%[b]
MSKCC *(62)*	39 (T1, T2, T3)	RT 50.4 Gy; 5-FU in 20 pts.	8 (21%)	70% (5-yr)

[a]RT = radiation therapy, 5-FU = 5-fluorouracil.
[b]5-yr relapse-free survival.

histologic grade as likely candidates for local excision. Full-thickness excision can be achieved by a transanal approach or a posterior transcoccygeal (Kraske procedure) approach, which permits better exposure but has greater morbidity. Well-differentiated T1 lesions without blood vessel or lymphatic invasion are associated with a low risk of nodal involvement and a local failure rate typically less than 10% with adequate margins, and may be safely managed without additional treatment. Patients with tumors exhibiting adverse pathologic features should receive additional chemoradiation to address the significant chance of local-regional recurrence. Patients who are found to have pathologic T3 disease or positive margins should undergo standard operative procedures.

Only recently have these criteria for local excision been applied in a prospective, multi-institutional setting. The Cancer and Leukemia Group B organized a single-arm prospective study (CALGB 8984) using standardized criteria for local excision: ≤4 cm, ≤40% of bowel wall circumference, and ≤10 cm from dentate line *(59)*. Of 180 registered patients, 110 patients with pathologic T1 or T2 lesions with negative margins remained on-study; those with T2 lesions underwent adjuvant pelvic irradiation (54 Gy) with bolus 5-FU chemotherapy. Local failure occurred in three (5%) patients with T1 lesions, and one was successfully salvaged with APR. Among patients with T2 lesions, seven (14%) experienced local failure, and four were successfully salvaged. After a median follow-up of 48 mo, 6-yr overall and failure-free survival was 85% and 78%, respectively. This study indicates that, by applying stringent guidelines, local excision and adjuvant combined modality therapy can successfully manage most patients with early stage distal rectal carcinomas with results similar to those reported in single-institution studies (Table 8).

5. FUTURE TRENDS IN COMBINED MODALITY THERAPY FOR COLORECTAL CARCINOMA

Investigative efforts are underway to further improve the results of multimodality therapy of colorectal carcinoma. In addition to previously discussed phase III trials, other studies are incorporating novel chemotherapeutic agents to improve systemic control and radiosensitization, optimizing physical delivery of radiation, and performing risk stratification with current molecular and genetic techniques.

5.1. Novel Chemotherapeutic Agents

A number of newer chemotherapeutic and biologic agents have shown activity in colorectal cancer in the metastatic setting. Clinical trials have been performed using irinotecan (CPT-11, Camptosar®) and oxaliplatin as a single-agent or in combination with 5-FU. Other studies are investigating the use of oral fluoropyrimidines such as capecitabine, uracil-tegafur (UFT)/leucovorin, and S-1, which may mimic the effect of continuous-infusion 5-FU. The combination of irinotecan, 5-FU, and leucovorin was shown to be a superior first-line agent in metastatic colorectal cancer compared to 5-FU and leucovorin alone *(63)*. This three-drug combination is being tested in the adjuvant setting for high-risk colon carcinoma in a rapidly accruing CALGB trial. A similar trial is being conducted with the three-drug combination of 5-FU, leucovorin, and oxaliplatin by the NSABP.

Trials incorporating these newer agents with radiation therapy for rectal carcinoma either preoperatively or adjuvantly are ongoing or under development. The maximum tolerated dose of weekly irinotecan was determined to be 50 mg/m^2 when added to a preoperative regimen of continuous-infusion 5-FU and 45 Gy of pelvic radiation therapy for locally advanced rectal cancer *(64)*. Other trials are adding oxaliplatin in novel combinations with 5-FU, leucovorin, and radiation therapy. There is also great interest in combining radiation therapy and oral fluoropyridimines, as these prodrugs behave pharmacologically similar to protracted-infusion 5-FU without the inconvenience and complications of long-term central line infusion. Phase I dose-escalation trials have reported that capecitabine or UFT/leucovorin concurrent with radiation therapy is well tolerated and appears to have promising activity in locally advanced rectal cancer *(65–67)*. Additional research will be necessary before any of these combination can be considered standard therapy.

5.2. Chronomodulation

Continuous-infusion 5-FU and radiation therapy offers a disease-free and survival advantage over bolus 5-FU, but diarrhea and stomatitis remain significant treatment-limiting toxicities. Rather than a flat infusion of 5-FU, trials are evaluating a circadian-shaped infusion of 5-FU with the greatest proportion of dose delivered between 20:00 and 04:00 h. This chronomodulation of 5-FU appears to incorporate the circadian cycles of gut and mucosal cell proliferation and 5-FU pharmacodynamics, and may result in fewer toxicities. A phase I study from the University of Florida has shown that chronomodulated infusions of 5-FU at a dose of 275 mg/m^2/d during pelvic irradiation is well tolerated *(68)*. Chronomodulated combination of oxaliplatin, 5-FU, and leucovorin resulted in higher response rates and less stomatitis and neuropathy in metastatic colorectal carcinoma *(69)*, and may become a viable option for treatment of primary disease.

5.3. Prognostic and Predictive Factors in Outcome and Response to Treatment

Traditionally, TNM staging and other histopathologic factors have guided prognostic predictions and treatment decisions. A number of molecular markers and genetic abnormalities have been described which may have further prognostic significance beyond histopathologic staging. Many of these genetic alterations have been implicated in the pathogenesis of colon cancer. For example, allelic loss of the *DCC* (deleted in colon cancer) gene on chromosome 18q confers a significantly worse prognosis in colorectal cancer patients, particularly in stage B2 disease *(4)*. Assessment of *DCC* status in stage II patients may identify those who may benefit from adjuvant therapy. However, clinical trials are necessary to determine whether it is feasible to stratify patients by molecular methods, and whether higher risk patients benefit from adjuvant treatment.

Other molecular and genetic markers may allow clinicians to predict response to treatment. Cell proliferation markers as measured by Ki-67 and proliferating-cell nuclear antigen staining and mitotic index have been correlated with response to preoperative radiation therapy with or without 5-FU for rectal cancer *(70,71)*. Higher proliferative activity was associated with increased downstaging with preoperative treatment, and following radiation, improved survival. Others have correlated response to preoperative irradiation with p21 expression *(72)* or the presence of microsatellite instability *(73)*. Although the ability to identify patients who may respond favorably to preoperative chemoradiation is intriguing, further study of these tumor markers is required before relying on these for treatment decisions.

REFERENCES

1. Greenlee RT, Murray T, Bolden S, Wingo PA. Cancer Statistics, 2000. *CA Cancer J Clin* 2000; 50(1):7–33.
2. Compton CC, Fielding LP, Burgart LJ, et al. Prognostic factors in colorectal cancer. College of American Pathologists Consensus Statement 1999. *Arch Pathol Lab Med* 2000; 124:979–994.
3. Elsaleh H, Joseph D, Grieu F, et al. Association of tumour site and sex with survival benefit from adjuvant chemotherapy in colorectal cancer. *Lancet* 2000; 355(9217):1745–1750.
4. Shibata D, Reale MA, Lavin P, et al. The DCC protein and prognosis in colorectal cancer. *N Engl J Med* 1996; 335:1727–1737.
5. Galandiuk S, Wieand HS, Moertel CG, et al. Patterns of recurrence after curative resection of carcinoma of the colon and rectum. *Surg Gyn Obst* 1992; 174:27–32.
6. Wolmark N, Fisher B, Rockette H, et al. Postoperative adjuvant chemotherapy or BCG for colon cancer. Results from NSABP protocol C-01. *J Natl Cancer Inst* 1988; 80:30–36.
7. Laurie JA, Moertel CG, Fleming TR, et al. Surgical adjuvant therapy of large bowel carcinoma: an evaluation of levamisole and the combination of levamisole and 5-fluorouracil. *J Clin Oncol* 1989; 7:1447–1456.
8. Moertel CG, Fleming TR, Macdonald JS, et al. Fluorouracil plus levamisole as effective adjuvant therapy after resection of stage III colon carcinoma: a final report. *Ann Intern Med* 1995; 122:321–326.
9. Wolmark N, Rockette H, Wickerham DL, et al. The benefit of leucovorin modulated fluorouracil as postoperative adjuvant therapy for primary colon cancer: results from National Surgical Adjuvant Breast and Bowel Project Protocol C-03. *J Clin Oncol* 1993; 11:1879–1887.
10. Wolmark N, Rockette H, Mamounas EP, et al. The relative efficacy of 5-FU + leuocovorin (FU-LV), 5-FU + levamisole (FU-LEV), and 5-FU + leucovorin + levamisole (FU-LV-LEV) in patients with Dukes' B and C carcinoma of the colon: first report of the NSABP C-04 [Abstract]. *Proc Am Soc Clin Oncol* 1996; 15:205.
11. Haller DG, Catalano PJ, Macdonald JS, et al. Fluorouracil (FU), leuocovorin (LV) and levamisole (LEV) adjuvant therapy for colon cancer: five-year report of INT-0089 [Abstract]. *Proc Am Soc Clin Oncol* 1998; 17:256a.
12. Moertel CG, Fleming TR, Macdonald JS, et al. Intergroup study of fluorouracil plus levamisole as adjuvant therapy for stage II/Dukes' B2 colon cancer. *J Clin Oncol* 1995; 13:2936–2943.
13. International Multicentre Pooled Analysis of B2 Colon Cancer Trials (IMPACT B2) Investigators. Efficacy of adjuvant fluorouracil and folinic acid in B2 colon cancer. *J Clin Oncol* 1999; 17:1356–1363.
14. Mamounas E, Wieand S, Wolmark N, et al. Comparative efficacy of adjuvant chemotherapy in patients with Dukes' B versus Dukes' C colon cancer: results from four National Surgical Adjuvant Breast and Bowel Project adjuvant studies (C-01, C-02, C-03, and C-04). *J Clin Oncol* 1999; 17:1349–1355.
15. Willett CG, Fung CY, Kaufman DS, Efird J, Shellito PC. Postoperative radiation therapy for high-risk colon carcinoma. *J Clin Oncol* 1993; 11(6):1112–1117.
16. Martenson J, Willett C, Sargent C, et al. A phase III study of adjuvant radiation therapy (RT), 5-fluorouracil (5-FU), and levamisole (LEV) vs 5-FU and LEV in selected patients with resected, high risk colon cancer: initial results of INT 0130 [abstract]. *Proc Am Soc Clin Oncol* 1999; 235a.
17. Fabian C, Giri S, Estes N, et al. Adjuvant continuous infusion 5-FU, whole-abdominal radiation, and tumor bed boost in high-risk stage III colon carcinoma: a Southwest Oncology Group pilot study. *Int J Radiat Oncol Biol Phys* 1995; 32:457–464.
18. Allee PE, Tepper JE, Gunderson LL, Munzenrider JE. Postoperative radiation therapy for incompletely resected colorectal carcinoma. *Int J Radiat Oncol Biol Phys* 1989; 17:1171–1176.
19. Schild SE, Gunderson LL, Haddock MG, et al. The treatment of locally advanced colon cancer. *Int J Radiat Oncol Biol Phys* 1997; 37(1):51–58.
20. Rich T, Gunderson, LL, Lew R, et al. Patterns of recurrence of rectal cancer after potentially curative surgery. *Cancer* 1983; 52:1317–1329.
21. Minsky BD, Mies C, Recht A, et al. Resectable adenocarcinoma of the rectosigmoid and rectum: 1. Patterns of failure and survival. *Cancer* 1988; 61:1408–16.
22. Tepper JE, Cohen AM, Wood WC, et al. Postoperative radiation therapy of rectal cancer. *Int J Radiat Oncol Biol Phys* 1987; 13:5–10.
23. Gastrointestinal Tumor Study Group. Prolongation of the disease-free interval in surgically treated rectal carcinoma. *N Engl J Med* 1985; 312:1465–1472.
24. Fisher B, Wolmark N, Rockette H, et al. Postoperative adjuvant chemotherapy or radiation therapy for rectal cancer: results from NSABP protocol R-01. *J Natl Cancer Inst* 1988; 80:21–29.

25. NIH Consensus Conference. Adjuvant therapy for patients with colon and rectal cancer. *J Am Med Assoc* 1990; 264:1444–1450.
26. Krook JE, Moertel CG, Gunderson LL, et al. Effective surgical adjuvant therapy for high-risk rectal carcinoma. *N Engl J Med* 1991; 324:704–715.
27. Gastrointestinal Tumor Study Group. Radiation therapy and fluorouracil with or without semustine for the treatment of patients with surgical adjuvant adenocarcinoma of the rectum. *J Clin Oncol* 1992; 10:549–557.
28. O'Connell MJ, Martenson JA, Wieand HS, et al. Improving adjuvant therapy for rectal cancer by combining protracted-infusion fluorouracil with radiation therapy after curative surgery. *N Engl J Med* 1994; 331:502–507.
29. Wolmark N, Wieand HS, Hyams DM, et al. Randomized trial of postoperative adjuvant chemotherapy with or without radiotherapy for carcinoma of the rectum: National Surgical Adjuvant Breast and Bowel Project Protocol R-02. *J Natl Cancer Inst* 2000; 92(5):388–396.
30. Tepper JE, O'Connell MJ, Petroni GR, et al. Adjuvant postoperative fluorouracil-modulated chemotherapy combined with pelvic radiation therapy for rectal cancer: initial results of Intergroup 0114. *J Clin Oncol* 1997; 15(5):2030–2039.
31. Siani A, Cunningham D, Norman AR et al. Multicentre randomized trial of protracted venous infusion (PVI) 5 FU compared to 5 FU/folinic acid (5FU/FA) as adjuvant therapy for colorectal cancer [Abstract]. *Proc Am Soc Clin Oncol* 2000; 19:240a.
32. Paty PB, Enker WE, Cohen AM, et al. Long-term functional results of coloanal anastomosis for rectal cancer. *Am J Surg* 1994; 167:90–95.
33. MacFarlane JK, Ryall RD, Heald RJ. Mesorectal excision for rectal cancer. *Lancet* 1993 Feb 20; 341(8843):457–460.
34. Enker WE, Thaler HT, Cranor ML, Polyak T. Total mesorectal excision in the operative treatment of carcinoma of the rectum. *J Am Coll Surg* 1995; 181(4):335–346.
35. Heald RJ, Moran BJ, Ryall RD, et al. Rectal cancer: the Basingstoke experience of total mesorectal excision, 1978–1997. *Arch Surg* 1998; 133(8):894–899.
36. Arenas RB, Fichera A, Mhoon D, Michelassi F. Total mesenteric excision in the surgical treatment of rectal cancer: a prospective study. *Arch Surg* 1998; 133(6):608–612.
37. Kapiteijn E, Marijnen CAM, Nagtegaal ID, et al. Preoperative radiotherapy combined with total mesorectal excision for resectable rectal cancer. *N Engl J Med* 2001; 345(9):638–646.
38. Haller DG. Defining the optimal therapy for rectal cancer [letter]. *J Natl Cancer Inst* 2000; 92(5): 361–362.
39. Willett CG, Badizadegan K, Ancukiewicz M, Shellito PC. Prognostic factors in stage T3N0 rectal cancer: do all patients require postoperative pelvic irradiation and chemotherapy? *Dis Colon Rectum* 1999; 42(2):167–173.
40. Swedish Rectal Cancer Trial. Improved survival with preoperative radiotherapy in resectable rectal cancer. *N Engl J Med* 1997; 336:980–987.
41. Camma C, Giunta M, Fiorica F, et al. Preoperative radiotherapy for resectable rectal cancer: A meta-analysis. *J Am Med Assoc* 2000; 284:1008–1015.
42. Minsky BD, Cohen AM, Enker WE, et al. Preoperative 5-FU, low-dose leucovorin, and radiation therapy for locally advanced and unresectable rectal cancer. *Int J Radiat Oncol Biol Phys* 1997; 37(2):289–295.
43. Bosset JF, Magnin V, Maingon P, et al. Preoperative radiochemotherapy in rectal cancer: long-term results of a phase II trial. *Int J Radiat Oncol Biol Phys* 2000; 46(2):323–327.
44. Rich TA, Skibber JM, Ajani J, et al. Preoperative infusional chemoradiation therapy for stage T3 rectal cancer. *Int J Radiat Oncol Biol Phys* 1995; 32(4):1025–1029.
45. Mohiuddin M, Hayne M, Regine WF, et al. Prognostic significance of postchemoradiation stage following preoperative chemotherapy and radiation for advanced/recurrent rectal cancers. *Int J Radiat Oncol Biol Phys* 2000; 48:1075–1080.
46. Chari RS, Tyler DS, Anscher MS, et al. Preoperative radiation and chemotherapy in the treatment of adenocarcinoma of the rectum. *Ann Surg* 1995; 221(6):778–787.
47. Chan AKP, Wong AO, Langevin J, et al. Preoperative chemotherapy and pelvic radiation for tethered or fixed rectal cancer: a phase II dose escalation study. *Int J Radiat Oncol Biol Phys* 2000, 48:845–856.
48 Janjan NA, Khoo VS, Abbruzzese J, et al. Tumor downstaging and sphincter preservation with preoperative chemoradiation in locally advanced rectal cancer: the M. D. Anderson Cancer Center experience. *Int J Radiat Oncol Biol Phys* 1999; 44(5):1027–1038.

49. Minsky BD. Primary treatment of rectal cancer: present and future. *Crit Rev Oncol Hematol* 1999; 32:19–30.
50. Hyams DM, Mamounas EP, Petrelli N, et al. A clinical trial to evaluate the worth of preoperative multimodality therapy in patients with operable carcinoma of the rectum: a progress report of a national surgical adjuvant Breast and Bowel Project protocol R-03. *Dis Col Rectum* 1997; 40:131–139.
51. Wagman R, Minsky BD, Cohen AM, et al. Sphincter preservation in rectal cancer with preoperative radiation therapy and coloanal anastomosis: long term follow-up. *Int J Radiat Oncol Biol Phys* 1998; 42:51–57.
52. Valentini V, Coco C, Cellini N, et al. Preoperative chemoradiation for extraperitoneal T3 rectal cancer: acute toxicity, tumor response, and sphincter preservation. *Int J Radiat Oncol Biol Phys* 1998; 40:1067–1075.
53. Sauer R, Fietkau R, Martus P, et al. Adjuvant and neoadjuvant radiochemotherapy or advanced rectal cancer - first results of the German multicenter phase-III-trial [abstract]. *Int J Radiat Oncol Biol Phys* 2000; 48(3 Suppl):119a.
54. Francois Y, Nemoz CJ, Baulieux J, et al. Influence of the interval between preoperative radiation therapy and surgery on downstaging and on the rate of sphincter-sparing surgery for rectal cancer: the Lyon R90-01 randomized trial. *J Clin Oncol* 1999; 17(8):2396–2402.
55. Stahl TJ, Murray JJ, Coller JA, et al. Sphincter-saving alternative in the management of adenocarcinoma involving the distal rectum: 5-year follow-up results in 45 patients. *Arch Surg* 1993; 128:545–550.
56. Papillon J, Berard P. Endocavitary irradiation in the conservative treatment of adenocarcinoma of the low rectum. *World J Surg* 1992; 16:451–457.
57. Bleday R, Breen E, Jessup JM, et al. Prospective evaluation of local excision for small rectal cancer. *Dis Colon Rectum* 1997; 40:388–392.
58. Ota DM, Skibber J, Rich TA. M.D. Anderson Cancer Center experience with local excision and multimodality therapy for rectal cancer. *Surg Oncol Clin North Am* 1992; 1:147–152.
59. Steele GD, Herndon JE, Bleday R, et al. Sphincter-sparing treatment for distal rectal adenocarcinoma. *Ann Surg Oncol* 1999; 6:433–441.
60. Willett CG, Compton CC, Shellito PC, Efird JT. Selection factors for local excision or abdominoperineal resection of early stage rectal cancer. *Cancer* 1994; 73:2716–2720.
61. Chakravarti A, Compton CC, Shellito PC, et al. Long-term follow-up of patients with rectal cancer managed by local excision with and without adjuvant irradiation. *Ann Surg* 1999; 230(1):49–54.
62. Wagman R, Minsky BD, Cohen AM, et al. Conservative management of rectal cancer with local excision and postoperative adjuvant therapy. *Int J Radiat Oncol Biol Phys* 1999; 44:841–846.
63. Saltz LB, Cox JV, Blanke C, et al. Irinotecan plus fluorouracil and leucovorin for metastatic colorectal cancer. *N Engl J Med* 2000; 343:905–914.
64. Anne P, Mitchell EP, Ahmad N, et al. Radiosensitization in locally advanced adenocarcinoma of the rectum using combined modality therapy (CMT) with CPT-11, 5-fluorouracil concomitant irradiation [Abstract]. *Proc Am Soc Clin Assoc* 2000; 19:250a.
65. de la Torre A, Ramos S, Valcarcel FJ, et al. Phase II study of radiochemotherapy with UFT and low-dose oral leucovorin in patients with unresectable rectal cancer. *Int J Radiat Oncol Biol Phys* 1999; 45(3):629–634.
66. Hoff PM, Janjan N, Saad ED, et al. Phase I study of preoperative oral uracil and tegafur plus leucovorin and radiation therapy in rectal cancer. *J Clin Oncol* 2000; 18(20):3529–3534.
67. Dunst J, Reese T, Frings S. Phase I study of capecitabine combined with standard radiotherapy in patients with rectal cancer. *Proc Am Soc Clin Oncol* 2000; 19:256a.
68. Marsh RD, Chu NM, Vauthey JN, et al. Preoperative treatment of patients with locally advanced unresectable rectal adenocarcinoma utilizing continuous chronobiologically shaped 5-fluorouracil infusion and radiation therapy. *Cancer* 1996; 78(2):217–225.
69. Levi F, Zidani R, Misset JL. Randomized multicentre trial of chronotherapy with oxaliplatin, fluorouracil, and folinic acid in metastatic colorectal cancer. *Lancet* 1997; 350:681–686.
70. Willett CG, Warland G, Coen J, et al. Rectal cancer: the influence of tumor proliferation on response to preoperative irradiation. *Int J Radiat Oncol Biol Phys* 1995; 32:57–61.
71. Willett CG, Hagan M, Daley W, et al. Changes in tumor proliferation of rectal cancer induced by preoperative 5-fluorouracil and irradiation. *Dis Colon Rectum* 1998; 41:62–67.
72. Qiu H, Sirivongs P, Rothenberger M, et al. Molecular prognostic factors in rectal cancer treated by radiation and surgery. *Dis Colon Rectum* 2000; 43:451–459.
73. Anne PR, Edmonston TB, Rose D, et al. Microsatellite instability predicts for tumor response in a prospective trial of preoperative 5-FU, CPT-11, and radiation for locally advanced rectal cancer [Abstract]. *Int J Radiat Oncol Biol Phys* 2000; 48(3 Suppl):121.

15 Chemoradiotherapy in Muscle-Invasive Bladder Cancer

Bruce J. Roth, MD

Contents

1. INTRODUCTION

Transitional cell carcinoma of the bladder is diagnosed in approx 50,000 individuals in the United States each year, and accounts for 10,000 deaths annually. A majority of patients will present with nonmuscle-invasive disease, be treated adequately with transurethral resection (TURBT) with or without intravesical chemotherapy or immunotherapy, and will have only a 10–15% risk (higher for higher grades) of developing muscle-invasive disease. In contradistinction, the natural history of muscle-invasive disease is much more aggressive, with a 5-yr survival of only 50%.

2. SURGERY FOR MUSCLE-INVASIVE DISEASE

For decades the standard treatment approach for muscle-invasive disease has been a radical cystectomy. This therapy provides excellent local control with relatively few pelvic recurrences *(1)*. Aggressive surgical intervention also provides a significant cure rate, with an overall 5-yr survival for organ-confined disease of 65%, while those with extravesical extension 40% and for those with lymph-node positive disease 15% *(1–6)*. Over the past several decades, radical cystectomy has become a much safer procedure,

From: *Chemoradiation in Cancer Therapy*
Edited by: H. Choy © Humana Press Inc., Totowa, NJ

with minor complications occurring in <30% of patients and a perioperative mortality of approx 3% *(1)*.

Much of the patient aversion to this procedure stemmed from the requirement of a stomal appliance following an ileal conduit urinary diversion. This has prompted a number of approaches to preserve bladder function, including surgical approaches that create continent urinary diversions or orthotopic neobladders. Others have attempted to preserve native bladders by attempting to substitute a combination of chemotherapy and radiotherapy for radical cystectomy, and that approach is the focus of this chapter and will be discussed at length. However, since the creation of continent urinary diversions is rapidly becoming the standard of care, the potential quality-of-life (QOL) improvements achieved with bladder-sparing approaches will need to be compared to these new approaches to urinary diversion and not to a classic ileal conduit. The QOL of many patients has been improved by the use of continent diversions such as the Indiana, Mainz, or Kock pouches, which require intermittent catheterization but avoid the need for an external appliance. Other patients prefer to avoid an abdominal stoma altogether, and opt for the creation of an orthotopic neobladder, which allows the patient to continue to void through a native urethra, albeit with some additional effort (via Valsalva) and provides excellent functional voiding outcomes, although a minority of patients will continue to require intermittent catheterization due to high residual urinary volumes *(7–9)*.

3. RADIOTHERAPY FOR MUSCLE-INVASIVE DISEASE

Although cystectomy has remained the preferred modality of treatment for muscle-invasive disease in the United States, the use of primary radiotherapy in place of surgery gained favor in Europe and the United Kingdom, as it has in many other malignancies. Studies have included a broad range of total doses, from 50 to 70 Gy, with higher doses apparently associated with improved results *(10–16)*. Overall survival rates for radiotherapy alone on the surface appear to be significantly inferior to those obtained with cystectomy, with 5-yr survival of approx 35% for patients with clinical T2 and T3 disease *(12,17–19)*, which fall off to only 25% for clinical T3 disease *(10,20,21)*. These results are particularly disappointing given the fact that many patients have had maximal transurethral resection (and frequently to clinical T0 status) prior to initiation of what becomes in effect "adjuvant" radiotherapy. However, a number of factors could potentially confound this apparent inferiority:

1. The results with radiotherapy are necessarily based on clinical staging, as opposed to the pathologic staging associated with cystectomy. The error rate of clinical staging may be as high as 50%, with approximately two-thirds of those being understaging errors. Thus, many patients receiving radiotherapy with clinical T2 disease may in fact have pathologic stage T3b or node-positive disease and get the inferior results that would be expected for that pathologic stage.
2. The group of patients receiving radiotherapy may be enriched for an older patient population or those with a higher number of significant comorbidities, as these patients may have been selected for nonsurgical treatment options by their urologist.
3. Urologists may also have selected other patients to receive radiotherapy, namely, those with known poor prognostic factors, including those with hydronephrosis at presentation, higher grade tumors, the presence of anemia, and patients with multifocal tumors.

Despite these obvious biases against the results of radiotherapy, analysis of the published data does suggest that the results with radiation are somewhat inferior to those obtained with surgery, particularly with respect to higher grade and higher T-stage tumors. The results appear to be different both in terms of local control as well as 5-yr survival. One attempt to overcome this inferiority has been the addition of systemic chemotherapy to radiation.

4. CHEMOTHERAPY IN ADVANCED DISEASE

Certainly a minimum requirement of the addition of systemic chemotherapy to a local therapy such as radiation is that chemotherapy has significant activity in metastatic disease, even if that therapy is not associated with either curative potential or significant prolongation of survival. Certainly, combination chemotherapy for transitional cell carcinoma is able to achieve this requirement. In the early 1980s, cisplatin and methotrexate were felt to be the most active single agents, and a series of cisplatin and methotrexate-based regimens were developed. The most common of these was the cisplatin + methotrexate + vinblastine (CMV) regimen developed by the Northern California Oncology Group *(22)*, and the same three drugs in combination with doxorubicin (M-VAC), utilized at Memorial Sloan-Kettering Cancer Center *(23)*. The phase II data with M-VAC at Memorial in over 120 patients suggested true clinical synergism with the regimen, with a response rate of 72%, a complete response rate of 36% (although only 18% from chemotherapy alone), and a median survival of 13 mo *(23)*. However, this proved to be a moderately toxic regimen, with significant mucositis, pancytopenia, and neutropenic fever as dose-limiting toxicities, as well as a 3% toxic death rate. Over the next several years, phase III trials tempered the enthusiasm for M-VAC, with response rates of 40%, a complete response rate of approx 12%, and overall survival of 12 mo *(24,25)*. However, in these same trials, M-VAC proved to be superior to both single-agent cisplatin or the combination of cisplatin + cyclophosphamide + doxorubicin in terms of response rate and even a modest survival advantage. While the empiric addition of G-CSF to M-VAC successfully reduced the incidence of neutropenia and severe mucositis *(26)*, attempts to increase the response rate and survival of standard-dose M-VAC by escalation of doses had mixed results, with most trials demonstrating only increased toxicity without an increase in efficacy *(27,28)*, although a recent European trial of dose-dense M-VAC suggested some modest improvements in outcome.

This plateau of results over the past few years stimulated efforts to identify new active single agents in this disease *(29)*, with pacitaxel and gemcitabine identified as being the most active. Paclitaxel is likely the most active single agent in advanced bladder cancer, with a response rate in excess of 40% and a complete response rate of >25% *(30)*. It is particularly attractive in patients with bladder cancer (who frequently have significant subclinical or clinical renal impairment) since it is not primarily excreted by the kidneys, and can be given in full dose even to patients with mild to moderate renal insufficiency. The single-agent response rate of gemcitabine in previously untreated patients is approx 25%, with minimal nonhematologic toxicity *(31,32)*. Although a number of two-drug and three-drug combinations utilizing these agents have been tested, the most commonly used are carboplatin + paclitaxel and gemcitabine + cisplatin. The combination of carboplatin + paclitaxel has been extensively tested in the phase II setting, and shows significant activity, with an overall response rate of >50%, and a significant number of responses in patients with visceral metastatic disease *(33,34)*. This regimen is currently being tested in a phase III trial in patients with advanced disease vs standard-dose M-VAC by the Eastern Cooperative Oncology Group. Gemcitabine + cisplatin had similar response rates of 50% in phase II trials *(35,36)*, but have demonstrated marked myelosuppression and are somewhat less attractive because of the requirement to utilize a nephrotoxic drug such as cisplatin. Nevertheless, a phase III trial of gemcitabine + cisplatin vs M-VAC has been completed, and showed an identical response rate and survival when compared to M-VAC, no differences in QOL assessments, and with less neutropenia and neutropenic fever, but more anemia and thrombocytopenia *(37)*. Thus, several new regimens have shown equivalent efficacy to older regimens, but with significantly less toxicity. Additional trials attempting to increase the efficacy of these regimens are underway.

5. CHEMOTHERAPY + RADIOTHERAPY

The inferior results with radiotherapy alone compared to cystectomy in patients with muscle-invasive disease have prompted a large number of trials adding systemic chemotherapy to radiotherapy in an attempt to increase local control and eliminate micrometastatic disease frequently present at the time of diagnosis of muscle-invasive disease. It is not easy to directly compare surgical series with trials of bladder-sparing approaches. A number of confounding factors can potentially complicate the interpretation of trials of chemoradiotherapy, including the effect of the TURBT on the natural history of this disease, the errors of clinical staging both before and after chemotherapy/radiotherapy, and the endpoints utilized to determine efficacy.

6. IMPACT OF TURBT

The first is attempting to estimate the impact of one or more transurethral resections in the course of initial diagnosis, restaging, and so on. It has long been known that when considering nonsurgical options that an attempt at complete endoscopic resection is necessary and the successful completion of this prior to radiation therapy improved results *(38)*. It is unclear, however, whether it is the potential to have a complete resection or the resection itself that confers the advantage, analogous to the issue of primary surgical debulking in ovarian carcinoma. For example, a patient with a larger primary lesion, ureteral obstruction, or significant comorbidities may have a biopsy alone as opposed to an attempt to render them clinically NED (no evidence of disease) with TURBT. However, it may be these other prognostic factors that ultimately determine outcome independent of the extent of TURBT. In some series, in a highly selected patient population (possibly the same highly selected patients in chemoradiotherapy series), TURBT alone provided impressive 5- and 10-yr survival results *(39,40)*. In one of these studies, the 5- and 10-yr disease-specific survivals were 80.5% and 74.5% and the bladder-preservation rates for those two intervals were 82.7% and 79.6% *(40)*. It might be that this is the appropriate group of control patients when evaluating the results of phase II trials of chemoradiotherapy with bladder-sparing intent, since many of the patients in those studies were T0 prior to the start of therapy. Others have selected patients based on the TURBT results to select alternative bladder-sparing approaches, such as partial cystectomy *(41)*. In fact, as many as 10–15% of patients have no residual tumor in the cystectomy specimen (pT0) following an aggressive TURBT *(42,43)*, although there is some debate regarding the independent prognostic significance of achieving pT0 status *(44)*.

7. INACCURACY OF CLINICAL STAGING

As is true for all nonsurgical approaches to therapy, reliance on clinical staging is a necessary evil. A generally accepted estimate of the error rate of clinical vs pathologic staging is 50%, with approximately two-thirds of that error represented by understaging. In one study of 462 bladder tumors felt to be clinically NED, residual tumor was detected in 35% of cases *(45)*. At its extreme, many cases of "non-muscle invasive" disease upon review have no muscle in the specimen to determine invasiveness. In other cases, if that residual tumor is in the base of the resection and, consequently, the depth of invasion has been underestimated, the outcome with subsequent therapy will be inferior and related directly to the actual T-stage as opposed to the recognized T-stage. In short, one man's T2 is another man's T3b, based on the aggressiveness and completeness of the TURBT.

If such understaging impacts on the selection of patients for bladder-sparing approaches (either on or off protocol), the problem is magnified when clinical restaging is performed following either chemotherapy or radiation therapy or both. The general schema for such an approach involves, after initial TURBT, several cycles of chemotherapy and radiation therapy prior to restaging with a repeat TURBT. Based on the findings at this restaging, a decision is made whether the patient proceeds to cystectomy (if persistent disease is detected), or consolidative chemoradiotherapy if the patient is a "clinical complete responder." Thus unrecognized persistent disease places the patient at an increased risk for local recurrence. The accuracy of postchemotherapy clinical staging has been evaluated in a group of patients at Memorial Sloan-Kettering Cancer Center who underwent primary chemotherapy followed by cystectomy *(46)*. In a group of 51 patients, the predictive accuracy of postchemotherapy TURBT was only 82% (42/51), with the other 18% (9/51) incorrectly staged (7 understaged and 2 overstaged). Overall, clinical understaging for muscle-invasive disease is in the range of 30–40%. Pooled data have shown that in patients felt to have no residual tumor (T0) or only residual carcinoma-*in-situ* (Tis), 32% in fact have residual muscle-invasive disease at the time of subsequent cystectomy *(46)*. Presumably a similar percentage of patients getting consolidative chemoradiotherapy in place of cystectomy also have residual muscle-invasive disease. In a similar group of patients (with T0 or Tis disease) who chose not to undergo cystectomy and who were followed clinically, 22% subsequently developed metastatic disease *(46)*. In terms of survival, the largest neoadjuvant trial published to date showed that patients undergoing chemotherapy prior to cystectomy had a 20% higher incidence of achieving T0 status (12% vs 32%), but this only translated to a survival benefit of 6% *(43)*. It certainly seems likely that actual volumetric tumor reductions with chemotherapy and radiation therapy might serve only to make it more difficult for the pathologist to detect residual disease of any kind, much less muscle-invasive persistent disease. Although it may seem to the casual observer that the predictive accuracy of TURBT under these circumstances is reasonably good at 82%, in fact the error rate is many times greater than the actual differences that have been observed in neoadjuvant trials.

Trials combining chemotherapy and radiation therapy have followed three basic models, including the use of single agents given simultaneously with radiotherapy and functioning as radiopotentiating agents, the use of several cycles of combination chemotherapy prior to radiation therapy (neoadjuvant chemotherapy), or both. Some trials have utilized these strategies prior to a planned definitive surgical approach, while more recent efforts have focused on the possibility of this strategy to replace cystectomy and spare the native bladder.

Early phase II trials evaluating the potential benefit of adding a single chemotherapeutic drug with reported radiosensitizing properties focused on 5-fluorouracil (5-FU) and cisplatin. Because of the perceived toxicity of cisplatin, trials with 5-FU were initiated first, and the results of this combination suggested an increased rate of downstaging, although there also appeared to be an increase in the incidence of the radiation-induced injury to both bladder and rectum *(47,48)*. Cisplatin appeared to be a more logical choice for combination with radiation, given its higher single-agent response rate in metastatic bladder cancer, as well as some preclinical evidence suggesting enhancement of radiotherapy's effect *(49,50)*.

Phase II clinical studies combining single-agent cisplatin and full-dose radiotherapy varied tremendously in the patient populations treated, including muscle-invasive disease alone, patients with locally advanced disease, as well as N1 and N2 disease *(51–58)*. Therefore it is difficult to combine results and have definitive conclusions. However, this approach appeared to be feasible, provided reasonable local control rates, and 4-yr survival for all patients in the 40% range, and for complete responders 50%, which appeared to be superior to radiotherapy alone. Despite some initial promising results utilizing both cisplatin and 5-FU *(59)*, subsequent trials failed to show any obvious advantage to this approach.

Despite some apparent improvement over radiotherapy alone with these approaches, the majority of patients continued to succumb to metastatic disease despite adequate local control. This prompted studies that included several cycles of full-dose chemotherapy in addition to radiation +/- a radiosensitizing agent. Based on the predominance of cisplatin-based regimens at the time that the majority of these trials were designed, most studies utilized either CMV or M-VAC. Summarizing the results of these trials *(60–64)*, significant response rates (40–50%) were noted after chemotherapy alone, local invasive recurrences began to appear (vs new primary lesions) *(65)*, and some patients survived 5-yr NED with their bladders intact. However, an important observation was the appearance of distant metastases without locoregional recurrence and subsequent death from metastatic disease. A multivariate analysis of prognostic factors has shown that low T-stage and the absence of CIS predicted for obtaining complete response, and tumor size and response to chemoradiotherapy were significantly predictive of distant metastatic disease *(66)*.

8. THE MGH EXPERIENCE

In 1993, investigators at the Massachusetts General Hospital (MGH) published the results of an institutional study, which became the model for several subsequent trials *(67)*. In this first report, 53 patients (T2-4, NXM0) underwent maximal TURBT, followed by two cycles of CMV, then 4000 cGy + two cycles of single-agent cisplatin. Patients then underwent endoscopic reevaluation and those who had an incomplete response to therapy and who were surgical candidates underwent cystectomy, whereas complete responders were consolidated with an additional 2480 cGy and one additional cycle of cisplatin. Following 11 dropouts, 42 patients completed therapy and there was no chemotherapy-related mortality. Radical cystectomy was required in 15 patients, including 4 who were intolerant of therapy, 8 who had incomplete responses to therapy, and 3 who had a salvage cystectomy. At 48 mo of follow-up, 28 patients (53%) were alive and 24 (42%) were NED. However, with this "bladder-sparing" approach, only 20 patients (38%) were alive, NED with their native bladders intact. Eight of those 20 patients required additional intravesical therapy for nonmuscle-invasive recurrences. In an updated report on 106 patients, these investigators reported similar results *(67)*, with 85 patients completing therapy with only minor deviations. Nineteen patients underwent cystectomy because of an incomplete response or intolerance of chemoradiotherapy, and 76 patients were consolidated with additional radiotherapy and cisplatin. Thirty-six (34%) patients ultimately required cystectomy, with 49% of patients alive, and 43% alive with their native bladders intact. Although patients with T2 lesions had a 62% rate of achieving T0 status with induction therapy, this dropped off to 41% of patients with T3 and T4 disease, and fell even further to 20% in patients who presented with ureteral obstruction. Finally, distant metastatic disease continued to be a significant source of failure, despite systemic therapy being administered. Of patients who achieved T0 status and did not recur locally, the 5-yr actuarial likelihood of developing distant metastatic disease was 20%, while in patients who did not achieve a complete response or who achieved T0 and recurred locally, the 5-yr chance of relapse was 55%. These are important observations and suggest that the apparent excellent results obtained in a patient who can have a complete resection via TURBT, has low T-stage, a small primary and no hydronephrosis may not be extrapolated to a patient with a higher T-stage lesion, large volume residual tumor following TURBT, or other poor prognostic factors.

9. RTOG 88-02

The Radiation Therapy Oncology Group (RTOG) conducted a confirmatory phase II study based on the data from the initial 53 patients reported at the MGH. This trial, 88-02, utilized the identical regimen as outlined above, enrolled 91 patients, and the final results were published in 1996 *(68)*. Eighty-five patients completed induction therapy, 68 (75%) achieved a complete response, and 14 patients required an immediate cystectomy. In the 70 patients who proceeded to consolidative therapy, 36 (51%) developed recurrences, including 23 (33%) recurrences that were muscle-invasive, requiring salvage cystectomy. Overall, 37 of 91 patients (40%) required a cystectomy. Four-year actuarial results were reported, including a 43% risk of muscle-invasive local recurrence, a 22% risk of developing distant metastatic disease, an overall survival rate of 62%, and the likelihood of surviving with an intact bladder was only 44%. One important point reinforced by this trial was the accuracy of clinical restaging postchemoradiotherapy. Nineteen patients developed "non-muscle-invasive" recurrences, but four of these patients developed metastatic disease, and three had already died by the time of the report. Advocates of this approach argue that the patient likely would have died with metastatic disease anyway, and with this approach they did not have to endure a cystectomy. However, given the information from other trials regarding the clinical staging error, isn't it also possible that at least some individuals have persistent muscle-invasive disease following induction therapy that is confined to the bladder but undetectable by the urologist/pathologist? If so, those patients are destined to ultimately recur with distant metastatic disease. It is at least theoretically possible that some fraction of those patients would have been cured with cystectomy. Of course, this information cannot be derived from any phase II trial, despite the size of that trial. Although a definitive phase III trial of surgery vs a bladder-conservation approach cannot be accomplished, other questions can be answered by this mechanism.

10. RTOG 89-03

As a follow-up to 88-02, the RTOG conducted a randomized phase III trial to evaluate the role of the induction chemotherapy given as per the previous trial. This trial, 89-03, randomized patients to a control arm (including two courses of CMV) as outlined in the previous phase II trial, or the identical therapy without the two cycles of CMV *(69)*. This trial was initially designed to accrue 174 patients, but the protocol was stopped after 123 patients because of severe complications from the chemotherapy and 5 patients who suffered treatment-related deaths. Five-year actuarial data were presented, with 49% of patients alive and 38% with a functioning bladder. There were no differences between the two groups in terms of distant metastases, pelvic failures, or overall survival. Twenty patients developed a nonmuscle-invasive recurrence and were treated with additional local measures. Twenty other patients required salvage cystectomy because of muscle-invasive recurrences (n = 11), or noninvasive recurrences which did not respond to conservative management (n = 9).

There are several "take-home" messages from this study. First, this was a highly selected patient population with almost 75% of patients NED at the time of entry, having successfully undergone complete resection via TURBT. This does not represent the population of bladder cancer patients as a whole, and those who are able to have complete resection are more likely to have a favorable outcome. Therefore, in 75% of patients in this study, chemoradiotherapy was essentially administered as an adjuvant. In that context, the results are somewhat disappointing. Although the survival is comparable to muscle-invasive disease patients as a whole undergoing cystectomy, they are probably not equivalent to a group of patients who can undergo complete resection at TURBT and who subsequently have a cystectomy.

The percentage of patients who are alive with an intact bladder at 5 yr is only 38% with this "bladder-sparing" approach. This is not surprising, given what we know about the difficulties with clinical staging and the recognition of transitional cell carcinoma (TCC) of the urothelium as a field defect. People who are offered this approach as an "equivalent" option to cystectomy should be informed of these results.

There are several possible reasons for the negative results of this trial. One possibility is that an insufficient amount of chemotherapy was administered. Few would argue that two cycles of chemotherapy is likely insufficient to eradicate microscopic metastatic disease. However, in a 975 patient trial conducted by the Medical Research Council and the European Organization for the Research and Treatment of Cancer, three cycles of CMV given prior to definitive therapy failed to provide the 10% improvement in survival that could have been detected by the trial *(43)*. Similarly, other trials of neoadjuvant chemotherapy to date have similarly not shown any obvious improvement in survival *(70–73)*, so it is unlikely that the number of cycles of therapy here had a significant impact on the outcome of the study. Even if more cycles could have had an impact, it should be remembered that this trial was stopped early because of chemotherapy-related treatment deaths with only two cycles of treatment. Others have argued that the absence of doxorubicin in the CMV regimen makes this regimen inferior. However, no such randomized data exist, and it seems unlikely that a single, low dose of an agent with inferior single-agent activity when compared to CMV, would make a significant impact on results. Also, once again, M-VAC is clearly a more toxic regimen, and this trial was already stopped early because of toxicity, and the addition of doxorubicin to a group of patients receiving significant doses of radiotherapy is unlikely to be well tolerated. The final possible conclusion is that the concept of neoadjuvant chemotherapy simply does not work in bladder cancer. We await the results of the US Intergroup trial which randomized patients to receive surgery alone or three cycles of M-VAC prior to surgery. All other trials of chemotherapy in early stage disease have not shown a survival benefit.

If we have shown that two cycles of neoadjuvant chemotherapy is ineffective in this setting, then we are assuming that two to three doses of single-agent cisplatin added to radiotherapy will make that radiotherapy equivalent to cystectomy. Although this may be reasonable in patients with small, completely resected tumors, it clearly does not apply to patients with large residual tumors or with other poor prognostic factors such as the presence of hydronephrosis. The claim that the results with chemoradiotherapy are equivalent to surgery cannot be supported by the literature outlined here. Although advocates of bladder-sparing therapy have assumed that patients with a native, irradiated bladder necessarily have a better satisfaction rate and overall QOL than patients with any artificial diversion, this may not necessarily be true. Certainly bladder-sparing provides an improved QOL compared to an ileal loop diversion, but the majority of patients with continent diversions or orthotopic neobladders are equally pleased with their outcome. One must also consider the psychological impact on QOL of a patient who must be told that there is a 40% risk of invasive local failure by 4 yr, not to mention the need for additional intravesical therapy for noninvasive recurrences. This approach can certainly be offered to patients who are not surgical candidates because of medical comorbidities, or in the occasional patient who refuses surgical intervention.

REFERENCES

1. Stein JP, Lieskovsky G, Cote R, et al. Radical cystectomy in the treatment of invasive bladder cancer: long-term results in 1.054 patients. *J Clin Oncol* 2001; 3: 666–675.
2. Montie JE, Straffon RA, Stewart BH. Radical cystectomy without radiation therapy for carcinoma of the bladder. *J Urol* 1984; 131:477–482.
3. Skinner DG, Lieskovsky G. Contemporary cystectomy with pelvic node dissection compared to preoperative radiation therapy plus cystectomy in management of invasive bladder cancer. *J Urol* 1984;131: 1069–1072.
4. Giuliani L, Giberti C, Martorana G, Bonamini A, Natta GD, Rovida S. Results of radical cystectomy for primary bladder cancer: retrospective study of more than 200 cases. *Urology* 1985; 3:243–248.
5. Pagano F, Bassi P, Galetti TP, Meneghini AM, Milani C, Artibani W, Garbeglio A. Results of contemporary radical cystectomy for invasive bladder cancer: a clinicopathological study with an emphasis on the inadequacy of the tumor, nodes and metastases classification. *J Urol* 1991; 145:45–50.
6. Soloway MS, Lopez AE, Patel J, Lu Y. Results of radical cystectomy for transitional cell carcinoma of the bladder and the effect of chemotherapy. *Cancer* 1994; 73:1926–1931.
7. Weijerman PC, Schurmans JR, Hop WC. Morbidity and quality of life in patients with orthotopic and heterotopic continent urinary diversion. *Urology* 1996; 51:51–56.
8. Hautmann RE, Miller K, Steiner U. The ileal neobladder: 6 years of experience with more than 200 patients. *J Urol* 1993; 150:40–45.
9. Studer UE, Zingg EJ. Ileal orthotopic bladder substitutes: what we have learned from 12 years' experience with 200 patients. *Urol Clin North America* 1997; 24:781–793.

10. Goffinet DR, Schneider MJ, Glatstein EJ, et al. Bladder cancer: results of radiation therapy in 384 patients. *Radiology* 1975; 117:149–153.
11. Yu WS, Sagerman RH, Chung CT, Dalal PS, King GA. Bladder carcinoma: experience with radical and preoperative radiotherapy in 421 patients. *Cancer* 1985; 6:1293–1299.
12. Shipley WU, Rose MA, Perrone TL, Mannix CM, Heney NM, Prout GR. Full-dose irradiation for patients with invasive bladder carcinoma: clinical and histologic factors prognostic of improved survival. *J Urol* 1985; 134:679–683.
13. Quilty PM, Duncan W. Primary radical radiotherapy for T3 transitional cell cancer of the bladder: an analysis of survival and control. *Int J Rad Oncol Biol Phys* 1986; 12:853–860.
14. Pollack A, Zagars GK, Swanson DA. Muscle-invasive bladder cancer treated with external beam radiotherapy: prognostic factors. *Int J Rad Oncol Biol Phys* 1994; 2:267–277.
15. Mameghan H, Fisher R, Mameghan J, Brook S. Analysis of failure following definitive radiotherapy for invasive transitional cell carcinoma of the bladder. *Int J Rad Oncol Biol Phys* 1995; 2:247–254.
16. Gospodarowicz MK, Hawkins NV, Rawlings GA, et al. Radical radiotherapy for muscle invasive transitional cell carcinoma of the bladder: failure analysis. *J Urol* 1989; 142:1448–1454.
17. Greiner R, Skaleric C, Veraguth P. The prognostic significance of ureteral obstruction in carcinoma of the bladder. *Int J Rad Oncol Biol Phys* 1977; 2:1095–1100.
18. Blandy JP, England HR, Evans SJ, et al. T3 bladder cancer: the case for salvage cystectomy. *Br J Urol* 1980; 6:506–510.
19. Goodman GB, Hislop TG, Elwood JM, Balfour J. Conservation of bladder function in patients with invasive bladder cancer treated by definitive irradiation and selective cystectomy. *Int J Rad Oncol Biol Phys* 1981; 5:569–573.
20. Bloom HJ, Hendry WF, Wallace DM, Skeet RG. Treatment of T3 bladder cancer: controlled trial of preoperative radiotherapy and radical cystectomy versus radical cystectomy. *Br J Urol* 1982; 54:136–151.
21. Morrison R. The results of the treatment of cancer of the bladder - a clinical contribution to radiobiology. *Clin Radiol* 1975; 26:67–75.
22. Harker WG, Meyers FJ, Freiha FS, et al. Cisplatin, methotrexate, and vinblastine (CMV): an effective chemotherapy regimen for metastatic transitional cell carcinoma of the urinary tract; a Northern California Oncology Group study. *J Clin Oncol* 1985; 3:1463–1470.
23. Sternberg CN, Yagoda A, Scher HI, et al. Methotrexate, vinblastine, doxorubicin, and cisplatin for advanced transitional cell carcinoma of the urothelium: efficacy and patterns of response and relapse. *Cancer* 1989; 64:2448–2458.
24. Loehrer PJ, Einhorn LH, Elson PJ, et al. A randomized comparison of cisplatin alone or in combination with methotrexate, vinblastine, and doxorubicin in patients with metastatic urothelial carcinoma: a cooperative group study. *J Clin Oncol* 1992; 7:1066–1073.
25. Logothetis CJ, Dexeus FH, Finn L, et al. A prospective randomized trial comparing MVAC and CISCA chemotherapy for patients with metastatic urothelial tumors. *J Clin Oncol* 1990; 8:1050–1055.
26. Gabrilove JL, Jakubowski A, Scher H, et al. Effect of granulocyte colony-stimulating factor on neutropenia and associated morbidity due to chemotherapy for transitional-cell carcinoma of the urothelium. *N Engl J Med* 1988; 318:1414–1422.
27. Loehrer PJ, Elson P, Dreicer R, et al. Escalated dosages of methotrexate, vinblastine, doxorubicin, and cisplatin plus recombinant human granulocyte colony-stimulating factor in advanced urothelial carcinoma: an Eastern Cooperative Oncology Group trial. *J Clin Oncol* 1994; 12:483–488.
28. Logothetis C, Finn L, Amato R, Hassan E, Sella A. Escalated MVAC +/- rhGM-CSF in metastatic transitional cell carcinoma. *Proc Am Soc Clin Oncol* 1992; 11:202.
29. Roth BJ, Bajorin DF. Advanced bladder cancer: the need to identify new agents in the post-M-VAC (methotrexate, vinblastine, doxorubicin and cisplatin) world. *J Urol* 1995; 153:894–900.
30. Roth BJ, Dreicer R, Einhorn LH, et al. Significant activity of paclitaxel in advanced transitional cell carcinoma of the urothelium: a phase II trial of the Eastern Cooperative Oncology Group (E1892). *J Clin Oncol* 1994; 11:2264–2270.
31. Moore MJ, Tannock IF, Ernst DS, Huan S, Murray N. Gemcitabine: a promising new agent in the treatment of advanced urothelial cancer. *J Clin Oncol* 1997; 12:3441–3445.
32. Stadler WM, Kuzel T, Roth B, Raghavan D, Dorr FA. Phase II study of single-agent gemcitabine in previously untreated patients with metastatic urothelial cancer. *J Clin Oncol* 1997; 11:3394–3398.
33. Vaughn DJ, Malkowicz SB, Zoltick B, et al. Paclitaxel plus carboplatin in advanced carcinoma of the urothelium: an active and tolerable outpatient regimen. *J Clin Oncol* 1998; 1:255–260.

34. Redman BG, Smith DC, Flaherty L, Du W, Hussain M. Phase II trial of paclitaxel and carboplatin in the treatment of advanced urothelial carcinoma. *J Clin Oncol* 1998; 5:1844–1848.
35. Moore MJ, Winquist EW, Murray N, et al. Gemcitabine plus cisplatin, an active regimen in advanced urothelial cancer: a phase II trial of the National Cancer Institute of Canada Clinical Trials Group. *J Clin Oncol* 1999; 9: 2876–2881.
36. Kaufman D, Raghavan D, Carducci M, et al. Phase II trial of gemcitabine plus cisplatin in patients with metastatic urothelial cancer. *J Clin Oncol* 2000; 9: 1921–1927.
37. von der Maase H, Hansen SW, Roberts JT, et al. Gemcitabine and cisplatin versus methotrexate, vinblastine, doxorubicin, and cisplatin in advanced or metastatic bladder cancer: results of a large, randomized, multinational, multicenter, phase III study. *J Clin Oncol* 2000; 17:3068–3077.
38. Shipley WU, Prout GR, Kaufman SD, Perrone TL. Invasive bladder carcinoma: the importance of initial transurethral surgery and other significant prognostic factors for improved survival with full-dose irradiation. *Cancer* 1987; 60:514–520.
39. Henry K, Miller J, Mori M, Loening S, Fallon B. Comparison of transurethral resection to radical therapies for stage B bladder tumors. *J Urol* 1988; 140:964–967.
40. Solsona E, Iborra I, Ricos JV, Monros JL, Casanova J, Calabuig C. Feasibility of transurethral resection for msucle infiltrating carcinoma of the bladder: long-term follow-up of a prospective study. *J Urol* 1998; 159:95–99.
41. Herr HW. Conservative management of muscle-infiltrating bladder cancer: prospective experience. *J Urol* 1987; 138:1162–1163.
42. Herr HW. Transurethral resection in regionally advanced bladder cancer. *Urol Clin North Am* 1992; 19:695–700.
43. Medical Research Council Advanced Bladder Cancer Working Party. Neoadjuvant cisplatin, methotrexate, and vinblastine chemotherapy for muscle-invasive bladder cancer: a randomised controlled trial. *Lancet* 1999; 354:533–540.
44. Thrasher JB, Frazier HA, Robertson JE, Paulson DF. Does a stage pT0 cystectomy specimen confer a survival advantage in patients with minimally invasive bladder cancer? *J Urol* 1994; 152:393–396.
45. Kolozsy Z. Histopathological "self-control" in transurethral resection of bladder tumours. *Br J Urol* 1991; 67:162–164.
46. Herr HW, Whitmore WF, Morse MJ, Sogani PC, Russo P, Fair WR. Neoadjuvant chemotherapy in invasive bladder cancer: the evolving role of surgery. *J Urol* 1990; 144:1083–1088.
47. Rotman M, Macchia R, Silverstein M, et al. Treatment of advanced bladder carcinoma with irradiation and concomitant 5-fluorouracil infusion. *Cancer* 1987; 4: 710–714.
48. Russell KJ, Boileau MA, Ireton RC, et al. Transitional cell carcinoma of the urinary bladder: histologic clearance with combined 5-FU chemotherapy and radiation therapy. *Radiology* 1988; 167:845–848.
49. Kyriazis AP, Yagoda A, Kereiakes JG. Experimental studies on the radiation-modifying effect of cis-diamminedichloroplatinum II (DDP) in human bladder transitional cell carcinomas grown in nude mice. *Cancer* 1983; 52:452–457.
50. Nag S, Blatnik A, Soloway M. Enhancement of high intensity iodine-125 brachytherapy by cis-platinum in a murine bladder tumor model. *J Urol* 1984; 131:1225–1228.
51. Herr HW, Yagoda A, Batata M, Sogani PC, Whitmore WF. Planned preoperative cisplatin and radiation therapy for locally advanced bladder cancer. *Cancer* 1983; 52:2205–2208.
52. Shipley WU, Coombs LJ, Einstein AB, Soloway MS, Wajsman Z, Prout GR. Cisplatin and full dose irradiation for patients with invasive bladder cancer: a preliminary report of tolerance and local response. *J Urol* 1984; 132:899–903.
53. Jakse G, Frommhold H, Nedden DZ. Combined radiation and chemotherapy for locally advanced transitional cell carcinoma of the urinary bladder. *Cancer* 1985; 55:1659–1664.
54. Sauer R, Schrott KM, Dunst J, Thiel H-J, Hermanek P, Bornhof C. Preliminary results of treatment of invasive bladder carcinoma with radiotherapy and cisplatin. *Int J Radiation Oncology Biol Phys* 1988; 15:871–875.
55. Sauer R, Dunst J, Altendorf-Hofmann A. Radiotherapy with and without cisplatin in bladder cancer. *Int J Rad Oncol Biol Phys* 1990; 19:687–690.
56. Dunst J, Sauer R, Schrott KM. Organ-sparing treatment of advanced bladder cancer: a 10-year experience. *Int J Rad Oncol Biol Phys* 1994; 30:261–266.
57. Chauvet B, Brewer Y, Felix-Faure C, Davin J-L, Choquenet C, Reboul F. Concurrent cisplatin and radiotherapy for patients with muscle-invasive bladder cancer who are not candidates for radical cystectomy. *J Urol* 1996; 156:1258–1262.

58. Coppin CML, Gospodarowicz MK, James K. Improved local control of invasive bladder cancer by concurrent cisplatin and preoperative or definitive radiation. *J Clin Oncol* 1996; 11: 2901–2907.
59. Housset M, Maulard C, Chretien Y, et al. Combined radiation and chemotherapy for invasive transitional-cell carcinoma of the bladder: a prospective study. *J Clin Oncol* 1993; 11: 2150–2157.
60. Wajsman Z, Marino R, Parsons J, Oblon D, McCarley D. Bladder-sparing approach in the treatment of invasive bladder cancer. *Sem Urology* 1990; 3: 210–215.
61. Farah R, Chodak GW, Vogelzang NJ, et al. Curative radiotherapy following chemotherapy for invasive bladder carcinoma (a preliminary report). *Int J Rad Oncol Biol Phys* 1991; 20:413–417.
62. Vikram B, Malamud S, Silverman P, Hecht H, Grabstald H. A pilot study of chemotherapy alternating with twice-a-day accelerated radiation therapy as an alternative to cystectomy in muscle infiltrating (stages T2 and T3) cancer of the bladder: preliminary results. *J Urol* 1994; 151:602–604.
63. Angulo JC, Sanchez-Chapado M, Lopez JI, Flores N. Primary cisplatin, methotrexate and viblastine aiming at bladder preservation in invasive bladder cancer: multivariate analysis on prognostic factors. *J Urol* 1996; 155:1897–1902.
64. Serretta V, Lo Greco G, Pavone C, Pavone-Macaluso M. The fate of patients with locally advanced bladder cancer treated conservatively with neoadjuvant chemotherapy, extensive transurethral resection and radiotherapy: 10-year experience. *J Urol* 1998; 139:1187–1191.
65. Herr HW, Bajorin DF, Scher HI. Neoadjuvant chemotherapy and bladder-sparing surgery for invasive bladder cancer: ten-year outcome. *J Clin Oncol* 1998; 4:1298–1301.
66. Fung CE, Shipley WU, Young RH, et al. Prognostic factors in invasive bladder carcinoma in a prospective trial of preoperative adjuvant chemotherapy and radiotherapy. *J Clin Oncol* 1991; 9: 1533–1542.
67. Kaufman DS, Shipley WU, Griffin PP, Heney NM, Althausen AF, Efird JT. Selective bladder preservation by combination treatment of invasive bladder cancer. *N Engl J Med* 1993; 329:1377–1382.
68. Tester W, Caplan R, Heaney J. Neoadjuvant combined modality program with selective organ preservation for invasive bladder cancer: results of Radiation Therapy Oncology Group phase II trial 8802. *J Clin Oncol* 1996; 1:119–126.
69. Shipley WU, Winter KA, Kaufman DS. Phase III trial of neoadjuvant chemotherapy in patients with invasive bladder cancer treated with selective bladder preservation. *J Clin Oncol* 1998; 11:3576–3583.
70. Martinez-Pineiro J, Martin MG, Arocena F, et al. Neoadjuvant cisplatin chemotherapy before radical cystectomy in invasive transitional cell carcinoma of the bladder: a prospective randomized phase III study. *J Urol* 1995; 153:964–973.
71. Canobbio L, Curotto A, Boccardo F, et al. A randomized study between neo-adjuvant chemo-radiotherapy before radical cystectomy and cystectomy alone in bladder cancer. A 6 years follow-up. *Proc Am Soc Clin Oncol* 1995; 14:245.
72. Ghersi D, Stewart LA, Parmar MKB, et al. Does neoadjuvant cisplatin-based chemotherapy improve the survival of patients with locally advanced bladder cancer: a meta-analysis of individual patient data from randomized clinical trials. *Br J Urol* 1995; 75:206–213.
73. Cortesi E. Neoadjuvant treatment for locally advanced bladder cancer: a randomized prospective clinical trial. *Proc Am Soc Clin Oncol* 1995; 14:237.

16 The Role of Combined Chemotherapy and Radiation Therapy in the Treatment of Gynecologic Malignancies

Patricia J. Eifel, MD

Contents

1. INTRODUCTION

In women with lower-genital-tract carcinomas—cervical, vaginal, and vulvar carcinomas—hematogenous metastases are rarely present at diagnosis, and thus disease can frequently be controlled with local treatment. Small tumors can usually be treated with surgery alone, but cancers that penetrate deeply, particularly those that involve adjacent

From: *Chemoradiation in Cancer Therapy*
Edited by: H. Choy © Humana Press Inc., Totowa, NJ

tissues or regional lymph nodes, require radiation therapy. Although radiation therapy controls pelvic disease in many cases, local and regional recurrence frequently contributes to the death of patients who are not cured with local treatment. To reduce these recurrences and improve cure rates, investigators have sought effective ways of combining chemotherapy with radiation therapy.

Although combinations of chemotherapy and radiation therapy ("chemoradiation") have been used to treat a variety of gynecologic malignancies, the most intense interest has focused on the use of chemoradiation in the treatment of cervical cancer. Recent studies have convincingly demonstrated that concurrent chemotherapy can significantly improve the outcome of some patients who require radiation therapy for treatment of their disease. Controversies persist about the indications for chemoradiation and ideal drug regimens, but its fundamental value in patients with locoregionally advanced cervical cancer has been established.

This chapter will review trials of chemoradiation in cervical cancer, including the recent trials that established the value of this approach, and will discuss several questions that remain to be resolved regarding this treatment, including the ideal dose and schedule, and the effect of chemoradiation on compliance and complications. The last section of this chapter will briefly discuss the use of chemoradiation in the treatment of other gynecologic malignancies.

2. STUDIES OF HYDROXYUREA IN COMBINATION WITH RADIATION THERAPY

Until recently, hydroxyurea was prominent in most of the prospective randomized trials of chemoradiation for cervical cancer. One must understand the early trials of chemoradiation with hydroxyurea to understand the design of later chemoradiation trials.

In the late 1960s, Sinclair *(1)* published results of in vitro laboratory experiments suggesting that hydroxyurea might be an effective radiation sensitizer. Encouraged by these in vitro results and preliminary clinical results *(2)*, Piver and colleagues *(3–7)* began a series of clinical studies of the effectiveness of concurrent hydroxyurea and radiation therapy in women with carcinoma of the cervix (Table 1). The first of these studies *(3)* was a small trial of 41 patients (37 evaluable) with stages IIB-IIIB carcinoma of the cervix who were randomly assigned to receive hydroxyurea (80 mg/kg every 3 d) or placebo during external-beam irradiation. At a follow-up time of 2 yr, the authors reported disease control rates of 67% in the hydroxyurea arm and 32% in the placebo arm (Table 1).

By 1977, Piver and colleagues *(8)* had enrolled 148 patients in this study, and they published an updated analysis that included 117 of these patients. In this update, the authors did not provide an overall survival comparison but reported comparative survival rates in a number of subsets from the original study.

The authors were most encouraged by the results in the subset of 66 women with stage IIB disease: at 2 yr, rates of freedom from disease were 74% in the 27 women treated with hydroxyurea and 44% in the 39 women who had received the placebo. These results were encouraging, but the small number of patients, exclusions, and short follow-up may have compromised the analysis. Another concern about Piver and colleagues' studies was the high rate of severe complications, a number of which were fatal *(5)*. These deaths were excluded from the authors' calculations of disease-free survival.

Piver and colleagues did not find a survival benefit with hydroxyurea for patients with stage III disease who were treated in their studies *(4,7)*. However, they believed that a

Table 1
Studies of Hydroxyurea Combined with Radiation Therapy in Patients with Locally Advanced Carcinoma of the Cervix

				No. of patients		*Hydroxyurea*		*Alternate treatment*				
Author	*Year*	*Accrual dates*	*Tumor characteristics*	*Randomized*	*Analyzed*	*No.*	*Survival rate (%)*	*No.*	*Treatment*	*Survival rate (%)*	*Endpoint*	p
Piver et al. *(3)*	1974	Not stated	IIB (22), IIIB (15)	41	37	15	66.6	22	Placebo	31.8	Surviving, NED at 2 yr[a]	0.001
Piver et al. *(4)*	1977	Not stated	IIB (67), IIIB (50)	148	117							
			IIB[b]	Unknown	66	27	74	39	Placebo	44	Surviving, NED at 2 yr	<0.01
			IIIB[b]	Unknown	51	23	52	27	Placebo	33	Surviving, NED at 2 yr	0.22
			IIIB, PAN- (LND)[b]		28	14	50	14	Placebo	57	Surviving, NED at 2 yr	
Hreshchyshyn et al. *(9)*	1979	1970–1976	IIIB (84), IVA (13)	190	97	51	25	46	Placebo	13	3-yr disease-free survival[c]	0.05
Piver et al. *(5)*	1983	1972–1976	IIB PAN- (LND)	40	40	20	94	20	Placebo	53	5-yr survival[d]	0.006
Piver et al. *(6)*	1985	1977–1984	IIB (LAG-, no LND)	—	20	20	88				5-yr disease-free survival	
Piver et al. *(7)*	1987		IIIB PAN- (LND)	45	45	20	60	25	Placebo	52	5-yr freedom from progression	0.49
Stehman et al. *(11)*	1993	1981–1985	IIB (180), III (107), IVA (9)	308	294	137	53	157	Misonidazole	44	5-yr survival	0.07
Whitney et al. *(13)*	2000	1986–1990	IIB (228), III (128), IVA (13)	388	368	191	47	177	PF	57	5-yr freedom from progression	0.03[e]
Rose et al. *(12)*	1999	1992–1997	IIB (228), III (128), IVA (13)	575	526	177	47	176 173	P PF + HU	67 64	2-yr freedom from progression	<0.001[e] <0.001[e]

[a]Crude percentage calculations. [b]Subset analysis. [c]Estimated from curves. [d]Endpoint was "5-year life table survival" but deaths from complications (2 in control arm and 4 in hydroxyurea arm) did not appear to have been included as events in survival calculations. [e]Favoring the cisplatin-containing arm.

F = fluorouracil, HU = hydroxyurea, LAG = lymphangiogram, PAN = paraaortic node, LND = lymph node dissection, NED = no evidence of disease, P = cisplatin.

protracted radiation therapy schedule and undiagnosed para-aortic metastases in some patients who did not undergo lymphadenectomy had compromised the overall effectiveness of treatment. In 1987, the authors *(7)* reported results in 45 women with stage III disease who had negative para-aortic lymph nodes at lymphadenectomy. Again, there was no survival benefit for patients treated with hydroxyurea ($p = 0.49$). However, the authors were encouraged by a 92% disease control rate in a small subset of 17 patients who had received hydroxyurea with continuous (rather than split-course) irradiation.

In the 1970s, the Gynecologic Oncology Group (GOG) *(9)* conducted a multi-institutional trial in which patients with stage IIIB or IVA cervical cancer were randomly assigned to receive hydroxyurea or placebo during external-beam irradiation; lymphadenectomy was not required (Table 1). Although the final analysis suggested that there was a benefit from hydroxyurea, the difference between the two arms was only marginally significant, and flaws in the study raised questions about the generalizability of the results. The initial trial design called for enrollment of a modest number of patients, 190 were randomized, but because of protocol violations and other problems only 97 of these patients (51%) were included in the final analysis. The exclusion of more than half of the patients entered in the trial probably invalidated the initial randomization. The study was also criticized because of the poor survival rate in the control arm (13%) and the relatively low dose of radiation used (many received 70 Gy or less).

Although flaws in these studies of hydroxyurea left their results open to question, the GOG was convinced that the weight of the evidence supported inclusion of hydroxyurea in the control arms of future trials. In the early 1980s, 308 patients with stages IIB-IVA cervical cancer were randomly assigned to receive radiation therapy with concurrent hydroxyurea or radiation therapy with concurrent misonidazole. A preliminary review *(10)* revealed that patients treated with hydroxyurea had a slightly superior survival rate (median progression-free interval 42.9 vs 40.4 mo; $p = 0.08$). This difference persisted but there was still no significant difference in survival in a 1993 update (5-yr survival 53% vs 44%, $p = 0.07$) (Table 1) *(11)*. The authors concluded that this study provided additional evidence of the benefit of hydroxyurea. However, the small difference and the possibility that any difference reflected a harmful effect of misonidazole rather than a benefit from hydroxyurea left many clinicians with persistent doubts about the value of hydroxyurea.

Continued optimism led to the inclusion of hydroxyurea in the control arms of two subsequent GOG trials *(12,13)* in which hydroxyurea plus radiation therapy was compared with three different cisplatin-containing chemoradiation regimens (Table 1). All three cisplatin-containing regimens were superior to treatment with radiation and hydroxyurea, leading most gynecologic oncologists to abandon the use of hydroxyurea as a radiation sensitizer.

3. STUDIES OF CISPLATIN-CONTAINING CHEMOTHERAPY IN COMBINATION WITH RADIATION THERAPY

Cisplatin was first used to treat advanced cervical cancer shortly after the drug was introduced into clinical practice in the early 1970s. Although cisplatin continues to be one of the most active agents against cervical cancer, response rates are less than 30% for patients with recurrent or metastatic disease, and complete responses are rare and usually of short duration *(14)*.

In contrast, multiagent cisplatin-containing regimens have produced fairly high response rates in women with untreated locally advanced disease. Although complete responses to chemotherapy are uncommon, partial response rates of 60% or more led clinicians to investigate the sequential use of cisplatin-containing regimens and radiation.

3.1. Sequential Therapy

Unfortunately, none of the seven randomized trials that have compared radiation therapy alone vs neoadjuvant cisplatin-containing chemotherapy plus radiation therapy demonstrated an improvement in overall or disease-free survival with combined-modality therapy (Table 2). Two studies actually demonstrated poorer survival with neoadjuvant chemotherapy. Souhami et al. *(15)* reported a significantly poorer survival rate with neoadjuvant chemotherapy in a small trial of patients with stage IIIB disease. This outcome was partly due to increased toxicity and poor compliance in patients who received chemotherapy. Another trial of neoadjuvant epirubicin and cisplatin was closed early when interim analysis revealed a significantly higher recurrence rate in the chemotherapy arm *(16)*. These trials fail to provide any evidence that sequential cisplatin-containing chemotherapy and radiation therapy are of benefit. Possible explanations for the disappointing results include the effects of chemotoxicity, altered compliance, and possible accelerated repopulation of resistant clones after neoadjuvant chemotherapy.

3.2. Concurrent Therapy

Other groups have investigated the use of concurrent cisplatin-containing chemotherapy and radiation therapy. Within the past 3 yr, five multi-institutional randomized trials *(12,13,17–19)* have been reported that demonstrated highly significant improvements in disease-free survival when cisplatin-containing chemotherapy was given concurrently with radiation therapy (Table 3). These findings have significantly altered the standard of care for women with locoregionally advanced cervical cancer.

The first trial to address this question was a GOG trial *(13)* comparing concurrent hydroxyurea plus radiation therapy vs concurrent cisplatin and fluorouracil plus radiation therapy in patients with locally advanced disease who had negative para-aortic nodes at lymphadenectomy. An early analysis of this trial, which was completed in 1990, failed to yield definitive results. Publication of the study findings was delayed until more complete follow-up could be obtained. Ultimately, the study demonstrated a modest but significant advantage for the cisplatin-fluorouracil combination.

The final results of the initial GOG trial were not available when the GOG designed its next trial *(12)* for patients with locally advanced disease and negative para-aortic nodes at lymphadenectomy. In the second trial, hydroxyurea was again used in the control arm, but this time it was compared with two more aggressive cisplatin-containing chemotherapy regimens. Patients in one investigational arm received weekly cisplatin with radiation therapy, while those in the other investigational arm received a combination of hydroxyurea, cisplatin, and fluorouracil with radiation therapy. This time, both cisplatin-containing treatments were found to yield dramatic, highly significant improvements in local disease control and survival. The median duration of treatment was somewhat longer than most experts currently consider to be ideal but was similar in all three arms of the study.

While the GOG was conducting its three-arm trial, two other groups were also studying the value of concurrent cisplatin-containing chemotherapy and radiation therapy in

Table 2
Results of Prospective Randomized Trials that Compared Neoadjuvant Cisplatin-Containing Chemotherapy Followed by Radiation Therapy with Radiation Therapy Alone in Patients with Locally Advanced Cervical Cancer *(52)*

Author	*Year*	*No. of patients*	*Stages*	*Drugs*	*Survival rate (%)* CT + RT	*Survival rate (%)* RT alone	p	*Endpoint*
Kumar et al. *(53)*	1994	184	IIB–IVA	BIP	38	43	0.5	OS at 32 mo
Tattersall et al. *(16)*	1992	71	IIB–IVA	PVB	44[a]	40[a]	N.S.	OS at 48 mo
Chauvergne et al. *(54)*	1990	107	IIIB	MtxCVP	47[a]	50[a]	N.S.	OS at 48 mo
Tattersall et al. *(55)*	1995	260	IIB–IVA	EpP	50[a]	69[a]	0.02	OS at 36 mo
Sundfør et al. *(56)*	1996	94	IIIB–IVA	PF	34[a]	37[a]	0.9	OS at 48 mo
Leborgne et al. *(57)*	1997	96	IB2-IVA	BOP	38	45	0.4	DFS at 60 mo
Souhami et al. *(15)*	1991	107	IIIB	BOMP	23	39	0.02	OS at 60 mo

[a]Percentages were estimated from survival curves.

B = bleomycin, C = chlorambucil, CT = chemotherapy, DFS = disease-free survival, Ep = epirubicin, F = fluorouracil, I = ifosfamide, M = mitomycin C, Mtx = methotrexate, O = vincristine, OS = overall survival, P = cisplatin, RT = radiation therapy, V = vinblastine.

Table 3

Prospective Randomized Trials that Investigated the Role of Concurrent Radiotherapy and Chemotherapy for Patients with Locoregionally Advanced Cervical Cancer

Authors (trial group)	*Eligibility*	*No. of patients*	*CT in investigational arm*	*CT in control arm*	*Median duration of RT (d)*[f]	*Relative risk of recurrence (95% C.I.)*	p
Chemoradiation only							
Whitney et al. *(13)* (GOG)	FIGO IIB–IVA	368	Cisplatin 50 mg/m^2 5-FU 4 g/m^2/96 h (2 cycles)	HU 3 g/m^2 (2×/wk)	Not stated	0.79 (0.62–0.99)	0.03
Rose et al. *(12)* (GOG)	FIGO IIB–IVA	526	Cisplatin 40 mg/m^2/wk (up to 6 cycles)	HU 3 g/m^2 (2×/wk)	63	0.57 (0.42–0.78)	< 0.001
			Cisplatin 50 mg/m^2 5-FU 4 g/m^2/96 h HU 2 g/m^2 (2×/wk) (2 cycles)	HU 3 g/m^2 (2×/wk)	65	0.55 (0.40–0.75)	< 0.001
Morris et al. *(18)* (RTOG)	FIGO IB–IIA (≥ 5 cm), IIB–IVA or pelvic nodes involved	403	Cisplatin 75 mg/m^2 5-FU 4 g/m^2/96 h (3 cycles)	None[a]	58	0.48 (0.35–0.66)	< 0.001
Pearcey et al. *(20)* (NCIC)	FIGO IB–IIA (≥ 5 cm), IIB–IVA or pelvic nodes involved	259	Cisplatin 40 mg/m^2/wk (up to 6 cycles)	None	49	0.91 (0.62-1.35)[c]	0.43
Wong et al. *(28)*	FIGO IB–IIA (> 4 cm), IIB–III	220	Epirubicin 60 mg/m^2 then 90 mg/m^2 q 4 wk for 5 more cycles[d]	None	Not stated	~ 0.65	0.02
Thomas et al. *(22)*	FIGO IB–IIA (≥ 5 cm), IIB–IVA	234	5-FU 4 g/m^2/96 h × 2	None[e]			N.S.
Chemoradiation plus surgery							
Keys et al. *(17)* (GOG)	FIGO IB (≥ 4 cm)	369	Cisplatin 40 mg/m^2/wk (up to 6 cycles)	None[b]	50	0.51 (0.34–0.75)	0.001
Peters III et al. *(19)* (SWOG)	FIGO I–IIA after radical hysterectomy with nodes, margins, or parametrium positive	268	Cisplatin 50 mg/m^2 5-FU 4 g/m^2/96 h (2 cycles)	None	43	0.50 (0.29–0.84)	0.01

[a]Patients in control arm had prophylactic para-aortic irradiation. [b]All patients had extrafascial hysterectomy after radiation therapy. [c]Survival. [d]Chemotherapy was begun on d 1 and continued every 4 wk through and after radiation therapy. [e]Patients were also randomly assigned to receive standard or hyperfractionated radiation therapy in a four-arm trial. [f]In investigational arms. In no case was the median duration of RT significantly different between control and investigational arms.

C. I. = confidence interval, FIGO = International Federation of Gynecology and Obstetrics, HU = hydroxyurea, PA = para-aortic, RT = radiotherapy.

patients with locally advanced disease. The Radiation Therapy Oncology Group (RTOG) compared a combination of cisplatin and fluorouracil with pelvic irradiation vs pelvic and para-aortic (extended-field) irradiation alone in RTOG 90-01 (Table 3) *(18)*. Eligible patients were required to have either a lymphangiogram or retroperitoneal lymph node dissection demonstrating negative para-aortic lymph nodes. The control arm was based on an earlier study that demonstrated an improvement in outcome when prophylactic para-aortic irradiation was added to standard pelvic irradiation. The RTOG trial was published ahead of schedule when an interim analysis revealed highly significant improvements in overall survival, disease-free survival, local disease control, and rates of freedom from distant metastases in the investigational arm.

Most recently, the National Cancer Institute of Canada Clinical Trials Group (NCIC) completed a randomized trial comparing standard pelvic radiation therapy vs concurrent chemoradiation using weekly cisplatin *(20)*. This is the only major randomized trial of cisplatin-containing chemotherapy that has not yet demonstrated a significant improvement in outcome with the addition of concurrent cisplatin. Although this trial was somewhat smaller than the others, the median follow-up duration was long (65 mo). The authors have suggested that the shorter duration of radiation therapy in their study improved the outcome with radiation therapy alone, explaining the failure of cisplatin to improve the results. However, the 12-mo local control rate was similar to that of the control arm of RTOG 90-01, suggesting that the margin for improvement was similar in the two studies.

Two trials have compared radiation therapy and chemoradiation in combination with surgery. The GOG conducted a trial in which patients with bulky stage IB carcinomas of the cervix were treated with external-beam radiation therapy followed by intracavitary radiation therapy and extrafascial hysterectomy *(17)*. Patients were randomly assigned to receive or not receive weekly cisplatin during external-beam irradiation. Other studies suggest that adjuvant extrafascial hysterectomy may not be necessary for these patients. However, the addition of chemotherapy to the regimen significantly increased both the pathologic complete response rate and the overall survival rate. The Southwest Oncology Group (SWOG) also found a benefit from concurrent chemotherapy in women who required adjuvant radiation therapy after radical hysterectomy *(19)*. In that study, women who received concurrent chemotherapy during adjuvant radiation therapy also received two additional cycles of chemotherapy after radiation therapy was finished.

4. STUDIES OF FLUOROURACIL IN COMBINATION WITH RADIATION THERAPY

The value of fluorouracil as a radiation sensitizer in patients with gynecologic cancer has not yet been clearly determined. The GOG recently completed a trial comparing weekly cisplatin with a chronic continuous infusion of fluorouracil alone, but results of this trial have not been reported. No study has yet compared the two most successful cisplatin-containing regimens described to date—specifically, weekly cisplatin (used in several GOG trials and the NCIC trial) vs three or four cycles of higher-dose cisplatin with fluorouracil (used in the RTOG and SWOG trials). The inclusion of hydroxyurea and the relatively low dose of cisplatin in the three-drug arm of the GOG trial reported by Rose et al. *(12)* make it impossible to ascertain the contribution of fluorouracil to the benefit and toxicity of that regimen. A recent update of an early trial from The University of Texas M. D. Anderson Cancer Center study *(21)* of fluorouracil given as a chronic continuous intra-arterial infusion with radiation provided anecdotal evidence of the efficacy of the drug. That review revealed that several patients with massive stage IIIB disease who were treated with only 50 Gy of pelvic irradiation and fluorouracil survived for more than 5 yr. More recently, a small prospective randomized trial exploring the use of concurrent continuous-infusion fluorouracil and radiation yielded encouraging but inconclusive results *(22)*.

5. STUDIES OF OTHER CYTOTOXIC AGENTS IN COMBINATION WITH RADIATION THERAPY

North American prospective trials of radiation sensitizers for cervical cancer have focused on the use of cisplatin, fluorouracil, and hydroxyurea. However, a number of other drugs also hold promise as effective radiation sensitizers for cervical cancer, including mitomycin C, epirubicin, paclitaxel, and carboplatin.

Citing the success of mitomycin-C in the treatment of anal cancer, a number of investigators have explored the use of this drug, usually in combination with fluorouracil, in patients treated with radiation for cervical and vulvar carcinomas *(23–27)*. Roberts et al. *(27)* recently reported results of an interim analysis of a randomized trial, conducted in Venezuela, in which women with locally advanced cervical cancer were treated with radiation therapy with or without mitomycin. At the time of this interim analysis (published while the authors were continuing to accrue patients to the study), the authors noted a significant improvement in disease-free survival ($p = 0.01$) with chemotherapy but no significant difference in overall survival ($p = 0.1$).

Although neoadjuvant epirubicin has not been found to benefit women with locally advanced cervical cancer, Wong et al. *(28)* reported significant improvements in disease-free and overall survival ($p = 0.03$ and $p = 0.04$, respectively) when the drug was given during and after radiation therapy in patients with stages IB2-III cervical cancer. In this study, epirubicin was given for six cycles, starting at the beginning of radiation therapy. For the first cycle the drug was given at a dose of 60 mg/m^2 and then at 90 mg/m^2 for five more cycles at 4-wk intervals.

Other potential radiation sensitizers for cervical cancer are being explored in phase I and II trials. Paclitaxel has been combined with cisplatin in several small phase I studies. Pignata et al. *(29)* found that 50 mg/m^2 per week of paclitaxel could be combined with weekly cisplatin (30 mg/m^2) and radiation therapy with acceptable toxicity, although 10 of 18 patients in their study had grade 3–4 hematologic toxicity. Chen et al. *(30)* also were able to give weekly paclitaxel at a dose of 50 mg/m^2 (in this case combined with 50 mg/m^2 of cisplatin every three weeks) with tolerable toxicity and minimal delay in planned radiation therapy. In both studies, the dose-limiting side effect appeared to be diarrhea. It should be noted that the total dose of cisplatin delivered in these trials was lower than that used in the most successful prospective trials of cisplatin or cisplatin and fluorouracil (Table 3).

Muderspach et al. *(31)* reported the results of a pilot study of concurrent carboplatin (30 mg/m^2 twice weekly) with radiation in 22 patients with stage IIA (>4 cm) to IIIB disease. The most significant chemotherapy-related side effects were grade 3 neutropenia and anemia. The authors reported 19 complete responders to this regimen, although only 11 patients were alive and disease-free at the time of their report. Because cisplatin has consistently been found to be the most active single agent in women with advanced and recurrent cervical cancer and because of the drug's proven activity as a radiation sensitizer, it has been preferred over carboplatin in most studies. However, a significant number of cervical cancer patients are ineligible to receive cisplatin because of renal failure secondary to cancer-related hydronephrosis. There is an important need to demonstrate whether less nephrotoxic agents such as carboplatin are effective radiation sensitizers in this setting.

Although a number of other agents are of interest as possible radiation sensitizers, most investigators find it difficult to justify testing them in potentially curable cervical cancer patients without including cisplatin because of the dramatic improvements documented when cisplatin was used in the prospective randomized trials described earlier in this chapter.

6. IMPORTANCE OF DRUG DOSE, SCHEDULE, AND MODE OF ADMINISTRATION

The studies of chemoradiation that have been completed in patients with carcinoma of the cervix provide little specific guidance about the importance of chemotherapy dose and schedule.

The dose of cisplatin in the RTOG regimen (two to three cycles of 75 mg/m^2) *(18)* and the dose used in the GOG weekly schedule (four to six cycles of 40 mg/m^2) *(12,17)* resulted in the highest total doses of cisplatin described to date in trials of chemoradiation for cervical cancer—an average total dose of more than 200 mg/m^2 (Table 2). Patients treated in the SWOG postoperative trial also received a high total dose of cisplatin, although some of the drug was delivered after radiation therapy was completed *(19)*. It has been tempting to suggest that the somewhat smaller reduction in risk seen for patients treated in the early GOG trial published by Whitney et al. *(13)* reflected the lower total dose of cisplatin used in that trial. However, the negative preliminary result reported for the NCIC trial *(20)*, in which the dose of cisplatin was relatively high, underscores the danger of attempting to compare results between trials to assess the relative benefit of different schedules.

So far, the available evidence probably supports the use of either the GOG weekly cisplatin regimen or the RTOG schedule of cisplatin and fluorouracil. As yet, no data support the use of weekly cisplatin at doses below the 40 mg/m^2/wk given in the GOG studies. The only randomized trial to investigate a lower dose of weekly cisplatin was an early study reported by Wong et al. *(32)* They were unable to demonstrate a benefit when 25 mg/m^2/wk of cisplatin plus radiation therapy was compared to radiation therapy alone. It must be noted, though, that the study was compromised by the small number of patients (fewer than 30 in each arm).

The literature strongly suggests that concurrent chemoradiation is superior to neoadjuvant chemotherapy followed by radiation therapy. However, the effect of continuing chemotherapy after radiation is complete is uncertain. Two of the positive trials (the SWOG postoperative trial *[19]* and a study of concurrent epirubicin *[28]*) involved additional cycles of chemotherapy after concurrent chemoradiation was completed. In their report, Peters et al. *(19)* suggested that postradiation chemotherapy contributed importantly to their patients' good outcomes because those who completed the full course of treatment appeared to have a better outcome than those who received only the concurrent chemoradiation. However, it may be impossible to determine whether termination of chemotherapy before the full planned course correlated with some other difference in the patients' disease or in their ability to cooperate with other important aspects of treatment. The weight of the literature still suggests that the concurrent component of treatment is most important, and further studies will be needed to determine the importance of additional chemotherapy.

All of the prospective studies cited in Table 3 involved delivery of chemotherapy throughout external-beam irradiation. However, only the RTOG trial *(18)* included a planned course of chemotherapy with the intracavitary irradiation. The trial by Wong et al. *(28)* also involved delivery of chemotherapy during intracavitary irradiation but did not specify the precise timing of the drugs with respect to intracavitary procedures. Patients who are treated with a combination of external-beam irradiation and low-dose-rate intracavitary therapy typically receive 50% or more of the dose to their primary tumor during 3–4 d of brachytherapy. This would seem to be an ideal time to give concurrent chemotherapy, but the value of this timing has not been proven. Today some clinicians are using high-dose-rate brachytherapy divided into 3- to 9-Gy fractions (to point A) to treat women with cervical cancer. The optimal timing of chemotherapy with respect to high-dose-rate intracavitary treatments in terms of tumor control and the potential for late effects is entirely unknown.

7. INFLUENCE OF CHEMORADIATION ON COMPLIANCE AND TREATMENT DURATION

Most locally advanced cervical cancers occur in women who have had limited or no experience with the medical care community. These women may have significant social, cultural, educational, and financial barriers to obtaining consistent care and may have difficulty complying with complex treatment regimens. Although compliance rates vary, some investigators have reported very high rates of incomplete or severely protracted treatment in patients with cervical cancer *(33,34)*. One of the factors thought to contribute to the disappointing results achieved with neoadjuvant chemotherapy was the higher likelihood that patients would fail to complete local treatment after a course of toxic chemotherapy.

The influence of concurrent chemotherapy on compliance is still incompletely understood. The average duration of treatment varied markedly between the randomized trials reported to date, although none of the trials reported a significant difference in the overall duration of radiation therapy between the regimens that were being directly compared (Table 3). Several of the trials reported a disturbingly high number of patients whose treatment was protracted beyond currently acceptable limits. In particular, in the large GOG trial reported by Rose et al. *(12)*, the median duration of treatment was 9 wk; 10% of patients required 12 wk or more, and 9% did not receive any brachytherapy. Because patients received chemotherapy in all three arms, it is impossible to estimate how many of these delays were related to compliance problems or side effects of chemotherapy. However, the long treatment duration and somewhat low average dose of radiation delivered to patients in this trial led some clinicians to question the generalizability of the trial until confirmatory results from other trials were revealed. Pearcey et al. *(20)* have argued that they may not have detected an advantage with weekly cisplatin in the NCIC trial because the duration of radiation therapy was shorter than that of other trials, resulting in more effective local treatment. However, a comparison of the 1-yr local control rates (78% and 77%, respectively) and 5-yr survival rates (66% and 58%, respectively) for patients in the control arms of the NCIC and RTOG trials suggests that the margins for improvement were similar in the two studies *(18,19)*.

Because patients with very severe social problems tend to be excluded from prospective trials, additional problems may emerge now that many clinicians have accepted chemoradiation as the standard treatment for locoregionally advanced disease. There is no evidence that the use of concurrent chemotherapy permits significant reductions in total treatment dose; there is also no evidence that chemoradiation overcomes the detrimental effects of treatment protraction. It is therefore critical that multidisciplinary teams work closely with patients and social services to educate patients and facilitate the timely and complete administration of this complex treatment.

8. INFLUENCE OF CHEMORADIATION ON ACUTE AND LATE COMPLICATIONS OF TREATMENT

The acute morbidity of chemoradiation is almost always greater than that of radiation therapy alone. With cisplatin, upper-gastrointestinal-tract symptoms occur in addition to the lower-gastrointestinal-tract symptoms usually seen with pelvic irradiation. Although cisplatin has relatively modest hematologic toxicity, only about half of patients are able to complete the full six courses of weekly cisplatin or the full three courses of the RTOG regimen *(18)*. An effort should be made to manage the dose and timing of chemotherapy to minimize the risk of severe neutropenia or thrombocytopenia, which could delay brachytherapy. Fluorouracil may increase the severity of acute lower-gastrointestinal-tract symptoms, particularly diarrhea, although grade 4 acute complications are still uncommon.

Trials of cisplatin-based chemoradiation have not yet demonstrated any dramatic increase in the incidence of major late complications with the addition of concurrent cisplatin. However, most of these trials did not have sufficiently mature follow-up at the time of publication to permit full evaluation of the comparative risks. Thomas et al. *(35)* reported a significantly higher rate of serious late bowel complications in patients who received mitomycin with or without fluorouracil than in patients who received fluorouracil alone ($p = 0.004$). However, Roberts et al. *(27)* have not yet reported an increased rate of late complications with chemotherapy in their Venezuelan study of radiation alone vs radiation plus mitomycin C and fluorouracil. Long-term follow-up of the randomized trials will be needed to improve our understanding of the influence of concurrent chemotherapy on late complications.

9. IS THE EFFECTIVENESS OF CHEMORADIATION RELATED TO DISEASE STAGE?

Thus far, all but one of the trials large enough to detect a 40–50% reduction in the risk of recurrence with cisplatin-based chemotherapy have been positive. The patients selected for these trials had overall recurrence rates that ranged between 25% and 60% at 5 yr; each trial also included patients with a range of disease presentations. Patients who were treated with radiation alone or with a combination of radiation and surgery benefited equally from the addition of chemotherapy during their radiation therapy. None of the randomized studies was large enough to permit reliable subset analyses even within the stratification groups. Preliminary analysis of the subset of 117 patients in RTOG 90-01 *(18)* who had stage III or IVA disease did not demonstrate a significant benefit with chemoradiation. It has been suggested that these patients may have had disease that was more resistant to the beneficial effects of concurrent cisplatin. However, the number of patients was too small and the analysis was too early to permit firm conclusions about the relationship between disease extent and the magnitude of risk reduction with chemotherapy. The GOG study reported by Rose et al. *(12)* that included only patients with stages IIB–IVA disease yielded a reduction in the risk of recurrence similar to that in the RTOG trial.

In general, the evidence suggests that patients who have a recurrence risk of more than 20–30% after radiation therapy alone are likely to benefit from concurrent chemotherapy if they have no major medical contraindications to chemoradiation.

10. CHEMORADIATION FOR OTHER GYNECOLOGIC MALIGNANCIES

A number of phase I and II trials of chemoradiation for gynecologic malignancies have included patients with vaginal or vulvar cancer, but the number of patients with these rare malignancies has been too small to support large randomized trials.

10.1. Vaginal Cancer

Vaginal cancers are so similar to cervical cancers with respect to epidemiology, behavior, and treatment response that many clinicians have chosen to treat vaginal cancers of stage II or greater with chemoradiation on the basis of results from cervical cancer trials. Unfortunately, only scattered published reports of chemoradiation are available for this rare tumor.

10.2. Vulvar Cancer

Vulvar carcinoma is also uncommon, but this tumor has been a focus of chemoradiation studies for a number of years because of the similarities between vulvar and anal cancer and the success of chemoradiation for anal cancer. Mitomycin C and fluorouracil, agents commonly used to treat anal cancer, have been particularly popular for use in chemoradiation regimens for vulvar cancer (Table 4). More recently, successful trials in patients with cervical cancer have added to clinicians' enthusiasm for chemoradiation in vulvar cancer and have probably contributed to the increasing use of cisplatin in phase II protocols. However, one important distinction of vulvar cancer patients is their relatively advanced age. Unlike cervical cancer, which commonly effects premenopausal women, vulvar cancer has its peak incidence in women over 70 yr of age, and more than half of affected women are more than 70 yr old at diagnosis. Many patients with vulvar cancer have significant intercurrent illnesses. The importance of this feature of the disease is emphasized in the results of early trials of concurrent chemoradiation with bleomycin, which was associated with a high chemotherapy-related mortality rate *(36,37)*. Recent trials have reduced severe toxicity by using less toxic chemotherapy regimens and by excluding patients with severe comorbid diseases.

In general, phase II trials of chemoradiation for vulvar cancer have yielded encouraging response rates (Table 4). Most studies of cisplatin or mitomycin C plus fluorouracil have yielded vulvar local control rates of better than 50% in women with advanced

Table 4
Concurrent Chemoradiation for Patients with Locally Advanced or Recurrent Carcinoma of the Vulva

Investigator	*Year*	*No. of patients*	*Chemotherapy drugs*	*RT dose (Gy)*	*No. of patients with recurrent or persistent local disease after RT ± surgery*	*Follow-up time (mo)*
Akl et al. *(38)*	2000	12	5-FU + Mito	30–36	1 (8%)[a]	8–125
Han et al. *(26)*	2000	14	5-FU ± CDDP or Mito	40–62	6 (43%)	7–120
Moore et al. *(46)*	1998	73	5-FU + CDDP	47.6	15 (21%)	22–72
Cunningham et al. *(40)*	1997	14	5-FU + CDDP	45–50	4 (29%)	7–81
Landoni et al. *(44)*	1996	58	5-FU + Mito	54	13 (22%)	4–48
Lupi et al. *(24)*	1996	31	5-FU + Mito	54	7 (23%)	22–73
Wahlen et al. *(49)*	1995	19	5-FU + Mito	45–50	1 (5%)	3–70
Eifel et al. *(41)*	1995	12	5-FU + CDDP	40–50	5 (42%)	17–30
Koh et al. *(43)*	1993	20	5-FU ± CDDP or Mito	30–54	9 (45%)	1–75
Russel et al. *(47)*	1992	25	5-FU ± CDDP	47–72	6 (24%)	4–52
Scheistroen et al. *(37)*	1992	42	Bleomycin	45	39 (93%)	7–60
Berek et al. *(39)*	1991	12	5-FU + CDDP	44–54	0	7–60
Thomas et al. *(48)*	1989	24	5-FU ± Mito	44–60	10 (42%)	5–43
Evans et al. *(42)*	1988	4	5-FU + Mito	25–70	2 (50%)	20–29
Levin et al. *(45)*	1986	6	5-FU + Mito	18–60	0	1–25
Iverson et al. *(36)*	1982	15	Bleomycin	15–40	11 (83%)[b]	4

[a]Vulva treated with electron-beam RT only; groins were managed by lymph node dissection without RT.
[b]Most patients had unresectable, stage IV lesions.
5-FU = fluorouracil, CDDP = cisplatin, Mito = mitomycin-C, RT = radiation therapy.

tumors, many of whom have unresectable or recurrent disease *(24,26,38–49)*. Although these data are encouraging, very few data regarding the response to radiation without chemotherapy are available for comparison.

Investigators have also been encouraged by the results of chemoradiation in women with vulvar cancer with positive or high-risk regional nodes *(50,51)*. Montana et al. *(51)* reported results of a GOG phase II trial of cisplatin and fluorouracil with radiation in 52 women with clinically suspicious inguinal lymph nodes; biopsy confirmation of inguinal node involvement was not required for entry. Of the 46 eligible patients, 37 went on to have a dissection of the clinically involved groin. Of these, 15 had no evidence of cancer in the specimen, and only one had an inguinal recurrence. However, only 12 of the patients in this study were alive and disease-free at the time of the report.

10.3. Ovarian Cancer

Although there have been some efforts to combine chemotherapy and radiation for patients with ovarian cancer, these cancers are usually advanced at presentation, limiting the role of local treatment. For patients with endometrial cancer, the possible role of combined adjuvant treatment is just beginning to be explored by the multi-institutional clinical trials groups.

REFERENCES

1. Sinclair W. The combined effect of hydroxyurea and x-rays on Chinese hamster cells in vitro. *Cancer Res* 1968; 28:198–201.
2. Hreshchyshyn MM. Hydroxyurea with irradiation for cervical carcinoma—preliminary report. *Cancer Chem Rep* 1968; 52:601–602.
3. Piver M, Barlow J, Vongtama V, et al. Hydroxyurea and radiation therapy in advanced cervical cancer. *Am J Obstet Gynecol* 1974; 120:969–972.
4. Piver M, Barlow J, Vongtama V, et al. Hydroxyurea as a radiation sensitizer in women with carcinoma of the uterine cervix. *Am J Obstet Gynecol* 1977; 129:379–383.
5. Piver MS, Barlow JJ, Vongtama V, et al. Hydroxyurea: A radiation potentiator in carcinoma of the uterine cervix. A randomized double-blind study. *Am J Obstet Gynecol* 1983; 147:803–808.
6. Piver MS, Krishnamsetty RM, Emrich LJ. Survival of nonsurgically staged patients with negative lymphangiograms who had stage IIB carcinoma of the cervix treated by pelvic radiation plus hydroxyurea. *Obstet Gynecol* 1985; 151:1006–1008.
7. Piver M, Vongtama V, Emtrich L. Hydroxyurea plus pelvic radiation versus placebo plus pelvic radiation in surgically staged stage IIIB cervical cancer. *J Surg Oncol* 1987; 35:129–134.
8. Piver MS, Barlow JJ. High dose irradiation to biopsy confirmed aortic node metastases from carcinoma of the uterine cervix. *Cancer* 1977; 39:1243–1246.
9. Hreshchyshyn MM, Aron BS, Boronow RC, et al. Hydroxyurea or placebo combined with radiation to treat stages IIIB and IV cervical cancer confined to the pelvis. *Int J Radiat Oncol Biol Phys* 1979; 5:317–322.
10. Stehman FB, Bundy BN, Keys H, et al. A randomized trial of hydroxyurea versus misonidazole adjunct to radiation therapy in carcinoma of the cervix. A preliminary report of a Gynecologic Oncology Group study. *Am J Obstet Gynecol* 1988; 159:87–94.
11. Stehman FB, Bundy BN, Thomas G, et al. Hydroxyurea versus misonidazole with radiation in cervical carcinoma: long-term follow-up of a Gynecologic Oncology Group trial. *J Clin Oncol* 1993; 11:1523–1528.
12. Rose PG, Bundy BN, Watkins J, et al. Concurrent cisplatin-based chemotherapy and radiotherapy for locally advanced cervical cancer. *N Engl J Med* 1999; 340:1144–1153.
13. Whitney CW, Sause W, Bundy BN, et al. A randomized comparison of fluorouracil plus cisplatin versus hydroxyurea as an adjunct to radiation therapy in stages IIB–IVA carcinoma of the cervix with negative para-aortic lymph nodes: A Gynecologic Oncology Group and Southwest Oncology Group study. *J Clin Oncol* 1999; 17:1339–1348.

14. Thigpen T, Shingleton H, Homesley H, et al. Cis-platinum in treatment of advanced or recurrent squamous cell carcinoma of the cervix. *Cancer* 1981; 48:899–903.
15. Souhami L, Gil R, Allan S, et al. A randomized trial of chemotherapy followed by pelvic radiation therapy in stage IIIB carcinoma of the cervix. *Int J Radiat Oncol Biol Phys* 1991; 9:970–997.
16. Tattersall MHN, Ramirez C, Coppleson M. A randomized trial comparing platinum-based chemotherapy followed by radiotherapy vs. radiotherapy alone in patients with locally advanced cervical cancer. *Int J Gynecol Cancer* 1992; 2:244–251.
17. Keys HM, Bundy BN, Stehman FB, et al. Cisplatin, radiation, and adjuvant hysterectomy for bulky stage IB cervical carcinoma. *N Engl J Med* 1999; 340:1154–1161.
18. Morris M, Eifel PJ, Lu J, et al. Pelvic radiation with concurrent chemotherapy compared with pelvic and paraaortic radiation for high-risk cervical cancer. *N Engl J Med* 1999; 340:1137–1143.
19. Peters WA, 3rd, Liu PY, Barrett RJ, 2nd, et al. Concurrent chemotherapy and pelvic radiation therapy compared with pelvic radiation therapy alone as adjuvant therapy after radical surgery in high-risk early-stage cancer of the cervix. *J Clin Oncol* 2000; 18:1606–1613.
20. Pearcey RG, Brundage MD, Drouin P, et al. Phase III trial comparing radical radiotherapy with and without cisplatin chemotherapy in patients with advance squamous cell cancer of the cervix. *J Clin Oncol* 2002; 20:966–972.
21. Chaney AW, Eifel PJ, Logsdon MD, et al. Mature results of a pilot study of pelvic radiotherapy with concurrent continuous infusion intra-arterial 5-FU for stage IIIB-IVA squamous cell carcinoma of the cervix. *Int J Radiat Oncol Biol Phys* 1999; 45:113–118.
22. Thomas G, Dembo A, Ackerman I, et al. A randomized trial of standard versus partially hyperfractionated radiation with or without concurrent 5-fluorouracil in locally advanced cervical cancer. *Gynecol Oncol* 1998; 69:137–145.
23. Christie DR, Bull CA, Gebski V, et al. Concurrent 5-fluorouracil, mitomycin C and irradiation in locally advanced cervix cancer. *Radiother Oncol* 1995; 37:181–189.
24. Lupi G, Raspagliesi F, Zucali R, et al. Combined preoperative chemoradiotherapy followed by radical surgery in locally advanced vulvar carcinoma. A pilot study. *Cancer* 1996; 77:1472–1478.
25. Rakovitch E, Fyles AW, Pintilie M, et al. Role of mitomycin C in the development of late bowel toxicity following chemoradiation for locally advanced carcinoma of the cervix. *Int J Radiat Oncol Biol Phys* 1997; 38:979–987.
26. Han SC, Kim DH, Higgins SA, et al. Chemoradiation as primary or adjuvant treatment for locally advanced carcinoma of the vulva. *Int J Radiat Oncol Biol Phys* 2000; 47:1235–1244.
27. Roberts KB, Urdaneta N, Vera R, et al. Interim results of a randomized trial of mitomycin C as an adjunct to radical radiotherapy in the treatment of locally advanced squamous-cell carcinoma of the cervix. *Int J Cancer* 2000; 90:206–223,
28. Wong LC, Ngan HY, Cheung AN, et al. Chemoradiation and adjuvant chemotherapy in cervical cancer. *J Clin Oncol* 1999; 17:2055–2060.
29. Pignata S, Frezza P, Tramontana S, et al. Phase I study with weekly cisplatin-paclitaxel and concurrent radiotherapy in patients with carcinoma of the cervix uteri. *Ann Oncol* 2000; 11:455–459.
30. Chen MD, Paley PJ, Potish RA, et al. Phase I trial of taxol as a radiation sensitizer with cisplatin in advanced cervical cancer. *Gynecol Oncol* 1997; 67:131–136.
31. Muderspach LI, Curtin JP, Roman LD, et al. Carboplatin as a radiation sensitizer in locally advanced cervical cancer: a pilot study. *Gynecol Oncol* 1997; 65:336–342.
32. Wong L, Choo Y, Choy D, et al. Long-term follow-up of potentiation of radiotherapy by cis-platinum in advanced cervical cancer. *Gynecol Oncol* 1989; 35:159–163.
33. Formenti SC, Meyerowitz BE, Ell K, et al. Inadequate adherence to radiotherapy in Latina immigrants with carcinoma of the cervix. Potential impact on disease free survival. *Cancer* 1995; 75:1135–1140.
34. Katz A, Eifel PJ, Moughan J, et al. Socioeconomic characteristics of patients with squamous cell carcinoma of the uterine cervix treated with radiotherapy in the 1992 to 1994 patterns of care study. *Int J Radiat Oncol Biol Phys* 2000; 47:443–450.
35. Thomas G, Dembo A, Fyles A, et al. Concurrent chemoradiation in advanced cervical cancer. *Gynecol Oncol* 1990; 38:446–451.
36. Iversen T. Irradiation and bleomycin in the treatment of inoperable vulval carcinoma. *Acta Obstet Gynecol Scand* 1982; 61:195–197.
37. Scheistroen M, Trope C. Combined bleomycin and irradiation in preoperative treatment of advanced squamous cell carcinoma of the vulva. *Acta Oncol* 1992; 32:657–661.

38. Akl A, Akl M, Boike G, et al. Preliminary results of chemoradiation as a primary treatment for vulvar carcinoma. *Int J Radiat Oncol Biol Phys* 2000; 48:415–420,
39. Berek JS, Heaps JM, Fu YS, et al. Concurrent cisplatin and 5-fluorouracil chemotherapy and radiation therapy for advanced-stage squamous carcinoma of the vulva. *Gynecol Oncol* 1991; 42:197–201.
40. Cunningham MJ, Goyer RP, Gibbons SK, et al. Primary radiation, cisplatin, and 5-fluorouracil for advanced squamous carcinoma of the vulva. *Gynecol Oncol* 1997; 66:258–261.
41. Eifel PJ, Morris M, Burke TW, et al. Preoperative continuous infusion cisplatinum and 5-fluorouracil with radiation for locally advanced or recurrent carcinoma of the vulva. *Gynecol Oncol* 1995; 59:51–56.
42. Evans LS, Kersh CR, Constable WC, et al. Concomitant 5-fluorouracil, mitomycin-C, and radiotherapy for advanced gynecologic malignancies. *Int J Radiat Oncol Biol Phys* 1988; 15:901–906.
43. Koh WJ, Wallace HJ, Greer BE, et al. Combined radiotherapy and chemotherapy in the management of local-regionally advanced vulvar cancer. *Int J Radiat Oncol Biol Phys* 1993; 26:809–816.
44. Landoni F, Maneo A, Zanetta G, et al. Concurrent preoperative chemotherapy with 5-fluorouracil and mitomycin C and radiotherapy (FUMIR) followed by limited surgery in locally advanced and recurrent vulvar carcinoma. *Gynecol Oncol* 1996; 61:321–327.
45. Levin W, Goldberg G, Altaras M, et al. The use of concomitant chemotherapy and radiotherapy prior to surgery in advanced stage carcinoma of the vulva. *Gynecol Oncol* 1986; 25:20–25.
46. Moore DH, Thomas GM, Montana GS, et al. Preoperative chemoradiation for advanced vulvar cancer: a phase II study of the Gynecologic Oncology Group. *Int J Radiat Oncol Biol Phys* 1998; 42:79–85.
47. Russell AH, Mesic JB, Scudder SA, et al. Synchronous radiation and cytotoxic chemotherapy for locally advanced or recurrent squamous cancer of the vulva. *Gynecol Oncol* 1992; 47:14–20.
48. Thomas G, Dembo A, DePetrillo A, et al. Concurrent radiation and chemotherapy in vulvar carcinoma. *Gynecol Oncol* 1989; 34:263–267.
49. Wahlen SA, Slater JD, Wagner RJ, et al. Concurrent radiation therapy and chemotherapy in the treatment of primary squamous cell carcinoma of the vulva. *Cancer* 1995; 75:2289–2294.
50. Leiserowitz GS, Russell AH, Kinney WK, et al. Prophylactic chemoradiation of inguinofemoral lymph nodes in patients with locally extensive vulvar cancer. *Gynecol Oncol* 1997; 66:509–514.
51. Montana GS, Thomas GM, Moore DH, et al. Preoperative chemo-radiation for carcinoma of the vulva with N2/N3 nodes: A Gynecologic Oncology Group study. *Int J Radiat Oncol Biol Phys* 2000; 48:1007–1013.
52. Eifel PJ. Chemoradiation for carcinoma of the cervix: Advances and opportunities. *Radiat Res* 2000; 154:229–236.
53. Kumar L, Kaushal R, Nandy M, et al. Chemotherapy followed by radiotherapy versus radiotherapy alone in locally advanced cervical cancer: A randomized study. *Gynecol Oncol* 1994; 54:307–315.
54. Chauvergne J, Rohart J, Héron JF, et al. Essai randomisé de chimiothérapie initiale dans 151 carcinomes du col utérin localement étendus (T2b-N1, T3b, MO). *Bull Cancer* 1990; 77:1007–1024.
55. Tattersall MHN, Larvidhaya V, Vootiprux V, et al. Randomized trial of epirubicin and cisplatin chemotherapy followed by pelvic radiation in locally advanced cervical cancer. *Am J Clin Oncol* 1995; 13:444–451.
56. Sundfør K, Trope CG, Hogberg T, et al. Radiotherapy and neoadjuvant chemotherapy for cervical carcinoma. A randomized multicenter study of sequential cisplatin and 5-fluorouracil and radiotherapy in advanced cervical carcinoma stage 3B and 4A. *Cancer* 1996; 77:2371–2378.
57. Leborgne F, Leborgne JH, Doldán R, et al. Induction chemotherapy and radiotherapy of advanced cancer of the cervix: A pilot study and phase III randomized trial. *Int J Radiat Oncol Biol Phys* 1997; 37:343–350.

IV

Specific Molecular Targeted Agents

17 Overview of Specific Molecular Targeted Agents for Combined Modality Therapy

Scott Saxman, MD, FACP *and Janet Dancey,* MD

CONTENTS

1. INTRODUCTION

Despite recent advances in the technology and techniques for delivering radiotherapy to patients with malignancies, the inability of maximally tolerated doses of radiation to locally eradicate all of the malignant cells remains a major clinical problem leading to failure of the overall treatment plan. As described by Rosen et al., there are a variety of reasons why tumors recur locally after radiotherapy *(1–3)*. A "geographic miss" occurs when a portion of the observable tumor volume is excluded from the radiotherapy port and those tumor cells receive a nominal dose of radiation. Frequently, the distribution of radiotherapy dose to the gross tumor is uneven, with the central portion of the targeted volume receiving a higher quantity of radiation than the cells at the peripheral tumor/normal tissue interface. These tumor cells at the edge of the radiation port therefore can receive a subtherapeutic or sublethal dose of radiation and retain the ability to regrow and repopulate. This is referred to as a "marginal miss." Irradiated tissues can also potentially be recolonized with tumor cells from regional anatomic sites or from hematogenous dissemination. This is referred to as "repopulation." However, the major cause of local recurrence is the inability of maximally tolerable dosages of radiation to completely eliminate the malignant cells within the tumor mass. Radioresistance in this sense is

From: *Chemoradiation in Cancer Therapy*
Edited by: H. Choy © Humana Press Inc., Totowa, NJ

relative, since presumably there is a dose of radiation that would kill all of the malignant cells if toxicity factors inherent to the host did not preclude its delivery.

The relationship between the optimal dose of radiation that results in the desired effect and the dose that produces undesired toxicity is referred to as the "therapeutic index." The goal of the radiation oncologist is to manipulate the therapeutic ratio such that there is maximal separation between the beneficial and the detrimental effects of the delivered therapy. This can be accomplished by either enhancing the impact of a given quantity of radiation on the malignant cell or by reducing the unfavorable damage to the normal tissues. Techniques that have been used with varying success include changes in time-dose relationships (hyperfractionation, accelerated fractionation), changes in the relative tumor/normal tissue volume exposed to radiation (three-dimensional conformal radiotherapy, stereotactic radiosurgery), and administration of radioprotective agents such as sulfhydryl compounds (amifostine). As described in previous chapters of this textbook, the concurrent or sequential administration of certain chemotherapeutic agents can also enhance the ability of radiotherapy to impact on the local control of a tumor and improve the therapeutic ratio. Although the mechanisms for this interaction are often poorly understood, prospective randomized trials have clearly demonstrated the benefit of agents such as cisplatin, taxanes, mitomycin-C, and 5-fluorouracil in the combined modality therapy of diseases such as squamous cell carcinomas of the head and neck, small cell and nonsmall-cell lung cancer (NSCLC), anal carcinoma, esophageal cancer, cervical cancer, and rectal cancer.

Over the past decade there has been a quantum increase in the understanding of the genetic and molecular mechanisms that underlie the process of oncogenesis, tumor development, growth, and metastasis. This has led to a growing awareness of mechanisms by which tumors and normal tissue are able to overcome damage from radiation injury. It is now known that mutations that affect tumor suppressor genes and oncogenes cause abnormalities in cellular growth and programmed cell death, as well as perturbations of the cell cycle, cytokine signaling pathways, and pathways of angiogenesis that can significantly impact on the ability of ionizing radiation to result in the death of the malignant cell. This knowledge has resulted in a vast amount of preclinical study into ways that these molecular abnormalities may be specifically targeted to result in clinical benefit, not only by potentially impacting on systemic disease, but by enhancing radiosensitivity. The remainder of this chapter will provide a brief overview of some of these agents and pathways; the following chapters in this textbook will describe these in much greater detail.

2. CYCLOOXYGENASE-2

COX-2, a key enzyme involved in the production of prostaglandins and other eicosanoids, is upregulated in a significant percentage of human cancers and is associated with invasive and metastatic tumor behavior *(4)*. Overexpression of COX-2 mRNA and protein has been demonstrated in a variety of tumor types including adenocarcinomas of the colon, breast and stomach, melanoma, and lung cancer *(5–7)*. There is also evidence that enhanced COX-2 expression is related to tumor grade, with well-differentiated lung and hepatocellular carcinomas having amplified expression when compared to more poorly differentiated tumors. Although COX-1 is constitutively expressed, COX-2 expression is highly inducible by a variety of cytokines and growth factors including

IL-1, tumor necrosis factor-alpha, epidermal growth factor, transforming growth factor beta, and oncogenes *ras* and *scr (4)*. The most important effect of COX-2 overexpression in malignant cells is inhibition of apoptosis; however, in some experimental models COX-2 overexpression also enhances cancer-induced angiogenesis and invasiveness. Several preclinical models have demonstrated that inhibition of COX-2 restores apoptosis, slows the growth of tumors, and enhances cell death. Cancer clinical trials in humans are underway, most of the clinical studies conducted to date have studied COX-2 inhibition in the context of chemoprevention. A notable example is a trial of celecoxib, a selective COX-2 inhibitor, in patients with familial adenomatous polyposis. When compared to placebo, 6 months of therapy with 400 mg twice daily of celecoxib resulted in a 28% reduction in the mean number of colorectal polyps and a 30.7% reduction in the polyp burden as compared with reductions of 4.5% and 4.9%, respectively, for placebo *(8)*. This difference was highly significant and suggests that COX-2 inhibition may be able to reverse the premalignant process and possibly reduce the incidence of malignancy in high-risk populations.

Little is known about the interactions of radiotherapy and COX-2 expression and inhibition. Investigators at Stanford have demonstrated that radiation induces upregulation of COX-2 in PC-3 cell lines, and that the induced protein is enzymatically active and results in elevated levels of prostaglandin *(9)*. The induction of COX-2 was also dose dependent, with an increase of 37% over controls seen following irradiation with 5 Gy, 80% at 10 Gy and 97% at 15 Gy. Cells radiated in the presence of a COX-2 inhibitor had reduced prostaglandin levels; however, they found no differences in cell cycle distribution or apoptosis between cells irradiated in the presence or absence of the COX inhibitor. Other investigators have shown that production of prostaglandin by animal tumors is associated with radioresistance, and that suppressing prostaglandin production with inhibitors of cyclooxygenase can enhance radiosensitivity of these tumors. Kishi et al. have looked at a selective COX-2 inhibitor, SC-236, in a murine sarcoma model *(10)*. When SC-236 was combined with radiotherapy, there was a significant increase in tumor growth delay and augmentation of tumor curability. They also found that the SC-236-induced enhancement of tumor radioresponse was associated with a decrease in the production of prostaglandins but there was no effect on COX-2 protein expression. They also determined in this model that the effect of COX-2 inhibition on normal tissue radioresponse was minimal. Petersen et al. demonstrated a similar enhancement of radioresponse when SC-236 was given in combination with radiation in a human glioma cell line grown both in monolayer culture as well as in nude mice tumor xenografts *(11)*.

Selective COX-2 inhibitors are currently being investigated in cancer patients in phase I and early phase II clinical trials. The currently available data would suggest that specific inhibitors of COX-2 have the potential to increase the therapeutic ratio of radiotherapy in tumors that express COX-2, and that clinical investigation of this interaction is warranted.

3. ANTIANGIOGENESIS AGENTS

The ability of tumors to co-opt existing blood vessels and induce growth of new vessels is considered essential for tumors to grow larger than a few millimeters in size. Angiogenesis is a complex, multistep process that is regulated by a balance between proangiogenic and antiangiogenic factors in the tumor and endothelial microenvironment. Endothelial cell growth and proliferation can be regulated by a number of growth factors including platelet-derived growth factor, vascular endothelial growth factor, fibroblast growth factor, and angiopoietins. There are currently a number of targeted inhibitors of angiogenesis that have been identified and are in various stages of clinical trials in a variety of malignancies.

Therapeutic irradiation is known to have multiple interactions with the vasculature of the irradiated tissue *(12)*. Radiation has direct cytotoxic effects on the vascular endothelium, likely due to induction of oxidative injury. Radiation-induced injury stimulates inflammation and influx of inflammatory cells in addition to creating a procoagulant state in the vascular space by the transcriptional induction of tissue factor with the subsequent activation of coagulation factors as well as von Willebrand factor and platelets. Experimental evidence suggests that the mechanism by which radiation initiates these responses is in part through the induction of cell-adhesion molecules including ICAM-1, E-selectin, and P-selectin and in part through local cytokine production and release *(13)*.

There is a theoretical concern when considering combining radiation with agents that inhibit angiogenesis. Because these agents may act by reducing blood vessel number and function within the tumor resulting in hypoxia, and because it is well known that the biologic effect of ionizing radiation is diminished in the presence of tissue hypoxia, it is possible that the administration of angiogenesis agents prior to or concurrently with radiotherapy may reduce the efficacy of radiation and result in inferior clinical outcome. There are a few preclinical experiments that have addressed this issue, and the results have been somewhat mixed. Teicher et al. demonstrated that the administration of antiangiogenic agents prior to chemotherapy or radiotherapy reduced the number and size of lung metastasis formed from the primary tumor in a Lewis lung carcinoma model when compared to either therapeutic modality alone *(14)*. Lund et al. examined the effect of TNP-470, a synthetic analog of fumagillin that inhibits endothelial cells, and radiotherapy on tumor growth vessel morphology and expression of angiogenic factors in a human glioblastoma line grown in the flank or intracranially in nude mice *(15)*. Compared to TNP-470 or radiotherapy alone, significant inhibition of tumor growth in the flank model was seen when the combination was given together. There was no effect of TNP-470 in the intracranial model, either when given alone or in combination with radiotherapy. Microscopic evaluation suggested that radiation-induced microvascular damage was prevented by concurrent TNP-470 administration. Murata et al. also studied TNP-470 with radiotherapy in a murine mammary carcinoma model *(16)*. In this experiment, 4–5 mm tumors were irradiated under hypoxic and oxygenated conditions. TNP-470 was administered subcutaneously twice a week during and/or after radiotherapy. Hypoxic tumors were not affected significantly when TNP-470 was started 24 h before radiotherapy; however, in the nonhypoxic group tumor control required higher doses of radiotherapy indicating that TNP-470 given during radiotherapy had a negative effect and decreased radiocurability. Other studies have examined angiostatin, a proteolytic fragment of plasminogen with antiangiogenic activity, in combination with radiotherapy. These studies suggest that there is an antitumor interaction between radiation and angiostatin in both cell cultures and xenograft models *(17,18)*.

There are several ongoing clinical studies that are addressing this issue. As an example, in NSCLC there are two phase III randomized trials in which antiangiogenesis agents are being given concurrently with radiotherapy and chemotherapy in patients with locally advanced disease. An Eastern Cooperative Oncology Group trial is testing the combination of carboplatin and paclitaxel and radiotherapy with and without thalidomide, while the MD Anderson CCOP program in cooperation with a consortium of Canadian investigators is testing the addition of a highly antiangiogenic shark cartilage extract to chemoradiation in the same clinical setting (*see* Website: http://www.cancer.gov). The results of clinical studies as well as continued preclinical investigation with other angiogenesis inhibitors will enhance our understanding of the radiobiology of this class of agents.

4. SIGNAL TRANSDUCTION INHIBITORS

Signal transduction refers to the biochemical steps that transmit extracellular and intracellular signals to the genome, ultimately altering gene expression and cell behavior. Signaling pathways are often complex, providing opportunity for cross-talk and branching between the cascades of cytoplasmic and nuclear protein kinases and phosphatases *(19)*. Although there are different pathways that transduce signals, a mechanism mediating the intracellular response involves changing the state of protein and lipid phosphorylation by either increasing or decreasing the activity of kinases or phosphatases. Given the importance of these signaling pathways in controlling cell behavior, it is not surprising that aberrant expression and/or phosphorylation of signaling molecules leads to dysfunctional signal transduction, which contributes to malignant transformation, autonomous growth, and resistance to chemotherapeutic agents and radiation *(20,21)*.

It is now known that oncogene products are frequently growth factors, growth factor receptors, or elements of growth factor signal transduction pathways and that inhibition of these membrane receptors or their downstream components can lead to tumor growth inhibition and regression *(22)*. In addition, human cells exhibit complex responses to DNA damage, including activation of genes involved in cell cycle arrest, DNA repair, and apoptosis *(23,24)*. Signal transduction pathways mediated by receptor tyrosine kinases and protein kinase C appear to be important for the induction of many of the genes related to key cellular functions that permit the cell to survive a dose of radiation. Specific blockade of these pathways in tumor cells may increase the cytotoxic effects of radiation.

The ErbB family of growth factor receptors is well characterized and has been generating increasing interest as a target for cancer therapeutics. The family, which consists of epidermal growth factor receptor (EGFR), HER-2, HER-3, and HER-4, is overexpressed in a significant proportion of human cancers *(25,26)*. In breast cancer, for example, 30% of tumors overexpress EGFR or HER-2, and 90% express HER-3. In addition, overexpression of the ErbB receptors is correlated with poorer prognosis and decreased survival compared to patients with tumors that are ErbB receptor negative. Most importantly, specific blockade of ErbB members EGFR and HER-2 has a number of antineoplastic effects. These effects include complete growth inhibition in vitro, a progressive diminution of colony-forming ability, and sensitization to the lethal effects of ionizing radiation.

Ionizing radiation activates both EGFR and downstream signaling involving the cytoprotective mitogen-activated protein kinase (MAPK) pathway *(27–29)*. MAPK cascade is a key cytoprotective pathway in A431 human squamous carcinoma cells that is activated in response to clinically relevant doses of ionizing radiation. Inhibition of this pathway potentiates the ability of low dose radiation to induce cell death in vitro. These results predict that blocking ErbB kinase activity would also sensitize cells to radiation.

One of the first of the signal transduction inhibitors proven to be therapeutically valuable for the treatment of cancer is the humanized anti-HER-2 murine monoclonal antibody trastuzumab (Herceptin™), which recognizes and blocks the p185^{HER2} growth factor receptor and is approved for the treatment of women with metastatic breast cancer. There is a strong rationale for evaluating Herceptin in combination with radiotherapy. Antisense oligonucleotides directed against HER-2 mRNA were able to reverse the radiation resistance of human tumor cell lines with HER-2 overexpression *(30)*. Anti-HER-2 receptor antibody enhances radiation-induced killing of naturally overexpressing SKBR3 human breast cancer cells as well as MCF-7 cells engineered to overexpress this receptor. Treatment with ionizing radiation combined with rhuMAb HER-2 was more effective compared to radiation or antibody alone in HER-2 overexpressing human breast cancer xenografts in nude mice. The combination of radiation and antibody therapy produced marked reductions in tumor growth, demonstrating a marked in vivo enhancement of radiation efficacy *(31)*.

EGFR is also an interesting potential therapeutic target. EGFR and its ligands EGF and T-cell growth factor (TGF)-alpha are important in cell proliferation as well as motility, adhesion, invasion, survival, and angiogenesis *(32)*. Its importance in the development and propagation of malignancies is supported by a number of observations. Overexpression of EGFR and its ligands leads to malignant transformation *(33)*. EGFR is overexpressed in epithelial malignancies such as glioma, nonsmall-cell lung, breast, head and neck, bladder, and ovarian carcinomas *(34–36)*. In some studies, EGFR overexpression was associated with poorer prognosis in bladder, head and neck, esophageal, nonsmall-cell lung, and breast cancer patients *(37–41)*. Treatment of tumor cells in vitro with anti-EGFR antibody typically induces arrest of cells in G1 with an increase in the cyclin-dependent kinase inhibitor p27kip1 and a decrease in retinoblastoma protein phosphorylation *(42)*. Although tumor growth delay is more typical, inhibitors of EGFR can induce regressions in certain tumor xenograft models suggesting that, for at least some tumors, EGFR pathway is important to cell survival *(43)*. Although the presence of EGFR was found to be necessary, but not sufficient, for in vitro response to EGFR inhibitors, the degree of EGFR expression may not be as important for antitumor effect as the reliance on this pathway for cell proliferation and survival *(44,45)*.

A number of studies have also shown a relationship between EGFR and sensitivity to chemotherapeutic drugs and radiation *(46–48)*. As an example, Wollman et al. demonstrated that adding EGF to MCF-7 mammary carcinoma cells increased radiation resistance and this effect was abrogated by antibody to EGFR *(49)*. There is evidence from in vitro studies that radiation stimulates proliferation by release of TGF-alpha by tumor cells. This autocrine stimulation could explain the accelerated repopulation that occurs during and following therapeutic radiation *(50,51)*. Thus, signaling through EGFR may increase the resistance of tumor cells to radiation and chemotherapeutic drugs, and antibodies that prevent the binding of ligand to the receptor or small molecules inhibiting receptor kinase activity can sensitize cells to radiotherapy by inhibiting EGF/TGF-alpha anti-apoptotic signaling. In addition to abrogating radiation resistance, inhibiting signaling through EGFR during the administration of fractionated radiotherapy may inhibit cellular proliferation during radiotherapy. Concerns that inhibiting proliferation during radiotherapy might also exacerbate radiation effects in rapidly proliferating normal tissues may be unfounded, as inhibiting EGFR gene expression has been shown to decrease proliferation in head and neck cancer cell lines without changing the proliferation rate of normal mucosal epithelial cells *(52)*.

Therapeutic agents targeting EGFR, including monoclonal antibodies against the extracellular domain of receptors and small molecules that inhibit receptor autophosphorylation and kinase activation, are being developed. A number of murine monoclonal antibodies against the EGFR extracellular ligand-binding domain inhibit ligand binding to receptor are also being developed *(53,54)*. The best characterized of these is mAb 225, which binds to EGFR with similar affinity to that of TGF-alpha and competes with the ligand for receptor binding. C225, a human/mouse chimeric of the mAb 225 antibody, binds to the EGF receptor extracellular domain. In vitro, this antibody blocks ligand-dependent proliferation of tumor cell lines and can induce tumor regression in xenografts. C225 potentiates the effects of ionizing radiation and, similar to trastuzumab, enhances the activity of doxorubicin and taxanes *(42,55)*. Preliminary results from a small phase I study have reported a response rate of 100% with the addition of C225 to radiation in patients with locally advanced head and neck carcinoma *(56)*. Based on these encouraging results, there is currently a phase III study designed to determine the additional benefit of C225 to radiation in this patient population.

Small-molecule inhibitors of the intracellular tyrosine kinase domain of EGFR are also under clinical evaluation. Currently available EGFR inhibitors belong to three chemical series: 4-anilinoquinazolines, 4-[ar(alk)ylamino]pyridopyrimidines, and 4-phenylaminopyrrolo-pyrimidines. Two quinazolines with in vivo anti-tumor efficacy and pharmacological properties desirable for clinical development are ZD 1839 and OSI-774 (previously known as CP 358 774). Collectively these small molecules competitively inhibit ATP binding to EGFR, induce tumor stasis and even tumor regression in some tumor xenograft models. In addition to their shared mechanism of action, these agents are both also administered orally on chronic schedules and have a similar spectrum of toxicity, with diarrhea and skin rash being the most common. More recently, potent, irreversible inhibitors of EGF receptor kinases have been developed such as PD 168 393/CI-1033. This compound binds to a cysteine residue near the ATP binding site. For further information, the reader is referred to selected reviews *(32,34,57,58)*.

Both antibodies and small molecules appear to be well tolerated, with promising results seen in early clinical trials. Current research goals include defining activity in a broader range of epithelial tumors, defining the optimal dose and schedule in combination with conventional chemotherapeutic agents and/or with radiation therapy, determining the best patient population in which to study and administer these agents, and expanding clinical trials to include other tumor types.

5. RAS FARNESYLATION INHIBITORS

The Ras family of small guanosine nucleotide binding proteins relay signals from activated growth factor receptors such as EGFR to downstream intracellular partners *(59)*. Following activation of transmembrane receptors, upstream Ras activators, such as Grb2-Sos nucleotide exchange factor complex, cause normal Ras to switch from its inactive guanosine 5'-diphosphate (GDP)-bound state to its active guanosine 5'-triphosphate (GTP)-bound state. Ras is inactivated by hydrolysis of bound GTP through its own intrinsic GTPase activity and by interaction with GTPase activation proteins. Importantly, posttranslational processing of Ras by prenylation is essential for membrane localization and Ras function. Activated membrane-bound Ras recruits such targets as serine/threonine kinases of the Ras family, which trigger the ERK/MAPK pathway as well as phosphoinositide 3-kinase, which activates other signal molecules *(60)*. Ras activation modulates the activity of nuclear factors such as FOS, JUN, and AP-1 that regulate transcription of genes required for proliferation *(61)*.

Given its pivotal role in a number of signaling pathways controlling cell proliferation, it is not surprising that mutations resulting in the persistent activation of Ras oncogenes are among the most frequent abnormalities found in human tumors *(62)*. Often, these mutations prevent the hydrolysis of GTP, so that the Ras protein in tumor cells is in a continually activated state; however, even wild-type Ras proteins may play a role in malignant transformation when oncogenic proteins or growth factors upstream of Ras drive this pathway *(63)*.

To function, Ras must be attached to the plasma membrane. Translocation from the cytoplasm to membrane requires a series of posttranslational modifications that begin with farnesylation of the cysteine residue, the fourth amino acid residue from the C terminus of the protein, by farnesyl protein transferase (FPTase) *(64)*. Attachment of the hydrophobic 15-carbon lipid farnesyl group allows Ras molecule insertion into the plasma membrane and is crucial for Ras signaling activity and transformation properties. As farnesylation is required for oncogenic Ras function, FPTase inhibitors (FTIs) are obvious candidate antineoplastic agents. Several drugs that inhibit Ras farnesylation are at various stages of clinical development *(65)*.

Although FTIs were identified by their ability to inhibit farnesylation Ras and cause tumor growth inhibition or regression, recent studies suggest that these two phenomena may not be directly related. Tumor cell lines display a range of sensitivity to FTIs which do not correlate with Ras mutational status suggesting that FTIs can function through mechanisms unrelated to Ras *(66)*. Other farnesylated proteins that may be FTI targets are members of the Rho and Rhe family. Treatment with FTIs results in the depleted farnesylated RhoB and favors accumulation of geranylgeranylated RhoB(gg-RhoB). GgRhoB accumulation correlates well with the anticancer activity of FTIs; however, the list of farnesylated proteins that could be targets continues to grow *(67,68)*. Although FTIs unequivocally inhibit tumor cell growth in preclinical models, FTIs illustrate the potential limitations of focusing on a single target at a time when our understanding of the molecular abnormalities in cancer cells and their potential as therapeutic targets is still naive.

Despite the uncertainties as to the mechanism of FTI inhibition of proliferation, FTIs radiosensitize tumor cells. This effect appears to be specific to Ras transformation *(69)*. Experimental evidence suggests that cells transformed with the activated Ras oncogene are often more resistant to cell killing by ionizing radiation *(70,71)*. Inhibition of farnesyltransferase with FTI-277 radiosensitizes human tumor cells with H-Ras mutations, and the combination of a geranylgeranyltransferase (GGTase) with an FTI radiosensitizes human tumor cells with K-Ras mutations but not tumor cells with wild-type Ras *(69,72)*. Thus Ras induced radioresistance can be reversed with FTIs *(73)*. As radiosensitization is not seen in cells with wild-type Ras , the combination of FTI and fractionated radiotherapy may result in improved therapeutic index through sparing of normal tissue relative to tumor tissue.

6. CELL CYCLE INHIBITORS

Signaling cascades ultimately converge to instruct the cell cycle machinery. In eukaryotic organisms, progression through the cell cycle depends on critically timed appearances/disappearances of cyclins and protein phosphorphylation/dephosphorphylation events *(74)*. Cyclins are proteins that accumulate and degrade at specific times during the phases of the cell cycle and they are required for activation of serine/threonine kinases, called cyclin-dependent kinases (CDKs), which regulate phosphorylation of proteins that control cell cycle progression. Despite the multiplicity of ligands, receptors, and effectors that form signaling pathways, most of the identified pathways converge on a few key genes required for G1 progression *(75)*. Most of these key molecules, including D-type cyclins, pRb, p16, and *p53*, are frequently mutated in human tumors.

Eukaryotic cells respond to DNA damage by eliciting multiple synchronous signals that can trigger both repair and apoptotic processes *(76)*. The specific intracellular pathways that trigger apoptosis and suppress DNA repair are unclear; however, one critical mediator of the cellular response to DNA damage is the tumor suppressor gene product *p53*, which is linked to cell cycle arrest, DNA repair, and programmed cell death after DNA damage due to ionizing radiation *(77–79)*. Among the downstream *p53*-regulated genes is *p21WAF1*, which inhibits cyclin/CDK complexes causing cell cycle arrest in G1 phase *(80)*.

Because ionizing radiation leads to G1 arrest and apoptosis by a *p53*-dependent pathway, reintroduction of functional wild-type *p53* genes into tumor cells is a potential strategy to improve radiation sensitivity. Using direct local delivery, recombinant viral vectors with wild-type *p53* have been successfully reintroduced into tumor cells in preclinical studies, and this strategy is being evaluated in clinical trials. In a phase I trial, intratumoral administration of an adenovirus vector containing wild-type *p53* complementary DNA was performed on 28 patients with NSCLC *(81)*. Expression of wild-type *p53* was seen in 46% of patients and two patients achieved partial tumor response. An alternative strategy was developed to use viruses to selectively target *p53* mutant cells. The 55-kDa E1B protein of adenovirus inactivates *p53*, allowing replication of virus in normal cells. Conversely, replication and cytopathogenicity of an E1B, 55-kDa gene-attenuated adenovirus, ONYX- 015, is blocked by functional *p53* and, therefore this attenuated virus selectively replicates and lyses *p53* mutant cells without harm to normal tissues. This claim to selective cytotoxicity against *p53* mutated cells has been disputed, as ONYX-015-induced cytotoxicity has also been seen in wild-type *p53* tumor cells suggesting there may be another mechanism for its antitumor effect *(82,83)*. Nonetheless, promising results have been reported from phase II trials in patients with head and neck carcinomas. Treatment by intratumoral injections of ONYX-015 either as a single agent or in combination with chemotherapy has been well tolerated and objective tumor responses have been seen *(84–86)*. Determining whether these approaches will be additive to radiotherapy will require further investigation.

The 7-hydroxy-staurosporine analog UCN-01 is another agent that targets a number of serine/threonine kinases that can cause G1 arrest and G2/M checkpoint abrogation. G1 arrest is associated with the accumulation of the dephosphorylated retinoblastoma protein, reduction in expression of cyclin A, and the induction of the CDK-inhibiting proteins p21 and p27 *(87)*. UCN-01 abrogates the G2 checkpoint by inhibiting Chk-1 kinase *(88)*. In preclinical studies, UCN-01 had potent cytostatic and cytotoxic effects against solid and leukemic tumor cell lines as a single agent and in combination with a number of DNA damaging agents including radiation *(89–94)*.

DNA damage-inducible cell cycle checkpoints are complex signal transduction networks that integrate the cellular responses to genotoxic insults by arresting cell cycle progression during the repair of DNA damage or the induction of apoptosis. The integrity of these checkpoint pathways is critical for maintenance of genomic stability and cellular recovery from genotoxic damage. In in vitro models, loss of the G2/M checkpoint leads to an increased sensitivity to DNA-damaging agents, suggesting that small-molecule inhibitors of the G2/M checkpoint response might be useful in cancer therapy as radio- and chemosensitizing agents. In cells where the G1-phase checkpoint is not active because of *p53* inactivation, irradiated cells accumulate in G2 phase because the G2 checkpoint is mediated by the inactivation of cyclin B/cdc2 by wee1 kinase. In contrast, UCN-01 induces the activation of cyclin B/cdc2 and thus promotes cells to enter early mitosis with the onset of apoptotic cell death *(95)*.

7. PROMOTORS OF APOPTOSIS

Tumor propagation requires an imbalance between those processes that promote cell proliferation and those that result in programmed cell death. These normally tightly controlled death pathways are often deranged in tumor cells due to imbalances in positive and negative regulators. Thus, complex interactions among many molecular factors determine the delicate balance between cell proliferation and cell death.

Among the modulators of apoptosis is Bcl-2, which influences the release of cytochrome C and/or modulates the Apaf1/caspase-9 interaction. Bcl-2 is the founding member of family of anti-apoptotic molecules such as Bcl-X_L as well as pro-apoptotic members such as Bax and Bcl-X_S *(96)*. Cell viability following an apoptotic stimulus is associated with the Bcl-2/Bax ratio *(97)*. These same genetic alterations that influence apoptosis during tumor development also modulate drug sensitivity and resistance. For example, loss of *p53* and overexpression of Bcl-2 have been shown to suppress apoptosis induced by cytotoxic drugs in certain cancers *(98,99)*. Many forms of drug resistance in cancer can be traced to a relative resistance of tumor cells to undergo apoptosis.

Alterations in proto-oncogenes like Bcl-2 that result in the overexpression of proteins are potentially excellent targets for antisense oligonucleotide therapies. Antisense deoxyribonucleotides complementary to specific RNA sequences bind and initiate degradation of message RNA, preventing the expression of a single, specific gene *(100)*. G3139 is an 18-mer Bcl-2 antisense oligonucleotide that has been evaluated in patients with low-grade non-Hodgkin's lymphomas, which overexpressed Bcl-2 *(101)*. It was administered as a 2-wk subcutaneous continuous infusion over a dose range of 4.6–147 mg/m^2/d. Drug-induced hematological toxicity was not seen and nonhematological toxicity included transient rise in nonfasting blood glucose levels and local skin reaction. Antitumor effects included improvement in symptoms, biochemical parameters, and minimal reductions in tumor bulk; however, six of eight patients who were treated with chemotherapy following antisense treatment went on to achieve partial remissions suggesting that modulating the anti-apoptotic effects of Bcl-2 may increase tumor sensitivity to subsequent cytotoxic treatment *(102)*.

Considering the redundancy of most signaling pathways controlling cell viability and proliferation, these new classes of target-specific drugs are likely to be most effective when combined with one another or in combination with existing cytotoxic agents. Signals that promote proliferation are simultaneously protecting cells from apoptosis. If the newer anticancer drugs block proliferation-promoting signals, they may lower the apoptosis threshold for cytotoxic agents. Antisense compounds that inhibit Bcl-2 expression and angiogenesis inhibitors that directly and/or indirectly increase tumor cell apoptosis may increase tumor sensitivity to radiation and cytotoxic drugs. In fact, there is extensive preclinical evidence of synergy between various classes of agents. Identifying effective combinations among different types of drugs with different mechanisms of action adds to the complexity of drug evaluation and it is possible that molecular targeted therapies will need to be evaluated in combination regimens even in the absence of single-agent anticancer activity. Developing preclinical models that predict for synergy with radiation and improved therapeutic index are clearly needed to prioritize agents for evaluation in combination with radiotherapy. Efficient clinical development will require defining the optimal biologically active dose in combination with radiotherapy, and identifying appropriate surrogate phase II efficacy endpoints. Possible surrogate endpoints include clinical endpoints of response duration or time to progression, possible biological endpoints include changes in tumor markers, target inhibition and/or functional imaging *(103)*. Ultimately, only phase III trials which show improvements in survival or quality of life will prove the value of these agents and the surrogate endpoints used to estimate their activity in early clinical trials.

8. CONCLUSIONS

Advances in science and biotechnology have created many opportunities to potentially prevent, diagnose, and treat cancer. Many new classes of agents are being developed to block effects of oncogene products and reinduce functional tumor suppressor proteins. In only a few years, the number of potential targets that can be exploited for clinical benefit has grown exponentially. Many of these agents appear to behave synergistically with radiotherapy and may improve clinical outcome. Given the rapidly expanding number of potential targets and agents, better preclinical models which predict how these drugs will function in combination with radiation in humans as well as better clinical trial designs to efficiently evaluate these agents are urgently needed.

REFERENCES

1. Rosen E, Fan S, Rockwell S, et al. The molecular and cellular basis of radiosensitivity: implications for understanding how normal tissues and tumors respond to therapeutic radiation. *Cancer Invest* 1999; 17:56–72.
2. Rosen EM, Fan S, Goldberg ID, et al. Biological basis of radiation sensitivity. Part 1: Factors governing radiation tolerance. *Oncol (Huntingt)* 2000; 14:543–550.
3. Rosen EM, Fan S, Goldberg ID, et al. Biological basis of radiation sensitivity. Part 2: Cellular and molecular determinants of radiosensitivity. *Oncol (Huntingt)* 2000; 14:741–757; discussion 757–758, 761–766.
4. Fosslien E. Molecular pathology of cyclooxygenase-2 in neoplasia. *Ann Clin Lab Sci* 2000; 30:3–21.
5. Soslow RA, Dannenberg AJ, Rush D, et al. COX-2 is expressed in human pulmonary, colonic, and mammary tumors. *Cancer* 2000; 89:2637–2645.
6. Ristimaki A, Honkanen N, Jankala H, et al. Expression of cyclooxygenase-2 in human gastric carcinoma. *Cancer Res* 1997; 57:1276–1280.
7. Denkert C, Kobel M, Berger S, et al. Expression of cyclooxygenase 2 in human malignant melanoma. *Cancer Res* 2001; 61:303–308.
8. Steinbach G, Lynch P, Phillips R, et al. The effect of celecoxib, a cyclooxygenase-2 inhibitor, in familial adenomatous polyposis. *N Engl J Med* 2000; 29:1946–1952.
9. Steinauer KK, Gibbs I, Ning S, et al. Radiation induces upregulation of cyclooxygenase-2 (COX-2) protein in PC-3 cells. *Int J Radiat Oncol Biol Phys* 2000; 48:325–328.
10. Kishi K, Petersen S, Petersen C, et al. Preferential enhancement of tumor radioresponse by a cyclooxygenase-2 inhibitor. *Cancer Res* 2000; 60:1326–1331.

11. Petersen C, Petersen S, Milas L, et al. Enhancement of intrinsic tumor cell radiosensitivity induced by a selective cyclooxygenase-2 inhibitor. *Clin Cancer Res* 2000; 6:2513–2520.
12. Hallahan D, Chen A, Teng M, et al. Drug-radiation interactions in tumor blood vessels. *Oncology* 1999; 13:71–77.
13. Hallahan D, Kuchibhotla J, Wyble C. Cell adhesion molecules mediate radiation-induced leukocyte adhesion to the vascular endothelium. *Cancer Res* 1996; 56:5150–5155.
14. Teicher BA, Sotomayor EA, Huang ZD. Antiangiogenic agents potentiate cytotoxic cancer therapies against primary and metastatic disease. *Cancer Res* 1992; 52:6702–6704.
15. Lund EL, Bastholm L, Kristjansen PE. Therapeutic synergy of TNP-470 and ionizing radiation: effects on tumor growth, vessel morphology, and angiogenesis in human glioblastoma multiforme xenografts. *Clin Cancer Res* 2000; 6:971–978.
16. Murata R, Nishimura Y, Hiraoka M. An antiangiogenic agent (TNP-470) inhibited reoxygenation during fractionated radiotherapy of murine mammary carcinoma. *Int J Rad Oncol Biol Phys* 1997; 37:1107–1113.
17. Gorski DH, Mauceri HJ, Salloum RM, et al. Potentiation of the antitumor effect of ionizing radiation by brief concomitant exposures to angiostatin. *Cancer Res* 1998; 58:5686–5689.
18. Mauceri HJ, Hanna NN, Beckett MA, et al. Combined effects of angiostatin and ionizing radiation in antitumour therapy. *Nature* 1998; 394:287–291.
19. Pawson T, Saxton TM. Signaling networks—do all roads lead to the same genes? [comment]. *Cell* 1999; 97:675–678.
20. Cole K, Kohn E. Calcium-mediated signal transduction: biology, biochemistry, and therapy. *Cancer Metastasis Rev* 1994; 13:31–44.
21. Christen RD, Isonishi S, Jones JA, et al. Signaling and drug sensitivity. *Cancer Metastasis Rev* 1994; 13:175–189.
22. Haimovitz-Friedman A, Kan CC, Ehleiter D, et al. Ionizing radiation acts on cellular membranes to generate ceramide and initiate apoptosis. *J Exp Med* 1994; 180:525–535.
23. Lichter AS, Lawrence TS. Recent advances in radiation oncology. *N Engl J Med* 1995; 332:371–379.
24. Canman CE, Gilmer TM, Coutts SB, et al. Growth factor modulation of p53-mediated growth arrest versus apoptosis. *Genes Development* 1995; 9:600–611.
25. Gullick WJ, Srinivasan R. The type 1 growth factor receptor family: new ligands and receptors and their role in breast cancer. *Breast Cancer Res Treat* 1998; 52:43–53.
26. Pegram MD, Pauletti G, Slamon DJ. HER-2/neu as a predictive marker of response to breast cancer therapy. *Breast Cancer Res Treat* 1998; 52:65–77.
27. Schmidt-Ullrich RK, Mikkelsen RB, Dent P, et al. Radiation-induced proliferation of the human A431 squamous carcinoma cells is dependent on EGFR tyrosine phosphorylation. *Oncogene* 1997; 15:1191–1197.
28. Carter S, Auer KL, Reardon DB, et al. Inhibition of the mitogen activated protein (MAP) kinase cascade potentiates cell killing by low dose ionizing radiation in A431 human squamous carcinoma cells. *Oncogene* 1998; 16:2787–2796.
29. Contessa JN, Reardon DB, Todd D, et al. The inducible expression of dominant-negative epidermal growth factor receptor-CD533 results in radiosensitization of human mammary carcinoma cells. *Clin Cancer Res* 1999; 5:405–411.
30. Pirollo KF, Hao Z, Rait A, et al. Evidence supporting a signal transduction pathway leading to the radiation-resistant phenotype in human tumor cells. *Biochem Biophys Res Commun* 1997; 230: 196–201.
31. Pietras RJ, Poen JC, Gallardo D, et al. Monoclonal antibody to HER-2/neu receptor modulates repair of radiation-induced DNA damage and enhances radiosensitivity of human breast cancer cells overexpressing this oncogene. *Cancer Res* 1999; 59:1347–1355.
32. Woodburn JR. The epidermal growth factor receptor and its inhibition in cancer therapy. *Pharmacol Ther* 1999; 82:241–250.
33. Salomon DS, Brandt R, Ciardiello F, et al. Epidermal growth factor-related peptides and their receptors in human malignancies. *Crit Rev Oncol Hematol* 1995; 19:183–232.
34. Fry DW. Inhibition of the epidermal growth factor receptor family of tyrosine kinases as an approach to cancer chemotherapy: progression from reversible to irreversible inhibitors. *Pharmacol Ther* 1999; 82:207–218.
35. Fox SB, Smith K, Hollyer J, et al. The epidermal growth factor receptor as a prognostic marker: results of 370 patients and review of 3009 patients. *Breast Cancer Res Treat* 1994; 29:41–49.

36. Neal DE, Mellon K. Epidermal growth factor receptor and bladder cancer: a review. *Urol Int* 1992; 48:365–371.
37. Diedrich U, Lucius J, Baron E, et al. Distribution of epidermal growth factor receptor gene amplification in brain tumours and correlation to prognosis. *J Neurol* 1995; 242:683–688.
38. Maurizi M, Almadori G, Ferrandina G, et al. Prognostic significance of epidermal growth factor receptor in laryngeal squamous cell carcinoma. *Br J Cancer* 1996; 74:1253–1257.
39. Ohsaki Y, Tanno S, Fujita Y, et al. Epidermal growth factor receptor expression correlates with poor prognosis in non-small cell lung cancer patients with p53 overexpression. *Oncol Rep* 2000; 7:603–607.
40. Dong M, Nio Y, Guo KJ, et al. Epidermal growth factor and its receptor as prognostic indicators in Chinese patients with pancreatic cancer. *Anticancer Res* 1998; 18:4613–4619.
41. Giatromanolaki A, Koukourakis MI, O'Byrne K, et al. Non-small cell lung cancer: c-erbB-2 overexpression correlates with low angiogenesis and poor prognosis. *Anticancer Res* 1996; 16:3819–3825.
42. Huang SM, Bock JM, Harari PM. Epidermal growth factor receptor blockade with C225 modulates proliferation, apoptosis, and radiosensitivity in squamous cell carcinomas of the head and neck. *Cancer Res* 1999; 59:1935–1940.
43. Gibbs JB. Anticancer drug targets: growth factors and growth factor signaling. *J Clin Invest* 2000; 105:9–13.
44. Baguley BC, Marshall ES, Holdaway KM, et al. Inhibition of growth of primary human tumour cell cultures by a 4-anilinoquinazoline inhibitor of the epidermal growth factor receptor family of tyrosine kinases. *Eur J Cancer* 1998; 34:1086–1090.
45. Sirotnak FM, Zakowsky MF, Miller VA, et al. Potentiation of cytotoxic agents against human tumors in mice by ZD1839 (IRESSA), an inhibitor of EGFR tyrosine kinase, does not require high levels of expression of EGFR. *Proc Ann Meet Am Assoc Cancer Res* 2000; 41:Abstract 3076.
46. Baselga J, Norton L, Masui H, et al. Antitumor effects of doxorubicin in combination with anti-epidermal growth factor receptor monoclonal antibodies. *J Natl Cancer Inst* 1993; 85:1327–1333.
47. Fan Z, Baselga J, Masui H, et al. Antitumor effect of anti-epidermal growth factor receptor monoclonal antibodies plus cis-diamminedichloroplatinum on well established A431 cell xenografts. *Cancer Res* 1993; 53:4637–4642.
48. Akimoto T, Hunter NR, Buchmiller L, et al. Inverse relationship between epidermal growth factor receptor expression and radiocurability of murine carcinomas. *Clin Cancer Res* 1999; 5:2884–2890.
49. Wollman R, Yahalom J, Maxy R, et al. Effect of epidermal growth factor on the growth and radiation sensitivity of human breast cancer cells in vitro. *Int J Radiat Oncol Biol Phys* 1994; 30:91–98.
50. Dent P, Reardon DB, Park JS, et al. Radiation-induced release of transforming growth factor alpha activates the epidermal growth factor receptor and mitogen-activated protein kinase pathway in carcinoma cells, leading to increased proliferation and protection from radiation-induced cell death. *Mol Biol Cell* 1999; 10:2493–2506.
51. Maciejewski B, Withers HR, Taylor JM, et al. Dose fractionation and regeneration in radiotherapy for cancer of the oral cavity and oropharynx: tumor dose-response and repopulation. *Int J Radiat Oncol Biol Phys* 1989; 16:831–843.
52. Grandis JR, Chakraborty A, Zeng Q, et al. Downmodulation of TGF-alpha protein expression with antisense oligonucleotides inhibits proliferation of head and neck squamous carcinoma but not normal mucosal epithelial cells. *J Cell Biochem* 1998; 69:55–62.
53. Gill GN, Kawamoto T, Cochet C, et al. Monoclonal anti-epidermal growth factor receptor antibodies which are inhibitors of epidermal growth factor binding and antagonists of epidermal growth factor binding and antagonists of epidermal growth factor-stimulated tyrosine protein kinase activity. *J Biol Chem* 1984; 259:7755–7760.
54. Mendelsohn J. Epidermal growth factor receptor inhibition by a monoclonal antibody as anticancer therapy. *Clin Cancer Res* 1997; 3:2703–2707.
55. Prewett M, Rockwell P, Rockwell RF, et al. The biologic effects of C225, a chimeric monoclonal antibody to the EGFR, on human prostate carcinoma. *J Immunother Emphasis Tumor Immunol* 1996; 19:419–427.
56. Bonner JA, Ezekiel MP, Robert F, et al. Continued Response Following Treatment with IMC-C225, an EGFr MoAb, Combined with RT in Advanced Head and Neck Malignancies. *Proc Am Soc Clin Oncol* 2000; 19:Abstract 5F.
57. Traxler P, Furet P. Strategies toward the design of novel and selective protein tyrosine kinase inhibitors. *Pharmacol Ther* 1999; 82:195–206.

58. Klohs WD, Fry DW, Kraker AJ. Inhibitors of tyrosine kinase. *Curr Opin Oncol* 1997; 9:562–568.
59. Grunicke HH, Maly K. Role of GTPases and GTPase regulatory proteins in oncogenesis. *Crit Rev Oncog* 1993; 4:389–402.
60. Magee T, Marshall C. New insights into the interaction of Ras with the plasma membrane [comment]. *Cell* 1999; 98:9–12.
61. Lopez-Ilasaca M, Crespo P, Pellici PG, et al. Linkage of G protein-coupled receptors to the MAPK signaling pathway through PI 3-kinase gamma. *Science* 1997; 275:394–397.
62. Zachos G, Spandidos DA. Expression of ras proto-oncogenes: regulation and implications in the development of human tumors. *Crit Rev Oncol Hematol* 1997; 26:65–75.
63. Spiegel AM. Mutations in G proteins and G protein-coupled receptors in endocrine disease. *J Clin Endocrinol Metab* 1996; 81:2434–2442.
64. Zhang FL, Casey PJ. Protein prenylation: molecular mechanisms and functional consequences. *Annu Rev Biochem* 1996; 65:241–269.
65. Lobell RB, Kohl NE. Pre-clinical development of farnesyltransferase inhibitors. *Cancer Metastasis Rev* 1998; 17:203–210.
66. Nagasu T, Yoshimatsu K, Rowell C, et al. Inhibition of human tumor xenograft growth by treatment with the farnesyl transferase inhibitor B956. *Cancer Res* 1995; 55:5310–5314.
67. Du W, Lebowitz PF, Prendergast GC. Cell growth inhibition by farnesyltransferase inhibitors is mediated by gain of geranylgeranylated RhoB. *Mol Cell Biol* 1999; 19:1831–1840.
68. Lebowitz PF, Casey PJ, Prendergast GC, et al. Farnesyltransferase inhibitors alter the prenylation and growth-stimulating function of RhoB. *J Biol Chem* 1997; 272:15,591–15,594.
69. Bernhard EJ, McKenna WG, Hamilton AD, et al. Inhibiting Ras prenylation increases the radiosensitivity of human tumor cell lines with activating mutations of ras oncogenes. *Cancer Res* 1998; 58:1754–1761.
70. McKenna WG, Weiss MC, Bakanauskas VJ, et al. The role of the H-ras oncogene in radiation resistance and metastasis. *Int J Radiat Oncol Biol Phys* 1990; 18:849–859.
71. Miller AC, Kariko K, Myers CE, et al. Increased radioresistance of EJras-transformed human osteosarcoma cells and its modulation by lovastatin, an inhibitor of p21ras isoprenylation. *Int J Cancer* 1993; 53:302–307.
72. Bernhard EJ, Kao G, Cox AD, et al. The farnesyltransferase inhibitor FTI-277 radiosensitizes H-ras-transformed rat embryo fibroblasts. *Cancer Res* 1996; 56:1727–1730.
73. Cohen-Jonathan E, Muschel RJ, Gillies McKenna W, et al. Farnesyltransferase inhibitors potentiate the antitumor effect of radiation on a human tumor xenograft expressing activated HRAS. *Radiat Res* 2000; 154:125–132.
74. Morgan DO. Principles of CDK regulation. *Nature* 1995; 374:131–134.
75. Roussel MF. Key effectors of signal transduction and G1 progression. *Adv Cancer Res* 1998; 74:1–24.
76. Rich T, Allen RL, Wyllie AH. Defying death after DNA damage. Nature 2000; 407:777–783.
77. Kastan MB, Onyekwere O, Sidransky D, et al. Participation of p53 protein in the cellular response to DNA damage. *Cancer Res* 1991; 51:6304–6311.
78. Clarke AR, Purdie CA, Harrison DJ, et al. Thymocyte apoptosis induced by p53-dependent and independent pathways. *Nature* 1993; 362:849–852.
79. Smith ML, Chen IT, Zhan Q, et al. Involvement of the p53 tumor suppressor in repair of u.v.-type DNA damage. *Oncogene* 1995; 10:1053–1059.
80. El-Deiry WS, Tokino T, Velculescu VE, et al. WAF1, a potential mediator of p53 tumor suppression. *Cell* 1993; 75:817–825.
81. Swisher SG, Roth JA, Nemunaitis J, et al. Adenovirus-mediated p53 gene transfer in advanced non-small-cell lung cancer. *J Natl Cancer Inst* 1999; 91:763–771.
82. Rothmann T, Hengstermann A, Whitaker NJ, et al. Replication of ONYX-015, a potential anticancer adenovirus, is independent of p53 status in tumor cells. *J Virol* 1998; 72:9470–9478.
83. Harada JN, Berk AJ. p53-Independent and -dependent requirements for E1B-55K in adenovirus type 5 replication. *J Virol* 1999; 73:5333–5344.
84. Kirn D, Hermiston T, McCormick F. ONYX-015: clinical data are encouraging [letter; comment]. *Nat Med* 1998; 4:1341–1342.
85. Khuri FR, Nemunaitis J, Ganly I, et al. A controlled trial of intratumoral ONYX-015, a selectively-replicating adenovirus, in combination with cisplatin and 5-fluorouracil in patients with recurrent head and neck cancer. *Nat Med* 2000; 6:879–885.

86. Heise CC, Williams A, Olesch J, et al. Efficacy of a replication-competent adenovirus (ONYX-015) following intratumoral injection: intratumoral spread and distribution effects. *Cancer Gene Ther* 1999; 6:499–504.
87. Akiyama T, Yoshida T, Tsujita T, et al. G1 phasc accumulation induced by UCN-01 is associated with dephosphorylation of Rb and CDK2 proteins as well as induction of CDK inhibitor p21/Cip1/WAF1/Sdi1 in p53-mutated human epidermoid carcinoma A431 cells. *Cancer Res* 1997; 57:1495–1501.
88. Yu L, Graves P, Tempcyzk A, et al. The checkpoint kinase Chk1 is a target of the anticancer agent UCN-01. *Proc Am Assoc Cancer Res* 1999; 40:Abstract 2019.
89. Seynaeve CM, Kazanietz MG, Blumberg PM, et al. Differential inhibition of protein kinase C isozymes by UCN-01, a staurosporine analogue. *Mol Pharmacol* 1994; 45:1207–1214.
90. Wang Q, Fan S, Eastman A, et al. UCN-01: a potent abrogator of G2 checkpoint function in cancer cells with disrupted p53. *J Natl Cancer Inst* 1996; 88:956–965.
91. Monks A, Harris E, Connelly J, et al. Enhancement of fludarabine and gemcitabine toxicity by UCN-01 in a variety of human tumor cell lines. *Proc Am Assoc Cancer Res* 1999; 40:Abstract 45.
92. Shao RG, Cao CX, Shimizu T, et al. Abrogation of an S-phase checkpoint and potentiation of camptothecin cytotoxicity by 7-hydroxystaurosporine (UCN-01) in human cancer cell lines, possibly influenced by p53 function. *Cancer Res* 1997; 57:4029–4035.
93. Shao RG, Shimizu T, Pommier Y. 7-Hydroxystaurosporine (UCN-01) induces apoptosis in human colon carcinoma and leukemia cells independently of p53. *Exp Cell Res* 1997; 234:388–397.
94. Akinaga S, Nomura K, Gomi K, et al. Enhancement of antitumor activity of mitomycin C in vitro and in vivo by UCN-01, a selective inhibitor of protein kinase C. *Cancer Chemother Pharmacol* 1993; 32:183–189.
95. Tsuchida E, Urano M. The effect of UCN-01 (7-hydroxystaurosporine), a potent inhibitor of protein kinase C, on fractionated radiotherapy or daily chemotherapy of a murine fibrosarcoma. *Int J Radiat Oncol Biol Phys* 1997; 39:1153–1161.
96. Shimizu S, Narita M, Tsujimoto Y. Bcl-2 family proteins regulate the release of apoptogenic cytochrome c by the mitochondrial channel VDAC. *Nature* 1999; 399:483–487.
97. Rosse T, Olivier R, Monney L, et al. Bcl-2 prolongs cell survival after Bax-induced release of cytochrome c. *Nature* 1998; 391:496–499.
98. Rafi MM, Rosen RT, Vassil A, et al. Modulation of Bcl-2 and cytotoxicity by licochalcone-A, a novel estrogenic flavonoid. *Anticancer Res* 2000; 20:2653–2658.
99. Eliopoulos AG, Kerr DJ, Herod J, et al. The control of apoptosis and drug resistance in ovarian cancer: influence of *p53* and Bcl-2. *Oncogene* 1995; 11:1217–1228.
100. Ho SP, Britton DH, Stone BA, et al. Potent antisense oligonucleotides to the human multidrug resistance-1 mRNA are rationally selected by mapping RNA-accessible sites with oligonucleotide libraries. *Nucleic Acids Res* 1996; 24:1901–1907.
101. Webb A, Cunningham D, Cotter F, et al. Bcl-2 antisense therapy in patients with non-Hodgkin lymphoma. *Lancet* 1997; 349:1137–1141.
102. Kuss B, Cotter F. Antisense—time to shoot the messenger. *Ann Oncol* 1999; 10:495–503.
103. Gelmon KA, Eisenhauer EA, Harris AL, et al. Anticancer Agents Targeting Signaling Molecules and Cancer Cell Environment: Challenges for Drug Development? *J Natl Cancer Inst* 1999; 91:1281–1287.

18 Receptor Tyrosine Kinases as Therapeutic Targets in Solid Tumors

Stacy L. Moulder, MD, MSCI
and Carlos L. Arteaga, MD

CONTENTS

1. INTRODUCTION

The introduction of nonspecific cytotoxic chemotherapeutic agents has provided palliation of symptoms, increased survival, and sometimes cure in patients with metastatic cancer. Unfortunately, patients with metastatic disease that are most likely to receive significant survival benefits from chemotherapy include those with less common malignancies, such as testis cancer and lymphoid neoplasms. In other more common malignancies, such as metastatic colon cancer or nonsmall-cell lung cancer (NSCLC), cytotoxic chemotherapy serves to palliate symptoms and has little or no role in prolonging life. Because of the nonspecific action of most current cytotoxic anticancer drugs, side effects such as bone marrow suppression, renal toxicity, and myocardial toxicity can often limit a patient's eligibility for and tolerance to therapy.

Recently, the development of rationally designed agents that target molecules differentially expressed in tumor but not in nonmalignant cells have provided new prospects for the treatment of common neoplasms such as breast, lung, head and neck, and colon carcinomas. Because these agents are in general tumor selective, they are likely to be substantially less toxic at clinically effective doses than traditional FDA-approved chemotherapeutic drugs *(1)*. Some of the most promising agents include inhibitors of receptor tyrosine kinases such as HER-2/neu, epidermal growth factor receptor (EGFR, HER-1), platelet-derived growth factor receptor (PDGFR), and the vascular endothelial growth factor receptors Flk-1/KDR (VEGFR-2) and Flt-1 (VEGFR-1).

From: *Chemoradiation in Cancer Therapy*
Edited by: H. Choy © Humana Press Inc., Totowa, NJ

2. RECEPTOR TYROSINE KINASES AND THEIR ROLE IN MALIGNANCY

Several families of tyrosine kinases have been identified since their initial discovery more than 20 yr ago. In general, tyrosine kinases play a fundamental role in normal cellular regulatory processes. However, the fact that many cellular proto-oncogenes encode for proteins with tyrosine kinase activity as well as the rare presence of phosphotyrosine in nontransformed cells, both argue persuasively that tyrosine phosphorylation is an important event in cellular transformation and tumor maintenance. Although there are several intracellular tyrosine kinases with oncogenic potential, the most novel therapeutic approaches currently in development target transmembrane receptor tyrosine kinases, which are vital for the transduction of extracellular signals into intracellular responses *(2,3)*.

Tyrosine kinase receptors exist as transmembrane glycoproteins that are composed of three major regions: an amino-terminal extracellular region, a hydrophobic transmembrane region, and a carboxy-terminal intracellular region that contains the tyrosine kinase domain and regulatory phosphorylation sites *(3,4)*. The receptor's ectodomain provides the ligand binding site for a range of polypeptides that, upon binding, activate the receptor's tyrosine kinase causing autophosphorylation of the receptor in specific C-terminal residues, and the recruitment to those C-terminal phosphotyrosines of specific second messengers that activate intracellular signaling pathways involved in enhanced proliferation, cell motility, dedifferentiation, and/or survival.

Most oncogenic receptor tyrosine kinases, such as the EGFR and its homologous receptor HER-2/neu, are critical in embryological development, normal epithelial cell proliferation, and tissue repair processes. However, their overexpression can lead to tumorigenesis as well as contribute to tumor progression and metastases *(4,5)*. Alternatively, some tumors take advantage of cellular responses in normal adjacent nontumor tissue. Such is the case with tumors that overexpress vascular endothelial growth factor (VEGF), a ligand that binds to receptors such as Flt-1 (VEGFR-1) and Flk-1/KDR (VEGFR-2). These receptors are located on the surface of normal endothelial cells and their activation results in endothelial cell proliferation and migration that leads to the increased neoangiogenesis necessary for tumor growth and induction of metastases *(6–9)*. Overexpression of both HER-2 and EGFR has been established as poor prognostic indicators in women with both early-stage and metastatic breast cancer *(4,5)*, and VEGF overexpression has been linked to early recurrence and decreased survival in patients with early-stage lung, gastric, breast, and ovarian cancers *(10–15)*. Many other tyrosine kinases are also involved in tumor maintenance and progression and are thus the target of molecular therapies in different stages of preclinical and clinical development. In this section, we will focus on the background and clinical status of inhibitors of EGFR, HER-2, and VEGFR signaling.

3. TARGETING THE EPIDERMAL GROWTH FACTOR RECEPTOR FAMILY

Both EGFR (HER-1, erbB1) and HER-2/neu (erbB2) are members of a family of transmembrane tyrosine kinases that also includes HER-3 (erbB3) and HER-4 (erbB4). The ectodomain of each EGFR, HER-3, and HER-4 interacts with a specific set of soluble ligands, whereas no ligand has been identified thus far for the orphan HER-2 receptor *(4)*. Based on transfection studies with fibroblasts, it is generally accepted that HER-2 is the most transforming of these tyrosine kinases. Binding of ligands to EGFR, HER-3, or HER-4 results in the formation of homodimeric and heterodimeric complexes into which HER-2 is recruited as a preferred signaling partner. In general, the HER-2-containing heterodimers exhibit enhanced stability and a more robust signaling potency *(4)*. Furthermore, inactivation of HER-2 function has been shown to impair signaling induced by activating ligands of EGFR, HER-3, or HER-4, suggesting a critical role for HER-2 in the overall function of the HER receptor network.

Abundant epidemiological data indicate that tumors that overexpress EGFR and/or HER-2 exhibit a worse outcome than tumors that do not overexpress these receptors. In addition, inhibition of these receptors with monoclonal antibodies has been shown to reverse transformation in preclinical models. Moreover, the measurable overexpression of EGFR and HER-2 in tumor diagnostic tissue and the lack of an obvious role for these tyrosine kinases in normal host tissues, all together, support the notion that these tumor cell surface molecules provide a therapeutic window that can be exploited in the treatment of carcinomas that overexpress EGFR and/or HER-2.

4. CLINICAL TRIALS WITH ANTI-HER-2 STRATEGIES

Trastuzumab (Herceptin™), a humanized IgG_1 raised against the ectodomain of HER-2, has been one of the first biologic agents available for use in clinical trials in patients with HER-2-overexpressing cancers. Preclinical laboratory studies have suggested several possible mechanisms of action. First, binding of the antibody stabilizes HER-2 homodimer formation and prevents the receptor from interacting with other HER coreceptors. Second, antibody binding induces phosphorylation of specific C-terminal residues, which recruit chaperon proteins that lead to receptor ubiquitination and degradation *(16)*. Third, the antibody reduces cyclin D1 and increases steady-state levels of the cyclin-dependent kinase inhibitor p27, leading to cell cycle arrest *(17)*. Fourth, it may reduce the expression and secretion of critical angiogenic factors by the cancer cells depriving them of an important mechanism for tumor maintenance in vivo *(18)*. Finally, binding of trastuzumab to tumor cells may recruit Fc receptor-expressing immune effector cells leading to antibody-dependent cell-mediated cytotoxicity (ADCC) and tumor eradication *(19)*.

Three phase I/II trials were performed to evaluate the safety and tolerability of trastuzumab. The drug was given intravenously to ensure consistent delivery and was administered on a weekly schedule based on the clearance of the antibody in preclinical studies. Trastuzumab was well tolerated with repeated weekly administration of doses ranging from 10 to 500 mg. Based on preclinical data showing a synergistic effect with the combination of trastuzumab with cisplatin *(20)*, one of the phase II trials utilized concomitant trastuzumab plus cisplatin in patients with chemoresistant metastatic breast cancer *(21)*. Adverse events encountered with the combination therapy were similar to those previously described with single-agent cisplatin and neither drug affected the pharmacokinetic profile of the other one.

Initial phase I and II trials with trastuzumab were done in patients with metastatic breast cancer with documented HER-2 overexpression as measured by immunohistochemistry. The first phase I/II study reported by Baselga et al. *(22)* enrolled patients heavily pretreated with chemotherapy and demonstrated an objective response rate of 11%. Side effects were minimal and consisted of occasional fever and chills acutely associated with the intravenous infusion of the antibody. Larger nonrandomized trials have validated these results with single-agent response rates of 20% in patients previously treated with chemotherapy or hormonal therapy *(23)* and 40% in patients with no prior therapy for metastatic disease *(24)*. In this last study, the median time to tumor progression in the responding patients was >18 mo. Preliminary data suggest that the clinical responses in these studies were limited to those tumors with the highest immunohistochemical levels of HER-2 and/or HER-2 gene amplification as measured by fluorescent *in situ* hybridization *(25)*. Adverse events noted in the larger trials included rare hypersensitivity reactions and an even rarer, unexpected side effect of reversible cardiomyopathy especially in those patients with a prior history of heart disease.

A recently published randomized phase III trial investigated the combination of standard chemotherapy with or without trastuzumab in patients with metastatic breast cancer that overexpress HER-2 *(26)*. The trial involved randomization of patients into four treatment groups. Those patients who had no history of adjuvant anthracycline were randomized to trastuzumab plus adriamycin/cytoxan (AC) or to AC alone. Patients who had received previous adjuvant anthracycline therapy were randomized to trastuzumab plus paclitaxel or paclitaxel alone. Although higher response rates were seen in patients treated with AC plus trastuzumab compared with AC alone (65% vs 42%), there was also a significant increase in cardiomyopathy (18% vs 3%) with the combination. Combination therapy with paclitaxel also produced higher response rates than single-agent therapy (57% vs 25%) with fewer cases of cardiomyopathy (2%). Remarkably, overall survival was improved by the addition of trastuzumab compared to those patients treated with chemotherapy alone *(26)*. These studies lead to FDA approval for the use of trastuzumab as single-agent therapy or in combination with paclitaxel in patients with metastatic breast cancer known to overexpress HER-2. Because of the incidence of cardiomyopathy, combination therapy with anthracyclines was not approved and, although clinically effective against metastatic breast cancer, it is considered contraindicated.

Trastuzumab has recently been combined with vinorelbine with a response rate of 71% in a single-arm phase II trial involving patients with HER-2 overexpressing metastatic breast cancer *(27)*. In another study, Pegram et al. *(21)* reported the ability of the antibody to sensitize breast tumors previously resistant to chemotherapy to cisplatin. These results seem very promising but await validation in larger randomized studies. Randomized trials are currently underway to investigate trastuzumab's role as adjuvant therapy for patients with stage I/II breast cancers that overexpress HER-2. Other trials are currently investigating trastuzumab's role in nonbreast malignancies by enrolling patients with metastatic lung, prostate, and bladder cancers that overexpress HER-2. Although the results of these trials have yet to mature, they represent trastuzumab's potential for therapy in a wide variety of tumor types. Of some concern, however, is the fact that the published rates of HER-2 overexpression and/or HER-2 gene amplification are much lower in carcinomas other than breast cancer, suggesting that clinical responses to Herceptin may be lower in these tumor types.

5. CLINICAL TRIALS TARGETING THE EGFR (HER-1)

As for HER-2, preclinical evidence exists to support targeting EGFR (HER-1) with a therapeutic intent in epithelial neoplasms. First, the expression of EGF receptors is elevated in many epithelial tumors and this overexpression has been associated with poor clinical outcome *(28)*. Second, coexpression of high levels of EGFR and its ligands, EGF or TGFα, results in a transformed cellular phenotype. Third, EGFR monoclonal antibodies and small-molecule inhibitors of the receptor's tyrosine kinase have been shown to inhibit growth of EGFR-overexpressing cancer cells in culture and in athymic nude mice *(29)*.

The mouse monoclonal IgG_2 mAb225 recognizes the ectodomain of the EGFR, competes for ligand binding, and induces receptor dimerization/downregulation, thus leading to inactivation of the receptor's tyrosine kinase activity *(30)*. The antibody also induces cell cycle arrest and tumor cell apoptosis in preclinical in vitro and in vivo models *(31,32)*. Initial phase I trials of single-dose mAb225 revealed selective tumor localization and drug safety profile in doses given up to 300 mg *(33)*. Unfortunately, all patients produced human antimouse antibodies (HAMA), which prevented further administration of the drug. A chimeric human-to-murine version of mAb225 (IMC C225) was produced in order to avert the human immune response and permit the continuous drug delivery that may be required for sustained antitumor action. Interestingly, the humanized antibody C225 was found to bind to the receptor with a higher affinity than mAb225 and was associated with greater antitumor effects against xenografts with high levels of EGFR *(34)*.

Preliminary safety data have been reported from phase I trials with C225, all in patients with locally advanced or metastatic or recurrent tumors of the upper aerodigestive tract and with detectable EGFR in tumor tissues as measured by immunohistochemistry *(35)*. One published trial investigated the combination of weekly cisplatin in patients with chemorefractory NSCLC or head and neck tumors. In this study, intravenous doses of 200–400 mg/m^2/wk resulted in steady-state serum concentrations of C225 that would have been predicted to saturate receptors in EGFR-dependent preclinical models and were thus judged to be adequate for phase II efficacy studies. Notably, this "optimal biological dose" was achieved before any dose-limiting toxicity or before reaching a maximally tolerated dose. C225 clearance did not change with the coadministration of cisplatin. Antibodies against C225 were detected in only 1 of 52 patients, and there was minimal toxicity associated with the antibody alone or the combination *(36)*. Disease stabilization was seen in a percentage of patients treated with C225 alone and two partial responses were documented in the last trial. Toxicities associated with C225 were in general well tolerated and included a 4% risk of grade 3 or 4 allergic reactions, a 2% incidence of grade 4 infusion-associated hypersensitivity reaction, and an 80% incidence of reversible, sterile folliculitis of the face, upper chest, and/or back.

Small single-institution trials have demonstrated a higher percentage of complete clinical responses in patients treated with advanced head and neck cancers treated with C225 and radiation therapy than would be expected from historical responses to radiation therapy alone *(37)*. Currently, ongoing phase II and III trials are studying the effects of C225 in combination with either radiation therapy or chemotherapy in patients with nonsmall-cell lung, locally advanced head and neck, and metastatic colon cancers. Preclinical studies have also demonstrated an additive effect when combining C225 with trastuzumab against HER-2-overexpressing breast cancer xenografts, thus providing a rationale for the use of combined anti-HER therapy (J. Baselga, personal communication).

An alternative approach to inhibiting the function of EGFR (HER-1) includes the use of small molecules identified by random screening of natural or synthetic compound libraries for specific protein kinase inhibitory activities. The selected compounds compete with ATP for binding to the receptor's ATP site in the n*M* range, thus blocking activation of its tyrosine kinase. Most of these reversible tyrosine kinase inhibitors belong to various classes of small molecules including dianilinophthalimides, pyrazolo-pyrrolopyridopyrimidines, and quinazolines *(38)*. In addition, some irreversible inhibitors bind covalently to specific residues in the ATP-binding pocket of the EGFR and may be able to achieve a more prolonged half-life inside a tumor cell target *(39)*.

ZD1839 (Iressa) is an orally active quinazoline that reversibly inhibits ATP binding to the receptor's tyrosine kinase with an in vitro IC_{50} of 1 μM *(40)*, thus preventing its activation and downstream signaling. Therapy with ZD1839 alone produces dose-dependent growth inhibition and apoptosis in human ovarian, breast, and colon cancer cell lines which coexpress EGFR and TGFα. Growth inhibition and induction of apoptosis are both enhanced when ZD1839 is combined with cytotoxic drugs such as cisplatin, paclitaxel, doxorubicin, and etoposide in the above mentioned cell lines. These effects have also been validated in xenograft models and do not seem to require high levels of HER-1 (EGFR) expression for antitumor activity *(41)*. Whether ZD1839 and other tyrosine kinase inhibitors work preferentially on EGFR that are activated by autocrine/paracrine ligands regardless of EGFR levels is a question with important clinical implications that requires further investigation.

Phase I trials have evaluated both intermittent administration (14 d of treatment followed by 14 d of observation) and continuous delivery (once daily for 28 d) of ZD1839. Oral dosing ranged from 50 to 1000 mg/d. Patients were eligible if they had tumors known to express EGFR (HER-1) such as NSCLC, breast, colon, ovarian, prostate, and head and neck cancers. Both schedules of administration were well tolerated with minor toxicities such as grade 1–2 skin rash, nausea, vomiting, and diarrhea. Dose-limiting toxicity was grade 3 diarrhea, which occurred at doses ≥700 mg/d. Although not a primary endpoint for these studies, objective responses as well as disease stabilization, especially in patients with NSCLC, were seen at several dose levels and were frequently associated with improvement of disease-related symptoms *(42,43)*.

Currently, large randomized trials in patients with NSCLC, prostate cancer, and bladder cancer are testing whether ZD1839 alters the response rate, time to tumor progression, and toxicity of standard chemotherapy. Preclinical laboratory data have indicated that ZD1839 is synergistic with ionizing radiation against breast cancer cell lines *(44)*. Preliminary data suggest that ZD1839 alone is also effective against HER-2-overexpressing breast cancer cells that also express EGFR and has an additive effect against these cells when combined with trastuzumab *(45)*. These observations imply a possible role for small molecule EGFR tyrosine kinase inhibitors in patients with breast cancer whose tumors overexpress HER-2.

6. RATIONALE FOR AND CLINICAL TRIALS WITH INHIBITORS OF ANGIOGENESIS

In addition to endogenous signaling pathways in tumor cells, tumor–host interactions also contribute to cancer progression. It is well established that the formation of new blood vessels, as a result of tumor-to-host cell crosstalk, is essential for the growth of primary and metastatic tumors *(7,46)*. Several receptor tyrosine kinases present in endothelial cells have been implicated in the endothelial cell migration and proliferation required for tumor-associated neoangiogenesis. As mentioned previously, VEGF and its associated receptors Flt-1 (VEGFR-1) and Flk-1 (VEGFR-2) are essential in generating neovascularization required for tumor growth and metastases.

Both receptors have seven immunoglobulin-like domains in their extracellular region, a single-membrane-spanning domain, and an intracellular split tyrosine kinase domain *(47)*. Ligands binding to these receptors, which are located predominantly in endothelial cells, induces upregulation of proteases, increases vascular permeability, and induces endothelial cell migration and proliferation *(48–50)*. Preclinical experiments have indicated a direct causal link between VEGF activity and tumor angiogenesis. Initially, anti-VEGF antibodies were found to suppress tumor growth in human tumor xenograft models *(51)*. Next it was reported that retrovirus-mediated expression of a dominant negative Flk-1 (VEGFR-2) mutant also suppressed tumor growth in nude mice *(52)*. Furthermore, antibodies against the Flk-1 (VEGFR-2) receptor also suppressed tumor angiogenesis and tumor growth *(53)*. Finally, small-molecule inhibitors of the VEGFR tyrosine kinase inhibited neovascularization and tumor growth *(54,55)*.

Clinical evidence also suggests an important role for VEGF in human tumor angiogenesis. First, VEGF m-RNA and VEGF protein are upregulated in a majority of human tumors when analyzed by *in situ* RNA hybridization or immunohistochemistry *(56)*. Second, quantitative analysis of tumor biopsy specimens has shown that VEGF overexpression is associated with a poorer prognosis and diminished survival *(10–15,46)*. Lastly, VEGF is highly expressed in ischemic cells proximal to areas of tumor necrosis, suggesting that angiogenesis is an important survival mechanism to overcome hypoxia-induced tumor cell death *(57)*.

Clinical trials are now underway to determine the role of several new compounds that target the tyrosine kinases involved in tumor neoangiogenesis, particularly Flk-1 (VEGFR-2) and Flt-1 (VEGFR-1). The rationale to support these novel approaches is robust. First, in the adult, new vessel formation is limited to ovulation, wound healing, and neoplastic tissues, leading to a potentially tumor-selective mechanism of action. Second, unlike traditional chemotherapeutic agents, these drugs do not damage DNA and target normal endothelial cells which lack the genetic plasticity and mutagenesis that usually leads to drug resistance in cancer cells, suggesting that resistance to anti-angiogenesis drugs may not occur rapidly in solid tumors *(58)*.

Initial efforts to inhibit angiogenesis focused on inhibition of the VEGF ligand with monoclonal antibodies to impede VEGFR activation. More recently, novel small-molecule VEGFR tyrosine kinase inhibitors have been introduced. SU5416 is a 3-substituted indolin-2-one that was found to potently inhibit Flk-1 (VEGFR-2), Flt-1 (VEGFR-1), and PDGFR tyrosine kinases *(54)*. SU5416 inhibits VEGF-induced mitogenesis of human endothelial cells but had no effect on tumor cell growth in vitro. On the contrary, intraperitoneal administration of 25/mg/kg/d of SU5416 was found to have antitumor activity against a large panel of human xenografts in athymic nude mice *(54)*.

Phase I studies with SU5416 continue to accrue heavily pretreated patients with a variety of tumor types. These trials have shown a favorable toxicity profile with documented cases of reduction in tumor size or stabilization of disease. Dose-limiting toxicity has been defined as headache with projectile vomiting, which occurred at a dose level of 190 mg/m^2/iv *(59)*. Current recommended phase II dosing for SU5416 is 145 mg/m^2/iv twice weekly. Oral inhibitors of VEGF receptor tyrosine kinases, such as SU6668 and ZD6474, have also demonstrated promising results in preclinical experiments *(60)*. Early reports of phase I trials with SU6668, an oral analog of SU5416, have revealed favorable toxicity profiles with some reports of disease stabilization *(61)*.

The study of the effects of aberrant signal transduction in malignancy has lead to a broad new field of biologically targeted therapy in oncology. The recent development of rationally designed agents that target tumor-specific tyrosine kinases offer the option of selective therapy that is likely to be substantially less toxic at clinically effective doses than traditional cytotoxic chemotherapy. Although these drugs offer new opportunities for target-based therapy, many of the pathways they affect, such as angiogenesis and cell cycle regulation, are involved in tumor growth, thus traditional clinical endpoints such as tumor response rates may not serve as accurate measurements of drug activity. Additionally, their dose–toxicity relationships are likely to be less steep than those of the nonspecific chemotherapeutic agents, thereby rendering such concepts as maximum tolerated dose less meaningful than alternatives such as the optimal biologic dose or the biologically effective dose *(1)*. In short, the development of rationally designed tyrosine kinase-based anticancer therapies has resulted in an exciting and clinically challenging future for oncologic research.

REFERENCES

1. Rowinsky EK. The pursuit of optimal outcomes in cancer therapy in a new age of rationally designed target-based anticancer agents. *Drugs* 2000; 60:1–14; discussion 41–42.
2. Noonberg SB, Benz CC. Tyrosine kinase inhibitors targeted to the epidermal growth factor receptor subfamily: role as anticancer agents. *Drugs* 2000; 59:753–767.
3. Hunter T. Signaling - 2000 and beyond. *Cell* 2000; 100:113–127.
4. Yarden Y, Sliwkowski MX. Untangling the ErbB network. *Nature Rev* 2001; 2:127–137.
5. Wells A. EGF receptor. *Int J Biochem Cell Biol* 1999; 31:637–643.
6. Neufeld G, Cohen T, Gengrinovitch S, et al. Vascular endothelial growth factor (VEGF) and its receptors. *Faseb J* 1999; 13:9–22.
7. Folkman J. Angiogenesis in cancer, vascular, rheumatoid and other disease. *Nat Med* 1995; 1:27–31.
8. Yeo KT, Wang HH, Nagy JA, et al. Vascular permeability factor (vascular endothelial growth factor) in guinea pig and human tumor and inflammatory effusions. *Cancer Res* 1993; 53:2912–2918.
9. Fukumura D, Xavier R, Sugiura T, et al. Tumor induction of VEGF promoter activity in stromal cells. *Cell* 1998; 94:715–725.
10. Volm M, Koomagi R, Mattern J. Prognostic value of vascular endothelial growth factor and its receptor Flt-1 in squamous cell lung cancer. *Int J Cancer* 1997; 74:64–68.
11. Maeda K, Chung YS, Ogawa Y, et al. Prognostic value of vascular endothelial growth factor expression in gastric carcinoma. *Cancer* 1996; 77:858–863.
12. Paley PJ, Staskus KA, Gebhard K, et al. Vascular endothelial growth factor expression in early stage ovarian carcinoma. *Cancer* 1997; 80:98–106.
13. Gasparini G, Toi M, Gion M, et al. Prognostic significance of vascular endothelial growth factor protein in node-negative breast carcinoma. *J Natl Cancer Inst* 1997; 89:139–147.
14. Linderholm B, Tavelin B, Grankvist K, et al. Vascular endothelial growth factor is of high prognostic value in node-negative breast carcinoma. *J Clin Oncol* 1998; 16:3121–3128.
15. Eppenberger U, Kueng W, Schlaeppi JM, et al. Markers of tumor angiogenesis and proteolysis independently define high- and low-risk subsets of node-negative breast cancer patients. *J Clin Oncol* 1998; 16:3129–3136.
16. Klapper LN, Waterman H, Sela M, et al. Tumor-inhibitory antibodies to HER-2/ErbB-2 may act by recruiting c-Cbl and enhancing ubiquitination of HER-2. *Cancer Res* 2000; 60:3384–3388.
17. Sliwkowski MX, Lofgren JA, Lewis GD, et al. Nonclinical studies addressing the mechanism of action of Trastuzumab (Herceptin). *Semin Oncol* 1999; 26(Suppl 12):60–70.
18. Viloria-Petit AM, Rak J, Hung M-C, et al. Neutralizing antibodies against epidermal growth factor and ErbB-2/neu receptor tyrosine kinases downregulate vascular endothelial growth factor production by tumor cells in vitro and In vivo. *Am J Pathol* 1997; 151:1523–1530.
19. Clynes RA, Towers TL, Presta LG, et al. Inhibitory Fc receptors modulate in vivo cytotoxicity against tumor targets. *Nature Med* 2000; 6:443–446.

20. Pietras RJ, Pegram MD, Finn RS, et al. Remission of human breast cancer xenografts on therapy with humanized monoclonal antibody to HER-2 receptor and DNA-reactive drugs. *Oncogene* 1998; 17:2235–2249.
21. Pegram MD, Lipton A, Hayes DF, et al. Phase II study of receptor-enhanced chemosensitivity using recombinant humanized anti-p185HER2/neu monoclonal antibody plus cisplatin in patients with HER2/neu-overexpressing metastatic breast cancer refractory to chemotherapy treatment. *J Clin Oncol* 1998; 16:2659–2671.
22. Baselga J, Tripathy D, Mendelsohn J, et al. Phase II study of weekly intravenous recombinant humanized anti-p185^{HER2} monoclonal antibody in patients with HER2/neu-overexpressing metastatic breast cancer. *J Clin Oncol* 1996; 14:737–744.
23. Cobleigh MA, Vogel CL, Tripathy D, et al. Multinational study of the efficacy and safety of humanized anti-HER2 monoclonal antibody in women who have HER2-overexpressing metastatic breast cancer that has progressed after chemotherapy for metastatic disease. *J Clin Oncol* 1999; 17:2639–2648.
24. Vogel C, Cobleigh MA, Tripathy D, et al. First-line, single-agent Herceptin(R) (trastuzumab) in metastatic breast cancer. a preliminary report. *Eur J Cancer* 2001; 37(Suppl 1):25–29.
25. Mass RD, Sanders C, Charlene K, et al. The concordance between the clinical trials assay (CTA) and fluorescence in situ hybridization (FISH) in the Herceptin pivotal trials. *Proc Am Soc Clin Oncol* 2000; 19:75 (abstr).
26. Slamon DJ, Leyland-Jones B, Shak S, et al. Use of chemotherapy plus a monoclonal antibody against HER2 for metastatic breast cancer that overexpresses HER2. *N Engl J Med* 2001; 344: 783–792.
27. Burstein HJ, Kuter I, Richardson PG. Herceptin and Vinorelbine for HER-2 positive metastatic breast cancer: a phase II study. *Proc Am Soc Clin Oncol* 2000; 19:102 (abstr).
28. Klijn JG, Berns PM, Schmitz PI, et al. The clinical significance of epidermal growth factor receptor (EGF-R) in human breast cancer: a review of 5232 patients. *Endocr Rev* 1992; 13:3–17.
29. Salomon DS, Brandt R, Ciardiello F, et al. Epidermal growth factor-related peptides and their receptors in human malignancies. *Crit Rev Oncol Hematol* 1995; 19:183–232.
30. Fan Z, Lu Y, Wu X, et al. Antibody-induced epidermal growth factor receptor dimerization mediates inhibition of autocrine proliferation of A431 squamous carcinoma cells. *J Biol Chem* 1994; 269:27,595–27,602.
31. Masui H, Kawamoto T, Sato JD, et al. Growth inhibition of human tumor cells in athymic mice by anti-epidermal growth factor receptor monoclonal antibodies. *Cancer Res* 1984; 44:1002–1007.
32. Wu X, Fan Z, Masui H, et al. Apoptosis induced by an anti-epidermal growth factor receptor monoclonal antibody in a human colorectal carcinoma cell line and its delay by insulin. *J Clin Invest* 1995; 95:1897–1905.
33. Divgi CR, Welt S, Kris M, et al. Phase I and imaging trial of indium 111-labeled anti-epidermal growth factor receptor monoclonal antibody 225 in patients with squamous cell lung carcinomas. *J Natl Cancer Inst* 1991; 83:97–194.
34. Goldstein NI, Prewett M, Zuklys K, et al. Biological efficacy of a chimeric antibody to the epidermal growth factor receptor in a human tumor xenograft model. *Clin Cancer Res* 1995; 1:1311–1318.
35. Cohen RB, Falcey JW, Paulter VJ, et al. Safety profile of the monoclonal antibody (MoAb) IMC-C225, an anti-epidermal growth factor receptor (EGFr) used in the treatment of EGFr-positive tumors. *Proc Am Soc Clin Oncol* 2000; 19:1862 (abstr).
36. Baselga J, Pfister D, Cooper MR, et al. Phase I studies of anti-epidermal growth factor receptor chimeric antibody C225 alone and in combination with cisplatin. *J Clin Oncol* 2000; 18:904–914.
37. Bonner JA, Ezekiel MP, Robert F, et al. Continued response following treatment with IMC-C225, an EGFr MoAb, combined with radiation therapy in advanced head and neck malignancies. *Proc Am Soc Clin Oncol* 2000; 19:5F (abstr).
38. Strawn LM, Shawver LK. Tyrosine kinases in disease: Overview of kinase inhibitors as therapeutic agents and current drugs in clinical trials. *Exp Opin Invest Drugs* 1998; 7:553–573.
39. Fry DW. Inhibition of the epidermal growth factor receptor family of tyrosine kinases as an approach to cancer chemotherapy: progression from reversible to irreversible inhibitors. *Pharmacol Ther* 1999; 82:207–218.
40. Woodburn JR, Kendrew J, Fennell M, et al. ZD1839 ('Iressa'), a selective epidermal growth factor receptor tyrosine kinase inhibitor (EGFR-TKI): inhibition of c-fos mRNA, an intermediate marker of

EGFR activation, correlates with tumor growth inhibition. *Proc Am Assoc Cancer Res* 2000; 41:2552 (abstr).
41. Sirotnak FM, Zakowsky MF, Miller VA, et al. Potentiation of cytotoxic agents against human tumors in mice by ZD1839 (Iressa) does not require high levels of expression of EGF receptors. *Proc Am Assoc Cancer Res* 2000; 41:3076 (abstr).
42. Baselga J, Herbst R, LoRusso P, et al. Continuous administration of ZD1839 (Iressa), a novel epidermal growth factor receptor tyrosine kinase inhibitor (EGFR-TKI), in patients with five selected tumor types: evidence of activity and good tolerability. *Proc Am Soc Clin Oncol* 2000; 19:177 (abstr).
43. Ferry K, Hammond L, Ranson M, et al. Intermittent oral ZD1839 (Iressa), a novel epidermal growth factor receptor tyrosine kinase inhibitor (EGFR-TKI), shows evidence of good tolerability and activity: final results from a phase I study. *Proc Am Soc Clin Oncol* 2000; 19:3 (abstr).
44. Rao GS, Murray S, Ethier SP. Radiosensitization of human breast cancer cells by a novel ErbB family receptor tyrosine kinase inhibitor. *Int J Radiat Oncol Biol Phys* 2000; 48:1519–1528.
45. Moulder SL, Yakes M, Bianco R, et al. Small molecule EGF receptor tyrosine kinase inhibitor ZD1839 (Iressa) inhibits HER2/neu (erbB-2) overexpressing breast tumor cells. *Proc Am Soc Clin Oncol* 2001; 20:8 (abstr).
46. Hanahan D, Folkman J. Patterns and emerging mechanisms of the angiogenic switch during tumorigenesis. *Cell* 1996; 86:353–364.
47. Schlaeppi JM, Wood JM. Targeting vascular endothelial growth factor (VEGF) for anti-tumor therapy, by anti-VEGF neutralizing monoclonal antibodies or by VEGF receptor tyrosine kinase inhibitors. *Cancer Metastasis Rev* 1999; 18:473–481.
48. Senger DR, Galli SJ, Dvorak AM, et al. Tumor cells secrete a vascular permeability factor that promotes accumulation of ascites fluid. *Science* 1983; 219:983–985.
49. Leung DW, Cachianes G, Kuang WJ, et al. Vascular endothelial growth factor is a secreted angiogenic mitogen. *Science* 1989; 246:1306–1309.
50. Keck PJ, Hauser SD, Krivi G, et al. Vascular permeability factor, an endothelial cell mitogen related to PDGF. *Science* 1989; 246:1309–1312.
51. Kim KJ, Li B, Winer J, et al. Inhibition of vascular endothelial growth factor-induced angiogenesis suppresses tumor growth in vivo. *Nature* 1993; 362:841–844.
52. Millauer B, Longhi MP, Plate KH, et al. Dominant-negative inhibition of Flk-1 suppresses the growth of many tumor types in vivo. *Cancer Res* 1996; 56:1615–1620.
53. Witte L, Hicklin DJ, Zhu Z, et al. Monoclonal antibodies targeting the VEGF receptor-2 (Flk-1/KDR) as an anti-angiogenic therapeutic strategy. *Cancer Metastasis Rev* 1998; 17:155–161.
54. Fong TAT, Shawver LK, Sun L, et al. SU5416 is a potent and selective inhibitor of the vascular endothelial growth factor receptor (Flk-1/KDR) that inhibits tyrosine kinase catalysis, tumor vascularization, and growth of multiple tumor types. *Cancer Res* 1999; 59:99–106.
55. Wood JM, Bold G, Buchdunger E, et al. PTK787/ZK 222584, a novel and potent inhibitor of VEGF receptor tyrosine kinases, impairs VEGF-induced responses and tumor growth after oral administration. *Cancer Res* 2000; 60:2178–2189.
56. Ferrara N, Davis-Smyth T. The biology of vascular endothelial growth factor. *Endocr Rev* 1997; 18:4–25.
57. Shweiki D, Itin A, Soffer D, et al. Vascular endothelial growth factor induced by hypoxia may mediate hypoxia induced angiogenesis. *Nature* 1992; 359:843–845.
58. Boehm T, Folkman J, Browder T, et al. Antiangiogenic therapy of experimental cancer does not induce acquired resistance. *Nature* 1997; 390:404–407.
59. Stopeck A. Results of a phase I dose-escalating study of the antiangiogenic agent, SU5416, in patients with advanced malignancies. *Proc Am Soc Clin Oncol* 2000; 19:206 (abst).
60. Laird AD, Vajkoczy P, Shawver LK, et al. SU6668 is a potent antiangiogenic and antitumor agent that induces regression of established tumors. *Cancer Res* 2000; 60:4152–4160.
61. Rosen L, Hannah A, Rosen P, et al. Phase I dose-escalating trial of oral SU006668, a novel multiple receptor tyrosine kinase inhibitor in patients with selected advanced malignancies. *Proc Am Soc Clin Oncol* 2000; 19:182 (abst).

19 Adenoviral *p53* Gene Therapy Strategies in Nonsmall-Cell Lung Cancer

Stephen G. Swisher, MD
and Jack A. Roth, MD

CONTENTS

1. INTRODUCTION

Lung cancer is a worldwide problem. In the United States, less than 15% of people presenting with lung cancer survive 5 yr. Early-stage lung cancer (Stage I and II) is curable with surgery. Unfortunately, the majority of patients present with locoregionally advanced (Stage III) or metastatic (Stage IV) lung cancer, which is seldom curable with surgery alone. Multimodality approaches with conventional therapies have been developed combining surgery, chemotherapy, and radiation therapy to improve survival. Unfortunately, despite these strategies, the 3-yr survival rates for patients with Stage III disease are still only 20% dropping to less than 5% for Stage IV patients. Additionally, many of the lung cancer patients now in treatment have failed currently available multimodality strategies, often because their tumors have proven remarkably resistant to the effects of radiation or chemotherapy. Although some progress has been made in combining conventional therapies, the increased toxicity is often unacceptable and median survival of nonsmall-cell lung cancer (NSCLC) patients has not markedly improved *(1)*. The identification of novel, less toxic cancer therapy strategies is there-

From: *Chemoradiation in Cancer Therapy*
Edited by: H. Choy © Humana Press Inc., Totowa, NJ

fore critical to improve on current treatment strategies, and it is becoming increasingly clear that rational development of these new therapies will depend on our understanding of the molecular biology of tumors.

2. GENETIC BASIS OF LUNG CANCER

In recent years it has become apparent that cancer is caused by mutations in DNA. Most malignant tumors are found to have several mutations that have occurred sequentially over time, eventually leading to transformation to the malignant phenotype. On first examination, the genetic link to cancer appears too complicated to exploit for therapeutic purposes. Analysis of tumor cell DNA reveals that different cancers as well as individual patients present varied genetic profiles. Further analysis, though, has uncovered some types of gene alterations that, although not expressed in all cancers, show up in a significant subset of patients.

The gene families most commonly implicated in the etiology of common cancers are the oncogenes and tumor suppressor genes. The protein products of these genes are critical to the cellular machinery that is responsible for the normal processes of signal transduction, DNA transcription, cell division, cell cycle arrest, and programmed cell death or apoptosis. The improper functioning of each of these processes plays a role in cancer. Thus, gene therapy strategies that inactivate critical oncogenes or replace critical tumor suppressor genes may lead to tumor regression by reversion of the malignant phenotype.

The *p53* gene is one of the most commonly mutated genes in all cancers and is felt to be a critical tumor suppressor gene *(2)*. The gene is mutated in 50–70% of patients with lung cancer. Additionally, in a large proportion of cases in which there is no mutation, *p53* is inactivated through binding by high levels of Mdm-2 protein or is functionally inactive because downstream genes such as the pro-apoptotic Bcl-2 family members which *p53* transactivates are mutated or transcriptionally inactive *(3)*. There is also evidence that the E6 protein of human papilloma virus can bind to and inactivate *p53* protein *(4)*. It has therefore been suggested that almost all lung cancer cells are *p53* defective and potentially targeted by gene transfer approaches with wild-type *p53*.

The protein product of the *p53* gene is a transcription factor with DNA binding capabilities that is responsible for the repair of damaged DNA, or the induction of apoptosis when repair is not appropriate or is not accomplished. Because the wild-type *p53* gene transactivates multiple other genes involved in growth control, gene therapy strategies designed to replace defective *p53* genes have the potential to suppress multiple genes driving the malignant cell toward uncontrolled cell growth and proliferation. Gene transfer of a single critical gene such as wild-type *p53* may therefore be able to offset multiple genetic mutations in the malignant cell.

Another potential clinical benefit of transferring wild-type *p53* is that only tumor cells appear to contain mutated or defective *p53* gene copies whereas normal cells continue to contain the wild-type *p53* genes. This allows a unique therapeutic window in which the gene transfer of wild-type *p53* induces apoptosis or cellular growth inhibition in tumor cells although leaving normal cells unaffected. Unlike conventional agents such as radiation therapy or chemotherapy where normal cells are also affected, wild-type *p53* gene transfer has the potential of being a selective therapeutic modality allowing it to be given alone or in combination with conventional agents in a relatively nontoxic fashion.

3. GENE TRANSFER TECHNIQUES

The concept of gene therapy is based on the simple premise of transferring a gene into a cell and having the transduced cell express the transferred gene. Various techniques are available to transfer genes into a cell, and can be broadly classified into viral and nonviral delivery systems. At the present time there is no perfect gene transfer technique. Each technique has its own inherent advantages and limitations. Because adenoviral delivery systems are some of the most commonly used especially in clinical trials, we will focus on this technology and explore the potential advantages and limitations of this technique for wild-type *p53* gene transfer in lung cancer.

4. ADENOVIRAL DELIVERY SYSTEMS

In contrast to nonviral delivery systems, viral vectors have shown much higher transduction efficiencies both in vitro and in vivo, which allows the potential for large-scale clinical trials. Recombinant adenovirus vectors are among the most popular delivery systems because they are easy to produce in vitro and can transduce nonreplicating cells safely and efficiently. Gene transfer is accomplished by creating adenovirus recombinants. The first generation adenoviral vectors, which are the most common type currently being used in lung cancer gene therapy trials, lack the E1 region of the viral genome. Into the E1 region the wild-type *p53* gene was inserted in conjunction with a cytomegalovirus (CMV) promoter to drive protein production. Because the E1 region is critical for replication, the E1-deleted adenoviral recombinants (*Ad-p53* alternatively called *Ad-CMVp53*) are capable of infecting cells but not replicating. Even though viral replication does not occur, the transferred gene is still expressed, leading to foreign protein production (i.e., wild-type *p53*) in the transduced cell.

The replication-incompetent adenoviral recombinant markedly increases the efficiency of gene transfer by enhancing cellular uptake and transcription of the transferred gene. Following transduction with *Ad-p53* in vitro and in vivo in lung cancer cells, a burst of wild-type *p53* gene expression occurs that peaks at 3 d and drops off dramatically over the next 2 wk. *Ad-p53* gene therapy strategies that utilize E1-deleted adenovirus recombinants must therefore take into account that gene expression is only transient and that high levels of transferred gene product are not present indefinitely probably requiring repeated deliveries for significant antitumoral activity. Delivery of the *Ad-p53* vector is most efficient when performed by direct intratumoral injection. Systemic delivery suffers from much lower transduction efficiency in the target tumors because the vector is delivered throughout the body and tends to concentrate in certain organs such as the liver. Also of concern is the potential immune response to viral vectors. Preclinical studies in an immunocompetent mouse model have demonstrated increased tumor regression and transgene expression despite elevated levels of circulating antiviral antibodies *(5)*. Other studies, however, have demonstrated cellular and humoral immune responses to adenoviral vectors *(6)*. Because a single dose of *Ad-p53* is unlikely to be effective, one major question for preliminary clinical lung cancer trials was the ability to repeatedly give *Ad-p53* doses safely and effectively in the face of augmented cellular and humoral responses.

5. *p53* GENE TRANSFER IN LUNG CANCER

5.1. Preclinical Studies

Antitumor activity after *p53* gene transfer has been demonstrated in preclinical studies in vitro and in vivo, in both immunodeficient and immunocompetent animal models. Fujiwara and colleagues *(7)* demonstrated a therapeutic effect in an orthotopic lung cancer model transduced with a retroviral wild-type *p53* expression vector. Zhang *(8)* achieved high-level gene transfer and expression using an adenoviral *p53* (*Ad-p53*) construct. Additionally, the growth of human lung cancer cells bearing multiple genetic lesions is suppressed by the introduction of wild-type *p53* genes but not by mutated *p53* genes *(9)* or control genes such as Actin suggesting the antitumoral effect is owing to the transfer of the wild-type *p53* gene rather than the adenoviral vector. The mechanism of cytotoxicity after *Ad-p53* gene transfer appeared to be due in large part to the induction of programmed cell death or apoptosis in part by upregulation of pro-apoptotic genes such as *Bak*, *Bax*, and *Fas* and downregulation of anti-apoptotic genes such as *Bcl-2* *(10)*. Unlike normal cells, cancer cells appear "primed" to undergo apoptosis after *Ad-p53* gene transfer leading to a selective therapeutic advantage.

During the course of the preclinical studies, a major concern was that only a small number of cells would be transduced in vivo, thereby limiting the therapeutic effect. The discovery by Fujiwara *(7)*; however, that viral vectors readily penetrate three-dimensional cancer cell matrices indicated that therapeutic genes would likely spread beyond the intratumoral injection site. *Ad-p53* gene transfer also induced significant "bystander" killing in which wild-type *p53* transduced cells mediated the killing of surrounding cells that had not themselves been transduced, possibly by mechanisms involving inhibition of angiogenesis *(11,12)* or induction of soluble Fas protein *(13)*, which traffic to neighboring cells. These preclinical observations all contributed to the pool of evidence demonstrating the feasibility of human clinical gene replacement trials in lung cancer patients through a strategy of a single intratumoral injection.

6. PRELIMINARY CLINICAL TRIALS WITH *p53* GENE TRANSFER IN LUNG CANCER

6.1. Retroviral p53 *Gene Transfer in NSCLC*

The first clinical trial involving transfer of wild-type *p53* into lung cancer used a retroviral vector containing a wild-type *p53* cDNA driven by a β-actin promoter that had been inserted into a modified LNSX retroviral vector. In the trial, retroviral wild-type *p53* supernatant was directly injected into endobronchial tumors under bronchoscopic guidance in four patients and CT guidance in five patients (four with chest wall tumors and one with an adrenal metastasis) *(14)*. The presence of wild-type *p53* was demonstrated in the biopsied tumor specimens of three patients by DNA amplification via the polymerase chain reaction (PCR). Antitumor activity was demonstrated in six of seven evaluable posttreatment tumor biopsies by terminal deoxynucleotidyl transferase (TT)-mediated biotin dUTP nick end-labeling (TUNEL) staining for apoptotic cells. In addition, three of seven evaluable patients showed evidence of tumor regression. This preliminary trial demonstrated the feasibility and safety of gene therapy strategies based on the restoration of wild-type *p53* gene function in advanced NSCLC. The use of retroviral vector in large-scale clinical trials was limited, however, by the inability to achieve high titers of virus (>10^7) and by the cumbersome need for a packaging cell line to produce retroviral vector on a large scale.

6.2. Adenoviral p53 *Gene Transfer in NSCLC*

Because of the limitations of retroviral constructs, the clinical efficacy of adenoviral vectors containing wild-type *p53* (*Ad-p53*) was evaluated. The advantage of adenoviral vectors was that they could be produced at substantially higher viral titers (>10^{12} viral particles) than retroviral vectors and could transduce both replicating and nonreplicating lung cancer cells at high efficiency with high levels of transgene protein. Adenoviral vectors do not integrate into the genome (they are maintained episomally for several cell divisions) and expression is therefore transient, necessitating multiple doses. Additionally, preclinical data suggested multiple doses of *Ad-p53* might elicit a humoral and cellular response to adenoviral antigens leading potentially to decreasing *p53* gene transfer and clinical side effects. The questions of safety and efficacy of repeated intratumoral *Ad-p53* gene transfer was therefore critical in the initial *Ad-p53* gene therapy trial in lung cancer.

The initial Phase I clinical trial performed at M. D. Anderson Cancer Center *(15)* utilized a first generation adenovirus vector containing wild-type *p53* complementary DNA (*Ad-p53*, INGN 201) in 28 patients with NSCLC whose tumors had failed to respond to conventional therapy. The *Ad-p53* vector was a replication-defective adenovirus serotype 5 vector, carrying a human *p53* expression cassette consisting of the CMV promoter, human wild-type *p53* cDNA, and the SV40 polyadenylation signal in place of the adenoviral E1 region. This study directly injected primary or metastatic lesions via bronchoscopy or computed tomography (CT) guidance. These treatments were repeated monthly up to 6 mo if there was no progression noted. Doses were escalated from 10^6 plaque forming units (pfu); approx 10^7 viral particles (vp) to 10^{11} pfu (10^{12} vp) in cohorts of 3. All tumors were biopsied 3 d after injection to assess gene transduction, *p53* mRNA expression and apoptosis induction. Clinical responses of the injected lesion were assessed by monthly CT scans. The first important finding of this study was that multiple doses of *Ad-p53* (INGN 201) could be safely administered in patients with advanced metastatic NSCLC. A total of 84 doses were administered to 28 patients with 56 of the doses repeated injections (up to six monthly). Despite sharp rises in neutralizing anti-adenovirus antibody levels after the first dose *(16,17)*, vector-related adverse events were minimal. There were no anaphylactic reactions or episodes and only one grade 3 vector-related adverse event. All other vector-related toxic effects were grade 1 or 2 and consisted primarily of transient fevers and chills treated with antipyretics. Repeated delivery of the vector by CT guidance or bronchoscopy was also feasible with six pneumothoraces observed during 84 injections. These pneumothoraces were able to be treated by observation in four patients and percutaneous pigtail catheter placement in two patients. The other most common adverse event was injection site pain in 13 out of 84 injections, which was successfully treated with analgesics and resolved within 24–48 h in the majority of cases. Because of the low toxicity, the last 10 patients were treated as outpatients without problems. The second important observation of this trial was that intratumoral delivery of *Ad-p53* (INGN 201) resulted in wild-type *p53* gene transfer in the injected tumor even in the face of neutralizing levels of anti-adenovirus antibody. Vector-specific primers that incorporated flanking regions of the adenovirus were used to ensure detection of adenovirally transferred *p53* mRNA rather than native *p53*. Gene transfer appeared to be dose dependent and could still be seen even with neutralizing anti-adenovirus antibodies present in the circulation. The third important finding of this study was that anti-tumoral activity was noted following *Ad-p53* gene transfer. Despite the fact that all patients had failed conventional therapy, 2/28 patients (7%) demonstrated a greater than 50% reduction in tumor size and 16/28 patients (57%) demonstrated stabilization of disease for periods of 2 to 24 mo off all other therapy. A prolonged time to progression was also noted in patients treated at the higher dose of *Ad-p53* vector (INGN 201) suggesting a relationship to gene transfer. It was also important to note that both patients who responded to therapy continued to regress after multiple doses despite elevated antiadenoviral antibodies. The mechanism of antitumor activity was assessed by evaluation of tumor biopsies obtained 3 d after treatment. These demonstrated increased TUNEL activity in 11 of 24 evaluable patients suggesting the induction of programmed cell death or apoptosis presumably through *p53* induction of pro-apoptotic pathways. Although immune-mediated responses have been reported after adenovirus treatment *(7)*, no significant increase in inflammatory cell infiltrate in posttreatment tumor biopsies was noted. Increases in cell-mediated immunity were noted in the peripheral blood to adenoviral antigens, but this was not demonstrated intratumorally *(16)*.

Schuler et al. *(18)* performed a Phase I study in 15 patients with Stage IIIB or IV NSCLC. A single intratumoral injection of *Ad-p53* (SCH 58500) was performed by bronchoscopy or CT guidance and was begun at 10^7 pfu (7.5×10^{10} vp) escalating to 10^{10} pfu (7.5×10^{12} vp). No clinically significant toxicity was observed and successful transfer of wild-type *p53* was demonstrated in posttreatment biopsies of six patients. Transient local disease control was observed in four of the six patients that had demonstrated wild-type *p53* gene transfer. This study demonstrated that intratumoral injection of *Ad-p53* (SCH 58500) was feasible and resulted in successful gene transfer at higher doses of *Ad-p53*. Perhaps because only one injection was performed and gene expression is transient with *Ad-p53* gene transfer, clinical responses were sustained only for short periods.

6.3. Adenoviral p53 *Gene Transfer with Chemotherapy in NSCLC*

The Phase I studies with *Ad-p53* alone demonstrated low toxicity possibly because of the tumor selective nature of action of wild-type *p53* as opposed to conventional antitumor agents. Several clinical limitations were also identified with *Ad-p53* alone. First, not all patients responded to *Ad-p53*. Second, perhaps because of the locoregional delivery, antitumor activity in systemic noninjected metastases was not observed. The clinical implications of this observation are that *Ad-p53* may require treatment in conjunction with other conventional agents to enhance response. The potential use of *Ad-p53* in combination with chemotherapy agents is supported by preclinical studies which demonstrate that the antitumor effects of *p53* gene transfer are enhanced by combined treatment with cisplatin, paclitaxel, CPT-11, 5-fluorouracil, and doxorubicin *(19–22)*. Because toxicity with *Ad-p53* is low, this may be a reasonable strategy especially if *Ad-p53* does not increase chemotherapy related toxicity. Another potential advantage of combining *Ad-p53* with chemotherapeutic agents is that it may allow treatment of distant as well as local disease.

Because of the preclinical observations, Nemunaitis et al. completed a Phase I trial of *Ad-p53* gene transfer in sequence with cisplatin in 24 NSCLC patients *(23)*. Intravenous cisplatin was administered on d 1 and the *Ad-p53* (INGN 201) vector was administered on d 4 by intratumoral CT or bronchoscopic injection. Up to a total of six monthly courses of treatment were carried out if toxicity or progression was not observed. The most common adverse effect attributable to *Ad-p53* treatment was fever, which occurred in 8 of 24 patients and was transient and self-limiting. This mild toxicity was not dose dependent. Following treatment, seventeen patients remained stable, two (both treated endobronchially) achieved partial responses, four continued to have progressive disease, and one was unevaluable due to progressive disease. Both patients achieving partial responses had previously shown progression on platinum-based chemotherapy combinations. Of the seven patients who received *Ad-p53* at endobronchial sites, five achieved reduction in the tumor mass to an extent that bronchial obstruction was relieved. Analysis of apoptosis in tumor biopsies from patients able to provide biopsies, showed an increased number of apoptotic cells (by the TUNEL assay) in 79% of the patients, a decrease in apoptosis in 7% of patients, and no change in the remaining 14%. Cisplatin alone has been shown to induce apoptosis to a small degree, but *Ad-p53* (INGN 201) or the combination of *Ad-p53* (INGN 201) and cisplatin, showed significantly more killing. This study suggested that antitumor strategies combining *Ad-p53* (INGN 201) with chemotherapy are feasible and potentially beneficial.

Schuler et al. recently completed a Phase II study in metastatic NSCLC evaluating three cycles of carboplatin (AUC 6) plus paclitaxel (175 mg/m^2) or cisplatin (100 mg/m^2) plus vinorelbine (25 mg/m^2) in combination with 7.5 × 10^{12} vp of *Ad-p53* (SCH 58500) on d 1 of each cycle *(24)*. Twenty-five patients were entered in the study and patients were required to have two lesions so that comparisons could be made (one which was injected and one which was observed). The first finding of this study was that the combination of these conventional chemotherapy agents and *Ad-p53* (SCH 58500) resulted in minimal vector-related toxicity (fever, nausea, fatigue, and injection site pain) and no increase in chemotherapy-related adverse events. Additionally, mean local tumor regression as measured by size was greater in the injected lesion compared to the control lesion especially with the cisplatin and vinorelbine regimen. Overall response rates and survival were not significantly different, but this may have been because of the small number of patients and the multiple regimens in the trial.

The implication of these trials is that the combination of *Ad-p53* and chemotherapy agents does not significantly increase overall toxicity and may be a reasonable strategy to pursue if therapeutic benefit can be demonstrated by the combination in randomized trials.

6.4. Adenoviral p53 *Gene Transfer with Radiation Therapy in NSCLC*

At the present time, delivery of *Ad-p53* requires direct injection into the tumor with guidance by bronchoscopy or CT scan. This delivery system allows high concentrations of vector to be administered in and around the injected tumor but it is not able to target micrometastatic disease. Another strategy therefore would be to combine *Ad-p53* with radiation therapy to try to enhance locoregional control without increasing toxicity. Currently, despite improvements in radiation and chemoradiation, the locoregional control of locally advanced NSCLC remains poor. One- and 2-yr pathologic control rates following radiation or chemoradiation are estimated to be less than 20% *(25)*. Preclinical studies with *Ad-p53* indicate that delivery of wild-type *p53* to *p53*-deficient cells, in both in vitro and in vivo models, increases tumor sensitivity to ionizing radiation *(26–29)*. Because of these preclinical results, we evaluated the potential impact of *Ad-p53* (INGN 201) in combination with radiation in a Phase II trial *(30)*. This trial was designed for locoregionally advanced, nonmetastatic patients who could not tolerate chemoradiation because of age, comorbidities, or completely obstructed bronchi. Additionally, patients with localized disease who were unable to tolerate resection because of poor pulmonary function were also eligible. The trial focused on a biopsy 3 mo following treatment to determine pathologic control rates. Patients were treated with three intratumoral injections of *Ad-p53* (INGN 201) on d 1, 18 and 32 in conjunction with radiation therapy (60 Gy). *Ad-p53* (INGN 201) doses were escalated from 3×10^{11} to 3×10^{12} vp and were injected directly into the primary tumor by bronchoscopy or CT guidance. Of the first 16 patients entered, 13 patients underwent 61 CT-guided biopsies or injections with 13 pneumothoraces. All pneumothoraces were managed as outpatients with observation (8 patients) or percutaneous pleural catheter (5 patients). No treatment-related mortality was observed and most patients were successfully treated as outpatients. Pathologic negative biopsies were noted in 8 out of 11 biopsied patients suggesting a high pathologic control rate at the primary tumor. One-year progression-free survival was 45.5% with most failures occurring because of metastatic progression rather than local failure *(30)*. Additionally, multiple biopsies were performed throughout the study and were evaluated with quantitative DNA and RT-PCR for changes in *p53* and *p53*-regulated genes (*Bak*, *MDM 2*, *p21*, and *Fas*). These biopsies demonstrated that there was a dramatic rise in wild-type *p53* DNA and mRNA, 24 h after gene transfer with associated increases in expression of the *p53*-regulated genes *Bak*, *p21*, and *MDM 2* but not *Fas (31)*.

This study shows that *Ad-p53* (INGN 201) can be given in conjunction with radiation therapy in a group of high risk patients with low toxicity in an outpatient setting. The high negative pathologic control rate is encouraging but the continued metastatic failure emphasizes the need to combine *Ad-p53* (INGN 201) in the future with chemotherapy agents to try to address the distant disease.

6.5. Future Role of Adenoviral p53 *Gene Transfer with Conventional Agents in NSCLC*

The clinical advantages of *Ad-p53* are its tumor-selective mechanism of action and low toxicity profile that allow combinations with conventional chemotherapy and radiation therapy. The limitations are the locoregional delivery and inability to target metastatic disease. Clearly, early-stage patients who cannot tolerate surgery because of poor pulmonary function or other comorbidities and would be treated with radiation therapy alone may represent a subset that would benefit from the addition of *Ad-p53* to radiation therapy.

The locoregional delivery and efficacy limit the potential therapeutic benefit of *Ad-p53* in metastatic Stage IV NSCLC patients except perhaps in a palliative role with low-dose radiation therapy. Currently, ECOG is evaluating the feasibility of *Ad-p53* (INGN 201) in combination with 30 Gy of radiation therapy for recurrent or previously radiated NSCLC. This trial initiated by Choy is the first *Ad-p53* study to be performed in a cooperative group setting.

The role of *Ad-p53* in locally advanced NSCLC (Stage III) needs to be further investigated. Although, metastatic disease plays a major role in determining survival in locally advanced NSCLC, there are several randomized studies which demonstrate that improved survival in Stage III NSCLC can be achieved with improved locoregional control. Saunders et al. *(32)* demonstrated that increased daily fractions of radiation in locally advanced NSCLC led to improved survival, although Schaake-Konig et al. *(33)* demonstrated that radiation sensitizing doses of chemotherapy improved survival by enhanced local control. Another therapeutic strategy therefore for *Ad-p53* would be to improve locoregional control by combining *Ad-p53* with concurrent or sequential chemoradiation. The low toxicity profile of *Ad-p53* might allow combinations with concurrent or sequential chemoradiation to further improve long-term survival benefits achieved with improved locoregional control. We plan to evaluate this strategy in an upcoming randomized Phase III study which will randomize high performance, unresectable Stage III NSCLC patients to concurrent chemoradiation vs concurrent chemoradiation and Ad-p53.

7. CONCLUSIONS

The poor overall survival of lung cancer patients treated with conventional therapies (surgery, radiation therapy, and chemotherapy) mandate novel approaches to treatment. Gene therapy strategies may ultimately lead to a new class of agents that target molecular abnormalities in lung cancer cells. At the present time, however, clinical trials utilizing gene therapy strategies are just beginning. Preliminary results from ongoing gene therapy trials suggest that toxicity is minimal and randomized Phase III studies are needed to determine potential survival benefits. In the future, such novel treatment strategies may complement conventional therapies and help to improve overall survival rates for patients with lung cancer.

ACKNOWLEDGMENTS

This work was partially supported by grants from the National Cancer Institute and the National Institutes of Health (P01 CA78778-01A1); SPORE (2P50-CA70970-04); by gifts to the Division of Surgery, from Tenneco and Exxon for the Core Laboratory Facility; by the UT M. D. Anderson Cancer Center Support Core Grant (CA 16672); by a grant from the Tobacco Settlement Funds as appropriated by the Texas State Legislature (Project 8), the W. M. Keck Foundation, and a sponsored research agreement with Introgen Therapeutics, Inc. (SR93-004-1). The authors wish to thank D.M. Smith for her assistance in the preparation of this manuscript.

REFERENCES

1. Parker SL, Tong T, Bolden S, Wingo PA. Cancer statistics, 1997. *CA Cancer J Clin* 1997; 47:5–27.
2. Mukhopadhyay T, Maxwell SA, Roth JA. p53 Suppressor Gene. Austin, TX: R.G. Landes Co., 1995.
3. Rampino N, Yamamoto H, Ionov Y, et al. Somatic frameshift mutations in the Bax gene in colon cancers of the microsatellite mutator phenotype. *Science* 1997; 275:967–969.
4. Seewaldt VL, Mrozek K, Dietze EC, Parker M, Caldwell LE. Human papillomavirus type 16 E6 inactivation of p53 in normal human mammary epithelial cells promotes tamoxifen-mediated apoptosis. *Cancer Res* 2001; 61:616–624.
5. Li Z, Rakkar A, Katayose Y, et al. Efficacy of multiple administrations of a recombinant adenovirus expressing wild-type p53 in an immune-competent mouse tumor model. *Gene Ther* 1998; 5:605–613.
6. Dai Y, Schwarz EM, Gu D, Zhang WW, Sarvetnick N, Verma IM. Cellular and humoral immune responses to adenoviral vectors containing factor IX gene: tolerization of factor IX and vector antigens allows for long-term expression. *Proc Natl Acad Sci USA* 1995; 92:1401–1405.
7. Fujiwara T, Cai DW, Georges RN, Mukhopadhyay T, Grimm EA, Roth JA. Therapeutic effect of a retroviral wild-type p53 expression vector in an orthotopic lung cancer model. *J Natl Cancer Inst* 1994; 86:1458–1462.
8. Zhang WW, Fang X, Mazur W, French BA, Georges RN, Roth JA. High-efficiency gene transfer and high-level expression of wild-type p53 in human lung cancer cells mediated by recombinant adenovirus. *Cancer Gene Ther* 1994; 1:5–13.
9. Takahashi T, Carbone D, Nau MM, et al. Wild-type but not mutant p53 suppresses the growth of human lung cancer cells bearing multiple genetic lesions. *Cancer Res* 1992; 52:2340–2343.

10. Pearson AS, Spitz FR, Swisher SG, et al. Up-regulation of the proapoptotic mediators Bax and Bak after adenovirus-mediated p53 gene transfer in lung cancer cells. *Clin Cancer Res* 2000; 6:887–890.
11. El-Deiry WS, Tokino T, Velculescu VE, et al. WAF1, a potential mediator of p53 tumor suppression. *Cell* 1993; 75:817–825.
12. Miyashita T, Reed JC. Tumor suppressor p53 is a direct transcriptional activator of human Bax gene. *Cell* 1995; 80:293–299.
13. Owen-Schaub LB, Zhang W, Cusack JC, et al. Wild-type human p53 and a temperature-sensitive mutant induce Fas/APO-1 expression. *Mol Cell Biol* 1995; 15:3032–3040.
14. Roth JA, Nguyen D, Lawrence DD, et al. Retrovirus-mediated wild-type p53 gene transfer to tumors of patients with lung cancer. *Nat Med* 1996; 2:985–991.
15. Swisher SG, Roth JA, Nemunaitis J, et al. Adenovirus-mediated p53 gene transfer in advanced non-small cell lung cancer. *J Natl Cancer Inst* 1999; 91:763–771.
16. Yen N, Ioannides CG, Xu K, et al. Cellular and humoral immune responses to adenovirus and p53 protein antigens in patients following intratumor injection of an adenovirus vector expressing wild-type p53 (Ad-p53). *Cancer Gene Ther* 2000; 7:530–536.
17. Roth JA, Swisher SG, Merritt JA, et al. Gene therapy for non-small cell lung cancer: a preliminary report of a phase I trial of adenoviral p53 gene replacement. *Semin Oncol* 1998; 25:33–37.
18. Schuler M, Rochlitz C, Horowitz JA, et al. A phase I study of adenovirus-mediated wild-type p53 gene transfer in patients with advanced non-small cell lung cancer. *Human Gene Therapy* 1998; 9:2075–2082.
19. Lebedeva S, Bagdasarova S, Tyler T, Mu X, Wilson DR, Gjerset RA. Tumor Suppression and Therapy Sensitization of Localized and Metastatic Breast Cancer by Adenovirus p53. *Hum Gene Ther* 2001; 12:763–772.
20. Seth P, Katayose D, Li Z, et al. A recombinant adenovirus expressing wild type p53 induces apoptosis in drug-resistant human breast cancer cells: a gene therapy approach for drug-resistant cancers. *Cancer Gene Ther* 1997; 4:383–390.
21. Osaki S, Nakanishi Y, Takayama K, Pei XH, Ueno H, Hara N. Alteration of drug chemosensitivity caused by the adenovirus-mediated transfer of the wild-type p53 gene in human lung cancer cells. *Cancer Gene Ther* 2000; 7:300–307.
22. Nielsen LL, Lipari P, Dell J, Gurnani M, Hajian G. Adenovirus-mediated p53 gene therapy and paclitaxel have synergistic efficacy in models of human head and neck. *Clin Cancer Res* 1998; 4:835–846.
23. Nemunaitis J, Swisher SG, Timmons T, et al. Adenovirus-mediated p53 gene transfer in sequence with cisplatin to tumors of patients with non-small cell lung cancer. *J Clin Oncol* 2000; 18:609–622.
24. Schuler M, Herrmann R, De Greve JL, et al. Adenovirus-mediated wild-type p53 gene transfer in patients receiving chemotherapy for advanced non-small-cell lung cancer: results of a multicenter phase II study. *J Clin Oncol* 2001; 19:1750–1758.
25. Le Chevalier T, Arriagada R, Quoix E, et al. Radiotherapy alone versus combined chemotherapy and radiotherapy in nonresectable non-small-cell lung cancer: first analysis of a randomized trial in 353 patients. *J Natl Cancer Inst* 1991; 83:417–423.
26. Bouvet M, Bold RJ, Lee J, et al. Adenovirus-mediated wild-type p53 tumor suppressor gene therapy induces apoptosis and suppresses growth of human pancreatic cancer. *Ann Surg Oncol* 1998; 5:681–688.
27. Jung M, Notario V, Dritschilo A. Mutations in the p53 gene in radiation-sensitive and -resistant human squamous carcinoma cells. *Cancer Res* 1992; 52:6390–6393.
28. Pardo FS, Su M, Borek C, et al. Transfection of rat embryo cells with mutant p53 increases the intrinsic radiation resistance. *Radiat Res* 1994; 140:180–185.
29. Lee JM, Bernstein A. p53 mutations increase resistance to ionizing radiation. *Proc Natl Acad Sci USA* 1993; 90:5742–5746.
30. Swisher S, Roth JA, Komaki R, et al. A phase II trial of adenoviral mediated p53 gene transfer (RPR/INGN 201) in conjunction with radiation therapy in patients with localized non-small cell lung cancer (NSCLC). *Am Soc Clin Oncol* 2000; 19:461a (abstract).
31. Swisher SG, Roth JA, Komaki R, et al. Induction of pro-apoptotic mediators and tumor regression following intratumoral delivery of adenoviral p53 (RTR/INGN 201) and radiation therapy in patients with non-small cell lung cancer (NSCLC). *Proc Am Soc Clin Oncol* 2001; 20:257a.
32. Saunders M, Dische BA, Harvey A, Gibson D, Parmar M. Continuous hyperfractionated accelerated radiotherapy (CHART) versus conventional radiotherapy in non-small cell lung cancer: a randomised multicentre trial. *Lancet* 1997; 350:161–165.
33. Schaake-Koning C, van den Bogaert W, Dalesio O, et al. Effects of concomitant cisplatin and radiotherapy on inoperable non-small cell lung cancer. *N Engl J Med* 1992; 326:524–530.

20 Tumor Microvasculature as a Therapeutic Target During Radiotherapy

Dennis E. Hallahan, MD *and Don Stacy,* MD

Contents

1. INTRODUCTION

The controversy surrounding the use of antiangiogenic agents during radiotherapy is based upon the concern that the resulting hypoxia will impair tumor response to radiation *(1)*. Tumor hypoxia is a therapeutic problem, as it makes solid tumors resistant to sparsely ionizing radiation and some forms of chemotherapy. Hypoxia also may increase the percentage of tumor cells in G1, resulting in greater resistance to therapy. Recent clinical studies suggest hypoxia can enhance malignant progression and increase aggressiveness through clonal selection and genome changes. In addition, hypoxia is an independent prognostic factor in cervix cancers, carcinomas of the head and neck, and soft-tissue sarcomas. Despite these concerns, recent preclinical studies have suggested that antiangiogenic agents enhance tumor control in response to fractionated irradiation.

From: *Chemoradiation in Cancer Therapy*
Edited by: H. Choy © Humana Press Inc., Totowa, NJ

2. RESPONSE OF TUMOR BLOOD VESSELS TO IONIZING RADIATION

The concept of the tumor microvasculature as a therapeutic target during radiotherapy can be supported by studies correlating the radiation response of tumor blood vessels to tumor regression. The response of tumor microvasculature to radiation is dependent upon the dose and time interval after treatment *(2–8)*. Tumor blood flow does not decrease unless high doses of 20–45 Gy are delivered *(2)*. However, blood volume increases if doses below 500 rad are administered *(6,8)*. Blood flow studies (interstitial Xe clearance) of irradiated mouse sarcoma show that blood flow increases within 3–7 d *(6)*. Most recent studies suggest this delayed increase in tumor blood flow may be in part due to radiation-induced vascular endothelial growth factor (VEGF) expression *(9)*.

Previous studies of tumor blood vessel response to radiation have relied upon the clearance of Xe and the quantity of RBCs (Cr-59) within tumors following treatment with radiation *(3,6,8)*. Currently available methods allow direct, longitudinal observation of tumor blood volume and blood flow *(10,11)*. More recent models include the tumor vascular window *(11)*, power Doppler sonography *(10)*, and histologic evaluation of tumor blood vessels *(12,13)*. These models permit characterization of the dose-dependent response in tumor blood vessels.

Power Doppler sonography displays the amplitude of the Doppler signal but lacks the velocity and directional information present in frequency-based color Doppler sonography *(10)*. However, power Doppler is more sensitive in the depiction of tumor vascularity *(14–16)*, specifically within small tumor vessels *(10,17)*. The hind limb tumor model and power Doppler can be utilized to measure the response of tumor blood vessels to radiation, providing longitudinal assessment of microvascular response within the same tumor without the need to section tumors for histology at various time intervals.

Power Doppler has been used to study the response of tumor blood vessels to ionizing radiation by utilizing amplitude to measure flow in microvasculature. For example, B16F0 melanoma, Lewis lung carcinoma (LLC), and GL261 glioma tumors were implanted in the hindlimb of C57BL6 mice, and D54 was implanted into nude mice. Tumors were grown to 1 cm in diameter and then irradiated with 2, 3, 6, or 10 Gy. Doppler analysis of tumor blood flow was performed on d 3 and 7. Figure 1 shows representative color Doppler images at d 3 of GL261 tumors treated with 0, 3, and 10 Gy. The flow in each pixel (power-weighted pixel) was accumulated to compare dose- and tumor-dependent changes in tumor blood flow over time. Figure 2 shows the dose-dependent tumor blood flow of all tumor models at d 3 after irradiation. Blood flow increased in all tumors receiving 2–3 Gy (Figs. 1B and 2), which is the fractionation scheme used during conventional radiotherapy. Doses used for stereotactic radiosurgery, intraoperative radiotherapy, and high-dose-rate (HDR) brachytherapy (6–10 Gy) resulted in a reduction in blood flow in all tumor types.

3. TUMOR VASCULAR WINDOW MODEL

The dorsal skin fold window model allows direct observation of tumor microvasculature *(11)*. This model also permits longitudinal assessment of the tumor vascular response to therapy. An accurate systematic measurement of tumor blood vessels in the window model is the linear summation of blood vessels using Optimas software. This approach corrects for vascular dilation and hemorrhage. Quantification of red

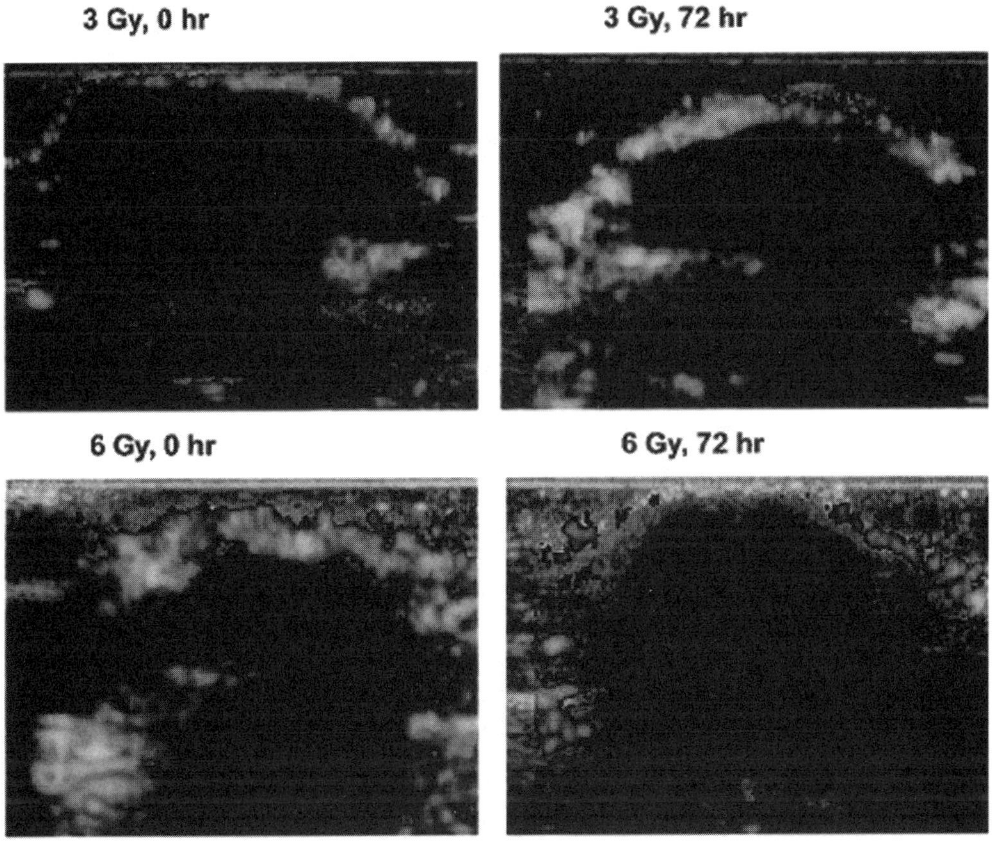

Fig. 1. GL261 and B16F0 tumor cell lines were pelleted and implanted into the hind limb of C57BL6 mice. Tumors were grown to diameters ranging from 0.7–1.1 cm and were irradiated. The vasculature of tumors was analyzed by power Doppler analysis. Shown are representative images acquired from power Doppler imaging of G1261 hindlimb tumors after 3 and 6 Gy irradiation.

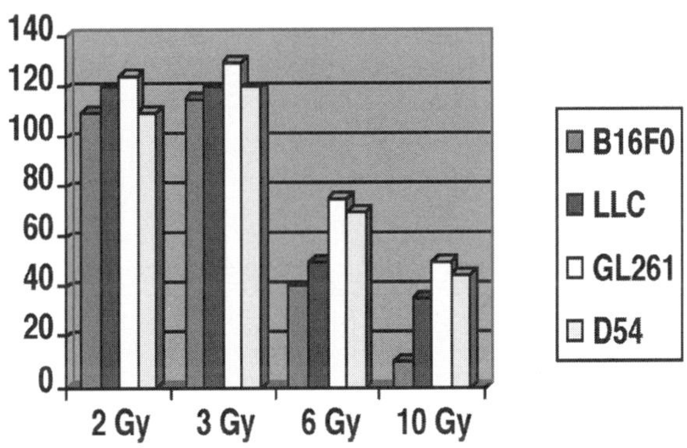

Fig. 2. Power weighted pixels Doppler (PWPD). Bar graph showing the change in GL261 and B1F60 tumor vascularity as measured by power Doppler after irradiation. The changes are compared with the vascularity of tumors measured immediately before irradiation.

pixels does not correlate with the manual counting of blood vessels in the microscopic field, because an increase in vascular diameter produces an increase in the number of pixels due to a dilatation of blood vessels, but not due to an increase in the number of blood vessels. Recent studies utilize linear summation of blood vessels in the window, correlating with results from histologic sections and Doppler blood flow studies of tumors following treatment.

The tumor vascular window model allows for measurement of tumor vascularity by use of fluorescent and light microscopy. A window is placed over the dorsal skin fold of a mouse and tumors are implanted within the window to allow microscopic visualization of tumor blood vessels (Fig. 3). The vascular window model facilitates direct measurement of the vascular response to ionizing radiation in several tumor models. Radiation induces dose- and time-dependent injury to tumor blood vessels within the window. Figure 3 shows blood vessels within GL261 (A and B) and B16F0 (C and D) implanted into the dorsal skin fold window model. Blood vessels developed over 1 wk, at which time they were treated with ionizing radiation. Figure 3E shows that the radioresistant GL261 tumor vessels had a minimal response to 6 Gy, whereas the radiosensitive B16F0 tumors showed elimination of microvasculature in response to 3 Gy.

The dose-dependent response of tumor blood vessels to radiation has been studied using the window model in C57BL6 mice. Tumor blood vessels were quantified by the use of vascular length density measurements using Optimas software, which quantifies the number of vessels showing fluorescent contrast *(18)* or hemoglobin, for either fluorescent or light microscopy, respectively. The quantification of tumor blood vessels within B16F0 melanoma tumor showed increased vasculature following treatment with 2 Gy. Treatment with 3 Gy reduced tumor vascularity within 48 h, while 6 Gy induced vascular obliteration within 24 h. Likewise, blood vessels within the GL261 glioma showed increased vascularity in response to 3 Gy. These preliminary results indicate the tumor vascular window is a useful method to study the role of tumor microvasculature in the host–tumor interaction. In Aims 1–3, the vascular window model will be utilized to study the role of Flk-1 receptor signaling in the resistance phenotype of tumor blood vessels.

4. GROWTH FACTORS CONTRIBUTE TO ENHANCED ENDOTHELIAL CELL VIABILITY

Growth factors contributing to enhanced endothelial cell viability include PDGF, FGF *(19)*, VEGF *(9)*, and EGFR. These growth factors bind to their respective receptors on the vascular endothelium. These receptors are tyrosine kinases (RTKs) that activate multiple signal transduction cascades within the endothelium. The signaling pathways mediate cell viability and proliferation through the induction of gene expression. Enhanced viability protects cells from radiation-induced cytotoxicity, and proliferation contributes to repopulation of injured cells. Therefore, new strategies to modify the radiation response include protection of normal endothelium by RTK agonists and reduced viability of irradiated tumor endothelium by RTK antagonists.

VEGF increases in tumors resistant to treatment such as malignant gliomas, and expression is also associated with worsened prognosis *(20)*. Blocking antibodies to VEGF have been shown to reduce angiogenesis in these receptors *(21)*. In addition, systemic administration of EGFR antibody with local radiation to SCC tumor xenografts demon-

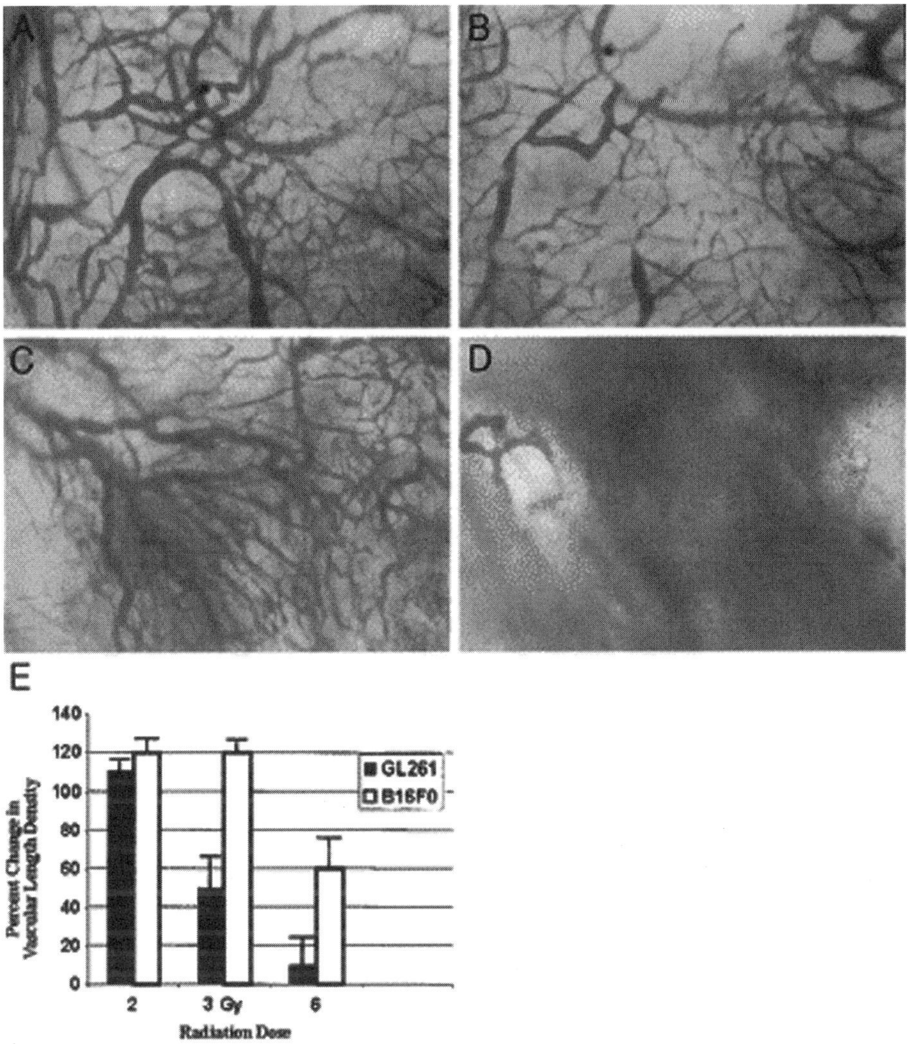

Fig. 3. The dorsal ventral window frame was applied to the skin fold of the flank of C57 BL6 mice after removal of the epidermis. Tumor cell lines GL261 and B16F0 were pelleted and implanted into the window skin fold. Angiogenesis into the implanted tumor occurred over the course of 7 d and were photographed by microscopy before irradiation (0 h). The same vascular windows were photographed daily. Shown are representative photographs of ×40 magnification of G1261 tumor vascular window models at 0 h (**A**) and 72 h (**B**) after treatment with 6 Gy. Vascular windows of B16F0 are shown at 0 h (**C**) and 72 h (**D**) after treatment with 3 Gy. (**E**) The length of tumor blood vessels photographed from the vascular window was summed on each of the days following irradiation. Changes in a quantity of blood vessels over time was compared with that observed at 0 h. Shown is the mean and SE of five experiments examining change in vascular length density in the dorsal window after irradiation of implanted tumors.

strates enhanced radiation response and inhibition of expression of tumor angiogenesis markers including VEGF *(22)*.

VEGF binds to endothelial receptors Flt-1 and Flk-1 to activate a signal transduction cascade (Fig. 4). Neutralizing antibodies to Flk-1 inhibit angiogenesis *(21)*. This inhibition of angiogenesis is most effective in glioblastoma xenographs and also reduces tumor

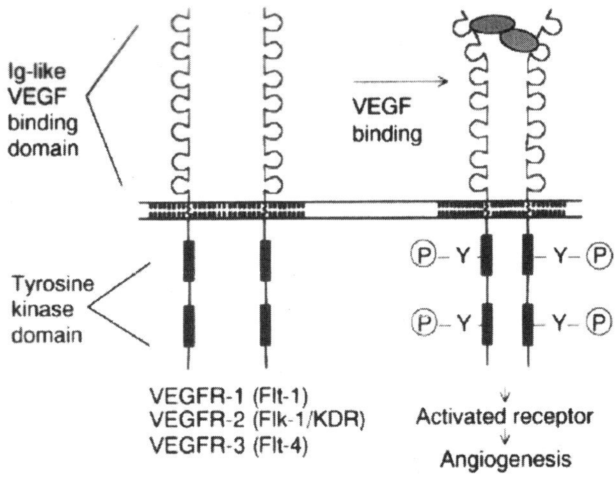

Fig. 4. VEGF binds to the Ig-like binding domain ligand of Flk-1, activating the intracellular tyrosine kinase domain and instigating a signal transduction cascade that leads to angiogenesis.

growth in several tumor models. A single chain antibody isolated from phage display library binds specifically to the extracellular domain of Flk-1 *(23)*. This antibody blocks the interaction between VEGF and Flk-1 and inhibits VEGF-stimulated activation of MAP kinase and P44/P42 of human endothelial cells *(23)*. These antibodies also neutralize VEGF-induced mitogenesis of human endothelial cells. These studies indicate Flk-1 is a receptor that activates proliferation of endothelial cells. Anti-VEGF antibody prolongs the growth delay achieved by radiation *(9)*. Endothelial cell proliferation and survival after in vitro irradiation are enhanced by supplementation of VEGF *(9)*. Anti-VEGF antibody enhances cytotoxic effects of irradiation in endothelial cells, and augments tumor radiation response under hypoxic and normoxic conditions *(24)*.

The importance of signal transduction through the VEGF receptors is illustrated by use of the truncated forms of receptors sFlt-1 and sFlk-1. These proteins bind to VEGF and sequester this ligand prior to its binding to cellular receptor *(11,25)*. These receptors also function as dominant negatives by forming inactive heterodimers with membrane-spanning VEGF receptors *(26)*. These specific inhibitors of VEGF prevent the mitogenic and migratory response of endothelial cells to VEGF. These studies show that VEGF-R1 (Flt-1) does not mediate a mitogenic or survival response in endothelial cells *(20)*. Experimental designs can therefore focus on Flk-1, whereas Flt-1 will serve as an alternative hypothesis to VEGF-mediated signaling in tumor endothelium.

VEGF-R2 (Flk-1/KDR) has a tyrosine kinase cytoplasmic domain that initiates signal transduction through multiple pathways *(20,27)*. Anti-VEGF R2 antibody decreases the dose of radiation needed to control small cell lung carcinoma and glioblastoma multiforme xenografts in mice *(28)*. The survival activity achieved by VEGF in the absence of serum may involve signal transduction through PI3-kinase since specific inhibitors of this kinase, LY294002 and Wortmannin, prevent this survival response *(29)*. This study also shows that VEGF induces phosphorylation of the serine-threonine kinase, Akt, in a PI3-kinase dependent manner. Constitutively active Akt is sufficient to promote the survival response of serum-starved endothelial cells, whereas the dominant negative form of Akt blocks survival effect of VEGF *(29)*. The role of Akt kinase and the survival response is supported by a study showing Flk-1 signaling through Akt kinase and Bcl-2 in a PI3 kinase-dependent manner *(30)*. In similar studies, PI3-kinase inhibition prevents Akt activation by VEGF-stimulated endothelial cells and dominant negative to Akt decreases endothelial cell viability response to VEGF *(29,31)*.

The VEGF-survival phenotype in endothelial cells is mediated by binding to the Flk-1/KDR receptor *(32,33)*. A potent and selective inhibitor of Flk-1/KDR blocks tyrosine kinase catalysis and inhibits tumor vascularization in growth *(34,35)*. The effectiveness of this Flk-1 inhibitor has been studied in gliomas *(36)*. This study suggests that inhibition of Flk-1 controls growth and progression of the angiogenesis-dependent neoplasms. A second Flk-1 antagonist is soluble Flk-1 receptor, which sequesters unbound VEGF, thereby preventing Flk-1 activation *(11)*. Preliminary data show that this signaling pathway generated by Flk-1 activation enhances the radiation response in tumor blood vessels.

5. APOPTOSIS OF VASCULAR ENDOTHELIAL CELLS

VEGF prolongs the survival of human endothelial cells, which is associated with increased expression of the anti-apoptotic protein Bcl-2 *(29,37,38)*. Enhanced endothelial cell survival is associated with a dose-dependent increase in Bcl-2 expression and decrease in expression of the processed forms of caspase-3 *(37)*. In addition to a 5.2-fold induction of Bcl-2 by VEGF, there is a 2.4-fold induction of A1 *(29)*. Over expression of Bcl-2 in HUVEC prevents apoptotic cell death in the absence of VEGF *(29)*. The signaling pathway required for VEGF inducing Bcl-2 expression includes the PI3 kinase-Akt/PKB signaling pathway *(38)*. This study shows that VEGF upregulates members of the anti-apoptotic proteins, inhibitors of apoptosis (IAP), in endothelial cells. VEGF stimulation leads to an induction of XIAP by threefold and survivin by 19-fold in HUVEC. Moreover, the VEGF-dependent upregulation of survivin is prevented by growth arrest indicating that the survival and mitotic functions of VEGF are more intrinsically related than previously anticipated *(38)*. Studies of the anti-apoptotic pathway in irradiated endothelial cells have also demonstrated the importance of PI3 kinase/Akt/Bad pathway *(39)*.

Expression of catalytically active mutants of Akt promotes the expression of Bcl-2 and c-Myc and inhibits apoptosis induced by cytokine deprivation. Bcl-2 interacts with several partners as well as itself. The ability to protect cells from activation of the caspase machinery is critically dependent upon the ratio of anti-apoptotic Bcl-2 like factors (Bcl-2, Bcl-XL, Mcl-1, and Bag) to pro-apoptotic factors (such as Bcl-XS, Bax, Bad, and Bak). These latter proteins can stabilize the protective effects of the Bcl-2 factors by dimerization. Bad is regulated by phosphorylation at two serine residues, Ser^{112} and Ser^{136} *(40,41)*. Phosphorylation of Bad is accompanied by association of the protein with 14-3-3 proteins, which recognize phosphoserine in the context of specific amino acid sequences *(42)*. Under these circumstances Bad phosphorylation correlates with survival, and agents that induce modification of Ser^{112} and Ser^{136} should provide a survival signal.

Akt is a downstream target of PI-3K activation *(43–45)*. PI-3K phosphorylates phosphoinositides (PtdIns) at the 3-position of the inositol ring, generating PtdIns*3*P, PtdIns(3,4)P_2, and PtdIns(3,4,5)P_3. The studies that elucidated these mechanisms were primarily based on the observation that growth-factor-induced Akt activation could be completely blocked by addition of Wortmannin, an inhibitor of PI-3K, and that growth-factor-receptor point mutations that prevent the activation of PI-3K also inhibit Akt.

Akt activity is induced in a PI-3K-dependent manner immediately suggesting that the phosphorylated lipid products of PI-3K mediate the activation. Incubation of purified Akt with purified 3-phosphorylated phospholipids results in various extents of activation *(44,46)*. These lipids, such as PtdIns*3*P, PtdIns(3,4)P_2, and PtdIns(3,4,5)P_3, specifically associate with PH domains in a number of proteins *(47)*. Furthermore, co-transfection of a dominant-negative form of PI-3K (delta-p85) also inhibits Akt activation *(43)*. It was later shown that introduction of constitutively active mutants of the catalytic subunit of PI-3K was sufficient to activate Akt in cells *(46,48)*. These studies strongly implicate Akt as a downstream effector of growth-factor-stimulated PI-3K activation in a variety of cell types.

6. ANTIANGIOGENIC AGENTS ENHANCE TUMOR CONTROL BY IONIZING RADIATION

Angiogenesis, the development of new blood vessels, is critical for human tumor growth. A single tumor blood vessel may feed as many as 10,000 tumor cells *(49,50)*. Tumor blood vessel endothelium is derived from genetically stable host cell endothelium and is unlikely to acquire resistance to antineoplastic therapy *(51)*. Antiangiogenic agents have been investigated as antineoplastic therapy in numerous preclinical trials. For example, antiintegrin alpha vs beta 3 inhibits breast cancer growth and angiogenesis in human skin *(52)*. Monoclonal antibody specific for vascular endothelial growth factor blocks human tumor growth in murine models *(53)*. The addition of tetrahydrocortisol, beta-cyclodextrin tetradecasulfate, and minocycline to standard cytotoxic treatment suppresses LLC growth *(54)*. TNP-470 alone or in association with minocycline represses murine FsaIIC fibrosarcoma and LLC growth in vivo when combined with cyclophosphamide *(55)*. TNP-470 also enhances the antitumor effect of ionizing radiation (IR) and prevents acute microvascular damage after IR in glioblastoma xenografts *(56)*, but provides no benefit for growth delay in tumor size when used in combination with combretastatin A-4 phosphate in rhabdomyosarcoma xenografts *(57)*. Furthermore, angiostatin and endostatin induce tumor dormancy in murine systems *(58,59)*. Statistical analysis of these preclinical trials reveals antiangiogenic therapy stabilizes neoplastic disease when used alone or concurrently with standard cytotoxic treatment. Investigators are currently testing antiangiogenic agents in combination with IR as antineoplastic therapy.

The antiangiogenic isocoumarin, NM-3, is cytotoxic to endothelial cells (HUVECs) but not to LLC cells or Seg-1, esophageal adenocarcinoma cells, in clonogenic survival assays. When HUVEC cultures are treated with NM-3 combined with IR, additive cytotoxicity is observed. In addition, the combination of NM-3 and IR inhibits HUVEC migration to a greater extent than either treatment alone. The effects of treatment with NM-3 and IR have also been evaluated in tumor model systems. C57BL/6 female mice bearing LLC tumors were given injections for four consecutive days with NM-3 (25 mg/kg/d) and treated with IR (20 Gy) for two consecutive days. Combined treatment with NM-3 and IR significantly reduced mean tumor volume compared with either treatment alone. Importantly, no increase in systemic or local tissue toxicity was observed after combined treatment (NM-3 and IR) when compared with IR alone. The bioavailability and nontoxic profile of NM-3 suggests the efficacy of this agent should be tested in clinical radiotherapy *(60)*.

Combined treatment with endostatin and radiation produces tumor growth inhibition in SQ20B and LLC tumors. By d 35, tumors receiving combined treatment with endostatin and IR are 47% smaller than tumors treated with endostatin alone. Histologic analyses demonstrate a reduction in microvascular density after combined treatment with endostatin and IR compared with endostatin treatment alone. Survival analyses confirm interactive cytotoxicity between endostatin and IR in both human aortic endothelial cells and human umbilical vein endothelial cells, but not in SQ-20B tumor cells. Combined treatment with endostatin and IR produce an increase in endothelial cell apoptosis compared with either treatment alone. The tumor regression observed after combined treatment with endostatin and IR suggests additive antitumor effects in both human and murine tumors. Importantly, the concentrations of endostatin employed produce little tumor regression when endostatin is employed as a single agent. The results from the clonogenic and apoptosis assays support the hypothesis that the endothelial compartment is the target for the endostatin/IR interaction *(61)*.

Angiostatin, a proteolytic fragment of plasminogen that was first isolated from the serum and urine of tumor-bearing mice, inhibits angiogenesis and thereby growth of primary and metastatic tumors *(62)*. Radiotherapy has been combined with angiostatin to target tumor vasculature that is genetically stable and therefore less likely to develop resistance. The results show an antitumor interaction between IR and angiostatin for four distinct tumor types at doses of radiation used in radiotherapy. The combination produces no increase in toxicity toward normal tissue. In vitro studies show radiation and angiostatin have combined cytotoxic effects on endothelial cells, but not tumor cells. In vivo studies show these agents, in combination, target the tumor vasculature. These results provide support for combining IR with angiostatin to improve tumor eradication without increasing deleterious effects *(63)*.

7. ANTAGONISTS OF RECEPTOR TYROSINE KINASES ENHANCE THERAPEUTIC RESPONSE TO RADIATION

To determine whether Flk-1 kinase inhibitors enhance radiation cytotoxicity, compound SU5416 kinases have been utilized *(34–36)*. SU5416 alone given as a single 0.75 mg intraperitoneal injection achieves a dose-dependent reduction in tumor blood vessels. The combination of subtherapeutic doses of radiation (2 Gy) with a minimally therapeutic dosage of SU5416 helps determine whether radiation responses can be modified by Flk-1 inhibition. B16F0, LLC, and GL261 tumors were implanted in the dorsal skin fold window in C57BL6 mice and angiogenesis was observed for 1 wk. Tumors treated with 2 Gy alone showed no vascular response to radiation. SU5416 showed a minimal regression of blood vessels and rapid restoration of vasculature. SU5416 administered 1 h prior to irradiation markedly enhanced the radiation effect with destruction of tumor blood vessels within 24 h of treatment. Assessment of blood vessels within the windows showed increased vascular destruction when tumors were treated with SU5416 prior to irradiation. The enhancement of the vasculitic effects of radiation was observed in all tumor models. The significance of these findings is that SU5416 alone has suboptimal therapeutic effect. However, when the endothelium is entirely destroyed in combination with radiation, the biological response is more pronounced and persistent.

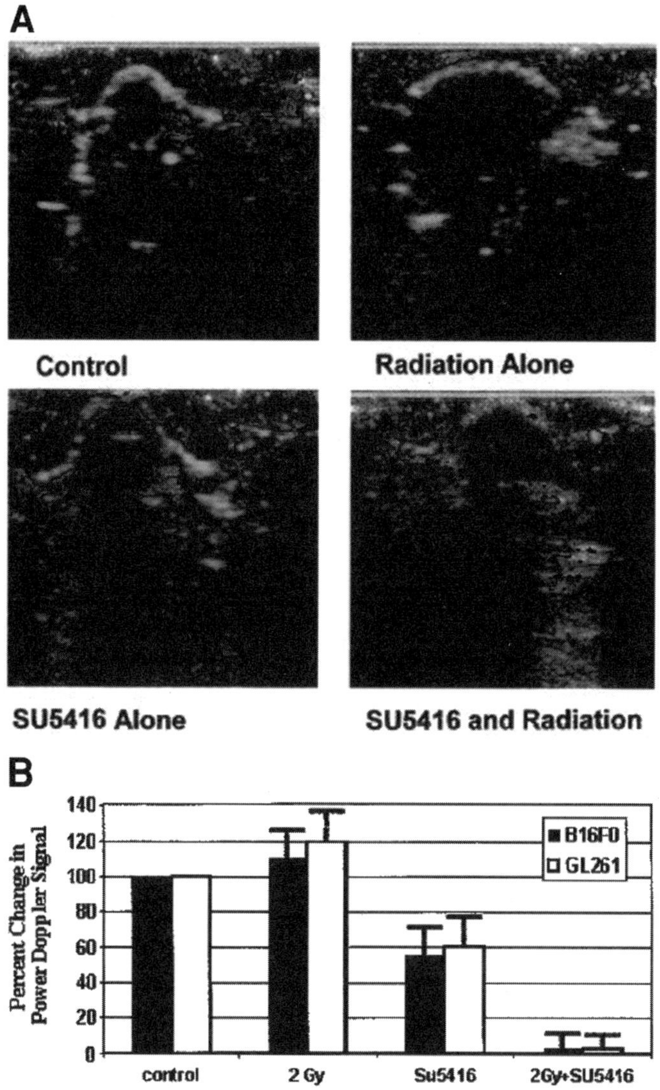

Fig. 5. Doppler blood flow of tumors on the indicated day after treatment with 6 Gy. Restoration of blood occurs in all tumors except those treated with Flk-1 antagonist SU5416 twice weekly for 2 wk (SU).

To determine whether inhibition of Flk-1-mediated signal transduction also enhances the cytotoxic effects of radiotherapy in established GL261 tumors, power Doppler can be used to quantify blood flow in 1 cm tumor models treated with Flk-1 inhibitors and radiation. GL261 tumors were selected because their vasculature is most resistant to radiation and these tumors require large radiation doses to achieve regression *(64,65)*. Animal models were then treated with a minimally effective dosage of SU5416 (0.75 mg) administered by intraperitoneal injection at 1 h prior to irradiation. SU5416 was injected every other fraction for a total of three doses. Tumors were treated with a minimally effective dose of 3 Gy per fraction given as six fractions to 18 Gy total in 10 d. Blood flow was quantified by power Doppler on d 4 and 7. Radiation alone and SU5416 alone achieved minimal reduction in tumor blood flow. Tumors treated with SU5416 1 h prior to irradiation showed significant reduction in tumor blood flow as compared to either agent alone (Fig. 5). These blood flow studies support the hypothesis that Flk-1-mediated signal transduction contributes to the resistance of tumor blood vessels to IR. The Flk-1-mediated survival phenotype has been shown to require the PI3 kinase/Akt pathway, which mediates Bcl-2 expression *(37,66)* and Bad phosphorylation. This signaling pathway thereby prevents the activation of intrinsic cell death mechanisms.

To determine whether Flk-1 antagonist enhances radiation-induced tumor volume regression, Gl261 glioma and LLC tumor models have been studied. Tumor bearing mice were treated with radiation using 3 Gy/d and three daily fractions/week for 2 wk. Mice received SU5416 0.75mg by intraperitoneal injection, administered 1 h prior to irradiation during fractions 1, 3, 4, and 6. Control mice received identical doses and schedule of either SU5416 alone or radiation alone. Tumors treated with radiation alone showed minimal growth delay. SU5416 alone achieved no growth delay in these tumors. However, the combination of SU5416 followed by radiation caused initial tumor regression and significant growth delay (Fig. 6). The schedule of administration of SU5416 was based upon the assumption that Flk-1 activity predetermines the tumor blood vessel survival phenotype.

8. ENDOTHELIAL REPAIR

A signal transduction pathway distinct from Akt regulates endothelial cell migration and motility *(67)*. VEGF prevents regression of capillary formation through the MAP kinase pathway but not the Akt signaling pathway *(67)*. A similar finding is that VEGF activates the protein kinase C-dependent Raf-MEK-MAPK kinase pathway resulting in DNA synthesis in endothelial cells *(68)*. This study also shows that Ras is not activated in this pathway. PKC-specific inhibitors reduce MEK phosphorylation and activation of MAP kinase. Unlike the Akt pathway, MEK signaling pathway is independent of PI3 kinase. This finding is supported by studies showing that MAP kinase P42/P44 phosphorylation occurs in VEGF stimulated endothelial cells.

CD34+ endothelial progenitor cells (EPCs) isolated from human peripheral blood differentiate into endothelial cells *(69,70)*. These progenitor cells develop foci of neovascularization in ischemic limbs at 4 wk after injection *(70)*. These circulating EPCs increase in sickle cell patients following ischemic episodes *(71)*. Signal transduction through VEGF participates in differentiation of pluripotent stem cells into endothelial cells *(72)*. Flk-1 receptors also participate in migration of these cells into ischemic tissue *(73)*. To determine the origin of these circulating EPCs, bone marrow stem cells containing the *Lac Z* reporter gene have been transplanted into tumor-bearing mice showing that EPCs from bone marrow origin are incorporated into tumor neovascularization *(69)*. VEGF increases the percentage of pluripotent hematopoietic stem cells staining positive for CD34 and Flk-1 *(74)*, including circulating stem cells.

Investigators hypothesize that the Flk-1-mediated signaling pathway also contributes to vascular repair following tumor irradiation. This hypothesis is supported by the findings that VEGF is induced by IR and that blocking antibodies to VEGF enhances tumor control in irradiated tumors *(9)*. As shown in Fig. 7, radiation-induced destruction of tumor vasculature resolves following irradiation. The study of vasculature by

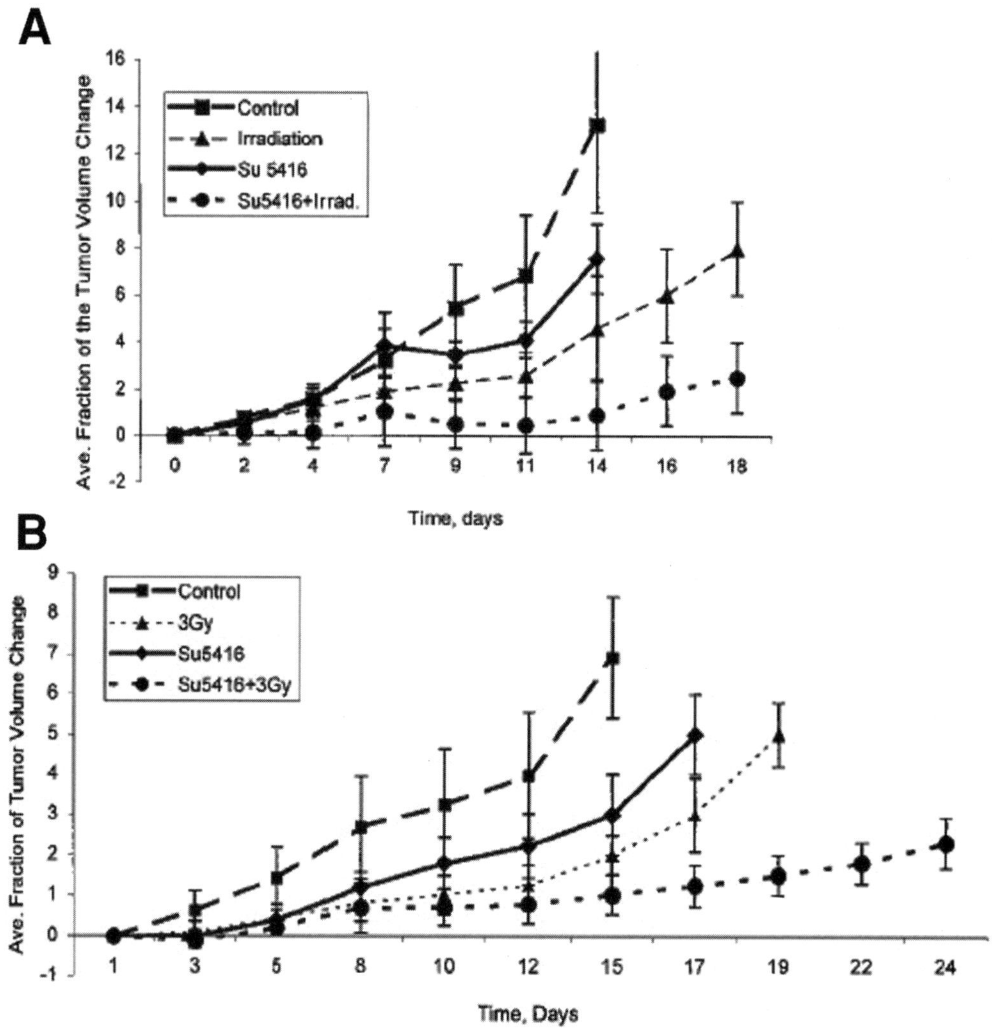

Fig. 6. GL261 tumor volume curves after treatment with SU5416 with or without radiation. GL261 cells were pelleted and implanted into the hind limb of C57BL6 mice. Tumors were grown to diameters ranging from 5–7 mm, at which time treatment was initiated (d 0). Tumor volumes were measured at the indicated time points for each of the treatment groups. Mice were sacrificed when tumor volume exceeded six times the original tumor volume. Control mice received no therapy. SU5416 was administered at 0.75 mg by ip injection given twice per week for a total of four treatments on d 0, 4, 7, and 11. Radiation was administered as 3-Gy fractions on eight occasions on days 0, 1, 2, and 3. **(A)** Shown are the mean and SE of six animals treated in each of the treatment groups. **(B)** A second group of 40 mice was studied, and 10 mice were stratified into the four treatment groups (control, radiation, SU5416 and radiation + SU5416). Shown are the mean and SE of 10 animals treated in each of the treatment groups.

both tumor windows shows both prevent regrowth of blood vessels into tumors. Doppler blood flow studies of GL261 glioblastoma tumors show blood flow increases on d 5 and 7 (Fig. 7). SU5416 eliminates this increase in tumor blood flow during radiotherapy of the GL261 models.

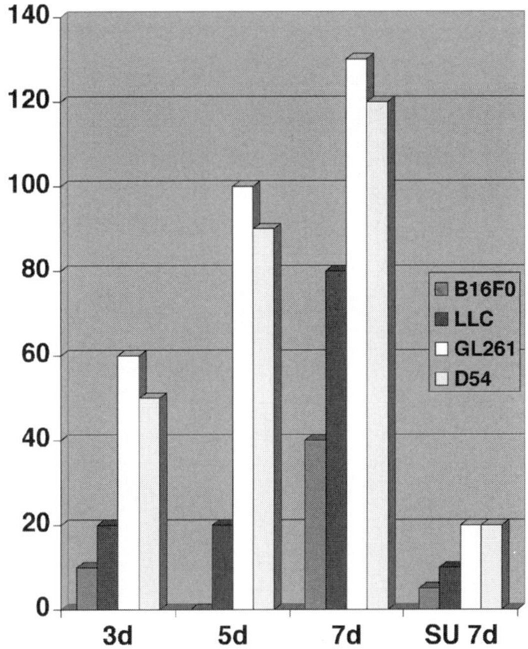

Fig. 7. Bar graph of blood flow vs time following irradiation. Radiation-induced destruction of tumor vasculature resolves following irradiation, except when SU5416 is administered concurrently.

9. GENE THERAPY APPROACH TO ANGIOLYTIC AND ANGIOSTATIC THERAPY IN CANCER

9.1. VEGF Antagonist Gene Therapy Enhances the Radiation Effect in Tumor Blood Vessels

The VEGF receptor, Flk-1, is a receptor tyrosine kinase that is specifically inhibited by the dominant negative expression of the mutant form of the receptor (soluble Flk-1) as previously described *(11)*. The soluble Flk-1 receptor is constructed by fusing the extracellular domain of murine flk-1 to the 6-histidine tag at the COOH terminus (ExFlk.6His). ExFlk.6His blocks activation of Flk-1 and forms heterodimers with endogenous cell surface Flk-1 in the presence of VEGF *(11)*. ExFlk.6His also inhibits VEGF-induced DNA synthesis and migration in HUVEC. To determine whether ExFlk.6His can inhibit angiogenesis in the dorsal tumor vascular window model, Ad.ExFlk.6His has been administered to mice by tail vein. Tumor blood vessels in GL261, B16F0, and LLC have been studied by use of the dorsal skin fold window model in C57BL6 mice. Tumors were implanted within the window and tumor blood vessels developed within 1 wk. Ad.ExFlk.6His was administered to the tumor bearing mice at 5×10^8 pfu. Vascular regression was visualized by use of the dorsal skin fold window model. Subtherapeutic doses of radiation (2 Gy) were given 16 h after a minimally therapeutic dosage of Ad.ExFlk.6His (2×10^8 pfu). The time course of vascular regression following treatment was studied. This showed that 2 Gy alone

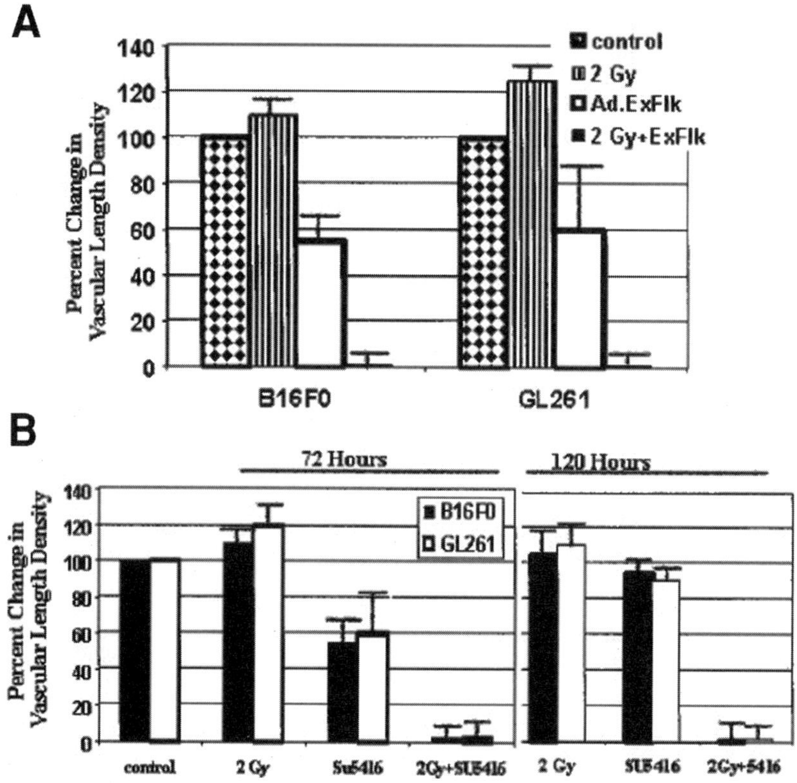

Fig. 8. (A) Soluble Flk-1 receptor enhances the response of tumor blood to radiation. GL261 and B16F0 tumors were implanted into the dorsal skin fold window following the development of tumor vasculature over the course of 1 wk; the adenovirus vector encoding the soluble Flk-1 (Ad. Ex Flk) was administered by tail vein injection. GL261 and B16F0 tumors implanted into vascular windows were treated with Ad. Ex Flk alone, radiation and control vector Ad. LacZ, or a combination Ad. Ex Flk, followed by radiation 24 h later. The vascular length density was summed and compared with the same blood vessels immediately before treatment. Changes in treated blood vessels were compared with the same blood vessels before treatment (100%). Shown are the mean and SE of changes in vascularity at 72 h after treatment. **(B)** Response of tumor blood vessels to Flk-1 antagonist SU5416 and irradiation. GL261 and B16F0 tumors were implanted into the dorsal skin fold window, and angiogenesis developed over the course of 1 wk. Blood vessels were photographed at the time of treatment (0 h) and then daily after treatment. Changes in the summed length of all blood vessels were determined and compared with that of the same blood vessels before treatment. Shown are the mean and SE of changes in tumor vascularity.

achieved no vascular regression (Fig. 8). Ad.ExFlk.6His alone at 2×10^8 pfu achieved minimal regression of tumor blood vessels, whereas the Ad.ExFlk.6His administered 16 h prior to irradiation resulted in regression of tumor blood vessels at a rate analogous to treatment with 6 Gy.

9.2. Radiation Combined with TNF Gene Therapy Induces Vascular Obliteration

Ionizing radiation induces von Willebrand factor expression *(75)*, and promotes platelet aggregation *(76)*. Radiation enhances platelet adhesion to the extracellular

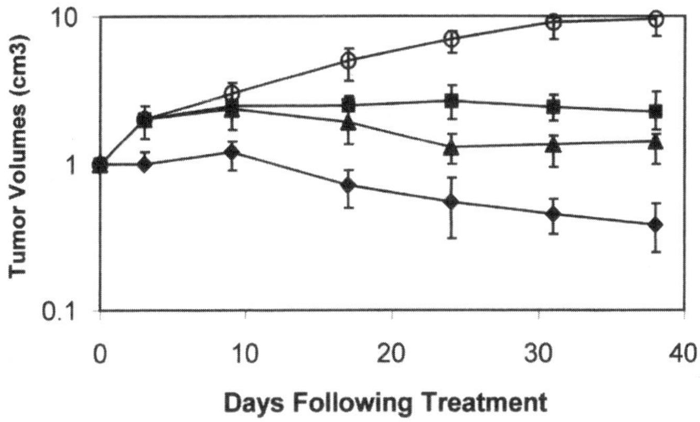

Fig. 9. Graph shows the logarithm of relative tumor volume as a function of days after treatment. Growth of tumors treated with adenovirus vector (dark square) or with radiation therapy (dark triangle) is diminished relative to that in the control group (light circle). Tumors receiving combined treatment (dark diamond) decreased in size over time. Error bars = SD.

matrix by an increase in the release of von Willebrand factor by endothelial cells *(77)*. Platelet aggregation can result in obliteration of tumor vasculature *(13)*. Radiation therapy alone, however, is often unsuccessful in treating tumors because of tumor cell resistance to radiation. Tumor necrosis factor (TNF) is a biological response modifier with antiangiogenic properties *(79)*. The combination of TNF and radiation therapy produces occlusion of tumor microvessels without significant damage to normal tissues *(80)*.

To study the effects of TNF gene therapy on tumor blood flow, mouse tumors have been treated with attenuated adenovirus containing TNF therapeutic gene (Ad.TNF). The control tumors continued to grow over time. Tumors treated with Ad.TNF alone plateaued 3 d following treatment. Tumors treated with radiation therapy alone decreased in size after 9 d. Tumors treated with both radiation therapy and TNF decreased in size below baseline after 9 d (Fig. 9) *(81)*. All tumors demonstrated neovascularity on power Doppler sonography. In all cases the majority of the color area was in the periphery of the tumor. The central portions of the tumor appeared relatively anechoic (Fig. 10). Color area of the total tumor decreased to 37% of control in mice treated with radiation therapy alone, 26% of control in mice treated with tumor necrosis factor alone, and 7.8% of control in those treated with both tumor necrosis factor and radiation. The combined treatment group showed a decrease to 25% of the average of the single-treatment groups. Because of the visible differences between the central and peripheral zones, similar analyses were performed on these areas. Similar trends were found in both the central and peripheral regions. In the peripheral region, color area decreased to 40% of control following radiation therapy, 28% of control following TNF, and 8% of control following combination therapy. The combined treatment group showed a decrease to 24% of the average of the single treatment groups. In the central region color area decreased to 26% of control following radiation therapy, 18% of control following TNF, and 7% of control following combination therapy. The combined treatment group showed a decrease to 32% of the average of the single treatment groups.

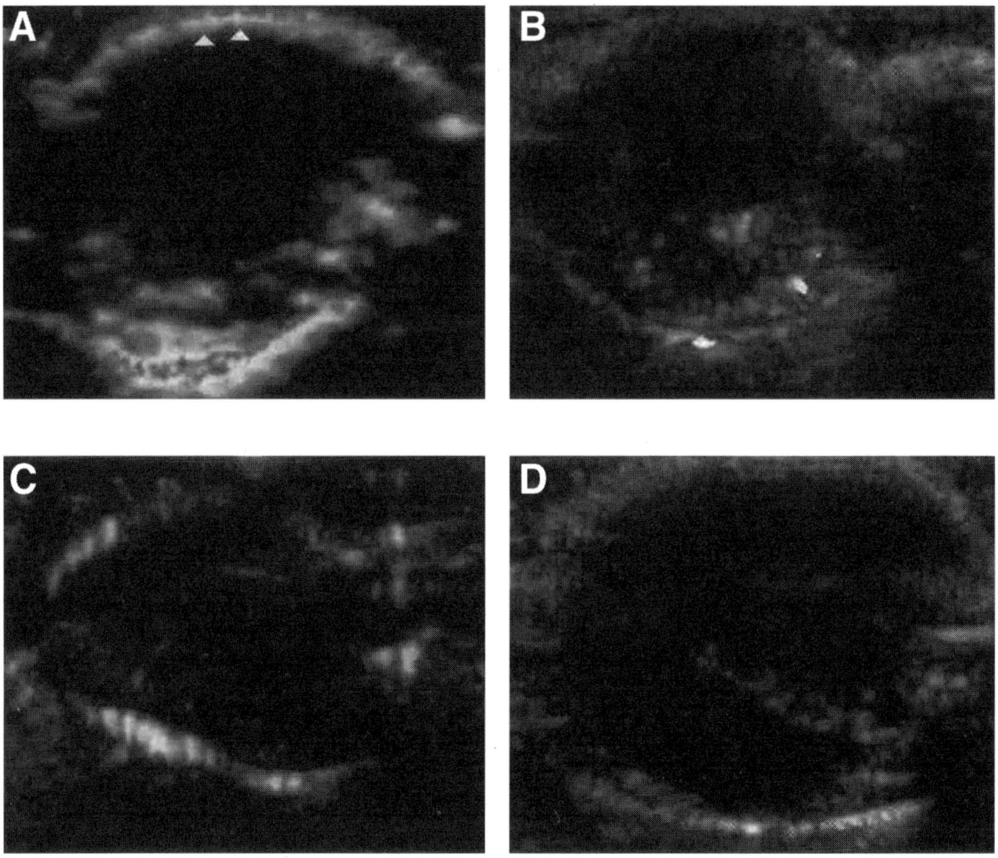

Fig. 10. Representative power Doppler US images from **(A)** tumors in the control group, **(B)** tumors treated with TNF, **(C)** tumors treated with radiation therapy, and **(D)** tumors receiving combined TNF and radiation therapy. Depicted blood vessels are greatest in the periphery of the tumors (arrowheads in A). Treatment with radiation alone or TNF alone results in a decrease in depicted blood vessels. Combined therapy results in a greater decrease in depicted blood vessels.

Ad.TNF gene therapy is presently in clinical trials in patients receiving radiotherapy. An open-label, phase I, dose-escalation study of tumor necrosis factor-alpha (TNFerade) gene transfer with radiation therapy for locally advanced, recurrent, or metastatic solid tumors is currently accruing patients and has several endpoints *(82)*, including toxicity and tolerable dose. Pharmacokinetics will be evaluated and biological correlates will determine the histologic response to therapy.

REFERENCES

1. Vaupel P, Kelleher DK, Hockel M. Oxygen status of malignant tumors: pathogenesis of hypoxia and significance for tumor therapy. *Semin Oncol* 2001; 28(2 Suppl 8):29–35.
2. Song C, Payne JT, Levitt SH. Vascularity and blood flow in x-irradiated Walker carcinoma 256 of rats. *Radiology* 1972; 104:693–697.
3. Song C, Sung JH, Clement JJ, et al. Vascular changes in neuroblastoma of mice following X-irradiation. *Cancer Res* 1974; 34:2344–2350.

4. Ting LL. Sarcoma blood perfusion change after x-irradiation. *Int J Radiat Oncol Biol Phys* 1991; 60:335–339.
5. Yamaura H, Yamada K, Matsuzawa T. Radiation effect on the proliferating capillaries in rat transparent chambers. *Int J Radiat Oncol Biol Phys* 1976; 30:179–187.
6. Kallman R,DeNardo GL, Stasch MJ. Blood flow in irradiated mouse sarcoma as determined by the clearance of xenon-133. *Cancer Res* 1972; 32:483–490.
7. Hilmas D, Gillette EL. Microvasculature of C3H/Bi mouse mammary tumors after x-irradiation. *Radiat Res* 1975; 61:128–143.
8. Johnson R. A thermodynamic method for investigation of radiation-induced changes in the microcirculation of human tumors. *Int J Radiat Oncol Biol Phys* 1976; 1:659–670.
9. Gorski DH, Beckett MA, Jaskowiak NT, et al. Blockade of the vascular endothelial growth factor stress response increases the antitumor effects of ionizing radiation. *Cancer Res* 1999; 59:3374–3378.
10. Fleischer AC. Sonographic depiction of tumor vascularity and flow. *J Ultrasound Med* 1999; 19:55–61.
11. Lin P, Sankar S, Shan S, et al. Inhibition of tumor growth by targeting tumor endothelium using a soluble vascular endothelial growth factor receptor. *Cell Growth Differ* 1998; 9(1):49–58.
12. Hallahan DE, Staba-Hogan MJ, Virudachalam S, et al. X-ray-induced P-selectin localization to the lumen of tumor blood vessels. *Cancer Res* 1998; 58(22):5216–5220.
13. Hallahan DE, Virudachalam S. Accumulation of P-selectin in the lumen of irradiated blood vessels. *Radiat Res* 1999; 152(1):6–13.
14. Lencioni R, Pinto F, Armillotta N, Bartolozzi C. Assessment of tumor vascularity in hepatocellular carcinoma: comparison of power Doppler US and color Doppler US. *Radiology* 1996; 201:353–358.
15. Choi B, Kim TK, Han JK, et al. Power versus conventional color Doppler sonography: comparison in the depiction of vasculature in liver tumors. *Radiology* 1996; 200:55–58.
16. Bartolozzi C, Lencioni R, Paolicchi A, et al. Differentiation of hepatocellular adenoma and focal nodular hyperplasia of the liver: comparison of power Doppler imaging and conventional color Doppler sonography. *Eur Radiol* 1997; 7:1410–1415.
17. Hosoki T, Mitomo M, Chor S, et al. Visualization of tumor vessels in hepatocellular carcinoma: power Doppler compared with color Doppler and angiography. *Acta Radiol* 1997; 38:422–427.
18. Leunig M, Yuan F, Menger MD, et al. Angiogenesis, microvascular architecture, microhemodynamics, and interstitial fluid pressure during early growth of human adenocarcinoma LS174T. *Cancer Res* 1992; 52:6553–6560.
19. Fuks Z. Intravenous bFGF protects the lung against radiation-induced apoptosis in vivo. *Cancer J* 1995; 1:62–72.
20. Valter MM, Hugel A, Huang HJ, et al. Expression of the Ets-1 transcription factor in human astrocytomas is associated with Fms-like tyrosine kinase-1 (Flt-1)/vascular endothelial growth factor receptor-1 synthesis and neoangiogenesis. *Cancer Res* 1999; 59(21):5608–5614.
21. Prewett M, Huber J, Li Y, et al. Antivascular endothelial growth factor receptor (fetal liver kinase 1) monoclonal antibody inhibits tumor angiogenesis and growth of several mouse and human tumors. *Cancer Res* 1999; 59(20):5209–5218.
22. Huang SM, Harari PM. Modulation of radiation response after epidermal growth factor receptor blockade in squamous cell carcinomas: inhibition of damage repair, cell cycle kinetics, and tumor angiogenesis. *Clin Cancer Res* 2000; 6:2166–2174.
23. Zhu Z, Lu D, Kotanides H, et al. Inhibition of vascular endothelial growth factor induced mitogenesis of human endothelial cells by a chimeric anti-kinase domain-containing receptor antibody. *Cancer Lett* 1999; 1(136):203.
24. Lee CG, Heijn M, di Tomaso E, et al. Anti-vascular endothelial growth factor treatment augments tumor radiation response under normoxic or hypoxic conditions. *Cancer Research* 2000; 60(19): 5565–5570.
25. Goldman C, Kendall RL, Cabrera G, et al. Paracrine expression of a native soluble vascular endothelial growth factor receptor inhibits tumor growth, metastasis, and mortality rate. *Proc Natl Acad Sci* 1998; 95:8795–8800.
26. Kendall RL, Thomas KA. Inhibition of vascular endothelial cell growth factor activity by an endogenously encoded soluble receptor. *Proc Natl Acad Sci* 1993; 90(22):10,705–10,709.
27. Seko Y, Takahashi N, Tobe K, et al. Vascular endothelilal growth factor (BEGF) activates Raf-1 mitogen-activated protein (MAP) kinases, and S6 kinase (p90rsk) in cultured rat cardiac myocytes. *J Cell Physiol* 1998; 3:239–246.

28. Kozin SV, Boucher Y, Hicklin DJ, et al. Vascular endothelial growth factor receptor-2-blocking antibody potentiates radiation-induced long-term control of human tumor xenografts. *Cancer Res* 2001; 61:39–44.
29. Gerber HP, McMurtrey A, Kowalski J, et al. Vascular endothelial growth factor regulates endothelial cell survival through the phosphatidylinositol 3-kinase/Akt signal transduction pathway: requirement for Flk-1/KDR activation. *J Biol Chem* 1998; 273(46):30,336–30,343.
30. Carmeliet P, Lampugnani MG, Moons L, et al. Targeted deficiency or cytosolic truncation of the VE-cadherin gene in mice impairs VEGF-mediated endothelial survival and angiogenesis. *Cell* 1999; 98(2):147–157.
31. Fugio Y, Walsh K. Akt mediates cytoprotection of endothelial cells by vascular endothelial growth factor in an anchorage-dependent manner. *J Biol Chem* 1999; 274(23):16,349–16,354.
32. Millauer B, Wizigmann-Voos S, Schnurch H, et al. High affinity VEGF binding and developmental expression suggest Flk-1 as a major regulator of vasculogenesis and angiogenesis. *Cell* 1993; 72(6):835–846.
33. Waltenberger J, Claesson-Welsh L, Siegbahn A, et al. Different signal transduction properties of KDR and Flt1, two receptors for vascular endothelial growth factor. *J Biol Chem* 1994; 269(43): 26,988–26,995.
34. Fong TL, Shawver LK, Sun L, et al. SU5416 is a potent and selective inhibitor of the VEGF receptor (Flk-1/KDR) that inhibits tyrosine kinase catalysis, tumor vascularization, and growth of multiple tumor types. *Cancer Res* 1999; 59:99–106.
35. Shaheen RM, Davis DW, Liu W, et al. Antiangiogenic therapy targeting the tyrosine kinase receptor for vascular endothelial growth factor receptor inhibits the growth of colon cancer liver metastasis and induces tumor and endothelial cell apoptosis. *Cancer Res* 1999; 59(21):5412–5416.
36. Vajkoczy P, Menger MD, Vollmar B, et al. Inhibition of tumor growth, angiogenesis, and microcirculation by the novel Flk-1 inhibitor SU5416 as assessed by intravital multi-fluorescence videomicroscopy. *Neoplasia* 1999; 1(1):31–41.
37. Nor JE, Christensen J, Mooney DJ, Polverini PJ. Vascular endothelial growth factor (VEGF)-mediated angiogenesis is associated with enhanced endothelial cell survival and induction of Bcl-2 expression. *Am J Pathol* 1999; 154(2): 375–384.
38. Tran J, Rak J, Sheehan C, et al. Marked induction of the IAP family antiapoptotic proteins surviving and XIAP by VEGF in vascular endothelial cells. *Biochem Biophys Res Commun* 1999; 264(3):781–788.
39. Zundel W, Giaccia A, et al. Inhibition of the anti-apoptotic PI(3)K/Akt/Bad pathway by stress. *Genes Dev* 1998; 12(13):1941–1946.
40. Gajewski TF, Thompson CB. Apoptosis meets signal transduction: elimination of a Bad influence. *Cell* 1996; 87(4):589–592.
41. Zha J, Harada H, Yang E, et al. Serine phosphorylation of death agonist Bad in response to survival factor results in binding to 14-3-3 not Bcl-X(L). *Cell* 1996; 87(4):619–628.
42. Yaffe MB, Rittenger K, Volinia S, et al. The structural basis for 14-3-3:phosphopeptide binding specificity. *Cell* 1997; 91(7):961–971.
43. Burgering BM, Burgering BM, Coffer PJ. Protein kinase B (c-Akt) in phosphatidylinositol-3-OH kinase signal transduction. *Nature* 1995; 376(6541):599–602.
44. Franke TF, Yang SI, Chan TO, et al. The protein kinase encoded by the Akt proto-oncogene is a target of the PDGF-activated phosphatidylinositol 3-kinase. *Cell* 1995; 81(5):727–736.
45. Kohn AD, Takeuchi F, Roth RA. Akt, a pleckstrin homology domain containing kinase, is activated primarily by phosphorylation. *J Biol Chem* 1996; 271(36):21,920–21,926.
46. Klippel A, Reinhard C, Kavanaugh WM, et al. Membrane localization of phosphatidylinositol 3-kinase is sufficient to activate multiple signal-transducing kinase pathways. *Mol Cell Biol* 1996; 16(8):4117–4127.
47. Takeuchi H, Kanematsu T, Misumi Y, et al. Distinct specificity in the binding of inositol phosphates by pleckstrin homology domains of pleckstrin, RAC-protein kinase, diacylglycerol kinase and a new 130 kDa protein. *Biochem Biophys Acta* 1997; 1359(3):275–285.
48. Didichenko SA, Tilton B, Hemmings BA, et al. Constitutive activation of protein kinase B and phosphorylation of p47phox by a membrane-targeted phosphoinositide 3-kinase. *Curr Biol* 1996; 6(10):1271–1278.
49. Harris AL. Anti-angiogenesis therapy and strategies for integrating it with adjuvant therapy. *Recent Results Cancer Res* 1998; 152:341–352.
50. Jones A, Harris AL. New developments in angiogenesis: a major mechanism for tumor growth and target for therapy. *Cancer J Sci Am* 1998; 4:209–271.

51. Boehm T, Folkman J, Browder T, et al. Antiangiogenic therapy of experimental cancer does not induce: Acquired drug resistance. *Nature (Lond)* 1997; 390:404–407.
52. Brooks PC Stromblad S, Klemke R, et al. Antiintegrin alpha v Beta 3 blocks human breast cancer growth and angiogenesis in human skin. *J Clin Investig* 1995; 96(4):1815–1822.
53. Kim KJ, Li B, Winer J, et al. Inhibition of vascular endothelial growth factor-induced angiogenesis suppresses tumour growth in vivo. *Nature (Lond)* 1993; 362:841–844.
54. Teicher BA, Sotmayor EA, Huang ZD, et al. Antiangiogenic agents potentiate cytotoxic cancer therapies against primary and metastatic disease. *Cancer Res* 1992; 52:6702–6704.
55. Teicher BA, Holden SA, Ara G, et al. Potentiation of cytotoxic cancer therapies by TNP-470 alone and with other anti-angiogenic agents. *Int J Cancer* 1994; 57:920–925.
56. Lund EL, Bastholm L, Kristjansen PE, et al. Therapeutic synergy of TNP-470 and ionizing radiation: effects on tumor growth, vessel morphology, and angiogenesis in human glioblastoma multiforme xenografts. *Clin Cancer Res* 2000; 6:971–978.
57. Landuyt W, Ahmed B, Nuyts S, et al. In vivo antitumor effect of vascular targeting combined with either ionizing radiation or anti-angiogenesis treatment. *Int J Radiat Oncol Biol Phys* 2001; 49(2):443–450.
58. O'Reilly M, Holmgren L, Shing Y, et al. Angiostatin: a novel angiogenesis inhibitor that mediates the suppression of metastases by a Lewis lung carcinoma. *Cell* 1994; 79:315–328.
59. O'Reilly M, Boehm T, Shing Y, et al. Endostatin: an endogenous inhibitor of angiogenesis and tumor growth. *Cell* 1997; 88:277–285.
60. Salloum R, Jaskowiak NT, Mauceri HJ, et al. NM-3, an isocoumarin, increases the antitumor effects of radiotherapy without toxicity. *Cancer Res* 2000; 60(24):6958–6963.
61. Hanna NN, Seetharam S, Mauceri HJ, et al. Antitumor interaction of short-course endostatin and ionizing radiation. *Cancer J* 2000; 6(5):287–293.
62. Folkman J. Seminars in medicine of the Beth Israel Hospital, Boston: Clinical applications of research on angiogenesis. *N Engl J Med* 1995; 333:1757–1763.
63. Mauceri HJ, Hanna NN, Beckett MA, et al. Combined effects of angiostatin and ionizing radiation in antitumor therapy. *Nature* 1998; 394:287–291.
64. Staba MJ, Mauceri HJ, Kufe DW, et al. Adenoviral TNF-α gene therapy and radiation damage tumor vasculature in a human malignant glioma xenografts. *Gene Ther* 1998; 5:293–300.
65. Advani S, Sibley GS, Song PY, et al. Enhancement of replication of genetically engineered Herpes Simplex Virus by ionizing radiation: a new paradigm for destruction of intractable tumors. *Gene Ther* 1998; 5:160–165.
66. Matsuzaki H, Tamatani M, Mitsuda N, et al. Activation of Akt kinase inhibits apoptosis and changes in Bcl-2 and Bax expression induced by nitric oxide in primary hippocampal neurons. *J Neurochem* 1999; 73(5):2037–2046.
67. Ilan N, Mahooti S, Madri JA. Distinct signal transduction pathways are utilized during the tube formation and survival phases of in vitro angiogenesis. *J Cell Sci* 1998; 111(Pt 24):3621–3631.
68. Takahashi T, Ueno H, Shibuya, M. VEGF activates protein kinase C-dependent, but Ras-independent Raf-MEK-MAP kinase pathway for DNA synthesis in primary endothelial cells. *Oncogene* 1999; 18(13):2221–2230.
69. Asahara T, Masuda H, Takahasi T, et al. Bone marrow origin of endothelial progenitor cells responsible for postnatal vasculogenesis in physiological and pathological neovascularization. *Circulation Res* 1999; 85:221–228.
70. Asahara T, Murohara T, Sullivan A. Isolation of putative progenitor endothelial cells for angiogenesis. *Science* 1997; 275:964–967.
71. Solovey A, Lin Y, Browne P, et al. Circulating activated endothelial cells in sickle cell anemia. *N Engl J Med* 1997; 337(22):1584–1590.
72. Kennedy M, Firpo M, Choi K, et al. A common precursor for primitive erythropoiesis and definitive haematopoiesis. *Nature* 1997; 386(6624):488–493.
73. Shalaby F, Rossant J, Yamaguchi TP, et al. Failure of blood-island formation and vasculogenesis in Flk-1-deficient mice. *Nature* 1995; 376(6535):62–66.
74. Ziegler-Heitbrock HW, Sternsdorf T, Liese J, et al. Pyrrolidine dithiocarbamate inhibits NF-kappa B mobilization and TNF production in human monocytes. *J Immunol* 1993; 151:6986–6993.
75. Jahroudi N, Ardekani AM, Greenberger JS, et al. Ionizing irradiation increases transcription of the von Willebrand factor gene in endothelial cells. *Blood* 1996; 88:3801–3814.
76. Hallahan DE, Chen AY, Teng M, et al. Drug-radiation interactions in tumor blood vessels. *Oncology (Huntingt)* 1999; 13(10 Suppl 5):71–77.

77. Verheij M, Dewit LG, Bloomgaard MN, et al. Ionizing radiation enhances platelet adhesion to the extracellular matrix of human endothelial cells by an increase in the release of von Willebrand factor. *Radiat Res* 1994; 137:202–207.
78. Old LD. Tumor necrosis factor. *Science* 1985; 230:630–636.
79. Mauceri HJ, Hanna NN, Wayne JD, et al. Tumor necrosis factor alpha (TNF-alpha) gene therapy targeted by ionizing radiation selectively damages tumor vasculature. *Cancer Res* 1996; 56:4311–4314.
80. Donnelly EF, Geng L, Wojcicki WE, et al. Quantified power Doppler US of tumor blood flow correlates with microscopic quantification of tumor blood vessels. *Radiology* 2001; 219:166–170.
81. Sharma A, Mani S, Hanna NN, et al. An open-label, phase 1, dose-escalation study of tumor necrosis factor-alpha gene transfer (TNFerade) with radiation therapy for locally advanced, recurrent, or metastatic solid tumors. *Hum Gene Ther* 2001; 12(9):1109–1131.

21 Cancer Drug Discovery and Development

Maximizing the Therapeutic Potential of Matrix Metalloproteinase Inhibitors for the Treatment of Cancer

Jeffrey S. Humphrey, MD, *Karen Price,* MS, *Elora Gupta,* PhD, *Andrew Baxter,* PhD, *John Bird,* PhD, *Daryl Sonnichsen,* PharmD, *and Joseph Naglich,* PhD

CONTENTS

1. INTRODUCTION

A significant amount of clinical research has been conducted with small molecules that inhibit matrix metalloproteinases (MMP), metal-containing enzymes that degrade the extracellular matrix and are implicated in tumor progression and angiogenesis *(1–3)*. The majority of matrix metalloproteinase inhibitors (MMPIs) are designed with a concept similar to protease inhibitors used in the treatment of acquired immunodeficiency syndrome. MMPIs are currently under development for the treatment of a variety of diseases most notably cancer *(3)*. Unlike conventional chemotherapy or radiation therapy, MMPIs are expected to slow tumor growth and prolong survival without causing detectable shrinkage of tumors. Because MMPIs are predicted to slow tumor growth but not shrink tumors, clinical development is not guided purely by objective tumor responses;

From: *Chemoradiation in Cancer Therapy*
Edited by: H. Choy © Humana Press Inc., Totowa, NJ

proving the therapeutic value of these molecules will therefore require randomized placebo-controlled trials with assessment of the impact of drug treatment compared to placebo. Proof that these compounds are effective cytostatic agents will require demonstrating a survival advantage when compared to a placebo in a randomized, controlled trial.

Additionally, MMPIs are not expected to replace currently used, proven-effective modalities of cancer treatment such as radiotherapy, hormonal/chemotherapy, or surgery. It is predicted that they will be clinically developed for use in combination with these agents. As expected, given nonoverlapping toxicities and differing mechanisms of action, MMPIs have been combined preclinically with radiation therapy *(4)*, cytotoxic *(5–9)*, resultant additive or supraadditive efficacy. With these data in mind, the ability to combine an MMPI with radiation therapy, chemotherapy, and hormonal therapy may become an important feature in the ultimate clinical success of these agents.

2. BACKGROUND

There is no "proof" currently that MMPIs as a class will prolong the survival of patients with cancer. Currently, three randomized trials of MMPIs have reported survival data: BAY 12-9566 vs gemcitabine in locally advanced or metastatic pancreatic cancer *(10)*, marimastat vs gemcitabine in locally advanced or metastatic pancreatic cancer *(11)*, and marimastat vs placebo in locally advanced or metastatic gastric cancer *(12)*.

The first trial, PA1 *(10)*, conducted by the National Cancer Institute of Canada, randomized 277 patients with previously untreated unresectable, recurrent or metastatic pancreatic cancer to BAY 12-9566 at 800 mg po bid or gemcitabine given at standard doses. The trial was closed prematurely after a planned interim analysis demonstrated a significant difference in overall survival. The 1-yr overall survival for patients randomized to BAY 12-9566 was 10% compared to a 1-yr overall survival of 25% for patients randomized to standard-dose gemcitabine ($p = 0.0001$). While BAY 12-9566 was clearly inferior to gemcitabine, it is important to interpret this survival result in the context of previous trials of gemcitabine in metastatic pancreatic cancer. The pivotal trial of gemcitabine randomized 126 patients with locally advanced or metastatic pancreatic cancer to 5-fluorouracil (5-FU) or gemcitabine. The 1-yr overall survival for patients randomized to 5-FU was 2% compared to a 1-yr overall survival of 18% for patients randomized to standard-dose gemcitabine ($p = 0.0009$). Thus, a 10% 1-yr survival rate for patients randomized to BAY 12-9566 may compare favorably to the 2% historical one-year survival rate for 5-FU.

In the second randomized trial of an MMPI (British Biotech Study 128) *(11)*, 414 patients with pancreatic cancer were randomized to one of four arms: marimastat 5 mg po bid, marimastat 10 mg po bid, marimastat 25 mg po bid, or standard dose gemcitabine. Patients randomized to a high dose (25 mg bid) of marimastat had a 20% 1-yr overall survival. The 1-yr overall survival of patients randomized to *high-dose* marimastat was numerically equivalent to the 20% 1-yr overall survival of patients randomized to standard-dose gemcitabine. The comparable survival of high-dose marimastat to gemcitabine in this trial stands in contrast to historical trials demonstrating inferior survival of patients randomized to 5-FU or to BAY 12-9566 compared to gemcitabine. Additionally, patients randomized to the *high dose* of marimastat had statistically superior overall survival compared to patients randomized to lower doses (10 mg or 5 mg bid), suggesting a dose-response effect of marimastat on overall survival. The principal toxic effect of marimastat was a dose-related, dose-limiting inflammatory polyarthritis resulting in interruption and discontinuation of marimastat dosing. The occurrence of this musculoskeletal toxic effect has been reported to be related to dose, substantially limiting administration of marimastat doses more than 10 mg twice a day *(13)*. These data suggest that marimastat has antitumor activity, but that activity is limited by limitations to dosing. Thus, dose-limiting arthritis and arthralgia reported for marimastat essentially limits efficacy for this agent.

In the third randomized trial of an MMPI (British Biotech Study 145) *(12)*, patients with locally advanced or metastatic gastric cancer were randomized in a double-blind fashion to a low dose (10 mg bid) of marimastat or matching placebo. Marimastat 10 mg po bid, which had inferior survival compared to the higher dose of marimastat, was presumably selected as the active control arm for this trial based on its superior tolerability compared to high-dose marimastat. Patients randomized to marimastat had a trend to better overall survival (167 d vs 135 d; $p = 0.07$) at the protocol stipulated endpoint of the study, and this statistical trend strengthened with an additional 6 mo of follow up ($p = 0.048$). Nevertheless, patients randomized to marimastat 10 mg po bid had statistically superior progression-free survival compared to patients randomized to placebo ($p = 0.027$). Marimastat 25 mg po bid, which was the most efficacious dose in British Biotech Study 128, was not tested in Study 145.

The available survival data, taken together, suggest that broad spectrum MMP inhibition can prolong progression-free and overall survival of patients with advanced solid malignancies, but that this beneficial effect is limited by constraints on optimal dosing due to adverse events. These clinical findings are consistent with preclinical data, which suggest that the optimal use of these agents requires administration in a dose and schedule sufficient to maintain plasma concentrations continuously above a certain minimum effective concentration. Thus, dose-limiting arthritis and arthralgia reported for marimastat limit efficacy for this agent. To be successful, future generations of MMPIs must minimize or eliminate these dose-limiting toxicities and maximize dose.

2.1. Maximizing the Potential of MMPI Therapy: Broad Spectrum Inhibitors That Minimize Toxicity and Maximize Dose

Matrix metalloproteinases are members of a large family of metalloproteases (Table 1) that require an essential zinc atom for activity. Other family members include the adamlysins (ADAMS), membrane secretases (sheddases), and others such as angiotensin converting enzyme (ACE). ACE inhibitors, such as captopril, are important examples of rationally designed small-molecule inhibitors that provide therapeutic benefit to patients. Captopril contains a sulfhydryl moiety as the zinc-binding group (ZBG), and it was originally shown to demonstrate oral activity in models of hypertension. In addition, captopril prolonged overall survival among patients with hypertension in randomized, controlled trials. To some extent, this example provides a precedent for successful development of MMPIs for patients with cancer, which, likewise, will require randomized trials demonstrating the ability of these agents to prolong overall survival.

Prolongation of survival by MMPIs is likely to be dependent upon a broad-spectrum inhibition of MMPs, similar to marimastat, given daily in high doses without interruption. A syndrome of dose-limiting arthritis has been reported for marimastat, prinomastat, and other hydroxamic acid-based MMPIs. This syndrome is primarily an inflammatory

Table 1
Matrix Metalloproteinase Family of Enzymes

MMPs:	Mammalian MPs:	Sheddases:
Collagenase 1 (MMP1)	ACE	*Adamalysin Related MPs:*
Collagenase 2 (MMP8)	ANP	TNFα Convertase
Collagenase 3 (MMP13)	Lysine Carboxypeptidase	ADAM-10 (MADM)
Matrilysin (MMP7)	Carboxypeptidase A	ADAM-15 (Metargidin)
Stromelysin 1 (MMP3)	Carboxypeptidase B	ADAM Family
Stromelysin 2 (MMP10)	Carboxypeptidase H	*Membrane Secretases:*
Stromelysin 3 (MMP11)	Endothelin Convertase	TNF R11 Sheddase
Gelatinase A (MMP2)	MP100 (α secretase?)	L-Selectin Sheddase
Gelatinase B (MMP9)		IL-1β RII Sheddase
Metalloelastase (MMP12)		APP α-Secretase
Aggrecanase		CD_{30} Sheddase
Membrane Type MMPs (MMP-MT1,MT2,MT3,MT4)		FasL Sheddase
MMP19		

Table 2
Comparison of Sheddase Activity

IC_{50} Values, μM (micromolar)

Compound	TNFα Release*	TNFα-RII Shedding	L-Selectin Shedding	IL1-RII Shedding	IL-6R Shedding
BMS-275291	*>100*	*>100*	*>100*	*>100*	*>100*
Marimastat	4	6	1	3.4	3.6
Prinomastat	1.6	14	0.8	1.8	12
CGS-27023B	8	7	11	5	6.5
BAY 12-9566	IA				

Comparison of sheddase selectivity profiles for BMS-275291 and earlier generation inhibitors as determined by cell based assays. Unlike marimastat, BMS-275291 spares the sheddases, a finding hypothesized to explain the lack of dose-limiting arthritis for this compound.

arthritis involving the shoulders and arms. The incidence and onset are related to the dose of MMPI being administered, with a higher incidence and severity of arthritis associated with higher doses. Two hypotheses are proposed to explain this toxicity. The first hypothesis is that toxicity is a result of inhibiting MMP-1 activities. This has yet to be proven conclusively, but recent clinical data suggest that the dose-limiting arthritis may be a side-effect unrelated to inhibition of MMP-1 activities (see below). The other proposed hypothesis is that the dose-limiting toxicity is a result of inhibiting the activities of closely related metalloproteases loosely referred to as "sheddases." These metalloproteases typically regulate the shedding of cytokines and cytokine receptors involved in mediating inflammatory processes. An example is tumor necrosis factor-α (TNF-α) converting enzyme (TACE), which regulates the shedding of TNF-α from the cell surface. Agents such as Enbrel selectively target TNF-α (a key mediator of inflammatory arthritis) and have demonstrated dramatic therapeutic success in the treatment of refractory rheumatoid arthritis in humans. Several hydroxamate-based MMPIs in clinical development (such as marimastat and prinomastat) are known to inhibit TACE and other sheddases (Table 1) as well as inhibit shedding of TNF-α from the cell surface at clinically relevant concentrations (Table 2). Consequently, a way of optimizing MMPI activities in humans is to rationally design a compound that effectively inhibits many MMP activities and is less active toward those of other metalloproteases such as the sheddases.

3. MAXIMIZING THE POTENTIAL OF MMPI THERAPY

The subset analyses of randomized controlled trial data for marimastat is consistent with a dose-response effect of MMP inhibition on survival, with higher doses of marimastat resulting in a greater effect on survival. However, in humans, the highest dose of marimastat tested in randomized controlled trials (25 mg bid) resulted in CTC grade 3 or 4 musculoskeletal toxicity in 12% of patients. Lower doses (e.g., 10 mg bid) were tolerated with less musculoskeletal toxicity but appeared less efficacious. These data suggest that broad-spectrum MMP inhibitors can prolong overall survival of patients with advanced solid malignancies and that the magnitude of therapeutic benefit is dependent upon dose in the absence of dose-limiting arthritis. Thus to maximize the potential of this class of anticancer agents, the next generation of MMPIs must minimize toxicity and maximize dose.

BMS-275291 is the first compound in clinical development from this new generation of MMPIs. BMS-275291 is a sulfhydryl-based broad-spectrum MMP inhibitor that is rationally designed to be less active toward the sheddases. Its chemical structure is shown in Fig. 1.

BMS-275291 contains a novel mercaptoamide ZBG (Fig. 1, dashed box) in marked distinction to the hydroxamic acid ZBG of other MMPIs such as marimastat and prinomastat. Hydroxamic-acid-based compounds are associated with potent zinc binding potential and poor oral activity. In contrast, in other types of inhibitors (such as inhibition of ACE) the zinc-binding function of the mercaptoamide group is known to be potent and associated with good oral activity (e.g., captopril). The portion of BMS-275291 depicted in the solid line box (Fig. 1) represents the peptidomimetic portion of the molecule that resembles natural polypeptide substrates of MMPs such as collagen. This region of BMS-275291 contains three peptide bonds and the amino acids leucine and *tert*-leucine and it is very similar in chemical structure to that of the broad spectrum MMPI, marimastat (Fig. 1). The similarity of these molecules undoubtedly contributes to their remarkably similar MMP selectivity profile. Both are potent nanomolar inhibitors of a broad spectrum of MMPs, and their activities for some MMPs are comparable to more selective, hydroximate-based MMPIs such as prinomastat and CGS-27023B. In vitro, BMS-275291 inhibits MMP-1 (IC_{50}-26 n*M*), MMP-2 (41 n*M*) and MMP-9 (25 n*M*), as well as MMP-3 (157 n*M*), MMP-7 (23 n*M*), MMP-8 (10 n*M*), MMP-13 (4 n*M*), and MMP-14 (40 n*M*). As can be seen, BMS-275291 has a very similar relative MMP selectivity profile as marimastat but it is less potent. Thus, BMS-275291 inhibits a broad

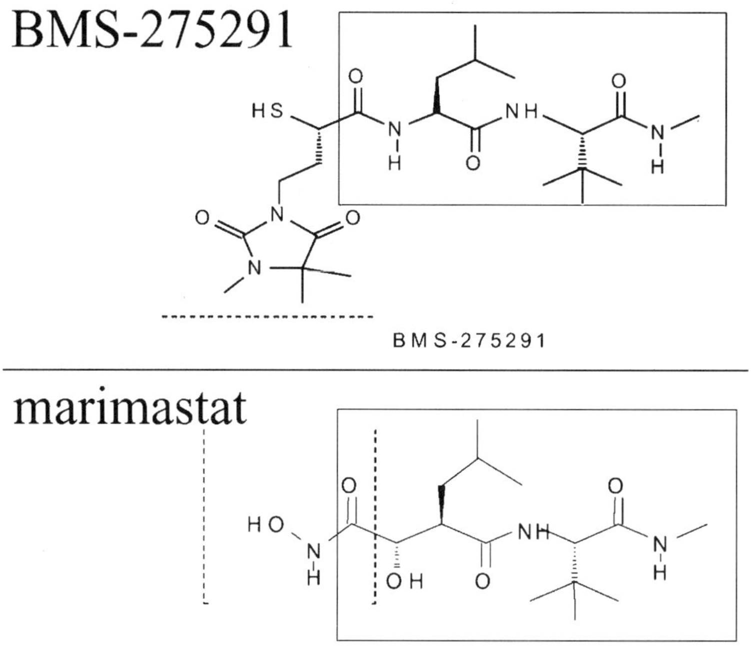

Fig. 1. Comparison of MMP Structures. Comparison of the chemical structures of BMS-275291 and marimastat. Solid-line box indicates peptidomimetic portion, dashed-line box indicates zinc-binding group.

spectrum of MMPs that include collagenases, stromelysins, gelatinases, matrilysin, and membrane-bound MMPs. In clinical trials, high doses of BMS-275291 taken after long durations has not caused dose-limiting arthritis in man. These data suggest that MMP-1 inhibition is not causative of the inflammatory arthritis and arthralgia associated with hydroxamate-based, sheddase-inhibiting MMPIs, in contradiction to prior hypotheses. As will be discussed further below, the lower potency of BMS-275291 compared to marimastat is compensated for by the 60–120-fold higher doses that can be chronically administered.

The MMP selectivity profile of BMS-275291 is similar to that of the other MMPIs in clinical development. What sets it apart from these is its activities toward the sheddases. Table 3 lists the IC_{50} micromolar values determined in a set of in vitro experiments designed to directly measure and compare the ability of BMS-275291, marimastat, prinomastat, or CGS-27023B to inhibit sheddase-mediated events that include the release of TNF-α, TNF-α receptor II, L-selectin, IL1-receptor II, or IL-6 receptor from the cell surface. As can be seen from the table, BMS-275291 did not inhibit the release of these molecules at concentrations exceeding 100 μ*M*. In contrast, marimastat, prinomastat and CGS 27023B inhibited these events at concentrations achievable in man. Consistent with the sheddase-sparing design, BMS-275291 given for a prolonged duration daily did not result in inflammatory arthritis or tendonitis in marmosets. This is in contrast to marimastat, which caused dose-dependent inflammation of tendons and joint ligaments when given for prolonged durations to marmosets *(14)*. Thus as designed, BMS-275291 inhibits many MMP activities and spares those of the sheddases.

Table 3
MMP Selectivity Profile

IC$_{50}$ Values, n*M* (nanomolar)[a]

Compound	MMP1	MMP8	MMP13	MMP7	MMP3	MMP2	MMP9	MMP14
BMS-275291	*26*	*10*	*4*	*23*	*157*	*41*	*25*	*40*
Marimastat	3	4	2	7	36	9	7	14
Prinomastat	17	7	0.2	60	30	2	4	8
CGS-27023B	24	2	25	250	18	17	7	25
BAY 12-9566	>5000	51	1470		134	11	301	

Comparison of MMP selectivity profiles for BMS-275291 and earlier generation inhibitors as determined by in vitro enzymatic assays. BMS-275291 is a broad spectrum MMP inhibitor similar to marimastat.

4. PHARMACOLOGY OF BMS-275291

Several MMPIs are known to inhibit tumor progression and angiogenesis in a variety of in vivo models *(1–3)*. BMS-275291 has been tested in a murine angiogenesis model -that measures endothelial cell migration into a subcutaneously implanted Matrigel plug. In this model, once daily oral BMS-275291 treatments (10–90 mg/kg) for 7 d resulted in a dose-dependent inhibition of endothelial cell migration or angiogenesis (Fig. 2). BMS-275291 has also been evaluated in a murine experimental lung metastases model where B16BL6 cells are implanted intravenously and subsequently form tumor foci in lung tissues. In this model, BMS-275291 oral treatment (30–90 mg/kg) inhibited the size and number of lung metastases formed compared to controls (Figs. 2 and 3). Together these in vivo data support the notion that BMS-275291 has the potential to inhibit those MMP activities critically involved in angiogenesis and tumor progression.

In rat embryo-fetal toxicology studies, doses of BMS-275291 were identified, which caused no clinical or histopathologic toxicity to the pregnant female adult rat and the fetus. Higher doses caused no clinical or histopathologic toxicity in the adult female, but resulted in toxicity to the fetus. Histopathologic examination of the femurs of the fetal rat demonstrated expansion of the epiphysial growth plate, impaired trabecular bone formation, and impaired blood vessel invasion of the chondrocyte zone (Figs. 4 and 5) *(15)*. These histopathologic findings are nearly identical to those reported for homozygous germline MMP-9 deletion in mice. These findings further validate the concept important to selection of the optimal doses for clinical development: Doses of BMS-275291 which are nontoxic to the fully formed adult animal may nonetheless inhibit MMP-dependent processes, such as osteogenesis and angiogenesis, as demonstrated by these data. In addition, inhibition of wound angiogenesis was demonstrated in patients in the phase I study of BMS-275291 at well-tolerated doses with relatively little toxicity. Thus, the dose selected for further clinical development should be based upon an estimation of the optimal biologic dose, and not the maximum tolerated dose as is often chosen for cytotoxic chemotherapeutic agents.

Epiphysial growth plate expansion is not only the pharmacologic phenotype of BMS-275291 activity, but has also been reported as the sole phenotype of mice treated with

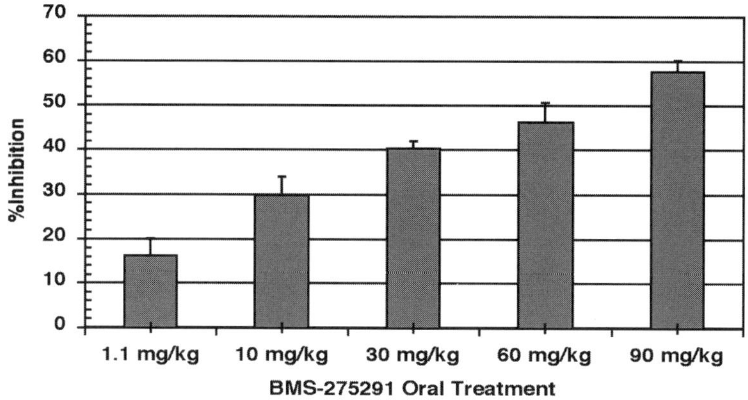

Fig. 2. Matrigel plug assay results. Matrigel™ was implanted subcutaneously into athymic mice on d 0 (8–10 mice per group). Daily BMS-275291 oral treatments began on d 0 and continued to d 6. Matrigel plugs were harvested on d 7 and processed for histochemical analyses. Results are expressed as % Inhibition ±SE (% Relative to Untreated Control).

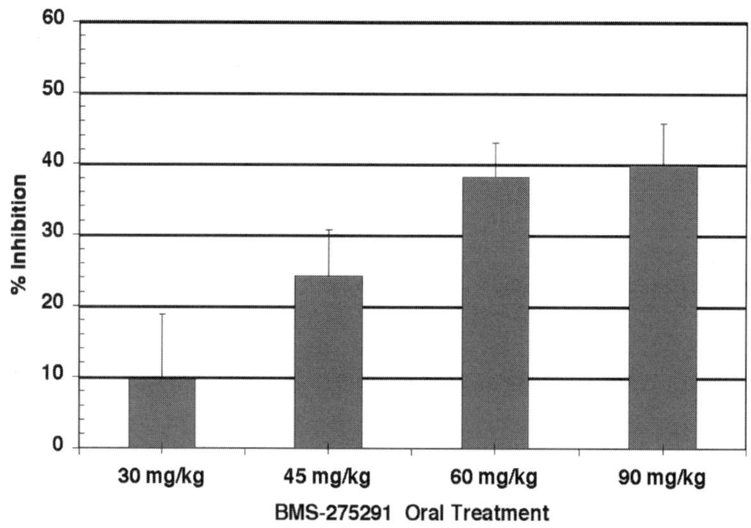

Fig. 3. B16BL6 metastases inhibition. Mice received B16BL6 melanoma cells intravenously at time 0 (8–10 mice per group). BMS-275291 or vehicle (water) were administered orally at –2 h, +2 h, +24 h, +48 h and +72 h relative to time of cell implantation (time 0). Mice were sacrificed 10 d after tumor cell implantation and the number of B16BL6 metastases counted. Results are expressed as % Inhibition ±SE (% Relative to Control).

murine anti-VEGF antibodies *(16,17)* and as the phenotype of mice treated with a small molecule inhibitor of VEGF receptor tyrosine kinase activity *(18)*. The identical phenotype seen for MMP inhibition by BMS-275291, homozygous MMP-9 gene deletion, anti-VEGF antibodies and VEGF receptor TK inhibitors may be explained in part by recent experiments demonstrating an important role for MMP-9 in VEGF signaling.

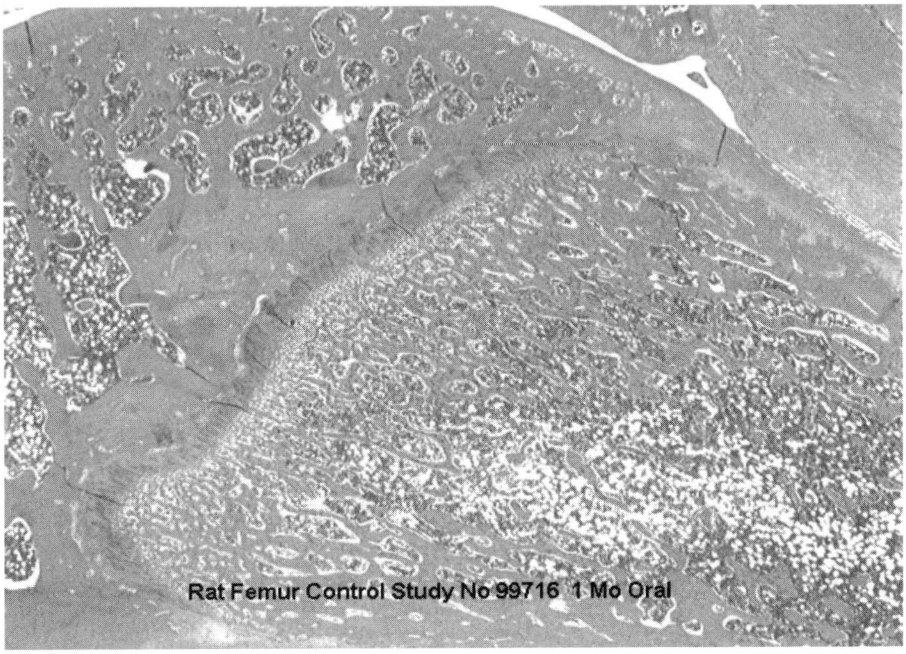

Fig. 4. Rat epiphysial growth place (control). Normal femur control for comparison.

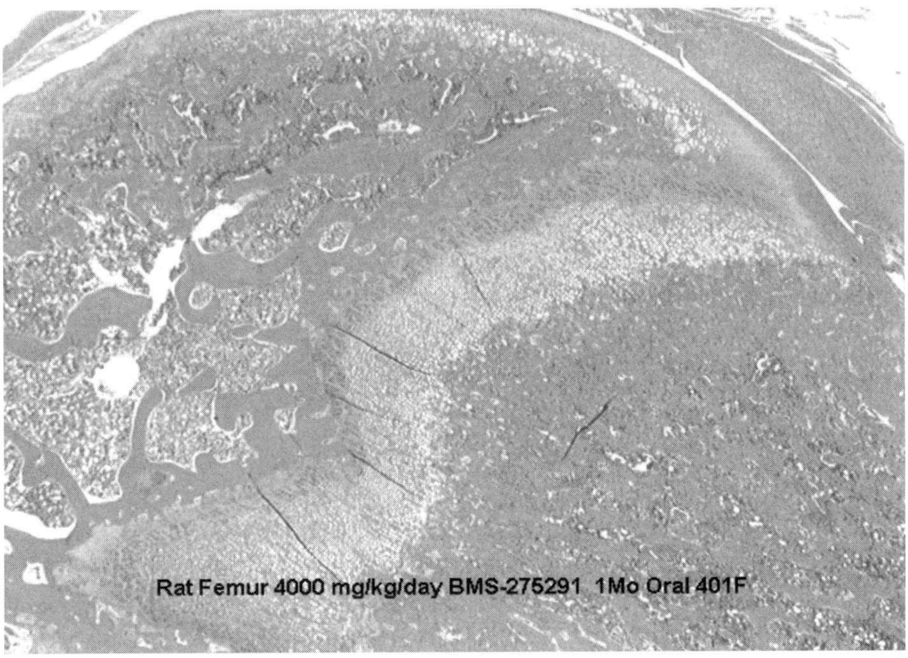

Fig. 5. Rat epiphysial growth rate (on-treatment). BMS-275291 treatment of young rats: induction of epiphysial growth plate expansion and suppressed blood vessel invasion in the femur of a rat given oral BMS-275291, 4000 mg/kg/d for 1 mo. This pharmacologic phenotype resembles reported phenotypes for mice with homozygous MMP-9 deletion as well as mice treated with inhibitors of VEGF signaling.

5. CLINICAL EXPERIENCE WITH BMS-275291

Preclinical toxicology data justified initial development of BMS-275291 in healthy subjects. Therefore, two trials of BMS-275291 were conducted in 65 healthy male subjects. In the first trial, subjects received single doses of orally administered BMS-275291 ranging from 25 mg up to 1200 mg as a single dose. These doses were well tolerated. Therefore, in a second trial, subjects received doses escalating from 300 to 1200 mg daily for 14 d *(19)*. Treatment was safe and very well tolerated across all dose levels. No dose-limiting adverse events were identified.

Note that the *starting* dose of BMS-275291 in these dose-escalation trials, 25 mg per day, already exceeded the phase III dose of marimastat, 10 mg twice per day and the phase III dose of prinomastat at 5 or 10 mg bid. The highest dose studied, 1200 mg daily, far exceeds the phase III doses of marimastat and prinomastat.

Based on pharmacokinetic data from these studies in healthy male subjects, a phase I trial was conducted in cancer patients with an initial dose level of 600 mg per day *(20)*. This daily dose was expected to result in plasma concentrations of parent BMS-275291 that would continuously exceed the IC_{50} determined in vitro for MMP-2 and MMP-9 by several-fold. Ultimately, 44 patients were enrolled to doses of 600, 900, 1200, 1800, and 2400 mg per day. The mean trough concentrations of parent BMS-275291 at the dose of 1200 mg/d were 8- and 13-fold greater than the IC_{50} values for MMP-2 and MMP-9 and exceeded the IC_{90} value for MMP-9. In comparison, trough concentrations of both prinomastat and marimastat would be about fivefold greater than the K_i/IC_{50} values for the relevant MMPs at the respective phase II/III doses. Consistent with data from marmoset toxicology studies and, as expected, given the sheddase-sparing design, prolonged daily oral administration of BMS-275291 was not associated with dose-limiting arthritis, arthralgia, or myalgia in this study, despite treatment durations exceeding 1 yr. Therefore, unlike marimastat or prinomastat at their phase III doses, no patient required interruption of daily therapy for arthritis, arthralgia or myalgia. At the highest dose tested, 2400 mg per day, there were no dose-limiting toxicities, thus maximum tolerated dose for BMS-275291 exceeds 2400 mg per day. Notably, this dose (2400 mg/d) exceeds by more than 100-fold the phase III doses of marimastat and prinomastat (10 mg twice per day), and was tolerated by all patients, with no patient experiencing dose-limiting toxicity or daily drug administration for any cause. In contrast, marimastat and prinomastat administration at phase III doses results in grade 3/4 musculoskeletal toxicity in patients, requiring dose reduction, dose interruption, or discontinuation of drug altogether.

Because angiogeneses induced by wounds and by tumors have mechanistic similarities, a wound angiogenesis assay was developed where a 4 mm punch biopsy was made in a patient's forearm *(21–23)*. Angiogenesis was observed directly in the normal skin at the periphery of the wound via video microscopy at 80× magnification at six timepoints over the 14 d following biopsy. Biopsies were performed both during pretreatment and while receiving treatment with BMS-275291, with each patient serving as his or her own control. For the first 13 patients assayed, the mean time for the appearance of early capillary loops within the skin surrounding the punch biopsy was delayed from a mean time of 5.1 ± 0.7 d pretreatment to 8.6 ± 1.0 d on treatment ($p = 0.02$). These data suggest that BMS-275291 inhibits wound angiogenesis in man and are consistent with the preclinical antiangiogenic activity of this compound. Randomized controlled trials are underway to assess the relevance of this biologic activity (delay in wound angiogenesis) to ultimate clinical benefit (prolongation of survival).

6. DEVELOPMENT ISSUES

Unlike cytotoxic chemotherapeutic agents, BMS-275291, as a single agent, is not expected to result in measurable shrinkage of established tumors. Development of cytostatic/antiangiogenic agents will require conduct of randomized controlled trials with relapse-free survival, progression-free survival, and overall survival as endpoints to attain clinical proof of principle. Based on considerations of preclinical data, nonoverlapping toxicity with conventional chemotherapeutics and radiation therapy, and a different mechanism of action from conventional chemotherapeutics and radiation therapy, the optimal development will involve administration of BMS-275291 in combination with radiation therapy and/or chemotherapy for patients with unresectable cancer or microscopic residual disease. Preclinical data and data from subset analyses of completed trials with early generation MMPIs suggest that clinical development plans should also focus on adjuvant treatment of patients with resected cancer.

7. SUMMARY

Oncology, as a field, is now faced with numerous, rationally designed agents that target biologic pathways felt to be relevant to tumor biology. As an inhibitor of MMFS, BMS-275291 was expected to inhibit angiogenesis and osteogenesis, as well as tumor progression and metastasis, in preclinical studies. BMS-275291 does, in fact, meet these expectations. Consistent with the sheddase-sparing design, phase I trials demonstrated that BMS-275291 could be administered to patients with cancer, without dose-limiting arthritis. BMS-275291 administration was associated with a delay in wound angiogenesis in man. A phase II clinical trial of this agent in nonsmall-cell lung cancer (NSCLC) is ongoing.

REFERENCES

1. Chambers AF, Matrisian LM. Changing views of the role of matrix metalloproteinases in metastasis. *J Natl Cancer Inst* 1997; 89:1260–1270.
2. Nelson AR, Fingleton B, Rothenberg ML, Matrisian LM. Matrix metalloproteinases: biologic activity and clinical implications. *J Clin Oncol* 2000; 18:1135–1149.
3. McCawley LJ, Matrisian LM. Matrix metalloproteinases: multifunctional contributors to tumor progression. *Molec Med Today* 2000; 6:149–156.
4. Shi Z, Raithatha S, Spencer D, Rewcastle, B, Brasher P, Morris D, et al. Enhanced effectiveness of a novel MMP inhibitor, prinomastat (AG3340) with radiotherapy (RT) in a glioma model. *Proc Am Assoc Cancer Res* 2000; 41:326 (2071a).
5. Herbst RS, Takeuchi H, Teicher BA. Paclitaxel/carboplatin administration along with antiangiogenic therapy in non-small-cell lung and breast carcinoma models. *Cancer Chem Pharm* 1998, 41: 497–504.
6. Anderson IC, Shipp MA, Docherty A, Teicher BA. Combination therapy including a gelatinase inhibitor and cytotoxic agent reduces local invasion and metastasis of murine lewis lung carcinoma. *Cancer Res* 1996; 56:715–718.
7. Shalinsky DR, Brekken J, Zou H, Bloom LA, McDermott CD, Zook S, et al. Marked antiangiogenic and antitumor efficacy of AG3340 in chemoresistant human non-small cell lung cancer tumors: single agent and combination chemotherapy studies. *Clin Cancer Res* 1999; 5:1905–1917.
8. Teicher BA. A systems approach to cancer therapy. *Cancer Metastasis Rev* 1996; 15:247–272.
9. Kakeji Y, Teicher BA. Preclinical studies of the combination of angiogenic inhibitors with cytotoxic agents. *Invest New Drugs* 1997; 15:39–48.

10. Moore MJ, Hamm P, Eisenberg P, Dagenais M, Hagan K, Fields A, et al. A comparison between gemcitabine (GEM) and the matrix metalloproteinase (MMP) inhibitor BAY 12-9566 (9566) in patients (pts) with advanced pancreatic cancer. *Proc Am Soc Clin Oncol* 2000; 19:240a (abstract).
11. Rosemurgy A, Buckels J, Charnley R. A randomized study comparing marimastat to gemcitabine as first line therapy in patients with non-resectable pancreatic cancer. *Proc Am Assoc Cancer Res* 1999; 18:261a (abstract).
12. Fielding J, Scholefield J, Stuart R, Hawkins R, McCulloch P, Maughan T, et al. A randomized double-blind placebo-controlled study of marimastat in patients with inoperable gastric adenocarcinoma. *Proc Am Soc Clin Oncol* 2000; 19:240a (abstract).
13. Ray JM, Stetler-Stevenson WG. Gelatinase A activity directly modulates melanoma call adhesion and spreading. *EMBO J* 1995; 14:908–917.
14. Wojtowicz PS, Torri J, Johnson M, Steen V, Marshall J, Ness E, et al. Phase I trial of Marimastat, a novel matrix metalloproteinase inhibitor, administered orally to patients with advanced lung cancer. *J Clin Oncol* 1998; 16:2150–2156.
15. Vu TH, Shipley JM, Bergers G, Berger JE, Helms JA, Hanahan D, et al. MMP-9/gelatinase B is a key regulator of growth plate angiogenesis and apoptosis of hypertrophic chondrocytes. *Cell* 1998; 93:411–422.
16. Gerber HP, Vu TH, Ryan AM, Kowalski J, Werb Z, Ferrara N. VEGF couples hypertrophic cartilage remodeling, ossification and angiogenesis during endochondral bone formation. *Nat Med* 1999; 5:623–628.
17. Ryan AM, Eppler DB, Hagler KE, Bruner RH, Thomford PJ, Hall RL, et al. Preclinical safety evaluation of rhuMAbVEGF, an antiangiogenic humanized monoclonal antibody. *Toxicol Pathol* 1999; 27:78–86.
18. Wedge SR, Ogilvie DJ, Dukes M, Kendrew J, Curwen JO, Hennequin LF, et al. ZD4190: an orally active inhibitor of vascular endothelial growth factor signaling with broad-spectrum antitumor efficacy. *Cancer Res* 2000; 60:970–975.
19. Daniels R, Gupta E, Kollias G, Huang MQ, Patel RN, Manning J, et al. Safety and pharmacokinetics of BMS-275291, a novel matrix metalloproteinase inhibitor in health subjects. *Proc Annu Meet Am Soc Clin Oncol* 2001; (abstract) submitted.
20. Hurwitz H, Humphrey J, Williams K, Ness E, Conway A, Bielefield M, et al. A phase I trial of BMS-275291: a novel, non-hydroxamate, sheddase-sparing matrix metalloproteinase inhibitor (MMPI) with no dose-limiting arthritis. *Proc Annu Meet Am Soc Clin Oncol* 2001; (abstract) submitted.
21. Lockhart AC, Braun RD, Dewhirst MW, Klitzman B, Humphrey JS, Yuan F, et al. Wound angiogenesis as a potential surrogate marker for anti-angiogenesis clinical trials. *Proc Am Assoc Cancer Res* 2000; 41:168 (abstract).
22. Hurwitz H, Lockhart AC, Dewhirst MW, Klitzman B, Yuan F, Grichnik JM, et al. Evaluation of wound angiogenesis in healthy volunteers: a potential surrogate marker for antiangiogenesis agents. *Proc Am Assoc Cancer Res* 2000; 41:168 (abstract).
23. Lockhart AC, Braun RD, Dewhirst MW, Humphrey J, Yuan F, Grichnik JM, et al. Wound angiogenesis inhibition as a marker for anti-angiogenic efficacy. *Exp Biol* 2000; (abstract).

22 The Role of Cyclooxygenase-2 Inhibitors in Combined Modality Therapy

Hong Pyo, MD, *Raymond N. DuBois*, MD, PhD, *and Hak Choy*, MD

CONTENTS

1. INTRODUCTION

Since the German chemist, Felix Hoffman, first developed a molecule with analgesic activity called acetylsalicylic acid or aspirin for his employer, the Bayer Company, in 1893, a class of drugs referred to as nonsteroidal antiinflammatory drugs (NSAIDs) has evolved that are now, 100 years later, among the most widely used therapeutic agents known to mankind *(1)*. In 1988, Kune et al. found an inverse association between aspirin use and the risk for colorectal cancer *(2)*. This unexpected finding occurred in the context of a case-control study that explored numerous potential associations with colorectal cancer risk. Although the authors speculated that this inverse association could be causal, general interest appeared to be limited until other studies reported similar findings in 1991 *(3,4)*. These early studies generated a great deal of interest in

From: *Chemoradiation in Cancer Therapy*
Edited by: H. Choy

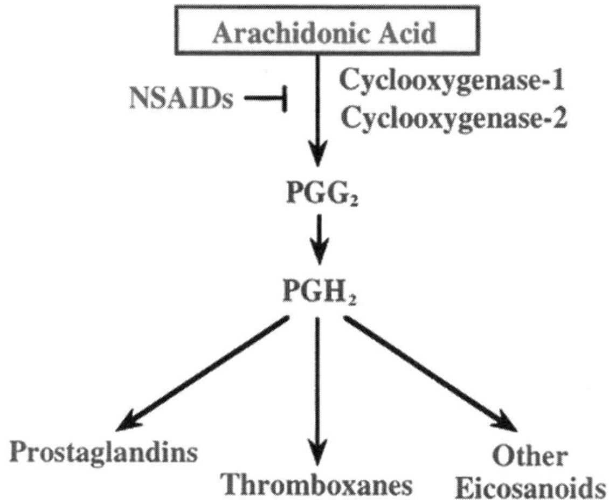

Fig. 1. Arachidonic acid metabolism (ref. *51*).

the possibility that aspirin or other NSAIDs could act as chemopreventive agents for colorectal cancer *(5)*.

It is well known that the main underlying action of NSAIDs is their inhibition of the cyclooxygenase (COX) enzymes, which may be the reason NSAIDs have a wide spectrum of pathophysiological activities, including analgesic and antiinflammatory effects, prophylaxis against cardiovascular disease, and cancer prevention. NSAIDs' long history of use over the past 100 yr may not be just an incidental phenomenon. Currently this class of drugs is being rediscovered as both chemopreventive and therapeutic agents for cancer.

2. PROSTAGLANDINS AND CYCLOOXYGENASE

Prostaglandins (PGs), thromboxanes, and leukotrienes, collectively known as eicosanoids, are metabolites of arachidonic acid that are involved in numerous biologic processes including inflammation, ovulation, implantation, angiogenesis, platelet aggregation, and immunologic function. Phospholipase enzymes cleave membrane-bound arachidonic acid, thus making it available for conversion to eicosanoids. The liberated arachidonic acid can be metabolized through one of three major pathways:

1. The COX pathway (prostaglandin endoperoxide synthase).
2. The lipoxygenase pathway.
3. The cytochrome P-450 monooxygenase pathway.

Additionally, free radical peroxidation can convert arachidonic acid nonenzymatically to yield isoprostanes *(6)*.

The COX pathway is the most extensively studied of these major pathways. COX converts arachidonic acid to PGG_2 and subsequently to PGH_2, which is the immediate substrate for a number of cell-specific PG and thromboxane synthases (Fig. 1) *(6)*. PGs are considered to be autocrine or paracrine hormones that display a wide range of pharmacological, physiological, and pathological effects. There are at least two isoforms of COX, which are referred to as COX-1 and COX-2. Although they catalyze the same enzymatic reaction, they are regulated independently *(1)*. COX-1 is constitutively

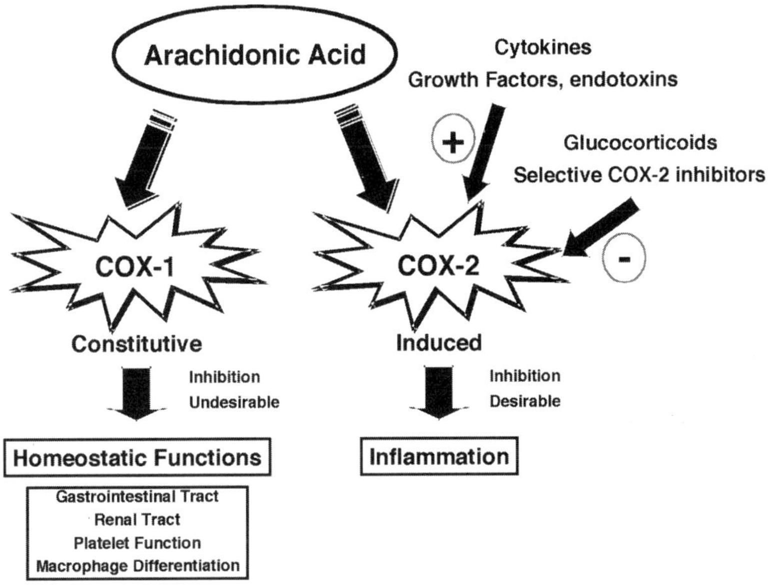

Fig. 2. Model for the role of COX-1 and COX-2.

expressed in many tissues (e.g., gastric mucosa) and acts in a variety of settings to produce homeostatic or maintenance levels of PGs. For example, COX-1 produces PGE_2 and PGI_2 in the gastrointestinal tract. These PGs stimulate gastric mucus formation, increase gastric mucosal blood flow, and reduce acid secretion to protect the mucosal lining from damage *(7)*. By contrast, COX-2 is usually undetectable in normal tissues (except for the brain, the macula densa of the kidney, and the placenta), but is rapidly induced in response to varied pathophysiological signals including those triggered by various types of cellular injury *(8)*. COX-2 is believed to be mainly responsible for the inflammatory processes, because it is rapidly induced at sites of inflammation and produces proinflammatory PGs (Fig. 2) *(7)*. However, more recent studies are beginning to reveal additional functions of COX-2: regulation of renal physicology; regulation of nerve and brain function; maintenance of gastrointestinal integrity; regulation of ovarian and uterine function; regulation of bone formation and resorption; and regulation of pain sensation and transmission *(1)*.

3. COX-2 EXPRESSION AND CANCER

There is an emerging body of data that indicates COX-2 upregulation may play a role in cancer growth and progression. Increased expression of COX-2 has been demonstrated in a number of different tumor types in humans *(9–41)*, although its production varies both quantitatively and qualitatively among tumors of different histological type and sites of origin (Table 1). It has also been found that although COX-2 is undetectable in normal colonic mucosa, it is elevated in about 85% of colorectal adenocarcinomas *(34,36,42)*. Similar findings have been reported with lung cancers *(13)*.

Epidemiological evidence reveals that individuals who take aspirin or NSAIDs have a 40–50% reduced risk of developing colon cancer and its nonmalignant precursor, the adenomatous polyp *(4,43–46)*. Familial adenomatous polyposis (FAP) is a disease inher-

Table 1
COX-2 Expression of Tumors According to Their Primary Sites of Origin

Primary sites	*Total number of samples*	*COX-2 expression (%)*	*Ref.*
Brain	100	58–100	*(9,10)*
Head and neck	22	100	*(11,12)*
Esophagus			*(13–16)*
Squamous	202	74–91	
Adeno	32	78–100	
Barrett's[a]	21	80	
Lung (NSCLC[b])	462	48–95	*(17,23)*
Breast	69	56–100	*(18,23,24)*
Stomach	161	47–100	*(25–27)*
Liver	82	54–97	*(28,29)*
Pancreas	159	58–100	*(30–33)*
Colorectum	150	71–100	*(18,23,34–37)*
Bladder	86	51–84	*(38,39)*
Prostate	63	83–100	*(23,40,41)*

[a]Barrett's; Barrett's metaplastic mucosa.
[b]NSCLC; nonsmall-cell lung cancer.

ited in an autosomal dominant fashion with variable phenotypic expression. The genetic mutation responsible for this disease occurs in the *adenomatous polyposis coli* (*APC*) gene, and somatic mutations in the *APC* gene have also been reported in over 50% of spontaneous colorectal cancers examined *(47,48)*. Clinical trials with NSAIDs in patients with FAP have demonstrated that NSAID treatment caused dramatic regression of preexisting adenomas, as well as prevention of new adenoma formation in these patients. NSAIDs, such as sulindac, are now commonly used in patients with FAP after a subtotal colectomy to prevent adenoma recurrence and facilitate surveillance of the remaining rectum *(49)*. Recently investigators found that celecoxib, a selective COX-2 inhibitor, also has a similar chemopreventive effect on patients with FAP *(50)*.

Preclinical experimental data appear to support the above findings. Studies in a variety of animal models (both genetic and carcinogen-induced) of colon cancer have also indicated a significant reduction in tumor multiplicity by NSAID treatment including the selective COX-2 inhibitor, celecoxib *(51,52)*. In fact, some of these studies have shown as much as an 80–90% reduction in tumor burden *(53)*. Another study has provided genetic evidence that directly links COX-2 expression to intestinal tumor promotion *(54)*. This report shows that $APC^{\Delta}716/+$ mice, which develop hundreds of tumors in their intestines, bred with COX-2 null mice have an 80–90% reduction in tumor multiplicity in the homozygous COX-2 null offspring. These results suggest that COX-2 may act as a tumor promoter in the intestine, and that increased levels of COX-2 expression may result directly or indirectly from disruption of the *APC* gene (Fig. 3) *(51)*. Tsujii and his colleagues performed experiments with rat intestinal epithelial cells that were programmed to express COX-2 constitutively *(55)*. The cells developed an altered phenotype including increased adhesion to the extracellular matrix and a resistance to undergo apoptosis. Both of these phenotypic changes are consistent with an increased malignant potential, and were made reversible by treatment with a selective COX-2 inhibitor.

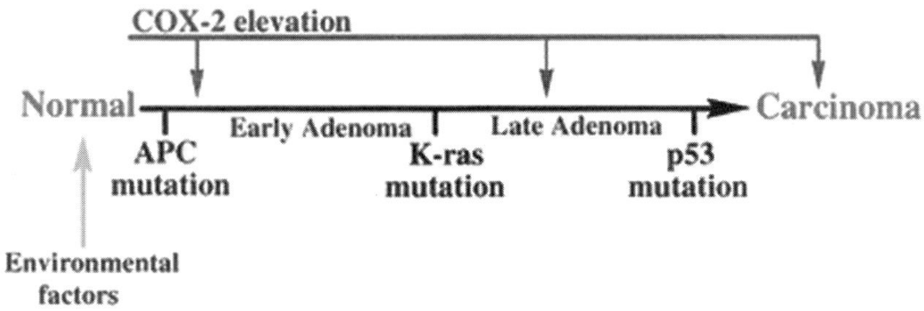

Fig. 3. Working hypothesis for the potential role of COX-2 in colorectal carcinogenesis (ref. *51*).

In addition, very recent work indicates that COX-2 may play a vital role in the regulation of angiogenesis associated with neoplastic tumor cells, hence COX-2 inhibitors may block the growth of blood vessels into developing tumors *(56)*. Thus, according to epidemiological, clinical, and experimental data, COX-2 appears to be intimately related to the development and growth of some types of cancer, especially of colorectal cancer.

There is some evidence that the level of COX-2 expression in tumors has prognostic significance for patients with various cancers. Increased COX-2 expression in tumors correlates with pathologically unfavorable findings such as larger tumor size, tumor dedifferentiation, increased number of metastatic lymph nodes, higher Dukes' stage, higher recurrence rate, and shorter survival time in patients with colorectal cancer *(57–59)*. In cases of patients with surgically resected adenocarcinoma of the lung, a significant relationship between elevated COX-2 expression in tumors and shortened patient survival was observed only in a cohort of patients with stage I disease *(20)*.

4. UNDERLYING MECHANISMS OF COX-2 ENZYME AND ITS INHIBITORS ON CANCERS

The underlying molecular mechanism responsible for the effect of COX-2 inhibitors on cancer cells is still unclear, although many hypotheses have been proposed. Increased levels of prostanoids in many human tumors have been verified, and a selective group of eicosanoids has been shown to increase the proliferative rate of human cancer cells *(60–63)*. Therefore, prostanoids may serve as autocrine or paracrine growth factors for a selective group of cancer cells. Although prostanoids can be produced by both COX-1 and COX-2, a comparison of neoplastic and adjacent tissue revealed no change in COX-1 expression but an upregulation of COX-2 in adenomas and adenocarcinomas compared with the normal mucosa *(64)*. Therefore, COX-2 inhibitors may inhibit the growth of cancer cells.

Induction of apoptosis is one of the most widely investigated and consistently supported potential mechanisms for the antineoplastic effect of COX-2 inhibitors. Cells overexpressing COX-2 tend to be resistant to undergo apoptosis *(55)*, and treatment with COX-2 inhibitors has been shown to induce apoptosis in these types of cells *(65–71)*. Bcl-2, which acts as a negative regulator of apoptosis, was also elevated in the transfected cell line that was forced to express COX-2 constitutively, but was undetectable in the parental cell line *(55)*. Many cancer chemotherapeutic drugs induce cell death through an apoptotic mechanism. In general, these drugs are thought to cause DNA damage that results in posttranscriptional induction of *p53* protein induction. Induction of *p53* protein expres-

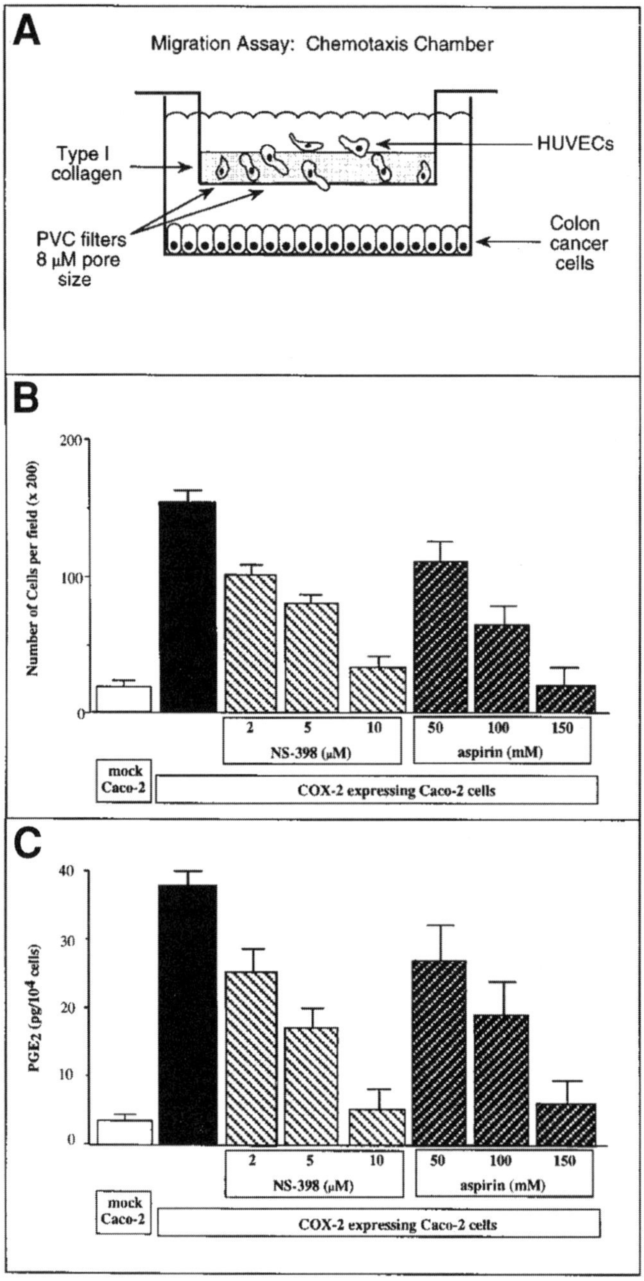

Fig. 4. Effect of COX-2 expression and COX inhibitors on prostaglandin production and migration of cocultured HUVECs. **(A)** Schematic diagram of the migration assay chamber. Colonic carcinoma cells were grown to confluence in the lower chamber, the medium was changed, and an upper chamber containing a monolayer of HUVECs plated onto a layer of type I collagen was inserted. The cells were incubated at 37°C for 4 h, and then the number of cells that had migrated through the collagen gel onto the filters in the bottom of the upper chamber were counted manually. **(B)** Migration of HUVECs cocultured with COX-2-expressing Caco-2 cells. Cell movement was evaluated by the number of cells that migrated toward conditioned medium of mock or COX-2-overexpressing Caco-2 cells in the outer chambers. Incubation was performed

(continued on next page)

sion causes cell cycle arrest and apoptotic cell death through regulation of other signaling pathways. Several researchers have shown that sulindac-induced apoptosis is not associated with increased *p53* expression at the mRNA or protein level, and that sulindac induces apoptosis in a cell line that has mutations of both *p53* alleles and no detectable *p53* protein *(72–74)*. These observations indicate that apoptosis induced by NSAIDs may not require *p53* induction and is therefore fundamentally different than apoptosis induced by chemotherapeutic agents *(49)*.

According to studies with COX-2-knockout mice bred with *APC* mutant Min-mice, a dramatic reduction occurred in the number and size of polyps in the COX-2 null mice compared with COX-2 wild-type mice. This suggests that the regulation of COX-2 appears to directly affect the promotion of colonic carcinogenesis, at least when through the *APC* gene initiated pathway *(54)*. However, several lines of evidence also suggest that some of the antineoplastic effect of NSAIDs, including the COX-2 inhibitors, may be independent of COX-2 inhibition. For example, the R isomer of flurbiprofen or the sulfone metabolite of sulindac do not inhibit COX-1 or COX-2, but they do inhibit adenoma or cancer formation in various in vivo carcinogenesis model systems *(49)*. However, it is known that the R isomer of flurbiprofen racemizes in rodents to form the active S isomer which does inhibit cyclooxygenase. Thus, whether NSAIDs block tumor progression solely through inhibition of COX-2 activity is a matter that is still being debated. Recently, it was shown that treatment of carcinoma cells with sulindac sulfone reduced prostaglandin levels by a noncyclooxygenase dependent mechanism (Williams et al. Neoplasia 1, 170–176, 1999).

COX-2 inhibitors have been found to have anti-angiogenic effects on tumors. COX-2 was expressed in the angiogenic vasculature present within tumors and in preexisting vasculature adjacent to malignant lesions as well as in the tumor cells themselves in colon, prostate, lung, and breast cancers. In contrast, COX-2 was not detected in normal colonic epithelium or stroma *(23,75)*. Newly vascularized endothelium in the basic fibroblast growth factor (FGF-2)–induced rat corneal angiogenesis model also expressed COX-2, whereas endothelial cells present in the established limbic vessels expressed only COX-1 *(23)*. Celecoxib inhibited the angiogenic response dose dependently; however, neither an inactive isomer of celecoxib nor a COX-1 specific inhibitor (SC-560) were able to block the development of angiogenesis in the rat cornea. These results suggest that PGs produced by the FGF-2 induction of COX-2 are essential to neovascularization *(23)*. COX-2 overexpressing cells produced high levels of proangiogenic factors (VEGF, bFGF, bFGF-binding protein, TBF-β, PDGF, endothelin-1, and iNOS), which stimulate both endothelial cell migration and tube formation in a model in which endothelial and cancer cells were co-cultured (Figs. 4 and 5). Selective COX-2 inhibitors reversed both the upregulation of the proangiogenic factors and the stimulation of the endothelial cell migration and tube formation *(56)*. Thus, COX-2 appears to play some role in angiogenesis as well as in tumor cell growth itself.

(continued from previous page)
at 37° for 4 h, and at the end of the incubation period, nonmigrated cells on the upper surface of the filter were removed, and the migrated cells were stained and counted manually. **(C)** PGE_2 production from mock and COX-2-expressing Caco-2 cells plus and minus aspirin and NS-398. COX-2-expressing Caco-2 cells were treated with NS-398 or aspirin at the indicated concentrations for 24 h prior to harvest. Medium was taken from mock or COX-2-expressing Caco-2 cells and used for ELISA assay (ref. *56*).

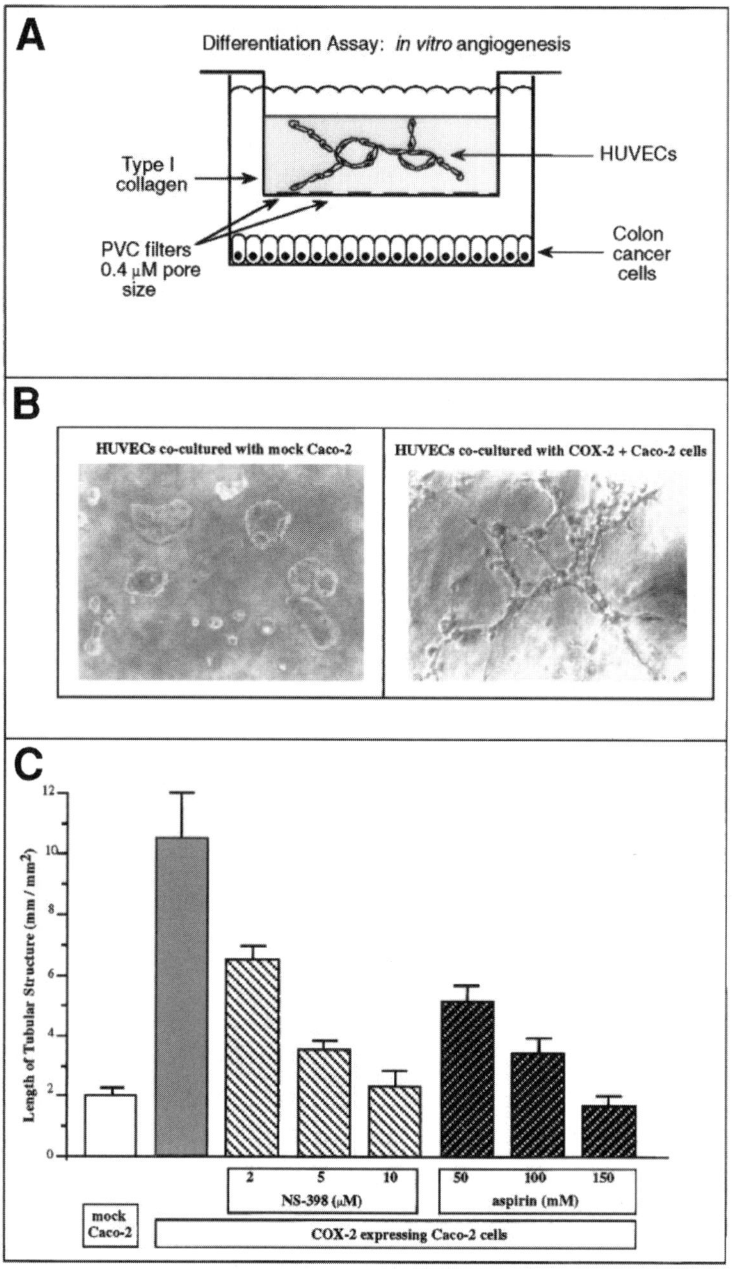

Fig. 5. Effect of COX-2 expression on angiogenesis in vitro. **(A)** Schematic diagram of the differentiation assay chamber. Colonic carcinoma cells were grown to confluence in the lower chamber, the medium was changed, and an upper chamber was inserted. The upper chamber was prepared by plating a monolayer of HUVECs onto a very thick layer of type I collagen followed by incubation at 37°C for 24 h. The HUVECs were then cocultured with the colonic carcinoma cells at 37°C for 4 d, and following incubation, the number of tube-like structures that formed in the gel were measured by total length per field (×200). **(B)** Phase contrast micrographs of HUVECs grown in collagen gel. (Left panel) HUVECs cocultured with mock Caco-2 cells did not form tubular structure, although a few HUVECs invade into collagen gel. (Right panel) HUVECs cocultured with COX-2-expressing Caco-2 cells showed tubular structure in the gel.

(continued on next page)

5. EFFECT OF COX OR SELECTIVE COX-2 INHIBITORS ON CANCER PREVENTION

NSAIDs or selective COX-2 inhibitors have been used as chemopreventive agents for patients with colorectal cancer. Kune *(76)* summarized and analyzed 22 epidemiologic or clinical studies that examined previous aspirin use and colorectal cancer risk. Of the 16 epidemiologic studies that examined previous regular aspirin use and colorectal cancer risk, 15 found a protective effect for aspirin, 14 of which were statistically significant. The degree of protection against colorectal cancer had a range of 21–70%, with a mean protection level of 40%. However, in a large randomized American trial designed to test cardiovascular disease protection, low-dose aspirin (325 mg on alternate days) had no effect on colorectal tumors after both 5 and 12 yr of follow-up *(77,78)*. The low dose of aspirin used in this study and the relatively short treatment period (5 yr) may account for this finding. In addition, all seven colorectal adenoma studies showed that previous aspirin use was associated with a statistically significant level of protection, and the range of protection was between 15% and 72%, with a mean protection level of 42% *(76)*. Although the precise dose schedule of aspirin treatment for prevention of colorectal cancer has not been determined, it is likely to be in the range of 150–300 mg per day for a minimum of 10 yr *(76)*. Several studies have shown that nonaspirin NSAIDs have effects similar to those of aspirin with respect to colorectal tumor chemoprevention *(76,79)*. However, the evidence for nonaspirin NSAID chemoprevention is less extensive and less consistent than that for aspirin. Recently, Torrance et al. conducted a study of a combined approach for the chemoprevention of intestinal tumors in *APCmin/+* mice *(80)*. They combined administration of sulindac, a prototypical NSAID, with EKI-569, a newly developed irreversible inhibitor of epidermal growth factor receptor (EGFR) kinase. All of the untreated *APCmin/+* mice developed approx 20 polyps, while nearly half the mice treated with these two agents developed no polyps at all (Table 2). This result suggests the possibility of developing a powerful chemopreventive strategy for patients with colorectal cancers.

Selective COX-2 inhibitors have also been shown to prevent early and late forms of colorectal neoplasia in rat models. Reddy et al. showed that administration of celecoxib inhibited aberrant colonic crypt foci (ACF) induction and multiplicity by about 40–49% in an azoxymethane-induced ACF rat model *(81)*. Later the same investigators also showed that dietary administration of celecoxib can inhibit both the incidence and multiplicity of colon tumors by about 93% and 97%, respectively in the same rat model *(82)*. Other researchers reported similar results with the Min mouse model *(52)*. There is little data on human clinical trials with selective COX-2 inhibitors for colorectal tumor prevention. Recently Steinbach et al. conducted a double-blind, placebo-controlled study with 77 patients with FAP, and reported that treatment with celecoxib, a selective COX-2 inhibitor, for 6 mo led to a significant reduction (28%) in the number of colorectal polyps in these patients *(50)*. Collectively, COX-2 nonspecific or specific NSAIDs appear to have chemopreventive activity against colorectal cancer development. Selective

(continued from previous page) **(C)** Quantitative analysis of angiogenesis in vitro by measuring the length of the tubular structures formed by HUVECs. The dose-dependent effect of NS-398 or aspirin treatment on endothelial tube formation was also assessed. The cell culture medium was changed daily with fresh addition of NS-398 or aspirin (ref. *56*).

Table 2
Effects of Sulindac and EKB-569 Treatment of $APC^{Min/+}$ Mice

Control (untreated) mean number of polyps (% of control)	*EKB-569, 20 mg/kg mean number of polyps (% of control)*	*Sulindac, 5 mg/kg mean number of polyps (% of control)*	*Sulindac + EKB-569 mean number of polyps (% of control)*
19.5 ± 14.1 (100%)	2.6 ± 1.6[a] (13%)	20.6 ± 11.8 (106%)	0.87 ± 1.1[b,c] (4%)

For each treatment arm, the values represent the means ± the standard deviation of the number of polyps per whole mouse intestine, as observed under a dissecting microscope. In each case, mice were fed the indicated diets for 60 d after weaning, then killed for determination of polyp number. Each group consisted of 14–15 mice.

[a] $p < 0.001$ compared with control diet, Students *t*-test (unequal variance).
[b] $p < 0.0001$ compared with control diet, Student *t*-test (unequal variance).
[c] $p < 0.001$ compared with diet containing EKB-569 alone, Student *t*-test (unequal variance) (ref. *80*).

COX-2 inhibitors may find a place in colorectal tumor chemoprevention, since they seem to have a better gastrointestinal safety profile than other nonspecific NSAIDs when given to patients for a long time. In addition, this approach for colorectal tumors may be able to be expanded to other COX-2 expressing human tumors.

6. EFFECT OF COX-2 INHIBITORS WITH CHEMOTHERAPEUTIC AGENTS OR RADIATION

The possibility of using COX-2 inhibitors as cancer-treatment agents for already developed neoplastic lesions has been proposed, since COX-2 expressing cancer cell lines are dependent on COX-2 activity for their tumorigenicity, and COX-2 inhibitors have been shown to reduce the growth rate of these cancer cells, in vitro and in vivo, as well as the growth rate of existing premalignant adenomas in human patients *(64)*. NSAIDs have been reported to produce synergistic growth inhibition against Lewis lung carcinomas when used in combination with various chemotherapeutic agents including cisplatin, cyclophosphamide, and carmustine (BCNU) *(83)*. Recently, a limited number of preclinical studies have been performed to investigate the effect of selective or non-selective COX-2 inhibitors on the chemosensitivity of cells from human cancers or normal tissues. Duffy et al. reported that a specific group of NSAIDs (indomethacin, sulindac, tolmetin, acemetacin, zomepirac, and mefenamic acid) significantly increased the cytotoxicity of the anthracyclines (doxorubicin, daunorubicin, and epirubicin), as well as teniposide, VP-16, and vincristine on human lung cancer and leukemia cell lines *(84)*. Soriano et al. have shown synergistic interactions for sulindac, exisulind, and nordihydroguaiaretic acid (NDGA) with paclitaxel, cisplatin, and 13-*cis*-retinoic acid using six NSCLC and small-cell lung cancer cell lines, and this was independent of the drug-resistance phenotype of the tumors *(85)*. Hida et al. tested the selective COX-2 inhibitor, nimesulide, with COX-2 overexpressing or low-expressing human lung cancer cell lines and with normal lung epithelial cell lines; 10–30 μM nimesulide reduced the IC_{50} values of various anticancer agents (including taxotere, VP-16, and cisplatin) by up to 77%. It was noted that lung cancer cell lines with high COX-2 expression levels were generally more sensitive to the combined treatment of nimesulide and anticancer agents than were low COX-2 expressing cells, and nimesulide showed almost no effect on the chemosensitivity of normal lung epithelial cell lines *(86)*. Thus, selective COX-2 inhibitors may have potential as chemosensitizers for the treatment of human cancers.

COX-2 nonspecific NSAIDs have been demonstrated to potentiate radioresponse of cancer cells grown in vitro *(87)* and in vivo *(88,89)*. Recently a limited number of preclinical studies have been performed to investigate the radiosensitizing effect of selective COX-2 inhibitors on tumor cells *(90–92)*. Milas et al. *(91)* have shown that SC-236, a selective COX-2 inhibitor, significantly enhanced the growth-inhibitory effect of radiation on murine COX-2 expressing tumors grown in vivo. SC-236 also significantly reduced the number of newly formed vessels seen in intradermal assay, which was associated with tumor growth retardation. Kishi et al. *(90)* confirmed this effect, and also showed that SC-236 does not affect the radioresponse of normal tissues, using jejunal mucosa as a model for acute damage, and the leg contracture model as being representative of late damage. Petersen et al. *(92)* have performed in vitro clonogenic cell survival analyses and have shown that SC-236 enhanced the effect of radiation on U251, a human glioma cell line, which constitutively expresses COX-2.

Pyo et al. *(93)* conducted in vitro radiation cell survival experiments with rat intestinal epithelial cells which were stably transfected with COX-2 cDNA, in the sense (RIE-S) and antisense (RIE-AS) orientations, to directly compare the radiation-enhancing effect of the NS-398, a selective COX-2 inhibitor, on COX-2 over-expressing (RIE-S) and low-expressing control (RIE-AS) cells. NS-398 enhanced radiosensitivity of RIE-S cells in a concentration-dependent manner; however, this effect was not shown in RIE-AS cells that are similar to normal intestinal epithelial cells (Fig. 6). In experiments with cancer cell lines, NS-398 enhanced the effect of radiation in NCI-H460 human lung cancer cells that overexpress COX-2, but not in HCT-116 cells that lack COX-2 expression (Fig. 7). NS-398 also enhanced radiosensitivity of H460 tumors grown in vivo; however, it did not enhance the radiosensitivity of HCT-116 tumors, although the effect was at least additive (Fig. 8). These in vitro and in vivo results suggest that selective COX-2 inhibitors enhance the effect of radiation on tumors that express COX-2, but not on normal tissues. Collectively, selective COX-2 inhibitors may have potential as radiosensitizers for the treatment of human cancers.

7. COX-2 INHIBITORS WITH COMBINED TREATMENT FOR PATIENTS WITH CANCERS

Selective COX-2 inhibitors are ideal agents to combine with chemoradiotherapy for several reasons. First, they have been shown to enhance the effect of various chemotherapeutic agents and radiation on cancer cells. Second, selective COX-2 inhibitors are relatively safe. They do not have severe gastrointestinal toxicity, which is common in many nonselective NSAIDs. For example, celecoxib, a selective COX-2 inhibitor which is currently being used for patients with arthritis, is 375-fold more selective for COX-2 compared to COX-1 *(94)*, and in large randomized, multicenter, placebo-controlled, double-blind trials conducted in patients with rheumatoid arthritis, celecoxib proved to be less toxic than nonselective inhibitors of COX-1 and COX-2, and no more toxic than a placebo *(95)*. Third, high-dose celecoxib (600 mg bid) has no effect on serum thromboxane or platelet function *(96)*. This is obviously important in patients receiving

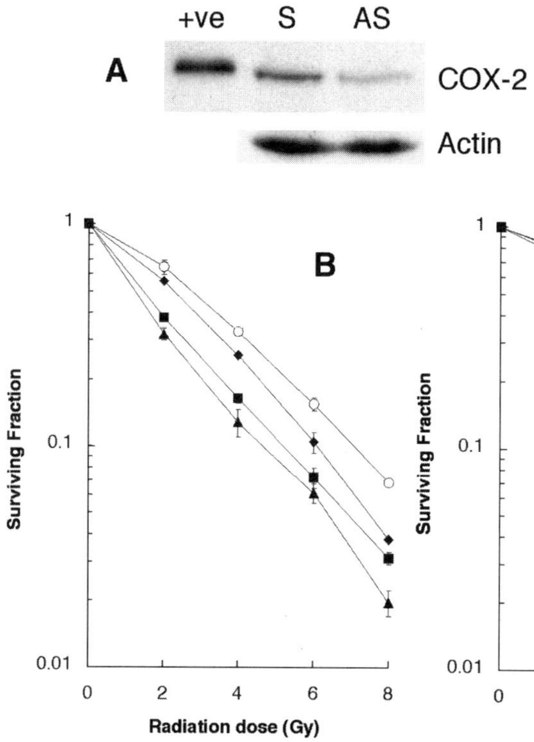

Fig. 6. (A) Western blot analysis of COX-2 levels in RIE-S and RIE-AS cells. +ve, COX-2 protein positive control. Survival curves for radiation plus NS-398 in RIE-S **(B)** and RIE-AS **(C)** cells. (○), radiation plus vehicle (DMSO) treatment; (◆), radiation plus 150 μ*M* NS-398 treatment; (■), radiation plus 300 μ*M* NS-398 treatment; (▲), radiation plus 400 μ*M* NS-398 treatment.

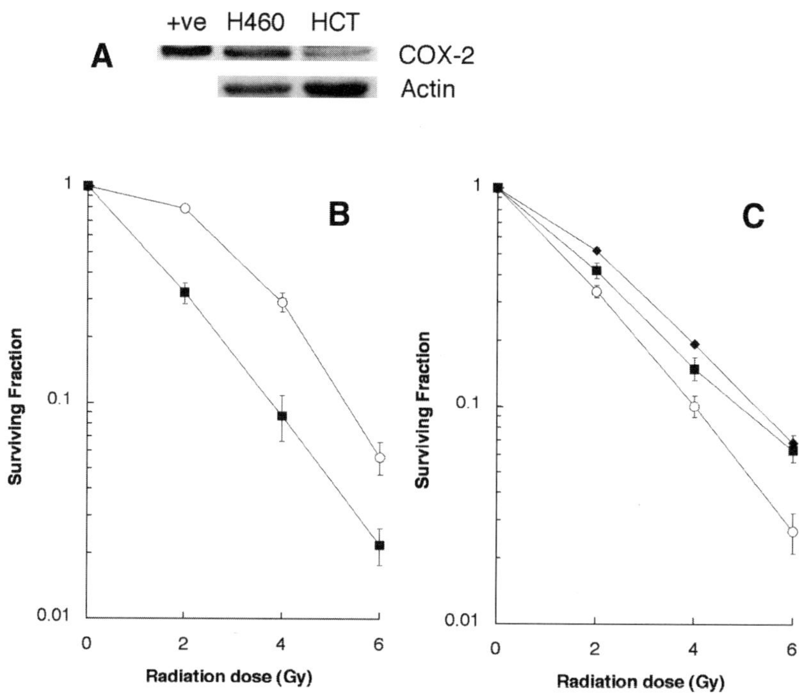

Fig. 7. *(Caption on next page)*

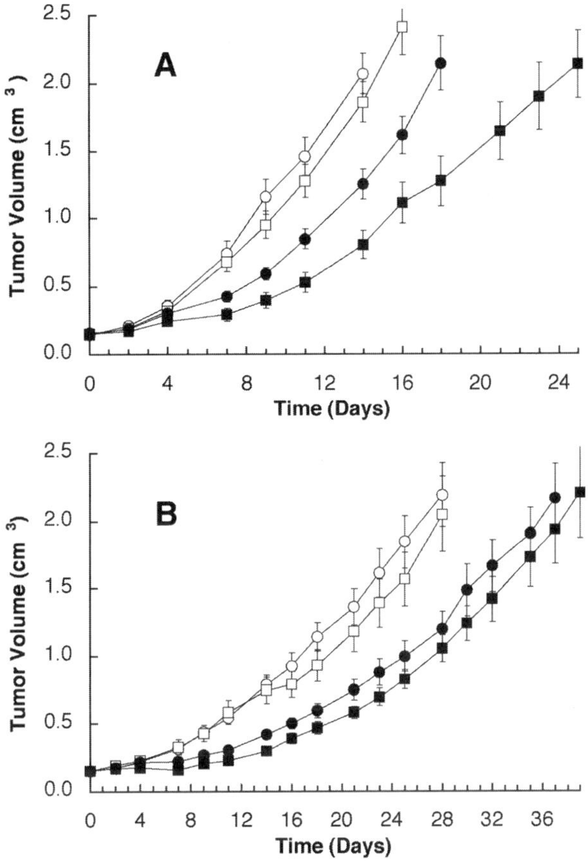

Fig. 8. Combined effect of fractionated NS-398 and radiotherapy on the tumor growth delay of H460 **(A)** and HCT-116 **(B)** human tumor xenografts in nude mice. Day 0 is defined as the first day of treatment. Tumors were treated with vehicle (DMSO) or 36 mg/kg NS-398 on d 1 through 7. Radiation fractions (2 Gy) were given 2 h after drug administration starting d 2, for 5 consecutive days. Error bars represent the ± SE from 8–9 mice. (○), vehicle treatment alone; (□), NS-398 treatment alone; (●), radiation plus vehicle treatment; (■), radiation plus NS-398 treatment.

myelosuppresive drugs in whom oncologists normally avoid agents that impair platelet function. Thus, selective COX-2 inhibitors may have a role for treatment in patients with cancers when combined with other therapeutic approaches; by enhancing the effect of chemotherapeutic agents and radiation without adding significant toxicity; or by reducing the total dose of chemotherapeutic agents or radiation without diminishing their effects. Several clinical trials are ongoing to investigate the effect of selective COX-2 inhibitors on chemoprevention or chemoradiosensitization for patients with cancer. Results from these trials will further define the role of COX-2 inhibitors for treatment of patients with cancer.

Fig. 7. *(from previous page)* **(A)** Western blot analysis of COX-2 levels in H460 and HCT-116 cells. +ve, COX-2 protein positive control. Survival curves for radiation plus NS-398 in H460 **(B)** and HCT-116 **(C)** cells. (○), radiation plus vehicle (DMSO) treatment; (◆), radiation plus 250 μ*M* NS-398 treatment; (■), radiation plus 300 μ*M* NS-398 treatment.

8. CONCLUSIONS AND FUTURE DIRECTIONS

Selective COX-2 inhibitors provide a distinct class of drugs in the history of evolution of NSAIDs, since they have basically removed the most disturbing, potentially fatal, complications of these drugs, thereby markedly enhancing the therapeutic ratio. Their use may provide a safe way to administer drugs long-term to reduce risks of suffering from several diseases including cancer. The use of this drug on a routine daily basis may be a revolutionary new way to reduce the risk of cancer. Ongoing preventive trials will define the role of this drug in the prevention of various cancers.

There are an increasing number of potential new therapeutic targets for cancer. These include inhibition of various oncogenic growth factors (e.g., epidermal growth factor, insulin-like growth factor, and nerve growth factor), inhibitors of invasion and metastases (e.g., matrix metalloproteinases inhibitors and antivascular endothelial growth factor antibodies), inhibitors of protein kinase C, replacement therapy of tumor suppressor genes (e.g., *p53* and *p16*), and inhibition of dominant oncogenes (e.g., *ras*, HER-2/neu, and cyclin D1) *(97)*. The combination of a selective COX-2 inhibitor with the use of one or more of these biologic therapies for sensitizing chemotherapeutic agents and radiation has a number of potential theoretic advantages. First, a markedly different mechanism of antitumor effect may result in therapeutic synergy. Second, it is likely that each treatment can be given at full dose, because the major side effects are nonoverlapping. As already discussed, selective COX-2 inhibitors have been shown to have chemo- or radiosensitizing effect, and several in vitro and in vivo studies have also shown that the combination of chemotherapeutic agents or radiation with monoclonal antibodies against autocrine growth factors or growth factor receptors produces a much greater effect than either treatment alone *(98–100)*. One promising result came from a chemoprevention study (already discussed above), which investigated the effect of a combination of an NSAID (sulindac) and an inhibitor of EGF (EKI-569) on intestinal tumor prevention in mice, and found that the effect of this combination was much stronger than that of either one alone *(80)*. Another recent study has shown directly that use of a selective COX-2 inhibitor plus a neutralizing antibody to the HER-2/neu receptor is much more effective than use of either agent alone at inhibiting the growth of colorectal carcinomas (Mann et al., Gastroenterology 120, 1713, 2001). Therefore, a combination of selective COX-2 inhibitors and other biologic therapies may further improve the treatment outcome of combined therapy in patients who are suffering from cancer.

REFERENCES

1. DuBois RN, Abramson SB, Crofford L, et al. Cyclooxygenase in biology and disease. *FASEB J* 1998; 12:1063–1073.
2. Kune GA, Kune S, Watson LF. Colorectal cancer risk, chronic illness, operations, and medications: case control results from the Melbourne Colorectal Cancer Study. *Cancer Res* 1988; 48:4399–4404.
3. Rosenberg L, Palmer J, Zauber A, et al. A hypothesis: non-steroidal anti-inflammatory drugs reduce the incidence of large-bowel cancer. *J Natl Cancer Inst* 1991; 83:355–358.
4. Thun MJ, Namboodiri MM, Heath CW Jr, et al. Aspirin use and reduced risk of fatal colon cancer. *New Engl J Med* 1991; 325:1593–1596.
5. Giovannucci E. The prevention of colorectal cancer by aspirin use. *Biomed Pharmacother* 1999; 53:303–308.
6. Williams CS, Mann M, DuBois RN. The role of cyclooxygenases in inflammation, cancer, and development. *Oncogene* 1999; 18:7908–7916.

7. Masferrer JL, Isakson PC, Seibert K. Cyclooxygenase-2 inhibitors. A new class of anti-inflammatory agents that spare the gastrointestinal tract. *Gastroenterol Clin North Am* 1996; 25:363–372.
8. Williams C, Shattuck-Brandt RL, DuBois RN. The role of COX-2 in intestinal cancer. *Ann NY Acad Sci* 1999; 889:72–83.
9. Joki T, Heese O, Nikas DC, et al. Expression of cyclooxygenase 2 (COX-2) in human glioma and in vitro inhibition by a specific COX-2 inhibitor, NS-398. *Cancer Res* 2000; 60:4926–4931.
10. Deininger MH, Weller M, Streffer J, et al. Patterns of cyclooxygenase-1 and -2 expression in human gliomas in vivo. *Acta Neuropathol* 1999; 98:240–244.
11. Mestre JR, Chan G, Zhang F, et al. Inhibition of cyclooxygenase-2 expression. An approach to preventing head and neck cancer. *Ann NY Acad Sci* 1999; 889:62–71.
12. Chan G, Boyle JO, Yang EK, et al. Cyclooxygenase-2 expression is up-regulated in squamous cell carcinoma of the head and neck. *Cancer Res* 1999; 59:991–994.
13. Zimmermann KC, Sarbia M, Weber AA, et al. Cyclooxygenase-2 expression in human esophageal carcinoma. *Cancer Res* 1999; 59:198–204.
14. Wilson KT, Fu S, Ramanujam KS, et al. Increased expression of inducible nitric oxide synthase and cyclooxygenase-2 in Barrett's esophagus and associated adenocarcinomas. *Cancer Res* 1998; 58:2929–2934.
15. Shamma A, Yamamoto H, Doki Y, et al. Up-regulation of cyclooxygenase-2 in squamous carcinogenesis of the esophagus. *Clin Cancer Res* 2000; 6:1229–1238.
16. Ratnasinghe D, Tangrea J, Roth MJ, et al. Expression of cyclooxygenase-2 in human squamous cell carcinoma of the esophagus; an immunohistochemical survey. *Anticancer Res* 1999; 19:171–174.
17. Marrogi AJ, Travis WD, Welsh JA, et al. Nitric oxide synthase, cyclooxygenase 2, and vascular endothelial growth factor in the angiogenesis of non-small cell lung carcinoma. *Clin Cancer Res* 2000; 6:4739–4744.
18. Soslow RA, Dannenberg AJ, Rush D, et al. COX-2 is expressed in human pulmonary, colonic, and mammary tumors. *Cancer* 2000; 89:2637–2645.
19. Hosomi Y, Yokose T, Hirose Y, et al. Increased cyclooxygenase 2 (COX-2) expression occurs frequently in precursor lesions of human adenocarcinoma of the lung. *Lung Cancer* 2000; 30:73–81.
20. Achiwa H, Yatabe Y, Hida T, et al. Prognostic significance of elevated cyclooxygenase-2 expression in primary, resected lung adenocarcinoma. *Clin Cancer Res* 1999; 5:1001–1005.
21. Wolff H, Saukkonen K, Anttila S, et al. Expression of cyclooxygenase-2 in human lung carcinoma. *Cancer Res* 1998; 58:4997–5001.
22. Hida T, Yatabe Y, Achiwa H, et al. Increased expression of cyclooxygenase 2 occurs frequently in human lung cancers, specifically in adenocarcinomas. *Cancer Res* 1998; 58:3761–3764.
23. Masferrer JL, Leahy KM, Koki AT, et al. Antiangiogenic and antitumor activities of cyclooxygenase-2 inhibitors. *Cancer Res* 2000; 60:1306–1311.
24. Brueggemeier RW, Quinn AL, Parrett ML, et al. Correlation of aromatase and cyclooxygenase gene expression in human breast cancer specimens. *Cancer Lett* 1999; 140:27–35.
25. Ratnasinghe D, Tangrea JA, Roth MJ, et al. Expression of cyclooxygenase-2 in human adenocarcinomas of the gastric cardia and corpus. *Oncol Rep* 1999; 6:965–968.
26. Uefuji K, Ichikura T, Mochizuki H, et al. Expression of cyclooxygenase-2 protein in gastric adenocarcinoma. *J Surg Oncol* 1998; 69:168–172.
27. Lim HY, Joo HJ, Choi JH, et al. Increased expression of cyclooxygenase-2 protein in human gastric carcinoma. *Clin Cancer Res* 2000; 6:519–525.
28. Kondo M, Yamamoto H, Nagano H, et al. Increased expression of COX-2 in nontumor liver tissue is associated with shorter disease-free survival in patients with hepatocellular carcinoma. *Clin Cancer Res* 1999; 5:4005–4012.
29. Shiota G, Okubo M, Noumi T, et al. Cyclooxygenase-2 expression in hepatocellular carcinoma. *Hepatogastroenterology* 1999; 46:407–412.
30. Koshiba T, Hosotani R. Miyamoto Y, et al. Immunohistochemical analysis of cyclooxygenase-2 expression in pancreatic tumors. *Int J Pancreatol* 1999; 26:69–76.
31. Molina MA, Sitja-Arnau M, Lemoine MG, et al. Increased cyclooxygenase-2 expression in human pancreatic carcinomas and cell lines: growth inhibition by nonsteroidal anti-inflammatory drugs. *Cancer Res* 1999; 59:4356–4362.
32. Okami J, Yamamoto H, Fujiwara Y, et al. Overexpression of cyclooxygenase-2 in carcinoma of the pancreas. *Clin Cancer Res* 1999; 5:2018–2024.

33. Tucker ON, Dannenberg AJ, Yang EK, et al. Cyclooxygenase-2 expression is up-regulated in human pancreatic cancer. *Cancer Res* 1999; 59:987–990.
34. Dimberg J, Samuelsson A, Hugander A, et al. Differential expression of cyclooxygenase 2 in human colorectal cancer. *Gut* 1999; 45:730–732.
35. Sheehan KM, Sheahan K, O'Donoghue DP, et al. The relationship between cyclooxygenase-2 expression and colorectal cancer. *JAMA* 1999; 282:1254–1257.
36. Eberhart CE, Coffey RJ, Radhika A, et al. Up-regulation of cyclooxygenase 2 gene expression in human colorectal adenomas and adenocarcinomas. *Gastroenterology* 1994; 107:1183–1188.
37. Sano H, Kawahito Y, Wilder RL, et al. Expression of cyclooxygenase-1 and -2 in human colorectal cancer. *Cancer Res* 1995; 55:3785–3789.
38. Shirahama T. Cyclooxygenase-2 expression is up-regulated in transitional cell carcinoma and its preneoplastic lesions in the human urinary bladder. *Clin Cancer Res* 2000; 6:2424–2430.
39. Mohammed SI, Knapp DW, Bostwick DG, et al. Expression of cyclooxygenase-2 (COX-2) in human invasive transitional cell carcinoma (TCC) of the urinary bladder. *Cancer Res* 1999; 15:5647–5650.
40. Kirschenbaum A, Klauner AP, Lee R, et al. Expression of cyclooxygenase-1 and cyclooxygenase-2 in the human prostate. *Urology* 2000; 56:671–676.
41. Gupta S, Srivastava M, Ahmad N, et al. Over-expression of cyclooxygenase-2 in human prostate adenocarcinoma. *Prostate* 2000; 42:73–78.
42. Kargman S, Charleson S, Cartwright M, et al. Characterization of prostaglandin G/H synthase 1 and 2 in rat, dog, monkey, and human gastrointestinal tracts. *Gastroenterology* 1996; 111:445–454.
43. Thun MJ. Aspirin and gastrointestinal cancer. *Adv Exp Med Biol* 1997; 400A:395–402.
44. Thun MJ. NSAID use and decreased risk of gastrointestinal cancers. *Gastroenterol Clin North Am* 1996; 25:333–348.
45. Giovannucci E, Egan KM, Hunter DJ, et al. Aspirin and the risk of colorectal cancer in women. *New Engl J Med* 1995; 333:609–614.
46. Vainio H, Morgan G, Kleihues P. An international evaluation of the cancer-preventive potential of non-steroidal anti-inflammatory drugs. *Cancer Epidemiol Biomarkers Prev* 1997; 6:749–753.
47. Miyaki M, Konishi M, Kikuchi-Yanoshita R, et al. Characteristics of somatic mutation of the adenomatous polyposis coli gene in colorectal tumors. *Cancer Res* 1994; 54:3011–3020.
48. Powell SM, Zilz N, Beazer-Barclay Y, et al. APC mutations occur early during colorectal tumorigenesis. *Nature* 1992; 359:235–237.
49. Ahnen DJ. Colon cancer prevention by NSAIDs: what is the mechanism of action? *Eur J Surg Suppl* 1998; 582:111–114.
50. Steinbach G, Lynch PM, Phillips RK, et al. The effect of celecoxib, a cyclooxygenase-2 inhibitor, in familial adenomatous polyposis. *New Engl J Med* 2000; 342:1946–1952.
51. Williams CS, Smalley W, DuBois RN. Aspirin use and potential mechanisms for colorectal cancer prevention. *J Clin Invest* 1997; 100:1325–1329.
52. Jacoby RF, Seibert K, Cole CE, et al. The cyclooxygenase-2 inhibitor celecoxib is a potent preventive and therapeutic agent in the min mouse model of adenomatous polyposis. *Cancer Res* 2000; 60:5040–5044.
53. Kawamori T, Rao CV, Seibert K, et al. Chemopreventive activity of celecoxib, a specific cyclooxygenase-2 inhibitor, against colon carcinogenesis. *Cancer Res* 1998; 58:409–412.
54. Oshima M, Dinchuk JE, Kargman SL, et al. Suppression of intestinal polyposis in $APC^{\Delta 716}$ knockout mice by inhibition of cyclooxygenase 2 (COX-2). *Cell* 1996; 87:803–809.
55. Tsujii M, DuBois RN. Alterations in cellular adhesion and apoptosis in epithelial cells overexpressing prostaglandin endoperoxide synthase 2. *Cell* 1995; 83:493–501.
56. Tsujii M, Kawano S, Tsujii S, et al. Cyclooxygenase regulates angiogenesis induced by colon cancer cells. *Cell* 1998; 93:705–716.
57. Masunaga R, Kohno H, Dhar DK, et al. Cyclooxygenase-2 expression correlates with tumor neovascularization and prognosis in human colorectal carcinoma patients. *Clin Cancer Res* 2000; 6:4064–4068.
58. Tomozawa S, Tsuno NH, Sunami E, et al. Cyclooxygenase-2 overexpression correlates with tumour recurrence, especially haematogenous metastases, of colorectal cancer. *Br J Cancer* 2000; 83:324–328.
59. Sheehan KM, Sheahan K, O'Donoghue DP, et al. The relationship between cyclooxygenase-2 expression and colorectal cancer. *JAMA* 1999; 282:1254–1257.

60. Karmali RA. Eicosanoids in neoplasia. *Prev Med* 1987; 16:493–502.
61. Zhang S, Fulton AM. Modulation of integrin-laminin receptor function on mammary tumor cells by prostaglandin E2 receptor antagonism. *Cancer Lett* 1994; 85:233–238.
62. Qiao L, Kozoni V, Tsioulias GJ, et al. Selected eicosanoids increase the proliferation rate of human colon carcinoma cell lines and mouse colonocytes in vivo. *Biochem Biophys Acta* 1995; 1258:215–223.
63. Bortuzzo C, Hanif R, Kashfi K, et al. The effect of leukotrienes B and selected HETEs on the proliferation of colon cancer cells. *Biochem Biophys Acta* 1996; 1300:240–246.
64. Gupta RA, DuBois RN. Aspirin, NSAID, and colon cancer prevention: mechanisms? *Gastroenterology* 1998; 114:1095–1100.
65. Crew TE, Elder DJE, Paraskeva CA. Cyclooxygenase-2 (COX-2) selective non-steroidal anti-inflammatory drug enhances the growth inhibitory effect of butyrate in colorectal carcinoma cells expressing COX-2 protein: regulation of COX-2 by butyrate. *Carcinogenesis* 2000; 21:69–77.
66. Hsu AL, Ching TT, Wang DS, et al. The cyclooxygenase-2 inhibitor celecoxib induces apoptosis by blocking Akt activation in human prostate cancer cells independently of Bcl-2. *J Biol Chem* 2000; 275:11,397–11,403.
67. Liu XH, Yao S, Kirschenbaum A, et al. NS398, a selective cyclooxygenase-2 inhibitor, induces apoptosis and down-regulates Bcl-2 expression in LNCaP cells. *Cancer Res* 1998; 58:4245–4249.
68. Hara A, Yoshimi N, Niwa M, et al. Apoptosis induced by NS-398, a selective cyclooxygenase-2 inhibitor, in human colorectal cancer cell lines. *Jpn J Cancer Res* 1997; 88:600–604.
69. Sheng H, Shao J, Morrow JD, et al. Modulation of apoptosis and Bcl-2 expression by prostaglandin E_2 in human colon cancer cells. *Cancer Res* 1998; 58:362–366.
70. Elder DJE, Halton DE, Hague A, et al. Induction of apoptotic cell death in human colorectal carcinoma cell lines by a cyclooxygenase-2 (COX-2)-selective nonsteroidal anti-inflammatory drug: independence from COX-2 protein expression. *Clin Cancer Res* 1997; 3:1679–1683.
71. Hsueh CT, Chiu CF, Kelsen DP, et al. Selective inhibition of cyclooxygenase-2 enhances mitomycin-C-induced apoptosis. *Cancer Chemother Pharmacol* 2000; 45:389–396.
72. Goldberg Y, Nassif II, Pittas A, et al. The anti-proliferative effect of sulindac and sulindac sulfide on HT-29 colon cancer cells: alterations in tumor suppressor and cell cycle-regulatory proteins. *Oncogene* 1996; 12:893–901.
73. Piazza GA, Rahm AL, Krutzsch M, et al. Antineoplastic drugs sulindac sulfide and sulfone inhibit cell growth by inducing apoptosis. *Cancer Res* 1995; 55:3110–3116.
74. Piazza GA, Rahm AK, Finn T, et al. Apoptosis fully accounts for the growth inhibitory properties of sulindac metabolites by a mechanism independent of cyclooxygenase inhibition, cell cycle arrest or p53 mediation. *Cancer Res* 1997; 57:2452–2459.
75. Masferrer JL, Koki A, Seibert K. COX-2 inhibitors. A new class of antiangiogenic agents. *Ann NY Acad Sci* 1999; 889:84–86.
76. Kune GA. Colorectal cancer chemoprevention: aspirin, other NSAID and COX-2 inhibitors. *Aust NZ J Surg* 2000; 70:452–455.
77. Gann PH, Manson JE, Glynn RJ, et al. Low-dose aspirin and incidence of colorectal tumors in a randomized trial. *J Natl Cancer Inst* 1993; 85:1220–1224.
78. Sturner T, Glynn RJ, Lee IM, et al. Aspirin use and colorectal cancer: post-trial follow-up data from the Physicians' Health Study. *Ann Intern Med* 1998; 128:713–720.
79. Smalley W, Ray WA, Dougherty J, et al. Use of non-steroidal anti-inflammatory drugs and incidence of colorectal cancer. *Arch Intern Med* 1999; 159:161–166.
80. Torrance CJ, Jackson PE, Montgomery E, et al. Combinatorial chemoprevention of intestinal neoplasia. *Nat Med* 2000; 6:1024–1028.
81. Reddy BS, Rao CV, Seibert K. Evaluation of cyclooxygenase-2 inhibitor for potential chemopreventive properties in colon carcinogenesis. *Cancer Res* 1996; 56:4566–4569.
82. Kawamori T, Rao CV, Seibert K, et al. Chemopreventive activity of celecoxib, a specific cyclooxygenase-2 inhibitor, against colon carcinogenesis. *Cancer Res* 1998; 58:409–412.
83. Teicher BA, Korbut TT, Menon K, et al. Cyclooxygenase and lipoxygenase inhibitors as modulators of cancer therapies. *Cancer Chemother Pharmacol* 1994; 33:515–522.
84. Duffy CP, Elliott CJ, O'Connor RA, et al. Enhancement of chemotherapeutic drug toxicity to human tumour cells in vitro by a subset of non-steroidal anti-inflammatory drugs (NSAIDs). *Eur J Cancer* 1998; 34:1250–1259.

85. Soriano AF, Helfrich B, Chan DC, et al. Synergistic effects of new chemopreventive agents and conventional cytotoxic agents against human lung cancer cell lines. *Cancer Res* 1999; 59:6178–6184.
86. Hida T, Kozaki K, Muramatsu H, et al. Cyclooxygenase-2 inhibitor induces apoptosis and enhances cytotoxicity of various anticancer agents in non-small cell lung cancer cell lines. *Clin Cancer Res* 2000; 6:2006–2011.
87. Palayoor ST, Bump EA, Calderwood SK, et al. Combined antitumor effect of radiation and ibuprofen in human prostate carcinoma cells. *Clin Cancer Res* 1998; 4:763–771.
88. Milas L, Furuta Y, Hunter N, et al. Dependence of indomethacin-induced potentiation of murine tumor radioresponse on tumor host immunocompetence. *Cancer Res* 1990; 50:4473–4477.
89. Furuta Y, Hunter N, Barkley T Jr, et al. Increase in radioresponse of murine tumors by treatment with indomethacin. *Cancer Res* 1988; 48:3008–3013.
90. Kishi K, Petersen S, Petersen C, et al. Preferential enhancement of tumor radioresponse by a cyclooxygenase-2 inhibitor. *Cancer Res* 2000; 60:1326–1331.
91. Milas L, Kishi K, Hunter N, et al. Enhancement of tumor response to γ-radiation by an inhibitor of cyclooxygenase-2 enzyme. *J Natl Cancer Inst* 1999; 91:1501–1504.
92. Petersen C, Petersen S, Milas L, et al. Enhancement of intrinsic tumor cell radiosensitivity induced by a selective cyclooxygenase-2 inhibitor. *Clin Cancer Res* 2000; 6:2513–2520.
93. Pyo H, Choy H, Amorino GP, et al. A selective cyclooxygenase-2 inhibitor, NS-398, enhances the effect of radiation in vitro and in vivo preferentially on the cells which express cyclooxygenase-2. Submitted for publication to *Clin Cancer Res* 2001.
94. Lipsky PE, Isakson PC. Outcome of specific COX-2 inhibition in rheumatoid arthritis. *J Rheumatol* 1997; 24(Suppl 49):9–14.
95. Simon LS, Weaver AL, Graham DY, et al. Anti-inflammatory and upper gastrointestinal effects of celecoxib in rheumatoid arthritis: a randomized controlled trial. *JAMA* 1999; 282:1921–1928.
96. Leese PT, Hubbard RC, Karim A, et al. Effects of celecoxib, a novel cyclooxygenase-2 inhibitor, on platelet function in healthy adults: a randomized, controlled trial. *J Clin Pharmacol* 2000; 40:124–132.
97. Bunn PA, Soriano A, Johnson G, et al. New therapeutic strategies for lung cancer: biology and molecular biology come of age. *Chest* 2000; 117:163S–168S.
98. Zhang L, Hung MC. Sensitization of HER-2/neu-over-expressing non-small cell lung cancer cell to chemotherapeutic drugs by tyrosine kinase inhibitor emodin. *Oncogene* 1996; 12:571–576.
99. Kroning R, Jones JA, Hom DK, et al. Enhancement of drug sensitivity of human malignancies by epidermal growth factor. *Br J Cancer* 1995; 72:615–619.
100. Pietras RJ, Poen JC, Gallardo D, et al. Monoclonal antibody to HER-2/*neu* receptor modulates repair of radiation induced DNA damage and enhances radiosensitivity of human breast cancer cells overexpressing this oncogene. *Cancer Res* 1999; 59:1347–1355.
101. Mann M, Sheng H, Shao J, Williams CS, Pisacane PI, Sliwkowski MX, DuBois RN. Targeting cyclooxygenase 2 and HER-2/neu pathways inhibits colorectal carcinoma growth. *Gastroenterology* 2001; 120(7):1713–1719.

INDEX

E

F

J

L

M

R

T

U

V